SCLEROTHERAPY

Treatment of
Varicose and Telangiectatic
Leg Veins

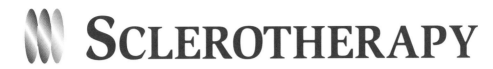

SCLEROTHERAPY

Treatment of Varicose and Telangiectatic Leg Veins

Mitchel P. Goldman, M.D.

Assistant Clinical Professor
Division of Dermatology
Department of Medicine
University of California, San Diego
San Diego, California

SECOND EDITION

With 555 illustrations, including 310 in color

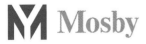 Mosby

St. Louis Baltimore Boston Carlsbad Chicago Naples New York Philadelphia Portland
London Madrid Mexico City Singapore Sydney Tokyo Toronto Wiesbaden

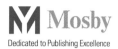

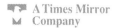

Editor: Susie H. Baxter
Developmental Editor: Ellen Baker Geisel
Editorial Assistant: Christy Stewart
Project Manager: John Rogers
Sr. Production Editor: Kathleen L. Teal
Designer: Amy Buxton
Manufacturing Manager: Betty Richmond
Cover Design: Renée Duenow

SECOND EDITION
Copyright © 1995 by Mosby–Year Book, Inc.

Previous editions copyrighted 1991

Printed in the United States of America
Composition by Graphic World, Inc.
Printing/binding by Walsworth Publishing Co.

Mosby–Year Book, Inc.
11830 Westline Industrial Drive
St. Louis, Missouri 63146

Library of Congress Cataloging in Publication Data

Goldman, Mitchel P.
Sclerotherapy: treatment of varicose and telangiectatic leg veins
/ Mitchel P. Goldman.--2nd ed.
p. cm.
Includes bibliographical references and index.
ISBN 0-8151-4011-8 (alk. paper)
1. Varicose veins--Treatment. 2. Injections, Sclerosing.
I. Title.
[DNLM: 1. Varicose Veins--therapy. 2. Sclerotherapy.
3. Telangiectasis--therapy. WG 620 G619s 1995]
RC695.G65   1995
616.1'43--dc20
DNLM/DLC
for Library of Congress   94-44914
                                                             CIP

95 96 97 98 99 / 9 8 7 6 5 4 3 2 1

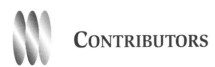

CONTRIBUTORS

JOHN J. BERGAN, M.D., F.A.C.S., F.R.C.S. (Hon.) Eng.

Scripps Memorial Hospital
La Jolla, California;
Professor of Surgery
Loma Linda University
Loma Linda, California;
Clinical Professor of Surgery
USCD Medical School
San Diego, California;
Clinical Professor of Surgery
USUHS
Bethesda, Maryland

HELANE S. FRONEK, M.D.

Attending Physician
Division of Cardiothoracic and Vascular Surgery
Scripps Clinic and Research Foundation
La Jolla, California;
Clinical Instructor in Medicine
University of California, San Diego
San Diego, California

.

To my family
Hedy, Risa, and **Melissa**

PREFACE TO FIRST EDITION

Varicose and/or telangiectatic leg veins occur in up to 80 million adults in the United States alone. Contrary to the popularly held belief among physicians, they are not merely a cosmetic nuisance, since over 50% of patients who seek treatment do so because of pain and discomfort. In addition, varicose veins have a real association with underlying venous hypertension and its resulting manifestations on the skin, which end in ulceration. Varicose veins are a predisposing factor in the development of superficial thrombophlebitis. Therefore, the treatment of this abnormal vascular condition is warranted for both medical and cosmetic reasons.

Up until the last few years, surgical ligation and stripping procedures were the only commonly recognized modalities for treating varicose veins in this country. Sclerotherapy treatment, which has been used for decades in Europe, primarily by dermatologists, was thought of disparagingly or ignored completely. The treatment of varicose veins within vascular surgery departments was relegated to the intern or first year resident, with veins thought of only as a nuisance within the surgical field.

Patients, usually women, who sought treatment from dermatologists for telangiectatic vessels on the legs were told most often that these did not require treatment or that treatment was not efficacious. At times these vessels were treated with various laser modalities or electrodesiccation, all fraught with complications including scarring. Sclerotherapy techniques, which have been largely ignored in dermatology and vascular surgery training, were used inappropriately in the past. High concentrations of strong sclerosing solutions were used to treat extremely thin-walled, delicate telangiectasias. This produced a number of complications and served to discredit this procedure.

While American physicians were either mistreating or inappropriately treating leg veins in this country, our European colleagues were perfecting sclerotherapy and other nonsurgical treatments of varicose and telangiectatic leg veins. In an effort to bridge the gap between our European and American colleagues, the North American Society of Phlebology was founded in 1986. Educational symposia sponsored by the society were phenomenally successful. All across the country among physicians in various specialties there proved to be a tremendous interest in learning how to treat these conditions. This was probably spurred on by an increasing public interest in and awareness of nonscarring techniques available to eliminate unsightly veins.

In 1989 the American Society for Dermatologic Surgery recognized the importance of phlebology training and invited the North American Society of Phlebology to be a member of the *Journal of Dermatologic Surgery and Oncology*. Also in 1989, the American Venous Forum was formed as an offshoot of the American Vascular Surgery Society. In 1990 the American Academy of Dermatology established a task force on phlebology to better define the curriculum for dermatology residency programs. These three organizations established a framework for the development of a phlebology curriculum.

What has been lacking is a reference source in the English language encompassing sclerotherapy treatment of varicose and telangiectatic leg veins. Most of the available scientific papers were published decades ago or are scattered among many different subspecialty journals. This textbook was written in an effort to present in a coherent fashion all of the available information necessary for the physician to obtain a working expertise in the treatment of varicose and telangiectatic leg veins. I have tried to incorporate as much of the non-English literature as is appropriate so that this textbook truly assumes a "worldly" stature.

It is my hope that this textbook will serve as an impetus for future research in the field of phlebology. This book has been written to be a readable resource for medical students, residents, and those physicians just beginning their training in phlebology, as well as to advance the training of those more expert in sclerotherapy techniques.

Mitchel P. Goldman, M.D.

PREFACE TO SECOND EDITION

Since publication of the first edition of *Sclerotherapy Treatment of Varicose and Telangiectatic Leg Veins* there has been an explosion of new textbooks, book chapters and scientific studies on all aspects of sclerotherapy and surgical treatment of varicose and telangiectatic leg veins. I have had the opportunity of editing two new texts on the treatment of varicose veins, *Varicose Veins and Telangiectasia: Diagnosis and Treatment** and *Ambulatory Treatment of Varicose and Telangiectatic Leg Veins: An Illustrated Guide†* I co-authored/edited *Ambulatory Phlebectomy: A Practical Guide‡* with Drs. Ricci and Georgiev. In addition, I was Guest Editor of Seminars in Dermatology issue on Diagnosis and Treatment of Varicose and Telangiectatic Leg Veins§, and Co-editor of the *Journal of Dermatologic Surgery and Oncology (Special Issue on Sclerotherapy Treatment of Varicose and Telangiectatic Leg Veins)‖* These Editorships have allowed me the opportunity of soliciting manuscripts from the leading physicians and surgeons in phlebology. Thus, this second edition incorporates their teaching which has led to the addition of over 625 new references, 160 new illustrations, and 6 new subsections.

Mitchel P. Goldman, M.D.

---

* Quality Medical Publishing, Inc., St. Louis, 1993
† Mosby, St. Louis, 1995
‡ Mosby, St. Louis, 1995
§ Saunders, Philadelphia, 1993
‖ Elsevier Science Publishing Co, New York, 1995

ACKNOWLEDGEMENTS

The first edition acknowledged those who helped me develop as a physician, researcher, author, and phlebologist. What was not acknowledged was the person who helped me develop as a person. In writing this text, as well as other works, I am continually reminded of motherhood. Although I will never be able to achieve that true enlightenment I believe that I have come to know some part of its meaning. Writing this text has allowed me the opportunity to know the subject as a lover would know his/her partner. The conception was easy, with immediate gratification. But after this event, came the hard work of building the foundation for the birth. In the *Second Edition* the foundation consisted of critically reviewing over 625 additional scientific manuscripts and attending an equal number of scientific presentations. It also consisted of critically evaluating the *First Edition* so growth could occur. Although this process took four years instead of nine months, the gestation period for the actual rewrite was nearly identical. After this nurturing experience the birth occurred as a joyous event. But, like parenthood, the final result, peer acceptance in the case of the text, will occur much later. This *Second Edition* is therefore dedicated to my mother, Betty Freedman Goldman, who brought me into this world, nurtured me both physically and mentally, and helped me become who I am today—I Love You Mom.

In addition to those mentioned in the *First Edition* I would like to acknowledge a few additional people who helped the development of the Second *Edition*. Robert and Margaret Weiss and John Bergan have been my sounding boards and mentors for advanced phlebology training. My overseas colleagues, Hugo Partsch, Paul Thibault, George Fegan, Mihael Geogiev, Leonardo Corcos, Dick Groenenweg, Martino Neumann, Dig Tazelaar, Andre Cornu-Thenard, Fredric Vin, Michel Sadick, Claude Guarde, Anita Fratilla, Ulrich Schultz-Ehrenburg, and Gebhard Sattler have provided a depth of knowledge and inspiration. In the States, Pauline Raymond-Martimbeau, Craig Feid, Neil Sadick, Walter de Groot and David Duffy continue to provide me with new ideas to advance my perpetual training in phlebology. Finally, I would like to thank John Bergan again for organizing the La Jolla Venous Lunch Group consisting of Helane and Arnost Fronek, Warner Bundens, Anton Butie, and Jay Murray. This informal monthly meeting serves as a source for interpreting daily problems in phlebology as well as reviewing the scientific work of others. Since formal training in phlebology is scarce or nonexistent, incorporation of an informal phlebology group into the routine of private and academic practice is encouraged for all those in this field.

I would also like to thank the editors and production team at Mosby for their hard work and dedication towards this project: Susie Baxter, Editor; Ellen Baker Geisel, Developmental editor; Christy Stewart, Editorial assistant; John Rogers, Project manager; and Kathleen Teal, Sr. production editor. I have been fortunate to keep most of the team together for my 4 Mosby projects. This cohesive group has made it a true joy to publish. Finally, at Mosby I would like to acknowledge my first editor, Eugenia Klein, who took a novice and taught him how to be an author. This *Second Edition* could not have flowed so easily if it had not been for your teaching and encouragement.

xiii

Finally, I have missed being with my family during these last few months. I would like to extend all my love and thanks to my wife Hedy, and daughters Risa and Melissa for their patience. This book as well as past and future works are dedicated to you.

M.P.G.

CONTENTS IN BRIEF

CONTENTS IN DETAIL

SCLEROTHERAPY

*Treatment of
Varicose and Telangiectatic
Leg Veins*

INTRODUCTION

A significant percentage of the population of the species *Homo sapiens* is known to develop varicose veins, emphasizing the great importance of the erect stance in the development of this condition. Varicose veins in four-legged animals are rare (Fig. A).[1] Why, then, do other erect species fail to develop varicose veins? The development of varicose veins is probably secondary to anatomic differences. Taller mammals, such as giraffes and humans, have relatively thick fascial layers enclosing the deep venous system; shorter mammals, such as rabbits and rats, do not.[2] Physiologic studies demonstrate that giraffe capillaries are highly impermeable to plasma proteins. In addition, their tight skin and fascial layers provide a functional "antigravity suit" to prevent venous hypertension. Finally, a prominent lymphatic system and precapillary vasoconstriction propel blood and lymphatic fluid against gravity. Therefore, with a disturbance in this complex system, the transmission of high venous pressure to superficial veins, which are not designed to contain that pressure, results in dilatation. The development of varicose veins is but one manifestation of "venous insufficiency."

As is discussed in detail below and in Chapter 2, varicose veins should be thought of as one clinical manifestation of venous hypertension. When chronic, venous hypertension results in a sequence of cutaneous complications: edema, cutaneous pigmentation, venous/stasis dermatitis, atrophie blanche, cutaneous ulceration, and malignant degeneration. Varicose veins alone may also be complicated by hemorrhage, thrombophlebitis, and pain.

The primary therapeutic procedure for all stasis complications, except malignant degeneration, is to normalize the underlying pathologic physiology that gives rise to cuticular venous hypertension: increased interstitial fluid and resultant decreased oxygenation and defective nutrition of the skin. Ideally, treatment is directed first to correcting cuticular venous hypertension. This may be accomplished through the treatment of the superficial or deep venous systems or their conduits.

Deep venous hypertension is usually managed with conservative compression therapy. In selected patients, vein valve transplantation or repair can also be efficacious. However, surgeons are understandably loathe to operate through eczematous skin that may be contaminated with bacteria. Thus, dermatologic treatment is extremely important in providing the optimal operative field. Alternatively, direct sclerotherapy of an underlying incompetent perforating vein through the ulcer may be performed. Sclerotherapy in this setting has been shown to markedly enhance ulcer healing.[3,4] Newer surgical techniques of perforating vein interruption utilizing endoscopic visualization can also normalize venous hypertension. Finally, in certain patients, treatment of the superficial venous system with either surgical intervention and/or sclerotherapy is also beneficial.

HISTORICAL ASPECTS OF TREATMENT

Hippocrates observed the association between varicose veins and leg ulceration more than 2000 years ago.[5] As with most physical diseases of that time, offerings to the gods for help comprised the earliest method of treating varicose veins,

1

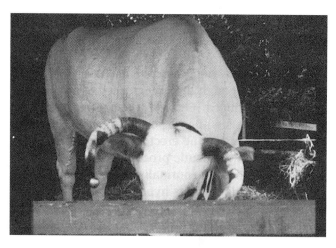

Fig. A   Brahma bull with a varicose vein on the right posterior medial leg. (Courtesy A. Butie, M.D.)

as shown in a votive relief found at the Greek Temple of Aesculapius in 400 BC (Fig. B). Physicians of the day, however, attempted to formulate more terrestrial treatments. Egyptian papyrus scrolls have been found that contain instructions for the treatment of leg disorders. Ebers, in his papyrus of 1550 BC, advised that surgery should not be performed on varicose veins.[6] The humoral theory of Hippocrates dictated bloodletting as a form of treatment for varicose veins, which remained the treatment of choice into the Middle Ages. The first description of medical treatment appears in the writings of Hippocrates in the fourth century BC. He describes treating varicose veins by traumatizing them with "a slender instrument of iron" to cause thrombosis.[7] Surgeons as well were developing various treatments for varicose veins. Stripping and cauterization were practiced by Celsus (30 BC to 30 AD). Antillus was the first to mention ligation of the vessels. In the second century AD, Galen recommended that varicose veins be torn out with a hook. Paulus of Aegina (circa 660 AD in Alexandria) performed ligation and stripping of the segments of the varicosity. After William Harvey's discovery of the true nature of circulation, surgical removal of the affected veins was rejected because the procedure could cause complications that were more dangerous than the disease itself. The modern history of surgical treatment began after the introduction of anesthesia and sterile techniques in the late nineteenth century. This is reviewed in Chapter 10.

Compression therapy was recognized very early as an effective form of therapy (see Chapter 6). Roman soldiers wrapped their legs in leather straps to minimize leg fatigue during long marches. Marianus Sanctus Barolitanus (1555), Pare Johnson (1678), and de Marque (1618) recommended the use of plaster bandages. Firm support was not widely used until Wiseman (1676) introduced the laced leather stocking for treating ulcers associated with varicose veins.[8] Although compression therapy may be quite effective for patients with limited venous disease,[9] when used alone it is associated with a high rate of ulcer recurrence.[10] This association may be related to the expertise of the medical practitioner applying compression and to the materials used. To be effective, a compression bandage must generate 40 to 70 mm Hg.[11] This means that the toes of a correctly bandaged leg must become slightly cyanotic when the leg is horizontal and return to a pink color on standing. Obviously, skill and experience are a prerequisite for proper compression treatment (see Chapter 6).

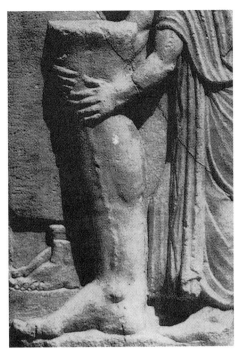

Fig. B   According to the inscription, this tablet found on the west side of the acropolis in Athens was dedicated to Doctor Amynos by Lysimachidis of Archarnes. This represents the earliest known depiction of varicose veins from the end of the fourth century BC. (From National Archaeological Museum of Greece.)

The first use of an intravenous injection in humans is attributed to Sigismund Eisholtz (1623-1688). He used an enema syringe to inject distilled plantain water into a branch of the crural vein to irrigate an ulcer with a small siphon.[12] In 1682, D. Zollikofer of St. Gallen, Switzerland, reported on the injection of an acid into a vein to create a thrombus.[12] This was the first attempt at "sclerotherapy," a term derived from the Greek word for "hard," made popular by H.I. Biegeleisen in 1939.[13]

Extravascular sclerotherapy of a hemangioma was first reported in 1836. The surgeon, Mr. Loyd, injected from 3 to 6 drops of nitric acid dissolved in a drachm of water. This solution was "thrown into the tumour by means of a syringe through a minute puncture at its base."[14] No mention was made of the outcome of this treatment, but the next reported case was instantly fatal.[15]

Intravascular sclerotherapy of an arterial malformation to produce a clot was first performed in 1840 on animals by Pravaz with a solution of absolute alcohol.[16] In 1851, a solution of ferric chloride was used to sclerose varicose veins.[17] This was made possible through modification of the syringe with the invention of a sharpened hollow needle capable of direct venous puncture.[18] In 1854, Desgranges reported the cure of 16 cases of varicose veins with the injection of a mixture of iodine 5 gm and tannin 45 gm in 50 ml of water.[19] Desgranges noted that this solution produced far fewer local reactions than those of ferric chloride. His patients were kept in bed for 10 to 12 days. Unfortunately, extended use of this solution and technique produced septic complications.

These intravascular sclerotherapy treatments were stimulated by Rynd's introduction of the hypodermic syringe in 1845.[20,21] The syringe of Rynd, an elaborate trocar and cannula, and the subsequently modified syringe of Pravaz, were both modifications of the lachrimal syringe developed by Anel in 1713.[22] It is interesting that the apparatus manufactured for Pravaz was unsatisfactory because when blood and coagulant/sclerosant mixed after the trocar had been withdrawn and the syringe was screwed on, blood clotted within the lumen of the cannula.[23] It was not until Wulfing Luer, in Germany, adopted the hollow needle onto a Ferguson syringe that a device approaching the modern syringe was used.

Between 1904 and 1910, P. Scharf utilized sublimate on himself and 90 patients with varicose veins.[24] Nathan Brann, founder of the first phlebology society, also recommended vein sclerosis with sublimate, which produced firm thrombosis of varicose veins.[25]

The foundation of modern sclerotherapy treatment of varicose veins began in 1916 when Linser reported many successful treatments using perchloride of mercury with an intravascular technique.[26] He emphasized ambulatory treatments limiting the maximal dose of sublimate to 1 to 2 ml per treatment session. He also inadvertently encouraged walking after treatment, noting that many "women had to walk for longer periods to their houses after treatment."[27] However, 1% to 3% of patients developed mercury intoxication with nephritis, stomatitis, and enteritis, and the procedure again was abandoned.[28] In 1916, Sicard noticed the sclerosing effect of Luargol solution used in the treatment of syphilis.[29] He reported his first series of cases in 1920 on the use of carbonate of soda but later found that salicylate of soda was best for sclerosing varicose veins.[30] The first pharmaceutically manufactured sclerosing solution was a mixture of saline and procaine. Thereafter, multiple solutions were produced by the German pharmaceutical industry. This stimulated research on both sides of the Atlantic for an ideal sclerosing solution and many different compounds were tried (see box on p. 5). These included the following: 50% grape sugar,[31] mercury biiodide,[32] 20% and 30% sodium salicylate,[33,34] sodium citrate,[35] 20% to 30% sodium chloride,[35] 1% bichloride of mercury,[36] 50% to 60% calorose (75% invert sugar with 5% saccharose),[37] and 12% quinine sulfate with 6% urethane.[37] These substances were widely used but resulted in unacceptable levels of allergic reactions, necrosis, pain, and even fatalities.[38,40] (A complete discussion of the development and properties of modern sclerosing solutions is found in Chapter 7.)

Tournay was instrumental in developing a school of sclerotherapy in France and refined the injection technique to include drainage of intravascular thrombi. McAusland popularized the technique in the United States in 1939 with his report of the successful treatment of 10,000 patients.[41] He promoted injection into empty veins to limit the degree of thrombosis, treatment of the incompetent saphenofemoral junction before sclerosing distal varices, the use of postsclerotherapy compression, and the use of minimal sclerosant concentrations (in the form of sodium morrhuate froth) for sclerosing telangiectasia. Brunstein further popularized injection into empty veins and the use of postsclerotherapy compression to produce cosmetic, painless, efficient sclerosis.[42] The advent of synthetic sclerosing agents in 1946 firmly established sclerotherapy (primarily in Europe) as a viable form of treatment for varicose veins. Still, many physicians perceived clinical results of sclerotherapy treatment to be less optimal than those obtained with surgical approaches.

Although the use of compression therapy for treatment of venous disease is mentioned in the Old Testament and was performed by Hippocrates in the fourth century BC, it has been used in sclerosing treatment of varicose veins only within the past 40 years.[43] Postsclerosis compression, initially described by Brunstein in the 1940s,[42] Sigg[44] and Orbach[45] in the 1950s, and Fegan in the 1960s,[46] is perhaps

HISTORICAL INTRODUCTION OF SCLEROSING AGENTS

1840	Absolute alcohol (Monteggio, Leroy D'Etiolles)
1851-1853	Ferric chloride (Pravaz)
1855	Iodo-tannic liquer (Desgranges)
1880	"Chloral" (Negretti)
1904	5% Phenol solution (Tavel)
1906	Potassium iodo-iodine (Tavel)
1910	"Sublime" (Scharf)
1917	Hypertonic glucose/calorose (Kausch)
1919	Sodium salicylate (Sicard and Gaugier)
1919	Sodium bicarbonate (Sicard and Gaugier)
1920	Bichloride of mercury (Wolf)
1922	12% Quinine sulfate with 6% urethane (Geneurier)
1922	Biiodine of mercury (Lacroix, Bazelis)
1926	Hypertonic saline with procaine (Linser)
1927	50% Grape sugar (Doerffel)
1929	Sodium citrate (Kern and Angel)
1929	20%-30% Hypertonic saline (Kern and Angel)
1930	Sodium morrhuate (Higgins and Kittel)
1933	Chromated glycerine (Sclermo) (Jausion)
1937	Ethanolamine oleate (Biegeleisen)
1946	Sodium tetradecyl sulfate (Sotradecol) (Reiner)
1949	Phenolated mercury and ammonium (Tournay and Wallois)
1959	Stabilized polyiodated ions (Variglobin) (Imhoff and Sigg)
1966	Polidocanol (Aetoxisclerol) (Henschel and Eichenberg)
1969	Hypertonic saline/dextrose (Sclerodex)

Modified from Goldman MP and Bennett RG: Treatment of telangiectasia: a review. J Am Acad Dermatol 17:167, 1987.

the most important advance in sclerotherapy treatment of varicose veins since the introduction of relatively safe synthetic sclerosing agents in the 1940s. With the advent of "compression" sclerotherapy, clinical results equal to surgical procedures are now reported.

In Europe, sclerotherapy has been fully accepted by the medical community since the 1960s and exists as a separate specialty (phlebology and/or angiology).[47] Even today, however, American physicians do not understand the technique or its indications, safety, and efficacy. Eighty-two percent of gynecologists recently surveyed did not have enough knowledge to advise patients who requested information on the treatment of varicose and telangiectatic leg veins. In fact, the gynecologists *incorrectly* perceived that sclerotherapy produced indiscriminate venous destruction; had a high risk of venous thrombosis and allergic reactions; caused permanent pigmentation or scarring; necessitated prolonged, repetitive, painful treatments; and had a low percentage of improvement.[48]

Patients seek therapy for telangiectasias or varicose veins principally because of their unsightly appearance. A recent survey has shown that American women are more concerned with lower extremity telangiectasia than with almost any other cosmetic problem.[49] However, proper treatment is frequently difficult to obtain because correct surgical intervention and sclerotherapy largely are not taught in medical schools or residency programs. Frequently, patients with telangiectasias of the legs are told that they must live with the problem. Treatment options, including sclerotherapy, either are not discussed or are mentioned disparagingly.

However, available evidence indicates that safe, effective forms of treatment other than surgery are possible and quite successful.

In addition to the cosmetic benefits of sclerotherapy, studies have demonstrated that sclerotherapy treatment of incompetent perforating veins increases the efficacy of the calf muscle pump, resulting in an improved clearance of extravascular fluid.[50] Lymphangiography of patients with chronic venous insufficiency who are treated with sclerotherapy also demonstrates normalization of lymphatic drainage, in addition to improvements in venous hemodynamics.[51,52] There also is a significant percentage of patients (28% to 85%) with chronic venous insufficiency who have superficial venous insufficiency alone or in combination with deep venous system abnormalities.[53,54,55] These patients show greater improvement with sclerotherapy and/or surgical treatment of the superficial veins combined with compression therapy than with compression therapy alone.[56] In addition, while the symptoms of heaviness and aching of the legs is often relieved by wearing a graduated compression stocking,[57] patients prefer to be rid of the veins to wearing a daily compression stocking, which may be difficult to apply, unsightly, and uncomfortable in warm, humid climates.

A common misconception of physicians is that knowledge of or dexterity in venipuncture confers expertise in sclerotherapy. True expertise in sclerotherapy, like all specializations in medicine and surgery, comes only after extensive postgraduate education, the observation of trained physicians using meticulous technique, and subsequent (preferably supervised) practice. Fortunately, physicians who specialize in the treatment of venous disease (phlebologists, dermatologists, and vascular surgeons) now can offer relatively simple treatments for this widespread medical ailment.

Hobbs,[3] Lofgren[58] and Beninson[59] have pointed out that the treatment of varicosities per se may have no effect on alleviating superficial venous pressure. It is the treatment of the underlying communicating or perforating veins draining the gaiter area that is important.[3,10,12,60,61] These vessels may be either surgically ligated,[10,12,60,61] or sclerosed.[3] Only then will the retrograde flow under high pressure via the calf muscle pump be diverted upstream and away from the skin. This succeeds in lowering the cuticular venous pressure with decreased capillary permeability and edema, thus increasing tissue oxygenation and nutrition. Wilson and Browse estimate that 40% to 50% of patients with venous ulceration have nonthrombotic and/or perforating vein incompetence that can be treated successfully with interruption of the abnormal veins, either through superficial ligation or sclerotherapy.[49]

PRESENT DAY TREATMENT

Sclerotherapy, as practiced today, has been shown to be as effective as comparable surgical procedures (ligation and stripping) in long-term follow-up studies of most types of varicose veins, excluding those with significant saphenofemoral incompetence.[62-65]

In patients with saphenofemoral reflux, sclerotherapy can be effective if surgical treatment is contraindicated. Wallois' recommendation is to treat these patients once or twice a year to maintain effective sclerosis of the varicose greater saphenous vein.[66] Although this method does not produce a cure, it maintains both cosmetic and symptomatic improvement. Finally, as discussed further in Chapter 10, sclerotherapy can complement surgical treatment, especially for varicose or perforating veins, and can prevent surgical recurrences.[67]

Modern sclerotherapy has also been demonstrated to result in a relief of symptoms in up to 85% of patients with both varicose[4] and telangiectatic veins.[68] In addition, sclerotherapy treatment has been demonstrated to be a more physiologic approach to eliminating abnormal varicose veins. One study of dissected cadaver legs demonstrated that more than 50% of the patients with significant varicose veins had a normal greater saphenous system, suggesting that vein stripping may be an inappropriate procedure in a significant percentage of patients.[69] This is especially important regarding utilization of the greater saphenous vein as a conduit for myocardial revascularization. Although the internal mammary artery is a better conduit for coronary artery bypass grafting, the greater saphenous vein is still necessary in a significant number of patients.[70] Most patients require multiple grafts and the internal mammary artery can accommodate only 1 to 2 graft segments.

Sclerotherapy of "varicose" (abnormal) veins does not impede the vascular surgeon from harvesting appropriate conduits for coronary artery bypass. The structural quality of vein grafts is of decisive importance for the maintenance of patency. Patency half-life with a good to excellent graft is 10.5 years vs. 0.5 years when fair and poor quality grafts (including those taken from varicose veins) are utilized.[71] A more recent study cites an incidence of graft failure at 30 months in 68% of patients grafted with diseased veins versus 27% when healthy veins are utilized.[72] Most important, treatment of "early" varicose veins is thought to halt their progression into larger, more severe varices.[73,74] Early treatment may prevent the development of valvular incompetence. Therefore, not only is sclerotherapy not detrimental to coronary bypass grafts, but it may help in providing better conduits for this procedure should the need arise.

Perhaps more significant in this age of cost control, sclerotherapy treatment has been demonstrated to be much less costly than surgical procedures in the treatment of varicose veins.[75,78] In lieu of the inpatient hospital ligation and stripping operation, sclerotherapy treatment is performed on an outpatient basis, permitting patients to return to work immediately after the procedure. Newer surgical techniques practiced in ambulatory surgical centers allow saphenofemoral junction ligation to be performed without general anesthesia. In this setting, the traditional expense of surgical procedures is lessened. However, even with the most modern surgical treatments, the morbidity and cost of surgery is greater than that of sclerotherapy.

However, when saphenofemoral incompetence is present, a limited ligation and stripping procedure, followed by immediate ambulatory phlebectomy or sclerotherapy 3 to 6 weeks later, may be necessary. Because of the "limited" nature of the procedure (as described in Chapter 10), hospitalization is usually not required and the procedure is performed in an outpatient surgical facility. In addition to cost savings, patients' preference for outpatient sclerotherapy has been a major reason for the modernization of varicose vein treatment.[75] This preference has occurred despite the recurrence of varicose veins (usually to a minor degree) in 88% of patients in whom sclerotherapy alone was performed.[75]

In summary, the presence of varicose and telangiectatic veins is not a normal physical finding, but a medical disease deserving of treatment. Varicose and telangiectatic veins may be symptomatic, representing an obvious manifestation of venous disease with its resultant complications, and may pose medical risks and complications in and of themselves. According to Hippocrates, the only advantages of having varicose veins are that "The bald are not subject to varicose veins; but should they occur, the hairs are reproduced," and "If varicose veins or hemorrhoids occur during mania, the mania is cured."[79]

Fortunately, the majority of patients with varicose and telangiectatic veins do not have a life-threatening problem. Therefore, treatment should be as simple as possible, with the least risk of significant side effects. Modern sclerotherapy treatment has been demonstrated to fulfill these requirements with efficacy that is comparable to operative procedures. This text examines the pathophysiology and practical application of sclerotherapy treatment for varicose veins and telangiectasias through a review of the world literature, presentation of experimental studies, and recommendations derived from my clinical practice and the practices of the contributing authors.

REFERENCES

1. Butie A: Personal communication, 1989.
2. Hargens AR et al: Gravitational haemodynamics and oedema prevention in the giraffe, Nature 329:59, 1987.
3. Hobbs JT: The problem of the post-thrombotic syndrome. Postgrad Med (Aug supp):48, 1973.
4. Fegan G: Varicose veins, London, 1967, William Heinemann.
5. Adams EF: The genuine works of Hippocrates, London, 1849, Sydenham.
6. Strandness DE Jr and Thiele BL: Selected topics in venous disorders. Mt Kisco, NY, 1981, Futura.
7. Benton W: Hippocratic writings on ulcers, Chicago, 1970, Brittanica Great Books.
8. Browse NL, Burnand KG, and Thomas ML: Diseases of the veins: pathology, diagnosis, and treatment, London, 1988, Edward Arnold.
9. Morris WT and Lamb AM: The Auckland Hospital varicose veins and venous ulcer clinic: a report on six years work, NZ Med J 93:350, 1981.
10. Negus D and Friedgood A: The effective management of venous ulceration, Br J Surg 70:623, 1983.
11. Leu HJ: Differential diagnosis of chronic leg ulcers, Angiology 14:288, 1963.
12. Kwaan JHM, Jones RN, and Connolly JE: Simplified technique for the management of refractory varicose ulcers, Surgery 80:743, 1976.
13. Biegeleisen HI: Am J Surg 44:622, 1939.
14. London Med Gazette 19:14, October 1, 1836.
15. Ibid. December 30, 1837.
16. Schneider W: Contribution to the history of the sclerosing treatment of varices and to its anatomopathologic study, Soc Fran de Phlebol 18:117, 1965.
17. Charles-Gabriel Pravas: Sur un nouveau myon d'operer la coagulation du sang dans les arteres applicable a la guerison des aneurismes, Compt Rend Hebd Seances Acad Sci 56:88, 1853.
18. Scholz A: Historical aspects. In W Westerhof, editor: Leg ulcers: diagnosis and treatment, 1993, Elsevier Science Publishers BV.
19. Desgranges: Injections Iodo-tanniques dans les varices, Mem de la Soc de Chir 4, 1985.
20. Garrison FH: An introduction to the history of medicine, Philadelphia, 1929, Saunder.
21. Rynd F: Neuralgia: introduction of fluid to the nerve. Dublin Med Press 13:167, 1845.
22. Anel D: Nouvelle methode de guerir les fistules lacrimales, on recueil de defferentes pieces pour et contre, et en faveur de la meme methode nouvellement inventee, Turin Zappatte, 1713.
23. Howard-Jones N: A critical study of the origins and early development of hypodermic medication, J Hist Med 2:201, 1947.
24. Scharf P: Ein neues Verfahren der intravenosen Behandlung der Varicositaten der Unterextremitaten, Berliner Klin Wochenschr 13:582, 1910.
25. Brann E: Die Varizenbehandlung mit Injektionen, Bit Beinhlkd 15:5, 1929.
26. Linser: Uber die Konservative Behandlung der Varicen, Med Klink 12:897, 1916.
27. Zirn C: Die Behandlung der Krampfadern mit intravenosen Sublimatinektionen. Eine Methode fur den praktische Arzt Inaug Diss Berlin, Karger, 1916.
28. Linser P: Die Behandlung der Krampfadern mit Sublimatinspritzung und ihre Erfolge, Med Klin 17:1445, 1921.
29. Stemmer R: Sclerotherapy of varicose veins, St. Gallen, Switzerland, 1990, Ganzoni & Cie, AG.
30. Sicard JA and Roger H: Traitment des Varices par Injections Intraveineuses Locales de Carbonate de Soude, Marseille Med 4:97, 1921.
31. Doerffel: Klinisches und Experimentelles uber Venenverodung mit Kochsalzlosung und Traubenzucker, Deutsche Med Wohnschr 53:901, 1927.
32. Bazelis R: Thesis de doctorate, Paris, 1924.
33. Schwartz E and Ratschow M: Experimentelle und Klinische erfahrungen bei der Kunstlichen Verodung von Varicen, Arch Klin Chir 156:720, 1929.
34. Meisen V: A lecture on injection-treatment of varicose veins and their sequelae (eczema and ulcus cruris), clinically and experimentally, Acta Scand 60:435, 1926.
35. Kern HM and Angle LW: The chemical obliteration of varicose veins: a clinical and experimental

study, JAMA 93:595, 1929.

36. Wolf E: Die histologischen Veranderungen der Venen nach intravenosen sub limatein Spritzungen, Med Klin 16:806, 1920.

37. Lufkin NH and McPheeters HO: Pathological studies on injected varicose veins, Surg Gynecol Obstet 54:511, 1932.

38. D'Addato M: Gangrene of a limb with complete thrombosis of the venous system, J Cardiovas Surg (Torino) 7:434, 1966.

39. Hohlbaum J: Todliche Embolie nach Varicenbehandlung mit Preglosung, Zentralbl Chir 7:218, 1922.

40. Hempel C: Erfahrungen mit Sublimatinjektichen bei Varizen, Deutsche Med Wochenschr 71:900, 1924.

41. McAusland S: The modern treatment of varicose veins, Med Press 201:404, 1939.

42. Brunstein IA: Prevention of discomfort and disability in the treatment of varicose veins. Am J Surg 54:362, 1941.

43. Orbach EJ: Compression therapy of vein and lymph vessel diseases of the lower extremities, Angiology 30:95, 1979.

44. Sigg K: The treatment of varicosities and accompanying complications, Angiology 3:355, 1952.

45. Orbach EJ: A new approach to the sclerotherapy of varicose veins, Angiology 1:302, 1950.

46. Fegan WG: Continuous compression technique of injecting varicose veins, Lancet 2:109, 1963.

47. Widmer LK: The time has come for vascular medicine: Angiology: a subspecialty of internal medicine and dermatology in Switzerland, Int Angiol 10:162, 1991.

48. Weiss RA, Weiss MA, and Goldman MP: Physicians' negative perception of sclerotherapy for venous disorders: review of a 7-year experience with modern sclerotherapy, South Med J 85:1101, 1992.

49. Wilson NM and Browse NL: Venous disease. In Clement DL and Shepherd JT, editors: Vascular diseases in the lower limbs, St. Louis, 1993, Mosby Yearbook.

50. Raso AM et al: Studio su 357 casi di flebite degli arti inferiori su due campioni interregionali, Minerva Chir 34:553, 1979.

51. Nitzche N and Petter O: Peripheres LymphabfluBsystem der unteren Extremitaten bei chronischer Veneninsuffizienz, Phlebologie 20:21, 1991.

52. Leu AJ et al: Microangiopathy in chronic venous insufficiency before and after sclerotherapy and compression treatment: results of a one-year follow-up study, Phlebology 8:99, 1993.

53. McEnroe CS, O'Donnell TF Jr, and Mackey WC: Correlation of clinical findings with venous hemodynamics in 386 patients with chronic venous insufficiency, Am J Surg 156:148, 1988.

54. Neglen P and Raju S: A rational approach to detection of significant reflux with duplex Doppler scanning and air plethysmography, J Vasc Surg 17:590, 1993.

55. Shami SK et al: Venous ulcers and the superficial venous system, J Vasc Surg 17:487, 1993.

56. Stacey MC et al: Calf pump function in patients with healed venous ulcers is not improved by surgery to the communicating veins or by elastic stockings, Br J Surg 75:436, 1988.

57. Chant ADB, Magnussen P, and Kershaw S: Support hose and varicose veins, Br Med J 290:204, 1985.

58. Lofgren EP: Leg ulcers: symptoms of an underlying disorder, Postgrad Med 76:51, 1984.

59. Gravatational eczema. In Rook A et al, editors: Textbook of dermatology, ed 4, Cambridge, Mass, 1986, Blackwell Scientific.

60. Cockett FB and Thomas ML: The iliac compression syndrome, Br J Surg 52:816, 1965.

61. Lim LT, Michuda M, and Bergan JJ: Therapy of peripheral vascular ulcers: surgical management, Angiology 29:654, 1978.

62. Hobbs JT: The treatment of varicose veins: a random trial of injection/compression versus surgery, Br J Surg 55:777, 1968.

63. Hobbs JT: Surgery and sclerotherapy in the treatment of varicose veins: a random trial, Arch Surg 109:793, 1974.

64. Chant ADB, Jones HO, and Wendell JM: Varicose veins: a comparison of surgery and injection/compression sclerotherapy, Lancet 2:1188, 1972.

65. Henry MEF, Fegan WG, and Pegum JM: Five-year survey of the treatment of varicose ulcers, Br Med J 2:493, 1971.

66. Wallois P: The conditions necessary to achieve an effective sclerosant treatment, Phlebologie 35:337, 1982.

67. Munn SR et al: To strip or not to strip the long saphenous vein? A varicose veins trial, Br J Surg 68:426, 1981.

68. Weiss R and Weiss M: Resolution of pain associated with varicose and telangiectatic leg veins after compression sclerotherapy, J Dermatol Surg Oncol 16:333, 1990.

69. Schwartz SI: Year book of surgery, Chicago, 1979, Year Book.

70. Nair UR, Griffiths G, and Lawson RAM: Postoperative neuralgia in the leg after saphenous vein

coronary artery bypass graft: a prospective study, Thorax 43:41, 1988.

71. Szilagyi DE et al: Autogenous vein grafting in femoropopliteal atherosclerosis: the limits of its effectiveness, Surgery 86:836, 1979.

72. Panetta TF et al: Unsuspected preexisting saphenous vein disease: an unrecognized cause of vein bypass failure, J Vasc Surg 15:102, 1992.

73. Gallagher PG: Major contributing role of sclerotherapy in the treatment of varicose veins, Vasc Surg 20:139, 1986.

74. Ludbrook J: Valvular defect in primary varicose veins: cause or effect? Lancet 2:1289, 1963.

75. Kistner RL et al: The evolving management of varicose veins, Postgrad Med 80:51, 1986.

76. Piachaud D and Weddell JM: Cost of treating varicose veins, Lancet 2:1191, 1972.

77. Doran FSA and White M: A clinical trial designed to discover if the primary treatment of varicose veins should be by Fegan's method or by operation, Br J Surg 62:72, 1975.

78. Beresford SAA et al: Varicose veins: a comparison of surgery and injection/compression sclerotherapy five-year follow-up, Lancet 1:921, 1978.

79. Coar T: The aphorisms of Hippocrates: with a translation into Latin and English, London, 1822, Longman.

1   ANATOMY AND HISTOLOGY OF THE VENOUS SYSTEM OF THE LEG

The venous system of the lower extremities functions as a conduit for carrying deoxygenated blood from the muscles and the cutaneous and subcutaneous tissues to the heart and also functions as a reservoir of blood. Although all veins have a similar structure, the particular functions of the venous system of the leg are imposed by their surroundings. When covered by muscle and fascia, the deep veins serve as a transport system. Depending on the tension of perivenous tissues, deep veins may either draw blood from the superficial veins or pump blood toward the heart. External to the fascia and muscles, superficial veins serve primarily as reservoirs with limited transport capability.

Nomenclature used throughout the text conforms to the Venous Consensus Conference Classification recently developed.[1] The long saphenous vein is referred to using the English-Latin term *greater,* the short saphenous vein is referred to using the English-Latin translation *lessor,* and those veins that "perforate" the fascia are termed *perforator veins.* Veins that connect to other veins within a fascial plane are referred to as *communicating veins.*

ANATOMY

The venous system of the lower limbs consists of two channels: one within the muscular system and one superficial to it (Fig. 1-1). Along most of their course, veins are intimately associated with both arteries and nerves. In certain locations this association assumes clinical and therapeutic importance. The lessor saphenous vein (LSV) is intimately connected with the tibial and sural nerves that are located equidistant either medial or lateral to the vein. This may explain the pain that occurs when this vein is varicose (Fig. 1-2).[2] When the LSV terminates into the greater saphenous vein (GSV) in the midthigh, it lies very close to the sciatic nerve. This is important because varicose veins in this location may press on the nerve and cause a "sciatica"-like pain[2] (Fig. 1-1, *C*).

Careless surgical exploration or excessive perivascular inflammation may cause a neuralgia to nearby nerves and damage to adjacent arteries. The saphenous nerve is intimately associated with the LSV or the GSV at the level of the knee joint after it emerges from the subsartorial canal (Fig. 1-3). The nerve lies along the vein anteriorly through the leg to the medial aspect of the dorsum of the foot before dividing into branches that supply the medial toes.[3,4] At times, the saphenous nerve is adherent to the GSV. In a study of 60 cadaver legs, four types of saphenous nerve/GSV associations were identified. Adhesion between the GSV and saphenous nerve was observed at the medial malleolus in 80% of dissections and at the midleg in 97% of dissections.[4] Just below the knee the nerve may lie anterior to the vein 40% to 80% of the time and posterior to it in 20% to 60% of dissections.[5,6] It may also be more common for the nerve to lie anterior to the vein in the lower third of the calf and posterior to the vein in the proximal half of the lower leg.[7,8]

Text continues on p. 16

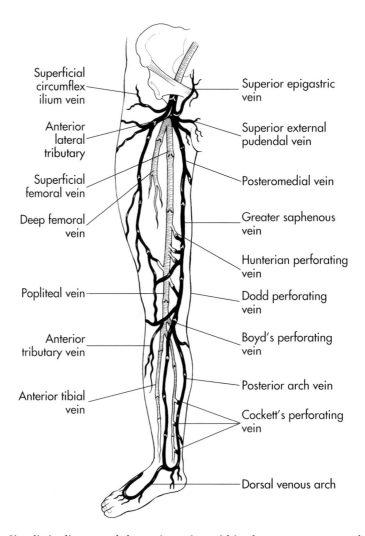

Superficial circumflex ilium vein

Anterior lateral tributary

Superficial femoral vein

Deep femoral vein

Popliteal vein

Anterior tributary vein

Anterior tibial vein

Superior epigastric vein

Superior external pudendal vein

Posteromedial vein

Greater saphenous vein

Hunterian perforating vein

Dodd perforating vein

Boyd's perforating vein

Posterior arch vein

Cockett's perforating vein

Dorsal venous arch

Fig. 1-1   Simplistic diagram of the major veins within the venous system of the lower limbs.

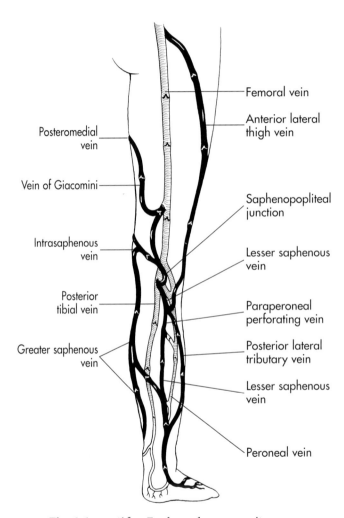

Fig. 1-1, cont'd For legend see opposite page.

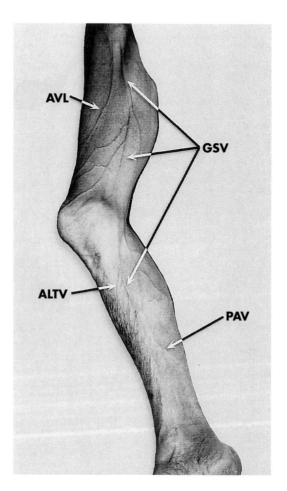

Fig. 1-1C   The GSV and its tributaries are occasionally well displayed on thin legs. (GSV, Greater saphenous vein; ALTV, anterolateral thigh vein; AVL, anterior vein of the leg [accessory saphenous vein]; PAV, posterior arch vein.) (Reproduced with permission from Somjen GM: Anatomy of the superficial venous system, J Dermatol Surg Oncol 1995 [in press].)

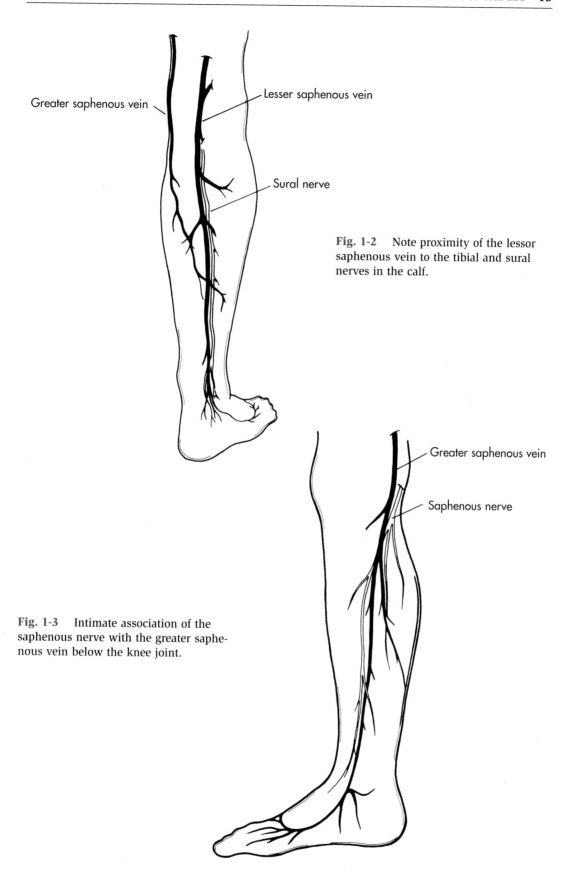

Greater saphenous vein

Lesser saphenous vein

Sural nerve

Fig. 1-2   Note proximity of the lessor saphenous vein to the tibial and sural nerves in the calf.

Greater saphenous vein

Saphenous nerve

Fig. 1-3   Intimate association of the saphenous nerve with the greater saphenous vein below the knee joint.

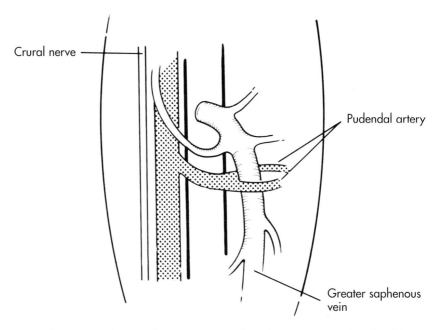

Crural nerve

Pudendal artery

Greater saphenous
vein

Fig. 1-4 Illustration of a possible association of a bifurcated external pudendal artery at the saphenofemoral junction.

Another area with potentially dangerous anatomy is the saphenofemoral junction (SFJ). The superficial external pudendal artery is intimately associated with the GSV at the SFJ, where it may bifurcate to enclose the GSV (Fig. 1-4). Twin gastrocnemius arteries and a smaller lessor saphenous artery also occur in intimate association with the GSV within the calf.

The principal deep veins are the femoral and popliteal/tibial veins. These begin in the foot as plantar digital veins. They lie unsupported within the loose connective tissue of the vascular bundle and not within the "muscle pump" as described below. These veins, as well as other deep veins in the body, contain one-way valves, located every few centimeters, that direct blood flow toward the heart (see Fig. 1-1). If the valve cusps do not meet and the blood therefore flows away from the heart as well as toward it, the valve is defined as incompetent. In addition, within the soleal muscle there are thin-walled, valveless venous reservoirs that number from 1 to 18. These reservoirs are linked to one another usually by venous channels (which contain valves) and empty high in the calf into the posterior tibial veins.[9] In addition to superficial veins, the deep muscle pump chamber is refilled by arterial inflow and distal deep veins. It should be emphasized that, through the action of muscular compression, almost 90% of all venous blood leaves the legs through the deep veins (Fig. 1-5).[2,10] Fluoroscopic study has demonstrated that, with muscular exercise, blood is drawn from the superficial veins through the perforating veins into the deep venous system (Fig. 1-6).[11] This system is correctly termed the *calf muscle pump* or *peripheral heart*.[12]

The only exception to the inward direction of blood flow is in the foot, where the perforating vein valves allow flow from the deep to the superficial veins.[13] It has been determined that at least 50% of pedal perforating veins do not contain valves.[14,15] In fact, occlusion of the superficial veins of the leg produces a flow of blood from the superficial to the deep pedal veins,[9] indicating that a muscle pump in the foot also provides an important mechanism for venous return. This has been confirmed with video-phlebography[16] and duplex scanning.[17] Therefore,

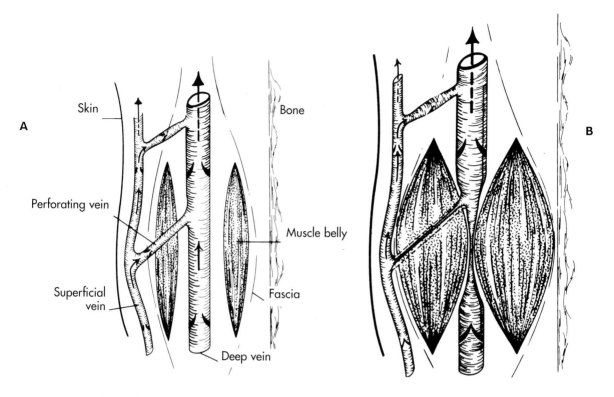

Fig. 1-5 Schematic diagram of the calf muscle pump. **A,** Relaxed state. All valves are open, allowing blood to flow in a proximal direction. Blood flows proximal to both the superficial vein and through the perforating vein into the deep veins. Note the fascial covering of the "deep system." **B,** With muscle contraction, the perforating veins are squeezed closed. Valves distal to the compression are closed to prevent distal blood flow.

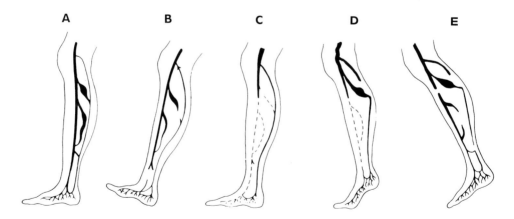

Fig. 1-6 Sequence of blood flow within the lower leg during walking. **A,** Resting. **B,** Early contraction with the heel pressed and gastrocnemius muscle beginning contraction. **C,** Full contraction of all muscles. **D,** Knee flexion with contraction of the soleus muscle and relaxation of the gastrocnemius. **E,** Relaxation of all muscles. (Redrawn from Almen T and Nylander G: Serial phlebography of the normal leg during muscle contraction and relaxation, Acta Radiol 57:264, 1962.)

PROXIMAL

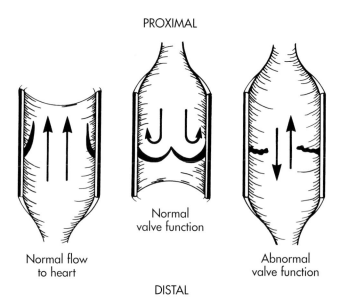

Normal valve function

Normal flow to heart

Abnormal valve function

DISTAL

Fig. 1-7   Diagram of normal and abnormal valvular function caused by venous dilation.

sclerotherapy of pedal veins could produce thrombosis in the deep veins fairly easily (see Chapter 8).[18]

Venous Valvular System

Fabricius of Aquapendente (1533-1620) was the first to detail the anatomy of veins and their valves. He suggested that valves " . . . ensure a fair distribution of the blood . . . prevent distention . . . and stop blood from flooding into the limb. . . ."[19] The valves appear on direct visualization as translucent, thin structures that vibrate with blood flow. Damaged valves appear cloudy and float haphazardly and/or freely within the lumen. Numerous bicuspid valves occur down to vein diameters less than 100 micrometers (μm),[20] with more recent studies demonstrating valves in venules as small as 40 μm in diameter.[21,22] Because venous valves comprise the weakest link in the calf muscle pump, an understanding of the pathophysiology of normal and diseased valves is crucial. Studies of the embryologic development of veins show that the number of venous valves decreases in utero with fetal maturity. It has been suggested that this disappearance continues, albeit at a reduced but variable rate, during childhood, adolescence, and adult life.[23,24] However, an autopsy study of 178 subjects without venous disorders and 70 subjects with primary varicose veins failed to demonstrate a decreased number of venous valves in advanced-age groups.[25] This was confirmed in a study of 50 cadaver GSVs.[26] Here, the mean number of valves (7.0) in 23 veins at ages 17 to 59 years was not significantly different from the mean number of valves (7.2) in 27 veins at ages 60 to 90 years. Therefore, aging in itself does not appear to produce a decrease in venous valves of the leg. Neither does there appear to be a difference in the number of venous valves between men and women.[2]

The number of venous valves has been found to be less in varicose veins than in normal veins. Because age and sex do not decrease valvular number, other factors must contribute to the loss of venous valves. Two potential sources of valvular dysfunction are fibrosis caused by turbulent high-pressure blood flow and a hereditary defect in vein wall and/or valvular support.

Competent venous valves can withstand pressures of up to 3 atmospheres[27]; therefore, for valvular damage to occur, the vein diameter must first dilate to ren-

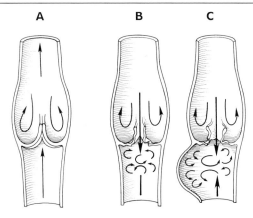

Fig. 1-8 **A,** Flow pattern in a normal superficial vein with competent valves. Note the eddies that occur beneath the valve cusps. **B,** Incompetent valves produces turbulent flow on the vein wall distal to the insertion of the valve cusps. **C,** Sideways thrust due to retrograde turbulence may eventually cause a "blow-out" of the vein wall, producing a sacule beneath the valve cusps as seen in the illustration and anatomic specimen.

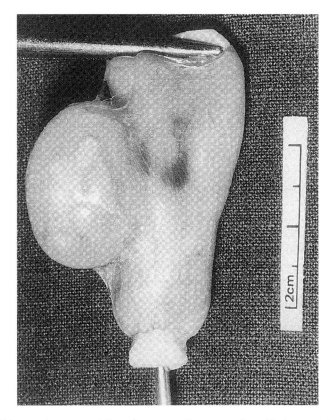

Fig. 1-9 This specimen was taken from a saphenous vein with incompetent valves 2.5 cm below its termination. (Reproduced with permission from Tibbs DJ: Varicose veins and related disorders, Oxford, 1992, Butterworth-Heinemann.)

der the valves incompetent (Fig. 1-7). This theory is supported by investigations that reveal no difference in visoelastic behavior in perivalvular vein wall tissue.[28] Chronic venous dilation may produce a strain on valves and lead to sclerosis. It is postulated that this occurs through the production of turbulent blood flow (Figs. 1-8, 1-9). Fegan[29] reasons that turbulence, once established, interferes with

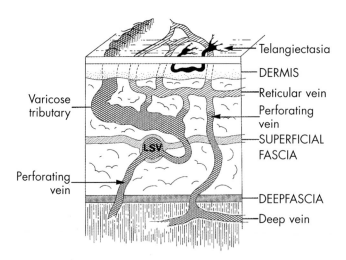

Fig. 1-10   Schematic diagram of subcutaneous venous anatomy showing 4 types of flow from subcutaneous veins (SCV). SCV to GSV/LSV to SFJ/SPJ to deep system; SCV to GSV/LSV to perforator to deep system; SCV to perforators to deep system; SCV to deep system. (Reproduced with permission from Somjen GM et al: Anatomical examination of leg telangiectasias with duplex scanning, J Dermatol Surg Gynecol 19:940, 1993.)

the blood supply to the vein wall via the vasa vasorum or subjects the collagen fibers to abnormal stress. Either or both of these changes lead to atrophic changes of the valves. This theory is supported by a study of 75 cadaver veins and 75 stripped veins from the medial malleolus to the saphenofemoral junction that demonstrated a statistically significant decrease in the number of valves in varicose veins (6.0 versus 1.7) compared with normal veins (7.3 versus 2.3).[26] Although 33 of 156 valves in varicose veins were sclerosed on examination after removal or autopsy, no evidence of sclerosis of the venous valves of normal veins was apparent.[26] However, sinus wall and valvular defects have been found in autopsy studies in up to 90% of adults without apparent varicosities.[30] Therefore, valve and valvular sinus abnormalities, at best, comprise only one factor in the development of varicose veins. A full explanation of the pathophysiologic significance of valvular deficiency and dysfunction is addressed in Chapter 3 in the section on primary valvular incompetence.

The Venous Network

The deep venous system is connected through multiple channels to superficial veins (Fig. 1-10). This has been demonstrated, both radiographically[31] and with duplex ultrasound, to occur with telangiectasia and reticular veins.[32] Thus, many alternate routes are available for blood to return to the heart after blockage of any main vein, such as the femoral vein. Superficial veins provide a pathway for venous return from the cutaneous and subcutaneous systems through the action of their one-way valves.[33] An anatomic study of the superficial venous system in 60 cadaver limbs disclosed a marked diversity in anatomy. No two limbs exhibited the same superficial venous arrangement.[34] Radiographic studies of cadaver legs also demonstrate a continuous network of arcades that follow the connective-tissue framework of the body in a manner similar to arterial networks.[35] The venous territories, termed *venosomes,* consist of a network of longitudinally oriented subdermal arcades that drain into a single perforator vein or other venosomes (Fig. 1-11); however, some consistent patterns do exist, as described in the following section.

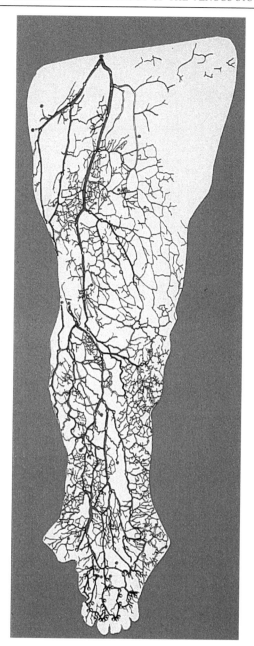

Fig. 1-11 Venous map of the lower limb based on a study of 6 fresh human cadavers evaluated with a radiopaque lead-oxide mixture injected into the integument and deep tissues. Valved veins are colored blue, oscillating veins are yellow, and perforator sites are highlighted by orange dots. (Reproduced with permission from Taylor GI et al: The venous territories [venosomes] of the human body: experimental study and clinical implications, Plast Reconstr Surg 86:185, 1990.)

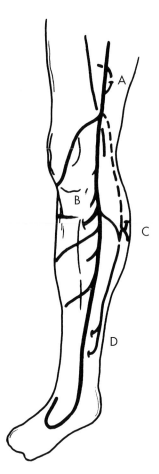

Fig. 1-12   Typical course of the GSV including its common tributaries and perforating veins. (**A**), Hunterian perforating vein; (**B**), posterior tibial perforating vein; (**C**), calf perforator in location of the intrasaphenous vein; (**D**), medial ankle or Cockett perforators. (Redrawn from Thompson H: The surgical anatomy of the superficial and perforating veins of the lower limb, Ann R Col Surg [Eng] 61:198, 1979.)

Greater saphenous vein. The most prominent superficial vein is the great (long) saphenous vein (GSV). (The term *saphenous* is derived from the Greek word for visible.) The average diameter of a normal GSV is 3.5 to 4.5 mm (range 1 to 7 mm).[36] The thick wall of the GSV allows it to be used as a conduit for arterial bypass surgery. This vein begins on the dorsum of the foot as a dorsal venous arch. It passes anterior to the medial malleolus and crosses the tibia obliquely, continuing along the medial aspect of the leg across the anteromedial thigh, to empty into the common femoral vein (Fig. 1-12). There are many variations in the termination of the GSV into the femoral vein (Fig. 1-13); these are discussed in Chapter 10. This termination point is referred to as the *saphenofemoral junction* (SFJ), but is also known as the *crosse,* which is the French description for its appearance as a shepherd's crook. In more than 80% of cases, the GSV lies on the deep fascia, enclosed by a loose compartment of fat and areolar tissue.[34] However, it may be so superficial that it resembles a collateral vein. Detailed dissection has noted only two perforating veins above the posterior tibial perforator connecting the GSV to the deep system.[34] Therefore, ligation at the SFJ

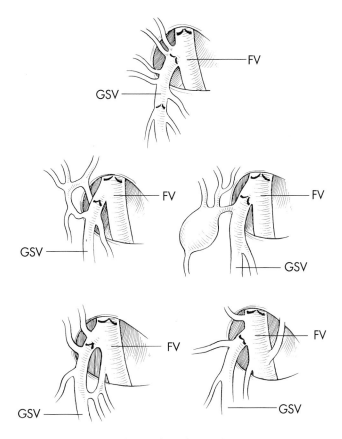

Fig. 1-13   The GSV terminates at the saphenofemoral junction in a variety of patterns. (GSV), greater saphenous vein; (FV), femoral vein; (ASV), accessory greater saphenous vein.

with a limited stripping (above or to the knee) is more anatomically correct than complete ligation and stripping to the ankle as was practiced formerly (see Chapter 10).

The GSV receives multiple tributaries along its course. These may lie in a less supported, more superficial plane to the membranous fascia. The posterior arch vein, the anterior superficial tibial vein, and the medial superficial pedal vein join the GSV in the lower leg. The posterior arch vein is a major tributary of the GSV. It terminates into the GSV below the knee and otherwise communicates with subfascial veins through multiple perforating veins. Two large tributaries from the posteromedial and anterolateral thigh join it proximally. These veins usually enter the GSV before it pierces the deep fascia. Both the medial and lateral superficial thigh veins may be so large that they are mistaken for the GSV itself.[37] A parallel, more superficial, thin-walled vein is seen frequently, directly over or just posterior to the GSV. These veins, which run anterior and posterior to the GSV, are called "accessory saphenous veins" (ASV).[38] These are sometimes double accessory veins and produce different varicose vein patterns that may be mistaken for GSV tributaries. Reticular or telangiectatic veins also may communicate directly with the GSV or bypass this superficial vein to connect directly with the femoral vein.[31,32] Finally, in the thigh the GSV may be duplicated in up to 10% of patients; the length of the duplication is variable.[39]

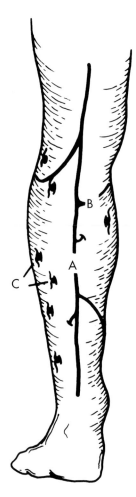

Fig. 1-14 Typical course of the lessor saphenous vein with termination above the popliteal fossae and associated perforator veins. (**A**), SSV; (**B**), intersaphenous vein with calf perforator; (**C**), paraperoneal perforating veins. (Redrawn from Thompson H: The surgical anatomy of the superficial and perforating veins of the lower limb, Ann R Col Surg [Eng] 61:198, 1979.)

The most constant perforating vein in the thigh connects the GSV to the femoral vein in the adductor (Hunter's) canal. A variable number of perforators connect the GSV to the femoral, posterior tibial, gastrocnemius, and soleal veins.[40]

The GSV is involved in varicose vein disease in approximately 60% of cases and is the only site of varicose changes in 12% of limbs.[41,42]

Lessor saphenous vein. The most prominent and physiologically important superficial vein below the knee is the lessor (short) saphenous vein (LSV). Like the GSV, the LSV has a thick wall and usually measures 3 mm in diameter when normal.[43] This major tributary begins at the lateral aspect of the foot and ascends posterior to the lateral malleolus as a continuation of the dorsal venous arch. It continues up the calf between the gastrocnemius heads to the popliteal fossa, ending in the popliteal veins or GSVs (Fig. 1-14).

The termination of the LSV is quite variable (Fig. 1-15), usually occurring in the popliteal vein. In 27% to 33% of the population, it terminates above the level

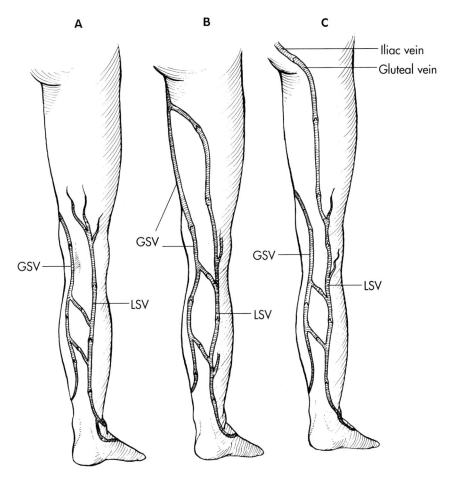

Fig. 1-15   Variations in the termination of the lessor saphenous vein *(LSV)*. **A,** Termination of the saphenopopliteal junction; **B,** termination into the greater saphenous vein *(GSV)*; **C,** termination into the gluteal vein.

of the popliteal fossae, either directly with the GSV or with other deep veins. In 15.3% patients, the LSV communicates with the popliteal vein, then continues terminating in the GSV. In 9% to 10%, the LSV empties into the GSV or the deep veins below the popliteal fossae.[44,45] The LSV may also join the GSV in the thigh via an oblique epifascial vein (Giacomini vein), or it may continue up under the membranous fascia of the thigh as the "femoropopliteal vein," joining the deep veins in the thigh at various locations.[46]

Like the GSV, the LSV runs on or within the deep fascia, usually piercing the deep fascia just below the flexor crease of the knee as it passes into the popliteal fossa. Gross incompetence of the LSV usually occurs only in areas where the LSV and its tributaries are superficial to the deep fascia, on the lateral calf and lower third of the leg behind the lateral malleolus. Tributaries of the LSV may be varicose without involvement of the LSV itself. It has been demonstrated that this is due to a competent valve below the tributaries that protects the vein from saphenopopliteal incompetence.[47]

The LSV often receives substantial tributaries from the medial aspect of the ankle, thereby communicating with the medial ankle perforators.[33] The LSV may also receive a lateral arch vein that courses along the lateral calf to terminate in the LSV distal to the popliteal fossae. It may also connect directly with the GSV.

Gastrocnemial veins. Varicose veins on the posterior calf are sometimes independent of saphenous veins that may appear clinically normal. These varicose veins may originate from incompetence of deep muscular veins, notably the gastrocnemial veins.[48,49,50] The gastrocnemial veins originate deep within the gastrocnemius muscle sinuses and drain into the popliteal vein. Multiple tributaries situated within the gastrocnemius muscle form the venous sinuses, which drain into the gastrocnemius vein 2 to 3 cm below its termination. Gastrocnemial veins communicate with the superficial venous system by perforating the fascia at the midcalf level. These veins may communicate with the posterior arch vein or superficial tributaries of the GSV or LSV, either directly or through tributary veins.

Like the LSV, terminations of the gastrocnemial veins are highly variable. Approximately one third of cases have a common termination with the LSV at the saphenopopliteal junction. One third of cases have a direct connection with the popliteal vein. The remaining one third of cases terminate in the femoropopliteal vein of Giacomini.[51]

Other superficial veins/collateral veins. The superficial collateral or communicating venous network consists of many longitudinally, transversely, and obliquely oriented veins. They originate in the superficial dermis, where they drain cuticular venules. These veins are normally of low diameter but when varicose, can dilate to more than 1 cm. They are usually more superficial than saphenous trunks and are thin-walled. They drain into deep veins through the saphenous veins; directly through perforating veins; or via anastomotic veins in the abdominal, perineal, and gluteal areas.[35] Therefore, collateral veins may become varicose either in combination with truncal varicose veins or independently.

Although many collateral veins are unnamed, prominent or consistent superficial veins are the Giacomini vein, which transfers reflux from the proximal GSV to the LSV; the accessory saphenous vein, which runs from the lateral knee to the saphenofemoral junction; the anterior crural veins, which run from the lower lateral calf to the medial knee; and the infragenicular vein, which drains the skin around the knee. Geniculate perforators, although small, may contribute significant reflux. Likewise, anterior tibial veins are the main draining vessels from the musculofascial compartment that contains extensors of the foot. With standing sports, such as tennis and running, these veins can become varicose through significant pressures generated with muscular activity. I term these varices *tennis veins.*

Unusual venous pathways may be associated with recurrent varicose veins after proper therapy. One drainage system has been termed the *sciatic venous pathway.* This connection runs from the internal iliac vein to the posterior thigh, as was noted in 7 of 1200 consecutive ascending phlebographies performed in the routine work-up of varicose veins.[52] This pattern is only one of many possible atypical pathways that must be sought in patients who do not respond to standard therapeutic techniques.

In addition, there are many unnamed tributaries to the saphenous vein that may become dilated and tortuous through an increase in venous pressure. These reticular or connecting branch veins are apparent clinically, especially in patients with light-colored skin (Fig. 1-16). They may represent a normal "reticular" network of subcutaneous veins, or when under high pressure they may be grossly varicose. They darken in color as they bulge from the cutaneous surface. Otherwise, infrared photography may be necessary to visualize their presence.[53] Differentiation of these veins from the major venous system is critical when planning

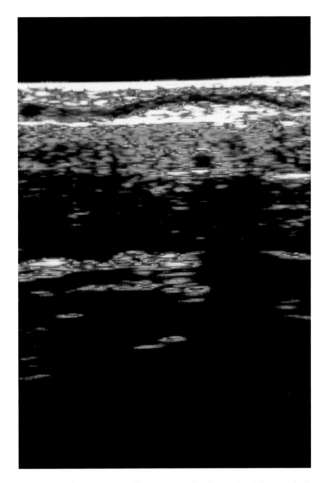

Fig. 1-16   Appearance of a 1.5 mm-diameter reticular vein 1.2 mm below the dermoepidermal junction as seen with the 20 MHz probe Cortex ultrasound (Cortex Technology ApS, Hadsund, Denmark.)

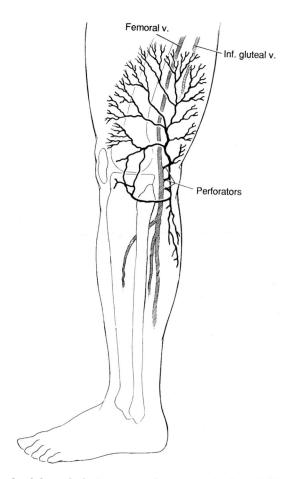

Fig. 1-17 Lateral subdermal plexis commonly seen on the lateral thigh arising from perforator veins from the femoral vein. (Reproduced with permission from Weiss RA and Weiss MA: Painful telangiectasias: diagnosis and treatment. In Bergan JJ and Goldman MP, editors: Varicose veins and telangiectasias: diagnosis and treatment, St. Louis, 1993, Quality Medical.)

treatment. Reticular veins in the thigh may connect with telangiectasia in up to 88% of patients examined with either Doppler or duplex ultrasound.[32,54]

A lateral subdermal plexus of reticular veins, first described by Albanese et al.,[55] has its origin through perforating veins at the lateral epicondyle of the knee (Fig. 1-17). It has been speculated to represent a remnant of the embryonic superficial venous system that fails to involute. This system of veins has its importance in the development of telangiectasia. These veins may become varicose even in the absence of truncal varicosities. They also may connect directly to the deep venous system through transfascial perforating veins.[56]

Perforating veins. Perforating veins were first described in 1803 by Van Loder.[57] They occur from the ankle to the groin, connecting the deep veins to the superficial veins; they "perforate" the aponeurotic fascia, giving them their name. Perforating veins usually communicate with the deep veins close to their junction with the soleal arcades, which dilate to form intramuscular soleal sinusoids. Therefore, incompetent perforators transmit high intramuscular pressure directly

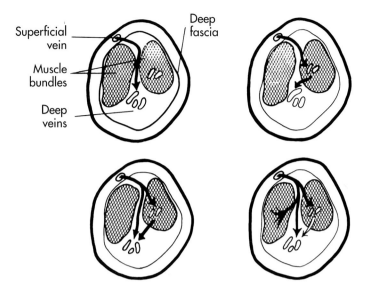

Fig. 1-18   Perforating veins can travel through the calf muscles connecting the deep to the superficial veins in various paths.

to their tributaries, which may not be visible until they dilate enough to produce a "corona phlebectasia." The corona phlebectasia is thus the most constant indication for perforator incompetence.[58]

The average number of perforating veins per leg has been found to be as high as 155[59] or as low as 64.[34] They are not distributed regularly along the limb's surface but increase in density from proximal to distal in a 1:2:8 proportion between the thigh, leg, and foot.[60]

Sixty percent of perforating veins are accompanied by an artery.[59] They usually contain one to three one-way valves, depending on their length. The one-way valves serve to prevent high venous pressure (from muscle contraction) from being transmitted to the superficial veins. Normally, perforating veins are thin-walled, varying in diameter from less than 1 mm to 2 mm.[57] They may also be valveless, especially when less than 1 mm in diameter.[61,62,63] In this case, their competence is maintained by their oblique orientation through muscle.

Anatomically, there are two types of perforating veins: direct and indirect. Direct perforators connect the superficial and deep veins without interruption. Indirect perforators connect the deep and superficial veins via muscular venous channels. Perforator veins empty into deep veins on a line between valve commissures, either just above the valve commissure or in the middle of the deep vein segment between two valves.[64,65] These veins usually run an oblique course through the deep fascia between muscle bundles. They are commonly located on either side of the sartorius and peroneal muscles, and between the vastus lateralis and hamstrings. However, their course beneath the deep fascia may be variable (Fig. 1-18).[66] With muscular movement, the deep fascia is tightened. This puts the perforator veins under tension, which closes the veins and prevents blood from escaping from the deep veins of the calf muscle pump into the superficial veins (see Fig. 1-5). Although variable in exact location, a number of perforating veins occur with marked regularity (Table 1-1).

Table 1-1 Distribution of incompetent perforator veins on 901 lower limbs

	Percent of limbs with incompetent veins	
Perforator veins	**Right limbs**	**Left limbs**
Saphenofemoral junction	100	100
Saphenopopliteal junction	15	15.5
Mid-Hunterian perforator	7	6.7
Genicular perforator	2.9	1.6
Lateral thigh perforators	1.8	1.3
13.5-cm midcalf Cockett	15.9	17.3
18.5-cm midcalf Cockett	34.3	35.2
24-cm midcalf Cockett	20	19.6
30-cm midcalf Cockett	13	12.7
35-cm midcalf Cockett	6.6	7
40-cm midcalf Cockett	4.2	3.1
Calf perforators (other)	12	11.2
Gastrocnemius/peroneal muscle perforator	25	24
Anterior tibialis/peroneal perforator	3.1	2.9
Lateral tibial perforators	0.02	0.04
Lateral foot perforators	2	2.4
Medial foot perforators	3.5	2.9

Modified from Sherman RS: Varicose veins: further findings based on anatomic and surgical dissections, Ann Surg 130:218, 1949.

Table 1-2 Clinically important perforator veins

Name	**Location**
Submalleolar	Medial; retromalleolar
Cockett's	Medial; 7, 12, and 18 cm above medial malleolus
Boyd's	Medial; 10 cm below knee joint
Lateral leg	Lateral; variable in location
Midcalf (soleus and gastrocnemius points)	Posterior; 5 and 12 cm above os calcis
Dodd's (Hunterian)	Medial thigh (mid or distal)

Perforator veins are presumed to play a fundamental role in the production of varicose veins.[67] An anatomic examination of 901 limbs found that the number of incompetent perforators in patients with varicose veins varied from 1 to 14.[67] The distribution of these perforators is detailed in Table 1-1, with clinically important perforating veins listed in Table 1-2. When perforator veins are incompetent, the resulting high pressure is transmitted directly from the deep veins of the calf muscle pump to the superficial veins. This causes dilation of the associated superficial veins (Fig. 1-19).[57,68] When incompetent, perforating veins become thick-walled and may reach a diameter of 5 mm or more (Fig. 1-20).[69] They also have a larger central diameter than peripheral diameter. This causes the reflux blood flow to enter the superficial veins at high velocity and may contribute to the development of localized fascial defects and bulging varicosities.[70]

There are one or two relatively constant perforating veins in the thigh associated with the medial intramuscular septum known as the Hunterian or Dodd's perforator(s) (Fig. 1-21). These connect the GSV to the femoral vein in the mid-

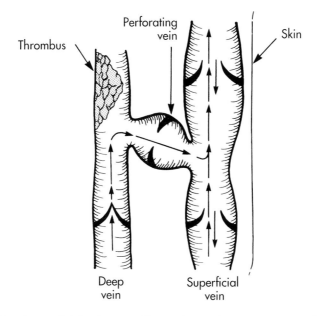

Fig. 1-19   Dilated superficial vein caused by perforator incompetence resulting from deep vein thrombosis blocking proximal flow of blood in the deep venous system. Note that with dilation of the superficial vein the valves are no longer competent.

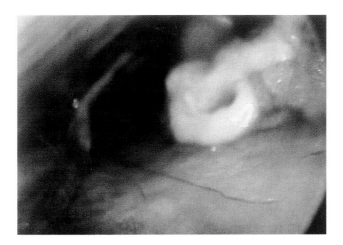

Fig. 1-20   A midcalf perforator from the posterior arch vein is visualized with the endoscope prior to interruption. Note its enlarged, thickened tortuosity. (Courtesy of JJ Bergan.)

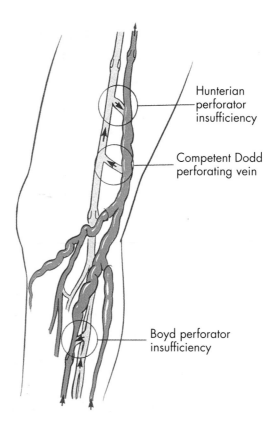

Hunterian
perforator
insufficiency

Competent Dodd
perforating vein

Boyd perforator
insufficiency

Fig. 1-21   The refluxing GSV in the distal thigh is seen to be dilated, whereas the refluxing GSV in the middle third and proximal third of the thigh is less involved but still shows
gross reflux. (Reproduced with permission from Bergan JJ: Common anatomic patterns of
varicose veins. In Bergan JJ and Goldman MP, editors: Varicose veins and telangiectasias:
diagnosis and treatment, St. Louis, 1993, Quality Medical.)

dle medial thigh and the middle lower third of the thigh.[71] These perforators are
found to be single in 50% to 80% of dissected limbs, with two or more midthigh
perforators occurring in 20% to 30% of limbs.[72,73] Many other perforators exist,
but, with the exception of the Hunterian perforator, they pierce muscles. The protection afforded by these muscles seems to preclude the possibility of these veins
becoming incompetent.[74] Incompetence of the Hunterian perforator is a common
cause for medial thigh varicose veins in patients with a competent saphenofemoral junction (Fig. 1-22).

Multiple smaller perforating veins may be present in the middle third of the
lateral aspect of the thigh and the midline of the posterior thigh. These connect
the GSV and its tributaries to the profunda femoris vein.

The posterior tibial perforator occurs in almost all limbs and connects the
GSV to the posterior tibial veins. It is found approximately 5 to 10 cm distal to the
knee on the medial calf.

Multiple perforating veins are also found with regularity along the medial
calf. These connect the LSV to the gastrocnemius veins. When they occur adjacent to the peroneal muscles, they are referred to as paraperoneal perforators.
Some authors state that there are 16 constant perforating veins that may become

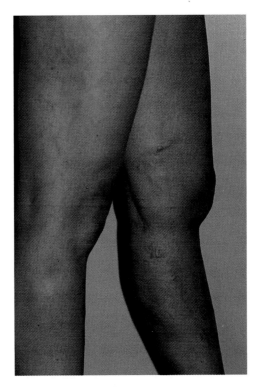

Fig. 1-22   Incompetent GSV with a competent saphenofemoral junction via incompetence of a Hunterian perforating vein demonstrated by venous Doppler examination.

incompetent. Eight of these drain into the posterior tibial vein and four into the gastrocnemius and soleal veins. It is thought that other smaller perforating veins that connect to the tibial vein rarely become incompetent because they are supported by muscles that take their origin from the deep surface of the fascia.

A group of perforating veins located from the medial ankle to the calf has been reported to occur 6 to 10 cm, 13.5 to 15 cm, 18.5 to 20 cm, and 24 to 25 cm above the sole of the foot along Linton's line.[67] This group is referred to as Cockett's perforators (Fig. 1-23). They connect the posterior arch vein with the posterior tibial veins but do not drain directly into the LSV.[75] Recently, a radiographic and surgical study found no predilection for their occurrence at any height.[76] In addition, it was found that these perforators did not occur at the level of Linton's line, but on a "lane" with a width of up to 3 cm. This latter study has dispelled some of the phlebologic dogma for predilection sites of perforating veins.

Perforating veins have also been described in the foot. Raivio has documented more than 40.[77] One is situated about 2.5 cm below the inferior tip of the medial malleolus. A second occurs approximately 3.5 cm below and anterior to the medial malleolus. The other two are on an arc approximately 3 cm anterior and below the medial malleolus. As previously mentioned, perforating veins in the foot are valveless or have one-way valves that are reversed to allow blood to flow from the deep to the superficial veins.[78] The great number of perforating veins and venous anastomoses of the foot allows for their safe removal.

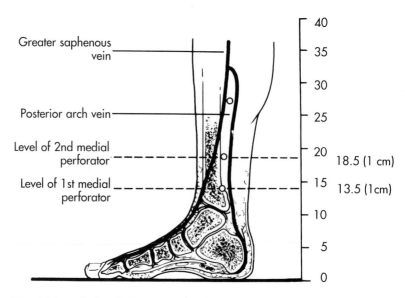

Fig. 1-23 Idealized illustration of the major Cockett perforating veins.

Fascial Envelope

The lower limb has a deep and a superficial fascia to contain the high-pressure calf muscle pump and support the deep venous system. The deep fascia is a dense fibrous membrane investing the entire lower limb like an elastic stocking and serves as a functional boundary between deep and superficial veins. The deep fascia is attached to the superficial fibers of the muscles it covers. The deep fascia is normally thin over the gastrocnemius muscles and is absent only over the perforating veins and fossa ovalis, the latter being protected by the cribriform fascia. Since the deep fascia surrounds the muscles of the limb and is relatively inextensible, contraction of the muscles causes a rise in pressure to all structures within its compartment.

The superficial fascia is composed of two layers: a superficial layer of loculated fatty tissues (Camper's fascia) and a deep layer of collagen and elastic tissue that provides stronger support (Scarpa's fascia).[29] The superficial fascia covers the saphenous trunks[79] (Fig. 1-24), and tributaries to the saphenous veins are superficial to this. Because they are not within its support, tributaries to the GSV are usually more grossly dilated than the GSV itself, even when proximal high venous pressure produces the varicosity.[80] The superficial fascia is homologous with Scarpa's fascia of the anterior abdominal wall and may be considered as a single unit.[29] The superficial fascia in four-legged animals is said to provide a firmer support than that found in bipeds.[81] The support of the superficial fascia may partly explain why varicose veins affect humans and not quadrupeds.

Although the preceding description seems simple, connections between the superficial and deep venous systems and their fascial coverings are actually much more complicated. Detailed anatomic studies by Raivio[77] provide some explanation for this variability, but the importance of the knowledge of the variations in the system explains the need for individualization of treatment in a given patient.

HISTOLOGY
Vein Walls

The first part of the venous system consists of the venule, which serves as a collecting tube for capillaries. The venule is approximately 20 μm in diameter and

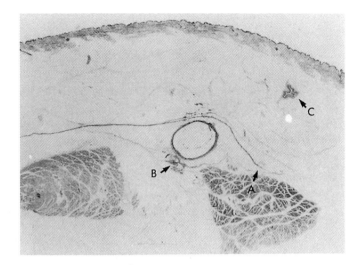

Fig. 1-24   Transverse section from the medial aspect of the thigh showing the fibrous envelope that ensheaths the GSV *(A)* and holds it against the deep fascia *(B)*. A superficial tributary vein external to the fascia is visible *(C)*. (Reproduced with permission from Thompson H: The surgical anatomy of the superficial and perforating veins of the lower limb, Ann R Col Surg [Eng] 61:198, 1979.)

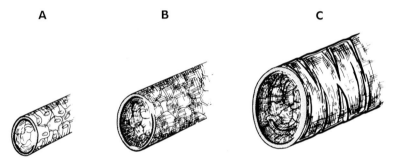

Fig. 1-25   Schematic illustration showing the walls of the blood vessels from capillary to vein. **A**, Capillary; **B**, venule; **C**, vein.

consists of an endothelium surrounded by a fibrous tissue composed of a thin layer of collagenous fibers. The venule increases in diameter, with smooth muscle cells appearing within the fibrous sheath when the diameter is approximately 45 μm. At a diameter of 200 μm, the muscular layer becomes better defined. At a clinically recognizable diameter consistent with small venectasia, the vessels are composed of a thick media with myocytes. Collagenous fibers are clearly organized into bundles and elastic fibers can be observed (see Chapter 3).[82] Larger diameters contain elastic fibers and a more organized structure (Fig. 1-25).

Microscopically, the normal young internal saphenous vein is a musculofibrous conduit with both passive and active functions. The normal vein is slightly oval, with the short axis perpendicular to the skin. In response to an increase in intraluminal pressure, the diameter increases and the vein loses its oval appearance. Veins tend to assume an elliptical shape, particularly at low transmural pressures (Fig. 1-26). These qualities of shape deformability allow veins to change volume with very little force, thus aiding their role as a high capacitance system.[83,84] With continued increases in venous pressure or progression of vari-

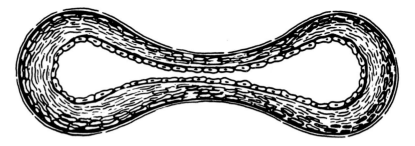

Fig. 1-26 Cross section of venous lumen. At high external pressures the vein collapses into an elliptical configuration. At low external pressures the vein assumes a circular to oval shape. (Modified from Moreno AH et al: Mechanics of distention of dog veins and other thin-walled tubular structures, Circ Res 27:1069, 1970. Permission granted by the American Heart Association, Inc.)

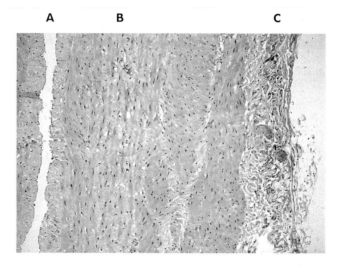

Fig. 1-27 Cross section of a fairly normal section from the varicose GSV of a 64-year-old man at the proximal thigh level. Three distinct layers are present. **A,** Intima; **B,** media; **C,** adventitia. (Hematoxylin-Eosin ×100.)

cose disease, the vein increases in both length and diameter and becomes tortuous. Whether normal or varicose, the saphenous vein is composed of three tunicas: intima, media, and adventitia (Fig. 1-27).

Intima

The intima is a thin structure consisting of a layer of endothelial cells and a deep fenestrated basement membrane bounded by a thin, fragmented elastic lamina (Fig. 1-28).[12] The central portion of the cell containing the nucleus bulges into the lumen and, on its free surface, exhibits multiple small microvilli. Although endothelial cells are easily destroyed by chemical and physical insults, they demonstrate a marked capacity for regeneration (see Chapter 7).[3]

Media

The media is composed of three layers of muscle bundles (Fig. 1-29). The inner layer consists of small bundles of longitudinally arranged muscle fibers. Loose connective tissue and small elastic fibrils separate the muscle bundles.[12] The middle layer is composed of wide bundles of smooth muscle in a circular orientation.

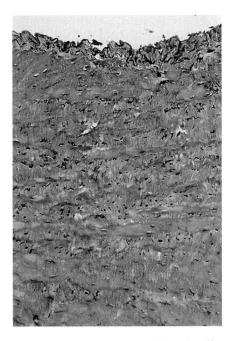

Fig. 1-28 Same specimen as Fig. 1-27 stained with Verhoeff-van Gieson (×150). Note some fragmentation of elastin fibers interspersed between muscle bundles with irregularity at the intima border. Elastic fibers stain black; collagen: red, muscle: brown-yellow.

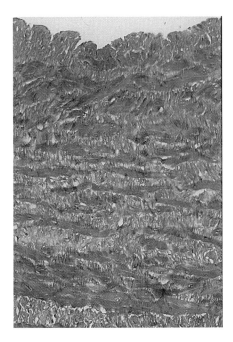

Fig. 1-29 Same specimen as Fig. 1-27 stained with Masson's trichrome (×150). Note the multiple layers of muscle bundles *(red)*.

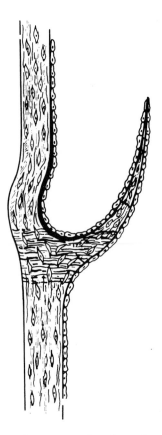

Fig. 1-30 Illustration of a cross section through a normal venous valve.

The muscle bundles may be separated by thin or thick layers of elastic fibrils.[12] In addition, the outer layer is quite variable, being composed of longitudinal muscle bundles spread out through thick fibrous tissue. The outermost cells of the circular layer interdigitate with the innermost cells of the longitudinal layer to improve contractile efficiency.[85]

The amount of muscle within the vein wall is not uniform throughout the venous system. There is an increasing smooth muscle content from the proximal to the distal and the deep to the superficial veins.[86] The obvious functional importance is to counteract hydrostatic pressure. In addition, the greatest extent of circular muscle occurs at the level of insertion of the valve leaflets. This composition helps to prevent valvular dilatation and incompetence and is the last region to dilate in a varicose vein.[87] This area is known to be dilated in primary valvular insufficiency (see Chapter 3).

Adventitia

The adventitia is the thickest portion of the vein wall. It is composed primarily of collagen, whose interlacing fibers are oriented in longitudinal, spiral, and circular fashions.[3] In larger vessels of the thigh, a considerable network of elastic fibers occurs and stretches from valve to valve.[29] The collagen layer merges with the perivenous connective tissue and contains the vasa vasorum and adrenergic nerve fibers.[88,89] The vasa vasorum composes the arteriovenous circulation in the wall of the blood vessel. These vessels arise as branches from arterioles present in perivenous connective tissue that are fed by neighboring arteries.[90] Venous capillaries of the vasa vasorum form venules that empty into veins that run in the loose perivenous connective tissue. As discussed in Chapter 3, alterations of the vasa vasorum may lead to the development of arteriovenous fistulas.

Venous Valves

Venous valves are composed of a thin layer of collagen and a variable amount of smooth muscle covered on both surfaces by endothelium (Fig. 1-30).[91] An increase in muscle fibers is found at the base of the valve cusp running circumferentially and longitudinally for a variable distance along the length of the valve cusp.[29,92] Elastic fibers extend along the whole length of the cusp and lie close to the endothelium. Collagen fibers are concentrated at the base, thinning out toward the free edge of the cusp. The valve is avascular and thus dependent on humeral blood for its oxygen supply.[93,94]

Fegan[29] proposes that the muscle fibers play an active role in regulating blood flow. Through an evaluation of anatomic dissection of multiple valves, he believes that contraction of the circular muscles at the base of the valve reduces the vein diameter, and contraction of the longitudinal fibers shortens and thickens the cusp. This type of coordinated muscle action maintains tone in the vein wall in the face of increased pressure from retrograde blood flow.

The valve cusp changes with age.[95] In the parietal layer, collagen becomes thicker and denser with an increase in the elastic lamellae. The luminalis develops deep, narrow depressions. The vein wall at the valve sinus thickens with an increase in adipose tissue, muscle cells, and connective tissue. These changes produce less flexibility of the valve cusp, which may produce abnormal blood flow currents and eddies that could lead to valvular incompetence (see Chapter 3).

Vein Wall Variations

The preceding description of the composition of vein walls is quite variable among various types and locations of veins. Depending on their location, veins assume many different functions. They are used as pumps and reservoirs and must withstand variations in gravitational and intravascular pressure demands. The muscular content of the vein wall also varies depending on the location of the vein. The percentage of smooth muscle increases with distal locations. Veins in the lower extremities are the only veins that are composed of greater than 40% smooth muscle, with veins in the foot having 60% to 80% smooth muscle, compared with 5% in axillary veins.[96] However, the hydrostatic pressure within the vein also correlates with smooth muscle content, with superficial veins having more smooth muscle than deep veins.[97] The differences in vein wall content may affect sclerotherapy treatment, as described in Chapter 7.

The function of the vein wall collagen is to prevent overdistention, whereas elastin produces elastic recoil. With advancing age, multiple changes may occur in the vessel wall. The intima thickens, increasing and disorienting elastic fibers.[12] The media develops a more disorganized arrangement of muscle bundles and hypertrophy of the outer muscular layer. Elastic fibers become more irregular and dystrophic. The elastic lamina becomes more fragmented, atrophic, thin, and irregular.[12] The adventitia becomes increasingly fibrous. Thus the lack of an organized elastic support and smooth muscle degeneration in an aged vein renders it more susceptible to pressure-induced distention.

Some histologic studies demonstrate that fibrotic wall changes are a common finding in the GSV in all age groups without venous disorders.[97] The incidence of fibrotic change increases from 25% to 50% in the population under 40 years of age to 100% in those over 70 years of age.[97]

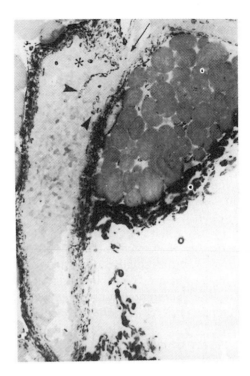

Fig. 1-31 Valve-containing venule at the dermal-fat interface. *Arrow* indicates presumed direction of blood flow. *Arrowheads* indicate valve leaflets. *Asterisk* indicates open valve sinus; other sinus is closed because valve leaflet is in contact with vessel wall (1 µ section, ×485). (Reproduced with permission from Braverman IM and Keh-Yen A: Ultrastructure of the human dermal microcirculation. IV. Valve-containing collecting veins at the dermal-cutaneous junction, J Invest Dermatol 81:438, © by Williams & Wilkins, 1983.)

Venules

Venules in the upper and middermis usually run in a horizontal orientation. The diameter of the postcapillary venule ranges from 12 to 35 µm. Collecting venules range from 40 to 60 µm in the upper and middermis and enlarge to 100 to 400 µm in diameter in the deeper tissues.[99] One-way valves are found at the subcutis (dermis)-adipose junction on the venous side of the circulation.[21] Valves are found usually in the area of anastomosis of small to large venules and also within larger venules unassociated with branching points. The free edges of the valves are always directed away from the smaller vessel and toward the larger and serve to direct blood flow toward the deeper venous system. The structure of these valves is identical to the valves found in deep and larger veins (Fig. 1-31).

Postcapillary venules are composed of endothelial cells covered by a basement membrane, some collagen fibers, and, rarely, smooth muscle cells. Collecting veins in the deep dermis gradually receive more muscle cells until they become veins with a continuous muscle coat (see Fig. 1-25).[100,101] The schematic representation of the normal vascular structure of the skin and subcutaneous tissues in Fig. 1-32 details the intimate connections between the cutaneous veins and their underlying drainage pathways.

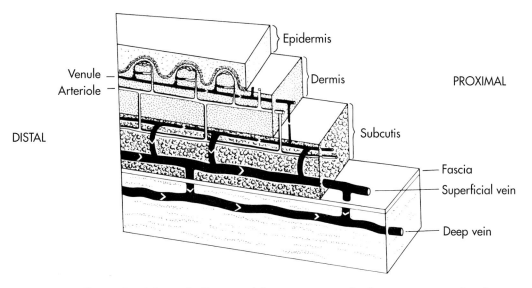

Fig. 1-32   Schematic diagram of the cutaneous and subcutaneous vascular plexus.

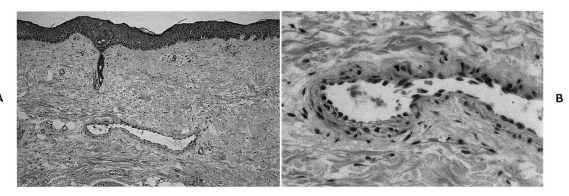

Fig. 1-33   Typical location and diameter of a linear telangiectasia on the thigh of a 45-year-old woman (hematoxylin − eosin; **A,** ×100; **B,** ×400).

Telangiectasias

Histologic examination of simple telangiectasias demonstrates dilated blood channels in a normal dermal stroma with a single endothelial cell lining, limited muscularis, and adventitia (Fig. 1-33).[102] Therefore, such vessels probably evolve from capillaries or early venules.

Blue-to-red arborizing telangiectasias of the lower extremities are probably dilated venules, possibly with intimate and direct connections to underlying larger veins of which they are direct tributaries (Fig. 1-34).[103-105] Electron microscopic examination of "sunburst" varicosities of the leg has demonstrated that these vessels are widened cutaneous veins.[82] They are found 175 to 382 μm below the stratum granulosum. The thickened vessel walls are composed of endothelial cells covered with collagen and muscle fibers. Elastic fibers are also present. Electron microscopy reveals an intercellular collagenous dysplasia, lattice

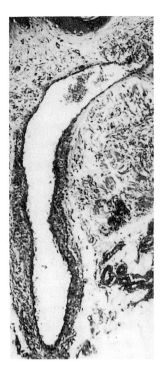

Fig. 1-34   Leg telangiectasia arising from a venule. (Reproduced with permission from de Faria JL and Moraes IN: Histopathology of the telangiectasias associated with varicose veins, Dermatologia 127:321, 1963.)

collagen, and some matrix vesicles. These findings suggest that telangiectatic leg veins, like varicose veins, have an alteration of collagen metabolism of their walls. Therefore, like varicose veins, these veins are dysplastic.

Alternatively, arteriovenous anastomoses may result in the pathogenesis of telangiectasias. Faria and Moraes[105] demonstrated arteriovenous anastomoses in 1 of 26 biopsy specimens of leg telangiectasia (Fig. 1-35).

Skin biopsy of more unusual forms of telangiectasia, such as unilateral nevoid telangiectasia, may show an accumulation of mast cells.[106] In these cases permanent vasodilation may be induced by the chronic release of one or more products of mast cells, particularly heparin.[107,108]

Innervation

Innervation of the vein plays an important part in the regulation of venous tone. Different stimuli are known to produce venous constriction: pain, emotion, hyperventilation, deep breathing, Valsalva maneuver, standing, and muscular exercise.[109] Although muscular veins have little or no sympathetic innervation, cutaneous veins are under hypothalamic thermoregulatory control and have both alpha- and beta-adrenergic receptors.[110] Because the outermost media and adventitia contain the nerve endings, myogenic conduction contributes to the neurogenic activation by coordinating venous contraction.[92,111] Even in the outer layers of the media, the separation of muscle cells from nerve endings is rarely less than 1000 Å.[112] Therefore, an intact smooth muscle layer is important in vein physiology.

Venous constriction and dilation occur through both central and local nervous stimuli.[113] This may be problematic when veins are used as arterial conduits. One report describes spasms of a vein graft 14 months after operation causing

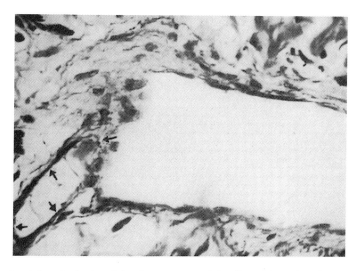

Fig. 1-35   Leg telangiectasia arising from an arteriole. (Reproduced with permission from de Faria JL and Moraes IN: Histopathology of the telangiectasias associated with varicose veins, Dermatologia 127:321, 1963.)

anginal symptoms.[114] Localized cooling provides both a potentiation of adrenergic stimulation and a direct stimulus for venous smooth muscle contraction.[115,116] Venoconstriction is reduced by warming.[116] Venoconstriction also occurs with infusions of norepinephrine,[117] epinephrine, phenylephrine, serotonin, and histamine.[118] Veins dilate in response to phenoxybenzamine, phentolamine, reserpine, guanethidine, barbiturates, and many anesthetic agents.[119] Therefore, circulating adrenergic and pharmacologic substances influence vein diameter. This may explain why central mechanisms may also be responsible for venous tone. Evidence for a central sympathetic control of venoconstriction has been demonstrated by the failure of such venoconstriction to occur with the tilting of sympathectomized patients.[120] Even the stress of mental arithmetic or unpleasant thoughts has been shown to activate adrenergic nerves connected to cutaneous veins.[109] Veins may become more distensible during sleep because of a change in either respiration or nerve stimulation.[121] This is one reason for recommending continuous compression of sclerotherapy-treated veins during the endosclerotic stages after treatment (see Chapter 8).

Local chemical changes produced through exercise also provide for the distribution of blood flow in accordance with local metabolic needs. Venous smooth muscle is also sensitive to endothelium-derived vasoconstrictor substances and peptides such as endothelin.[113] Finally, the increasing smooth muscle content from proximal to distal veins and a thicker muscular media in superficial veins as compared with muscular deep veins supports the physiologic concept of increasing venous contractility in the distal venous system.

REFERENCES

1. Venous Consensus Conference: Maui, February, 1994.
2. Kosinski C: Observation on the superficial venous system of the lower extremity, J Anat 60:131, 1926.
3. Farber EM and Bates EE: Pathologic physiology of stasis dermatitis, Arch Dermatol 70:653, 1954.
4. Holme JB, Holme K, and Sorensen LS: The anatomic relationship between the long saphenous vein and the saphenous nerve, Acta Chir Scand 154:631, 1988.
5. Price C: The anatomy of the saphenous nerve in the lower leg with particular reference to its relationship to the long saphenous vein, J Cardiovasc Surg 31:294, 1990.

6. Garnjobst W: Injuries to the saphenous nerve following operations for varicose veins, Surg Gynecol Obstet 119:359, 1964.

7. Last RJ: Anatomy regional and applied, ed 6, Edinburgh, 1978, Churchill Livingstone.

8. Anderson JE, editor: Grant's atlas of anatomy, ed 7, Baltimore, 1978, Williams & Wilkins.

9. Jacobsen BJ: The venous drainage of the foot, Surg Gynecol Obstet 131:22, 1970.

10. Klein Ronweler BJF, Kuiper JP, and Brakkee HJM: Venous flow resistance and venous capacity in humans with primary varicosis of the long saphenous vein, Phlebology 5:31, 1990.

11. McPheeters HO and Rice CO: Varicose veins: the circulation and direction of venous flow, Surg Gynecol Obstet 49:29, 1929.

12. Bouissou H et al: Vein morphology, Phlebology 3(suppl)1:1, 1988.

13. Kuster G, Lofgren EP, and Hollinshead WH: Anatomy of the veins of the foot, Surg Gynecol Obstet 127:817, 1968.

14. Lofgren EP, Myers TT, and Gustavokuster K: The venous valves of the foot and ankle, Surg Gynecol Obstet 2:107, 1965.

15. Gardner AMN and Fox RH: The return of blood to the heart, London, 1989, John Libbey.

16. Fox RH and Gardner AMN: Video-phlebography in the investigation of venous physiology and disease. In Negus D and Jantet G, editors: Phlebology 85, London, 1986, Libbey.

17. McMullin G et al: An assessment of the effect of the foot pump on venous emptying in chronic venous insufficiency. In Davy A and Stemmer R, editors: Phlebologie 89, Blanche, France, 1989, John Libbey Eurotext.

18. Askar O and Abdullah S: The veins of the foot, J Cardiovasc Surg 16:53, 1975.

19. Laufman H: Silvergirl's surgery: the veins, ed 1, Austin, Texas, 1986, Silvergirl.

20. Aharinejad S and Lametschwandtner A: Microvascular corrosion casting in scanning electron microscopy: techniques and applications, New York, 1992, Springer-Verlag.

21. Braverman IM and Keh-Yen A: Ultrastructure of the human dermal microcirculation. IV. Valve-containing collecting veins at the dermal-subcutaneous junction, J Invest Dermatol 81:438, 1983.

22. Dunn RM et al: Free flap valvular transplantation for refractory venous ulceration, J Vasc Surg 19:523, 1994.

23. Myers TT: Varicose veins. In Allen EV, Barker NW, and Hines EA, editors: Peripheral vascular diseases, ed 3, Philadelphia, 1962, WB Saunders.

24. Thurner J and Mar R: Probleme der Phlobopathologie mit besonderer Berucksichtigung der Phlebosklerose, Zentralblatt Fuer Phlebologie 6:404, 1967.

25. Villavicencio JL: Personal communication, 1989.

26. Cotton LT: Varicose veins: gross anatomy and development, Br J Surg 48:589, 1961.

27. Greenfield ADM: Physiology of the veins. In Luisada AA, editor: Cardiovascular functions, New York, 1962, McGraw-Hill.

28. Psaila JV et al: Do varicose veins have abnormal viscoelastic properties? In Davy A and Stemmer R, editors: Phlebologie 89, Blanche, France, 1989, John Libbey Eurotext.

29. Fegan G: Varicose veins: compression sclerotherapy, London, 1967, William Heinemann.

30. Eger SA and Wagner FB Jr: Etiology of varicose veins, Postgrad Med 6:234, 1949.

31. Bohler-Sommeregger K et al: Do telangiectases communicate with the deep venous system? J Dermatol Surg Oncol 18:403, 1992.

32. Somjen GM et al: Anatomical examination of leg telangiectases with duplex scanning, J Dermatol Surg Oncol 19:940, 1993.

33. Braverman IM and Keh-Yen A: Ultrastructure of the human dermal microcirculation. IV. Valve-containing collecting veins at the dermal-subcutaneous junction, J Invest Dermatol 81:438, 1983.

34. Thompson H: The surgical anatomy of the superficial and perforating veins of the lower limb, Ann R Col Surg Eng 61:198, 1979.

35. Taylor GI et al: The venous territories (venosomes) of the human body: experimental study and clinical implications, Plast Reconstr Surg 86:185, 1990.

36. Berry SM et al: Determination of a "good" saphenous vein for use in in situ bypass grafts by real-time B-mode imaging, J Vasc Surg 12:184, 1988.

37. Browse NL, Burnand G, and Thomas ML: Diseases of the veins: pathology, diagnosis, and treatment, London, 1988, Edward Arnold.

38. Dortu J: Anatomie clinique des collaterales variqueuses (varicoses essentielles), Phlebologie 42:553, 1989.

39. Shah DM et al: The anatomy of the greater saphenous venous system, J Vasc Surg 3:273, 1986.

40. Sherman RS: Varicose veins: anatomy re-evaluation of Trendelenburg tests and operating procedure, Surg Clin North Am 44:1369, 1964.

41. Georgiev M: Primary varicose veins: a topographic study. Presented at the IV European-American Symposium on Venous Disease, Washington, D.C., March 31-April 2, 1987.

42. Goren G and Yellin A: Primary varicose veins: topographic and hemodynamic considerations. J Cardiovasc Surg 31:672, 1990.

43. Kupinski AM: The lessor saphenous vein: an under-utilized arterial bypass conduit, J Vasc Technol 11:145, 1987.
44. Dodd H and Cockett FB, editors: The pathology and surgery of the veins of the lower limb, ed 2, Edinburgh, 1976, Churchill Livingstone.
45. Kubik S: Das venen system der enterem, Extremitat Dia-GM 4:32, 1985.
46. Hoffman HM and Straubesand J: Die venoesen Abflussverhaeltnisse des Musculus triceps surae, Phlebologie 20:164, 1991.
47. Hobbs JT: Errors in the differential diagnosis of incompetence of the popliteal vein and short saphenous vein by Doppler ultrasound, J Cardiovasc Surg 27:169, 1986.
48. Vandendriessche M: Association between gastrocnemial vein insufficiency and varicose veins, Phlebology 4:171, 1989.
49. Thiery L: La vena fossa poplitea, Phlebologie (Brussels) 2:649, 1983.
50. May R and Nissl R: Die phlebographie der unterern extemitat, Stuttgart, 1959, Thieme.
51. Giacomini G: di Acad di Med Torini, 14:1983.
52. Trigaux J-PF et al: Sciatic venous drainage demonstrated by varicography in patients with a patent deep venous system, Cardiovasc Intervent Radiol 12:103, 1989.
53. Zimmerman LM and Rattner H: Infra-red photography of subcutaneous veins, Am J Surg 27:502, 1935.
54. Weiss RA and Weiss MA: Doppler ultrasound findings in reticular veins of the thigh subdermic lateral venous system and implications for sclerotherapy, J Dermatol Surg Oncol 19:947, 1993.
55. Albanese AR, Albanese AM, and Albanese EF: The lateral subdermic venous system of the legs, Vasc Surg 3:81, 1969.
56. Goren G and Yellin AE: Primary varicose veins: topographic and hemodynamic correlations, J Cardiovasc Surg 31:672, 1991.
57. Bjordal RI: Circulation patterns in incompetent perforating veins in the calf and in the saphenous system in primary varicose veins, Acta Chir Scand 136:251, 1972.
58. Negus D: Leg ulcers, Oxford, 1991, Butterworth-Heinemann.
59. Limborgh J van: L'anatomie du systeme veineux de l'extremite inferieure en relatio avec la pathologie variqueuse, Folia Angiologica 8:240, 1961.
60. Thulesius et al: Blood flow in perforating veins of the lower extremity. In May R, Partsch H, and Staubesand J, editors: Perforating veins, Muenchen, 1981, Urban & Schwarzenberg.
61. Barber RF and Shatara FI: The varicose disease, NY State J Med 25:162, 1925.
62. Hadfield JIH: The anatomy of the perforating vein of the leg. In the treatment of varicose veins by injection and compression, Stoke Mandeville Symposium, 1971.
63. Sarin S, Scurr JH, and Coleridge-Smith PD: Medial calf perforators in venous disease: the significance of outward flow, J Vasc Surg 16:40, 1992.
64. Van Cleef J-F: A vein has a preferential axis of flattening, J Dermatol Surg Oncol 19:468, 1993.
65. Van Cleef J-F et al: Venous valves and tributary veins, Phlebology 6:219, 1991.
66. Stolic E: Terminology, division, and systematic anatomy of the communicating veins of the lower limb. In May R, Partsch H, and Straubesand J, editors: Perforating veins, Munich, 1981, Urban & Schwarzenberg.
67. Sherman RS: Varicose veins: further findings based on anatomic and surgical dissections, Ann Surg 130:218, 1949.
68. Arnoldi CC: Venous pressure in patients with valvular incompetence of the veins of the lower limb, Acta Chir Scand 132:628, 1966.
69. Linton R: Communicating veins of the lower leg and the operative technique for their ligation, Ann Surg 107:582, 1938.
70. Wupperman T, Mellimann J, and von Sclweder WJ: Morphometric characteristics of incompetent perforating veins in primary varicosis of the lower leg, Vasa 7:66, 1978.
71. Dodd H: The varicose tributaries of the superficial femoral vein passing into Hunter's canal, Postgrad Med J 35:18, 1959.
72. Papadakis K et al: Number and anatomical distribution of incompetent thigh perforating veins, Br J Surg 76:581, 1989.
73. Tung KT, Chan O, and Thomas ML: The incidence and sites of medial thigh communicating veins: a phlebographic study, Clin Radiol 41:339, 1990.
74. Sherman RS: Varicose veins: anatomic findings and an operative procedure based upon them, Ann Surg 120:772, 1944.
75. Cockett FB: The pathology and treatment of venous ulcers of the leg, Br J Surg 43:260, 1955.
76. Fischer R, Fullemann HJ, and Alder W: Zum phlebogischen Dogma der Pradilektionsstellen der Cockettschen Venae perforantes, Phlebo u Proktol 16:184, 1987.
77. Raivio EVL: Untersuchungen die Venen der unteren Extremitaten mit besonderer Bevuckgichtigunu der gegenseihgen Verbindugen zwischen den oberflachlichen und tiefen Venen, Ann Med Exp Fenn 26(suppl):1, 1948.

78. Askar O, Kassem KA, and Aly SA: The venographic pattern of the foot, J Cardiovasc Surg 16:64, 1975.

79. Kubik S: Anatomie der Beinvemen. In Wuppermann TW, editor: Varizen ulcus cruris und Thrombose, Berlin, 1986, Springer-Verlag.

80. Miller SS: Investigation and management of varicose veins, Ann Col Surg Eng 55:245, 1974.

81. Foote RR: Varicose veins, St Louis, 1949, CV Mosby.

82. Wokalek H et al: Morphology and localization of sunburst varicosities: an electron microscopic and morphometric study, J Dermatol Surg Oncol 15:149, 1989.

83. Moreno AH et al: Mechanics of distension of dog veins and other very thin-walled tubular structures, Circ Res 20:1069, 1970.

84. Strandness DE Jr and Thiele BI: Selected topics in venous disorders: pathophysiology, diagnosis, and treatment, New York, 1981, Futura.

85. Rhodin Johannes AG: Histology: a text and atlas, New York, 1974, Oxford University.

86. Kugelgen Av: Uber das Verhaltnis von Ringmuskulatur und Innendruck in menschlichen grossen Venen, Zeitschr Zellforsch 43:168, 1955.

87. Barrow DW: The clinical management of varicose veins, ed 2, 1957, Hoeber-Harper.

88. Vanhoutte PM: The role of systemic veins: an update, Phlebology 3(suppl)1:13, 1988.

89. Ehinger B, Falck B, and Sporrong B: Adrenergic fibers to the heart and to peripheral vessels, Bibl Anat 8:35, 1966.

90. O'Neill JP: The effects on venous endothelium of alterations in blood flow through the vessels in vein walls, and the possible relation to thrombosis, Ann Surg 126:270, 1947.

91. Edwards JE and Edwards AE: The saphenous valves in varicose veins, Am Heart J 19:338, 1940.

92. Butterworth DM et al: Light microscopy, immunohistochemistry and electron microscopy of the valves of the lower limb veins and jugular veins, Phlebology 7:27, 1992.

93. Hamer JD, Malone PC, and Silver IA: The Po² in venous valve pockets: its possible bearing on thrombogenesis, Br J Surg 68:166, 1981.

94. Saphir O and Lev M: Venous valvulitis, Arch Path 53:456, 1952.

95. Saphir O and Lev M: The venous valve in the aged, Am Heart J 44:843, 1952.

96. Kugelgen A: Uber des Verhaltnis von Ringmuskulatur und Innendruck in menschlichen grossen Venen, Z Zellforsch Mikrosk Anat 43:168, 1955.

97. Leu HJ, Vogt M, and Pfrunder H: Morphological alterations of nonvaricose and varicose veins, Basic Res Cardiol 74:435, 1979.

98. Braverman IM: Ultrastructure and organization of the cutaneous microvasculature in normal and pathologic states, J Invest Dermatol 93:28, 1989.

99. Miani A and Rubertsi U: Collecting venules, Minerva Cardioangiol 41:541, 1958.

100. Benninghoff, quoted by Moretti G. In Jadassho J, editor: Handbuch der Haut- und Geschlechtskrangheiten, Berlin, 1968, Springer-Verlag.

101. Bargmann W: Histologie und mikroskopische Anatomie des Meerschen, Stuttgart, 1956, Georg Thieme.

102. Goldman MP and Bennett RG: Treatment of telangiectasia: a review, J Am Acad Dermatol 17:167, 1987.

103. Bean WB: Vascular spiders and related lesions of the skin, Springfield, Ill, 1958, Charles C Thomas.

104. Bodian EL: Sclerotherapy, Sem Dermatol 6:238, 1987.

105. de Faria JL and Moraes IN: Histopathology of the telangiectasias associated with varicose veins, Dermatologia 127:321, 1963.

106. Fried SZ and Lynfield L: Unilateral facial telangiectasia macularis eruptiva perstans, J Am Acad Dermatol 16:250, 1987.

107. Azizkhan RG et al: Mast cell heparin stimulates migration of capillary endothelial cells in vitro, J Exp Med 152:931, 1980.

108. Folkman J: Regulation of angiogenesis: a new function of heparin, Biochem Pharmacol 34:905, 1985.

109. Shepherd JT: Reflex control of the venous system. In Bergan JJ and Yao JST, editors: Venous Problems, Chicago, 1978, Year Book.

110. Kaiser GA, Ross J Jr, and Braunwald E: Alpha and beta adrenergic receptor mechanisms in the systemic venous bed, J Pharmacol Exp Ther 144:156, 1964.

111. Johansson B and Ljung B: Role of myogenic propagation in vascular smooth muscle response to vasomotor nerve stimulation, Acta Physiol Scand 73:501, 1968.

112. Speden RN: Excitation of vascular smooth muscle. In Bulbring E et al, editors: Smooth muscle, Baltimore, 1970, Williams & Wilkins.

113. Vanhoutte PM: Venous wall and venous disease. In Vanhoutte PM, editor: Return circulation and norepinephrine: un update, Paris, 1991, John Libbey Eurotext.

114. Maleki M and Manley JC: Venospastic phenomena of saphenous vein bypass grafts: possible causes for unexplained postoperative recurrence of angina or early or late occlusion of vein bypass grafts, Br Heart J 62:57, 1989.
115. Vanhoutte PM and Shepherd JT: Thermosensitivity and veins, J Physiol (Paris) 63:449, 1970.
116. Vanhoutte PM and Shepherd JT: Effect of temperature on reactivity of isolated cutaneous veins of the dog, Am J Physiol 218:187, 1970.
117. Wood JE and Eckstein JW: A tandem forearm plethysmography for study of acute responses of the peripheral veins of man: the effect of environmental and local temperature change and the effect of pooling blood in the extremities, J Clin Invest 37:41, 1958.
118. Thulesius O and Gjores JE: Reactions of venous smooth muscle in normal men and patients with varicose veins, Angiology 25:145, 1974.
119. Mellander S: Operative studies on the adrenergic neuro-hormonal control of resistance and capacitance blood vessels in the cat, Acta Phys Scand 50:5, 1960.
120. Peterson LH: Some characteristics of certain reflexes which modify the circulation in man, Circulation 2:351, 1950.
121. Watson WE: Distensibility of the capacity blood vessels of the human hand during sleep, J Physiol (Lond) 161:392, 1962.

ADVERSE SEQUELAE AND COMPLICATIONS OF VENOUS HYPERTENSION

PATHOGENESIS

Venous insufficiency may be defined as relative impedance of venous flow back to the heart. When this occurs in the lower extremities, the normal reabsorption of perivascular fluids by osmotic and pressure gradients is impaired, resulting in accumulation of perivascular and lymphatic fluid. This leads to edema and impaired oxygenation of surrounding tissue (Figs. 2-1 and 2-2). This disruption of the normal vascular and lymphatic flow of the lower extremities may result in pain, cramping (especially at night), restless feelings, pigmentary changes, dermatitis, and ulceration (Fig. 2-3).[1-3] The association of abnormal venous flow with various signs and symptoms has been noted for centuries; it was first noted by Hippocrates in the fourth century BC[3] and was first reported by Wiseman in England in 1676.[4] It has been estimated that chronic venous insufficiency will develop in almost 50% of patients with major varicose veins.[5,6]

Several alterations of normal venous flow cause venous hypertension. Such hypertension in the lower extremities is usually caused by a loss or disruption of the normal one-way valvular system. This usually occurs because of deep vein thrombosis (DVT), thrombophlebitis, or a dilation of veins resulting from other causes.[7,8] When perforating vein valvular function becomes incompetent, there may be shunting of blood flow from the deep to the superficial venous system through incompetent perforating veins, with resultant adverse sequelae.[9-11] The superficial veins respond by dilating to accommodate the increased blood flow, which produces superficial valvular incompetence leading to the development of varicosities.[12] In addition, with muscular movement in the lower limbs, the high venous pressure normally occurring within the calf is transmitted straight to the superficial veins and subcutaneous tissues.[13,14] Venous pressure in the cuticular venules may greatly exceed the normal 100 mm Hg in the erect position.[15] This causes venular dilation over the whole area, resulting in capillary dilation, increased permeability,[16-19] and an increase in the subcutaneous capillary bed.[17,20] This is manifested as telangiectasia and venectasia (Fig. 2-4). Venous hypertension has also been demonstrated to destroy the venous valves, which are present in the subcuticular vascular system.[21] This destruction promotes persistent and progressive changes in the venous drainage system of the skin and subcutaneous tissues. The greater the degree of venous hypertension, the greater the risk of venous ulcer development.[22,23] Fortunately, both sclerotherapy and surgical treatment are capable of normalizing abnormal venous hypertension.

The lymphatic system also becomes overloaded because of interstitial edema, resulting from increased capillary filtration associated with venous hypertension.[24-26] Dilated lymphatics, resulting from venous obstruction, have been shown to fibrose.[24,27-29] In addition, lymphatic function in the leg has been demonstrated to decline with age.[30] Thus lymphatic stasis adds to venous stasis edema and may persist even after venous stasis has resolved. This may cause elephantiasis of the limb[12] or lymphostasis verrucosa cutis (Fig. 2-5).[31,32] Permanent disruption of the normal cutaneous and subcutaneous venous outflow ensues, producing poor

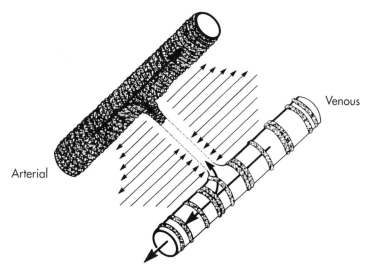

Venous

Arterial

Fig. 2-1   Schematic diagram showing the normal resorption of pericapillary fluid in response to precapillary and postcapillary pressure and interstitial pressure.

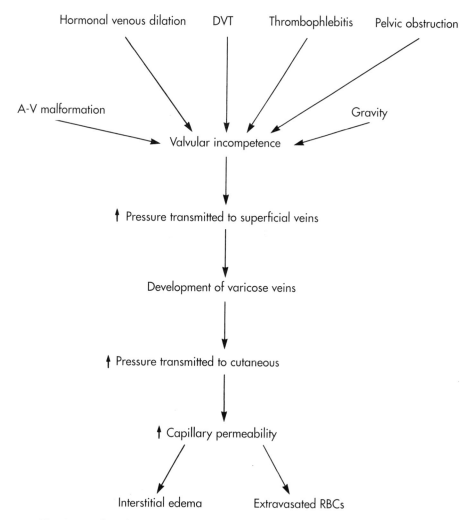

Hormonal venous dilation   DVT   Thrombophlebitis   Pelvic obstruction

A-V malformation

Gravity

Valvular incompetence

↑ Pressure transmitted to superficial veins

Development of varicose veins

↑ Pressure transmitted to cutaneous

↑ Capillary permeability

Interstitial edema   Extravasated RBCs

Fig. 2-2   Flowchart showing etiology of cutaneous venous hypertension.

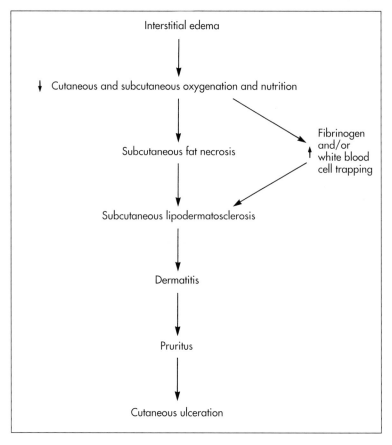

Fig. 2-3 Flowchart showing etiology of cutaneous manifestations of venous hypertension.

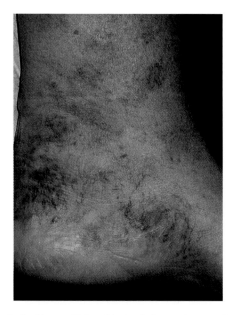

Fig. 2-4 Telangiectasia in the medial ankle/pedal area in a patient with chronic venous insufficiency referred to as *corona phlebectasia.*

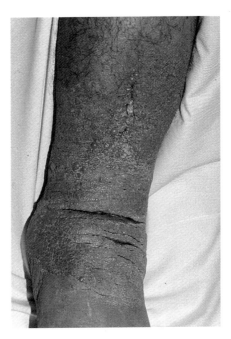

Fig. 2-5 Lymphostasis verrucosa cutis in a patient with long-standing venous hpyertension resulting from deep venous thrombosis and thrombophlebitis.

tissue nutrition and oxygenation.[2,33] Edema promotes dermatitis and infection[34] and may also impair wound healing.[35] Lymphatic damage may also be a component in the persistence of leg ulceration. Subcutaneous fat necrosis may develop, with subsequent reorganization of the subcutaneous tissue forming a hard plate.[25,36] The combined effects of venous hypertension and lymphatic stasis result in profound changes in the cutaneous and subcutaneous tissues. These changes are referred to collectively as *lipodermatosclerosis.*

The formation of subcutaneous lipodermatosclerosis is thought to be caused in part by an increase in the local and perivascular concentration of fibrinogen. Burnand et al.[17] have measured a high local concentration of fibrinogen and other macromolecules in the interstitial fluid after the production of increased venous pressure through an arteriovenous fistula in experimental animals. Hypercoagulability of the interstitial fluid then produces localized fibrin formation, which in turn may be responsible for the development of lipodermatosclerosis and subsequent cutaneous breakdown. Alternatively, perivascular fibrin cuffing (Fig. 2-6) may decrease diffusion of gases with resultant tissue hypoxia, which in turn may produce venous ulceration.[37,38] However, the fibrin cuff has not been proven to be a true barrier to oxygen diffusion,[39,40,41] thus casting some doubt on this theory. Fibrin cuffs may have a mechanical role in preventing vasodilation of capillaries and small vessels in response to exercise. This suggests a primary perfusion deficit in skin rather than an oxygen diffusion block.[42]

A new hypothesis to explain the cause of venous ulceration and cutaneous disease recently has been proposed.[39] Bollinger et al.[43] observed that patients with chronic venous insufficiency who demonstrated areas devoid of cutaneous blood flow had this flow restored with the use of graduated compression stockings. Multiple groups have demonstrated that capillary occlusion is a result of white blood cells sticking to the endothelial surface of intradermal capillaries, blocking blood flow.[39,44,45,46] It is thought that the trapped white blood cells release toxic

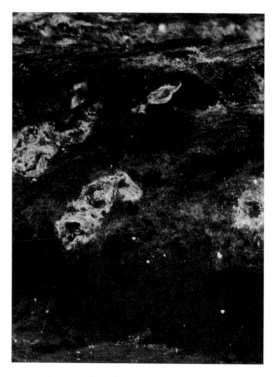

Fig. 2-6   Skin biopsy specimen taken from the edge of a venous ulceration. The tissue was stained by direct immunofluorescence with a polyclonal antifibrinogen antibody. There is intense pericapillary staining for fibrinogen and fibrin ($\times$ 250). (Courtesy Vincent Falanga, M.D., University of Miami School of Medicine.)

oxygen metabolites, free radicals, and proteolytic enzymes that damage capillaries, increasing their permeability and resulting in leakage of fibrinogen and other plasma proteins. This could lead to the formation of the fibrin cuff. This leakage also provokes an immunologic reaction that induces adhesion molecule expression, causing an increased adherence of leukocytes.[47] Trapped white blood cells may also prevent circulation in the subcutaneous capillary loops, which then increases tissue ischemia. Pentoxifylline (Trental, Hoechst-Roussel Pharmaceuticals, Inc., Somerville, NJ) has a potent effect on cytokine-mediated neutrophil activation. It has been shown to reduce white cell adhesion to endothelium and to reduce the release of superoxide free radicals from neutrophils.[48] This effect has clinical significance in accelerating the healing of leg ulcerations.[49]

Histologic examination of skin over areas of venous stasis demonstrates an increase in the number of dermal capillaries. These also appear elongated and tortuous.[18] Unlike cutaneous capillaries in the normal leg, these remain dilated in the supine position and do not change in caliber when subjected to pressure.[50] These capillaries also have been demonstrated to be encased in a fibrin cuff,[37] as described previously. Immunohistochemistry evaluation of patients with varicose veins and cutaneous venous stasis disease without ulceration demonstrated that the predominant infiltrating cell types were T-lymphocytes and macrophages. B cells and leukocytes were rarely seen. Tumor necrosis factor-alpha was not present. Interleukin (IL)-1 alpha and IL-1 beta was increased only in severely liposclerotic skin.[51] These findings suggest that hypoxia does not play a predominant role in preulcerative cutaneous venous hypertension. Capillary occlusion is probably not a major

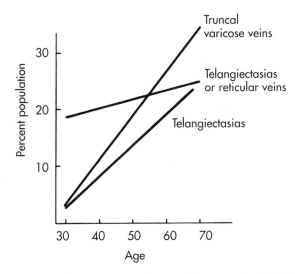

Fig. 2-7   Risk of varicosity by age. Increasing age best correlated with the development of varicose and/or reticular veins. (From Widmer L: Peripheral venous disorders: prevalence and socio-medical importance observations in 4529 apparently healthy persons. Basle Study III. Bern, Switzerland, 1978, Hans Huber.)

contributor to the development of lipodermatosclerosis. Cutaneous changes of venous insufficiency therefore may more likely be related to inflammation.

Advanced cutaneous changes of lipodermatosclerosis appear as an erythematous, telangiectatic, edematous plaque with mottled hyperpigmentation. Histologic examination shows advanced stasis changes, including zones of ischemic necrosis in the central part of fat lobules. Septal fibrosis, fat microcysts, membranous fat necrosis, and sclerosis occurs later. This advanced clinical/histologic change is termed *sclerosing panniculitis*.[52] With superficial venous insufficiency alone, changes in the histologic appearance of capillaries is moderate. The combination of deep venous insufficiency, with or without superficial venous insufficiency, produces more profound changes.[53,54]

Venous hypertension is not a benign condition. The cutaneous chain of events following the onset of venous stasis is thought to occur in the following temporal order: localized edema, induration, pigmentation, dermatitis, atrophie blanche, and, in untreated cases, eventual ulceration, infection, scarring, lymphatic obstruction, and sensitization to applied medications.

INCIDENCE

Varicose veins have been estimated to occur in 7% to 60% of the adult population in the United States.[5,15,55-58] Varicose veins have been noted to increase in incidence with age. Varicose veins occur in 8% of women between ages 20 and 29, increasing to 41% in the fifth decade, and 72% in the seventh decade of life.[56,59,60] A similar rate of increase in the incidence of varicose veins occurs in men: 1% in the third decade, increasing to 24% in the fourth decade, and 43% in the seventh decade.[56,59] The Basle Study III[5] found that the greatest correlation between age and incidence of varicose veins occurred in those with varicose veins only, rather than in those with the presence of telangiectasis (hyphenwebs) or reticular veins (Fig. 2-7). The Framingham study, curiously, shows no difference in the incidence of varicose veins with age.[61]

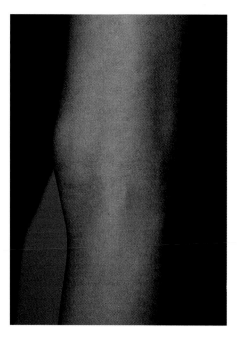

Fig. 2-8 Subtle, asymptomatic varicosity of the GSV at the junction in the popliteal fossa of an 11-year-old girl. There is no significant family history of varicose veins.

Varicosities in childhood are rare, occurring almost exclusively in association with congenital vascular malformations (see Chapter 3). When varicosities occur, they usually appear as a subtle physical finding, such as a slight bulge over the popliteal fossa (Fig. 2-8). One estimation on the incidence of telangiectasias in children was performed by Oster and Nielsen in Denmark.[62] Of 2171 Danish schoolchildren examined, 46.2% of the girls and 35.1% of the boys had telangiectasias on the nape of the neck; 1% of these children had pronounced telangiectasias elsewhere; that is, on the shoulders, thorax, cheeks, and ears. No mention was made of the occurrence of telangiectasias on the legs. An examination of 403 children, aged 8 to 18, in the former East Germany disclosed a 50% incidence of "very discrete" venous abnormalities of leg veins. Of the children examined, 15% had clear symptoms (without visible varices) that could be assigned to a prospective varicose disease. Only between the ages of 17 and 18 could reticular varicose veins be identified. In the 403 children studied by venous Doppler, 2.3% had incompetent communicating veins and 3.2% had an incompetent saphenofemoral junction.[63] An epidemiologic study of 419 Czechoslovakian children ages 8 to 13, with clinical examination plus digital photoplethysmography, showed clinically apparent varices in 8.7% and an impairment of venous function in 14.3% of the examined extremities.[64]

The most recent and complete study of 518 children aged 10 to 20 years, using photoplethysmography in addition to venous Doppler, is the Bochum I, II, and III studies. This continuing investigation initially demonstrated a 10.2% incidence of reticular varicose veins without other venous abnormalities in children 10 to 12 years of age.[65] When these children were examined 4 years later, the incidence of reticular veins was 30.3%; 2% of the children had developed varicose veins and 4% had developed incompetent communicating veins. When examined another 4 years later, the frequency of saphenous refluxes and large varices was still increasing (19.8% saphenous refluxes, 3.3% truncal varices, 5% tributary varices, and 5.2% incompetent perforators). The incidence of reticular veins increased to 35.5%, and the incidence of telangiectasia increased to 12.9%.[66] Therefore, venous disease can be demonstrated in a small number of children, its progression can be documented, and saphenous refluxes are a risk factor for the development of truncal varices.

SYMPTOMS

Varicose veins may be symptomatic in addition to being large and unsightly (see box below). A study of 4280 town and country inhabitants of Tubingen, Germany, found symptoms in 98% of patients with clinically relevant venous alterations.[67] Galen described the symptoms of varicose veins as "a heavy and depressing pain."[68] Pain is most likely related to pressure on the dense network of somatic nerve fibers present in the subcutaneous tissues adjacent to the affected nerve. Alternatively (or in addition), pain may occur from the dilated vein compressing adjacent nerves or from lactic acid accumulation that results from retrograde, circular, and/or slower venous blood flow/clearance. Symptoms may precede the clinical appearance of the varicosity and are proportional to the presence of intermittent edema. At this point, discomfort usually occurs during warm temperatures when the patient is standing for prolonged periods.[69] These patients may respond to systemic hydroxyrutosides, which decrease inflammation of the vein wall.[70,71,72] Paroven—a mixture that mainly consists of mono, di, tri, and tetra -0- beta-hydroxyethyl rutosides containing at least 45% troxerutin (Zyma, United Kingdom, Ltd.)—250 mg 3 or 4 times a day has been reported to help.[73] Reduction in the venous hypertension or excision of the involved segment usually results in prompt relief of pain.[4]

Almost all patients with postthrombotic obstruction complain of "bursting" calf pain that is exacerbated by exercise.[74] *Venous claudication* is an appropriate term to use in this situation to emphasize the relationship of exercise to pain. Pain during exercise may be due to nociceptor stimulation of the distended vein wall.[75] Alternatively, exercise pain may be due to an accumulation of tissue metabolites and/or an increase in interstitial pressure. Patients with acute DVT have an increased intramuscular pressure that is proportional to the degree of thrombosis.[76,77]

Kistner has found that perforator incompetence leads to indurated skin with ulceration, whereas incompetence of the tibial, popliteal, and/or superficial femoral system produces aching and swelling in the leg.[78] There are patients who have a significant amount of valvular incompetence without symptoms. Clinical symptoms vary based on the effectiveness of the calf muscle pump to compensate for venous hypertension. Young, thin, and more athletic patients have fewer symptoms than older and obese patients.

SYMPTOMS OF VARICOSE VEIN/VENOUS STASIS DISEASE (CHRONIC VENOUS INSUFFICIENCY)

Cosmetic	Dermatitis
Aches and pains	Ulceration
Night cramps	Hemorrhage
Edema	Superficial thrombophlebitis
Cutaneous pigmentation	

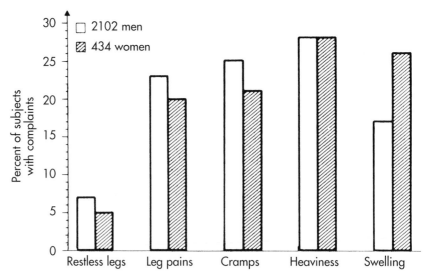

Fig. 2-9 Type of complaints according to sex. Except for an increase in the complaint of ankle swelling, men with varices have complaints similar to those of women. (From Widmer L: Peripheral venous disorders: prevalence and socio-medical importance observations in 4529 apparently health persons. Basle Study III. Bern, Switzerland, 1978, Hans Huber.)

Varicose vein pain is usually described as a dull aching of the legs, particularly after prolonged standing or during certain times of the menstrual cycle (especially during menses).[79] A small number of women also experience painful varicose veins after sexual intercourse.[80] It is proposed that the increase in venous pressure with distention of the varicose vein contributes to heaviness and tightness of the lower legs.[4,81] The Basle Study III[5] found a similar range of complaints in both men and women (Fig. 2-9) and also found an increased incidence of complaints among women and older patients. Many patients in the Basle Study III had complaints without evidence of peripheral vascular disease. Strandness and Thiele suggest that symptoms specifically caused by varicose veins improve with aging as the level of activity declines.[4]

Symptoms in varicose veins are often disproportionate to the amount of actual pathologic change. Patients with small, early-stage varices may complain more than those with large, long-standing varicosities.[26,49,50,82,83] A survey of 350 patients who presented for sclerotherapy treatment of veins that were less than 1 mm in diameter noted that 53% of these patients complained of swelling, burning, throbbing, and cramping of the legs, in addition to a "tired feeling."[84] A retrospective analysis of 401 patients who presented solely for treatment of telangiectasia disclosed 69% with various symptoms, including pain, heaviness, cramping, burning, throbbing, and heaviness.[85] These symptoms are so insidious that most patients fail to realize how good their legs can feel until after treatment of these blood vessels by either compression sclerotherapy or by wearing lightweight (20 mm Hg) graduated compression stockings.[58] One American health survey found that nearly 50% of those with varicose veins were bothered by their symptoms once in a while, and 18% noted frequent to continuous symptoms.[86]

The increased incidence of symptomatic varicose veins in women may have a hormonal etiology. It has been estimated that 27.7% of women with varicose veins have premenstrual pain in their varices.[87] Varicose veins during pregnancy appear to be more symptomatic than those unassociated with pregnancy. In a

---

DIFFERENTIAL DIAGNOSIS OF LEG PAIN

Varicose veins	Achilles tendonitis or tear
Thrombophlebitis	Intermittent (arterial) claudication
Osteoarthritis	Venous claudication
Rheumatoid arthritis	Spinal claudication
Malignancy	Myalgia
Osteomyelitis	Peripheral neuropathy
Meniscial tears	Lymphedema

From Browse NL, Burnand KG, and Thomas ML: Diseases of the veins: pathology, diagnosis, and treatment, London, 1988, Edward Arnold.

VENOUS STASIS DISEASE SIGNS

Ankle edema	Pigmentation
Dilated veins and venules	Venous dermatitis
Telangiectasias	Atrophie blanche
Corona phlebectasia	Ulceration

---

study of 150 pregnant women with varicose veins, 125 noted pain, and 26 were unable to stand for more than 1 to 2 hours because of the pain.[88]

Warm weather tends to increase the severity of pain, as does continual standing. Cooling the legs with water immersion or compresses or raising the legs relieves the symptoms.

The differential diagnosis of leg pain is extensive and not necessarily attributable to a patient's varicosities (see first box above). Symptoms derived from varicose veins can usually be distinguished from arterial symptoms. Pain associated with arterial diseases often disappears at rest and is exacerbated with walking. Pain associated with varicosities is dull, vague, and localized on the medial side of the legs. It is usually relieved with walking. In addition to the dull aching, varicose veins associated with venous hypertension may produce cramping or painful spasms of the legs and an increase in leg fatigue and restless legs, especially at night. Unfortunately, a patient's perception and reporting of pain is subjective in nature and is difficult to document. Browse, Burnand, and Thomas[89] advocate the use of compression hosiery as a diagnostic test to determine if the pain is of venous origin. I have found that if a patient's symptoms are alleviated with 20 mm Hg graduated compression stockings, sclerotherapy treatment also alleviates the symptoms.

SIGNS

In addition to the direct symptoms of varicose and telangiectatic veins, varicose veins may also be a cutaneous marker for venous insufficiency, where they occur in more than 50% of patients (see second box above).[27,90,91,92] Certainly, deep venous insufficiency secondary to valvular incompetence is the major etiologic factor for the cutaneous manifestations of chronic venous insufficiency. In fact, when descending venography was used to examine patients with chronic venous insufficiency, reflux occurred in the superficial system alone in only 2% of the 644 examined limbs. Eighteen percent of the limbs had combined deep and superficial reflux.[93] Studies utilizing ascending venography have shown that more than 20% of patients with chronic venous insufficiency have isolated perforator incompetence as the only demonstrable abnormality.[94] However, a significant group of patients has superficial venous insufficiency alone (13% to 38%) or in combination with deep venous insufficiency (28% to 78%).[92,95-100] In addition, Walsh et al. found that treating the incompetent superficial venous system with ligation and stripping the greater saphenous vein to the knee with stab avulsion of distal varices restored competency to the femoral vein.[101] Therefore, identification of patients with superficial venous insufficiency is important, because they may respond to sclerotherapy and/or surgical treatment of the superficial venous system alone.

It has been estimated that between 17% and 50% of the population with varicose veins has cutaneous findings.[102,2] Approximately 70% of limbs with chronic venous insufficiency have clinical findings.[96] There is a strong association between the severity of clinical signs (described below) and superficial venous incompetence.[96] Almost all patients with cutaneous abnormalities have incompetence of perforator veins. All patients with either active or healed venous ulcerations have evidence of perforator incompetence.[102] The cutaneous manifestation appears as edema, hyperpigmentation, dermatitis, or ulceration. More than 1 million Americans suffer from skin ulcers caused by abnormal circulation that results from varicose veins, and nearly 100,000 Americans are totally disabled by this condition.[56] Thus varicose and telangiectatic leg veins are not merely of cosmetic concern but represent a widespread and potentially serious medical problem.

Edema

Ankle edema is usually the first manifestation of chronic venous insufficiency.[103] Ankle edema tends to be worse in warm weather[2] and toward the end of the day.[58] It is especially common in persons who stand a great deal.[58] True "pitting" edema is rare,[26] resulting perhaps from increased dermal fibrosis present in lipodermatosclerosis. The edema usually found is restricted to a limited area drained by capillaries that empty directly into the varicose and/or incompetent perforating veins.[104] This area has been termed the *gaiter area* and refers to the ankle and lower calf. (In the 1800s it was commonly covered by a cloth or leather material [gaiter] to protect the ankle and instep from the environmental elements. Such protection is still used today by cross-country skiers.) Ankle edema caused by venous hypertension and varicose veins must be differentiated from that caused by other conditions (see box below). However, as previously de-

---

DIFFERENTIAL DIAGNOSIS OF ANKLE EDEMA

Cardiac failure
Renal failure
Deep vein thrombosis
Venous obstruction from other causes
Hypoalbuminemia
Fluid retention syndromes
Lymphedema
Lipodystrophy
Hemihypertrophy (Klippel-Trenaunay syndrome)
Venous valvular agenesis

scribed, lymphatic edema may also be present in patients with chronic venous leg ulcers.[30]

The protein-rich edema fluid stimulates fibroblastic activity, which entangles blood vessels and lymphatics into a fibrous mass.[105] Histologically, a microedema around capillaries is seen.[106] The edema, which contains fibrin, proteins, and neutral polysaccharides, is probably the main reason for the lack of nutrition of the skin.[107,108] The resulting lymphedema and the hypertrophy of the skin and subcutaneous tissues disrupts the flow of cutaneous nutrition. In women with venous stasis and fat, hairless, erythrocyanoid-type ankles, the resulting decrease in nutrition for the sizable fatty subcutaneous tissue and the decrease in local tissue oxygenation may result in sudden and massive fat necrosis of the subcutaneous tissue.[2,15] The affected area may then appear erythematous, indurated, and tender to the touch.

Treatment of ankle edema caused by increased venous pressure, with or without lipodermatosclerosis, is directed primarily toward the prevention of trauma and alleviation of superficial venous hypertension.[19] Temporizing treatments include leg elevation, systemic diuretics, and localized compression bandaging.[19] Graduated compression bandaging can normalize lymphatic flow over time. Thus this "conservative" form of treatment is actually therapeutic as well (see Chapter 6). Recently, fibrinolytic enhancement has reportedly been successful in improving symptoms, induration, and cutaneous thickening in patients with lipodermatosclerosis.[109] The authors of that report used stanozolol (5 mg by mouth, twice daily) in 14 patients with long-standing lipodermatosclerosis resulting from venous disease. Of these 14 patients, 11 noted improvement within 3 months. Long-term follow-up was not given, nor has this treatment been accepted elsewhere.

Pigmentation

Pigmentation (Fig. 2-10) is also a sign of venous stasis disease. The elongated, distended vascular system underlying areas of stasis is more susceptible to trauma

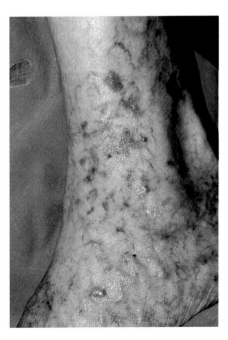

Fig. 2-10 Hyperpigmentation around dilated telangiectasias and venules in a 70-year-old man. There has been no history of cutaneous trauma.

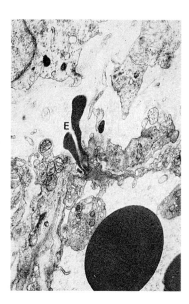

Fig. 2-11 Two deformed erythrocytes wind through an intercellular space (E) into the pericapillary tissue. IX/13. Osmium-cacodylate. ×18,100. (Reproduced with permission from Wenner A et al: Ultrastructural changes of capillaries in chronic venous insufficiency, Exp Cell Biol 48:1, 1980.)

than normal vessels. Even minor blunt injuries may cause rupture of the vascular wall with extravasation of erythrocytes into the cutis.[12,18,105] Histologically, cutaneous hyperpigmentation represents extravasated erythrocytes and hemosiderin-laden macrophages interspersed between dilated and tortuous capillaries.[12,110] Erythrocytes appear either intact or fragmented through their passage (Fig. 2-11). Extravasation appears to be due to increased intravascular pressure and not to chemotaxis as occurs with white blood cells.[110]

Extravasated erythrocytes may also be found in the deep dermis around adnexal structures (Fig. 2-12). When present clinically, it is a reliable guide to the existence of microangiopathy. A more acute "eruptive" cutaneous pigmentation has also been noted as a "blow-out" of erythrocytes into the dermis as a result of tremendous back pressure within the cutaneous microvasculature.[111] This phenomenon has been ascribed as the cause of lichen aureus (Fig. 2-13).[112] The only treatment for this condition is correction of the underlying venous hypertension (sclerotherapy and/or surgery), including graduated compression stockings and leg elevation. Fortunately, when venous hypertension is treated, pigment darkening gradually fades.

Venous (Stasis) Dermatitis

The next dermatologic manifestation to occur in the chain of events following venous hypertension/stasis is "stasis" dermatitis. This dermatitis has been given many names, including stasis eczema, varicose eczema, stasis syndrome, hypostatic eczema, congestive eczema, and dermatitis hypostatica. Because there may not be a true "stasis" in the lower leg with venous insufficiency, but rather venous hypertension, this condition is best referred to as "venous" dermatitis. Venous dermatitis occurs more frequently in women, obese people, middle-aged men and women, and in those with a history of deep venous thrombosis and thrombophlebitis.[3] Edema, which causes the change from the normal cutaneous venous

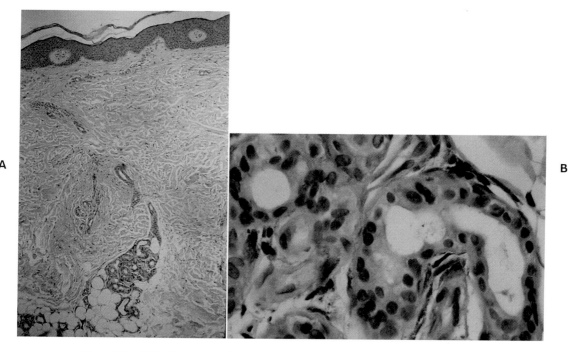

Fig. 2-12 Skin biopsy specimen taken from the medial malleolar area of a 38-year-old man with ankle/pedal telangiectasias and venulectases with associated hyperpigmentation. Note hemosiderin-laden macrophages interspersed among eccrine glands in the deep dermis. (Hematoxylin-eosin; **A,** ×50 ; **B,** ×200 .)

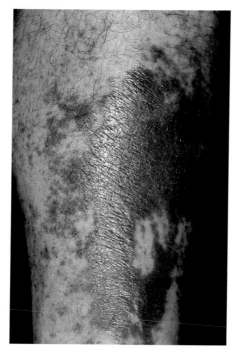

Fig. 2-13 Woman, 52 years old, with onset over 1 to 2 years of cutaneous hyperpigmentation of the anterior tibial and medial malleolar areas. Venous Doppler examination was diagnostic for an incompetent communicating vein.

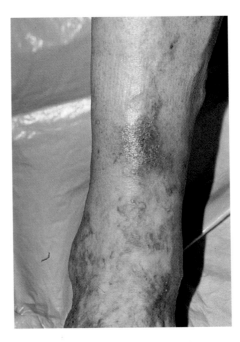

Fig. 2-14 Early venous eczema appearing as a nummular eczema overlying prominent dilated venules and reticular veins in a 58-year-old woman.

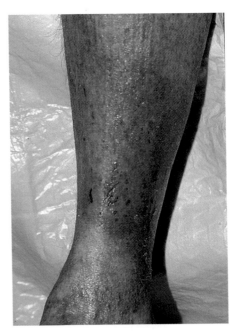

Fig. 2-15 Typical appearance of venous dermatitis. The affected area is erythematous, poorly marginated, and scaly with hyperpigmentation and excoriations.

circulation to a high pressure system with increased vascular permeability, is the precursor of this dermatitis.[113-115]

A random sample of 476 people over the age of 65 in Sheffield, England, found an incidence of "varicose dermatitis" in 21% of the men and 25% of the women.[116] In Denmark, the incidence of stasis dermatitis in a random sample of people in homes for the aged (55 to 106 years old, mean age of 80) was 6.9%.[117]

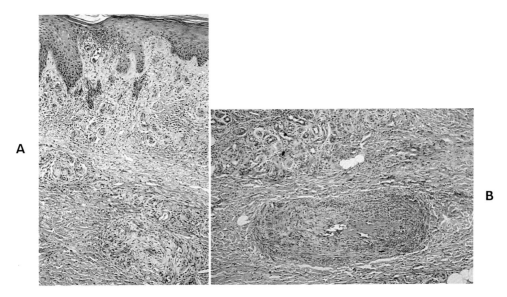

Fig. 2-16 Histologic examination of a patient with long-standing venous hypertension and overlying venous dermatitis. (For description see text.) (Hematoxylin-eosin; **A**, ×50; **B**, ×200.)

The authors speculated that the difference was due to better nutrition in the Denmark population. A similar incidence of stasis dermatitis (5.9%) was found in a randomized examination of noninstitutionalized volunteers aged 50 to 91 years (average age, 74 years) in Boston.[118] Interestingly, a survey of dermatologic patients in the Filipino population age 60 and over disclosed a 12% incidence of stasis dermatitis, with 49% of all patients having varicosities.[60] This is contrary to the popular belief (see Chapter 3) of a decreased incidence of venous disease in non-Western races.

The dermatitis usually begins in the medial paramalleolar region. This region is particularly vulnerable because the vascular supply, skin nutrition, and subcutaneous tissue are less abundant here than in other areas of the lower extremity.[119] Venous dermatitis appears clinically as a sharply marginated, erythematous, crusted plaque (Fig. 2-14). With time and cutaneous trauma resulting from pruritus, overlying lichenification may occur,[3] as well as exudation, depending on the extent of the inflammation and associated edema. However, an indolent venous flow may make the skin assume a much paler color with less moisture.[120] The color of the lesion darkens as a result of an increase in melanocytic postinflammatory hyperpigmentation and dermal hemosiderin (Fig. 2-15).[2,121] The dermatitis may also be complicated by a generalized systemic hypersensitivity or "ID" reaction.[2]

Histologic examination (Fig. 2-16) of the dermis demonstrates a diffuse homogenization of collagen, fragmentation or absence of elastic fibers, thickening and partial occlusion of arterioles, and atrophic changes of appendages.[12,122] There may also be an associated acanthosis and hyperkeratosis of the epidermis, which rarely results in pseudoepitheliomatous hyperplasia.[3] The lymphatic vessels are usually thickened and fibrotic, and there may be an associated dermal inflammatory infiltrate.[3] Because these changes are those of a nonspecific dermatitis, the histologic diagnosis of venous dermatitis can be certain only with clinical correlation.

Atrophie Blanche

Atrophie blanche is the descriptive name given to the appearance of porcelain-white scars seen on the lower extremities as a result of infarctive lesions of the skin (Fig. 2-17). This condition was originally attributed to syphilis or tuberculosis in 1929.[123] The white plaques are bordered by hyperpigmentation and telangiectasias. Histologically, meandering capillaries are detected at the border of lesions with their apex oriented toward the avascular center.[124]

The process usually occurs in middle-aged women with associated varicose veins and signs of venous insufficiency. However, this descriptive term represents the sequelae of many disease processes, including venous dermatitis, arteriosclerosis, dysproteinemia, diabetes mellitus, hypertension, systemic lupus erythematosus, scleroderma, juvenile rheumatoid arthritis, and idiopathic segmental hyalinizing vasculitis. Therefore, this physical condition is best thought of as an intermediate stage between venous dermatitis and varicose ulceration; the term *atrophie blanche* is best reserved for the idiopathic vasculitic condition.

Ulceration

Cutaneous ulceration represents the end-stage manifestation of venous stasis disease. This relationship has been noted for millenia. Hippocrates was the first to record the association.[125] More than 300 years ago, Wiseman noted that valvular incompetence caused by venous thrombosis could result in a circulatory defect leading to ulceration of the skin.[126]

The prevalence of varicose or postthrombophlebotic ulcers has been estimated to be as high as 1% of the United States population and 2% of the Swedish population (Fig. 2-18).[3,127,128] Although venous ulcers may have an onset in early adulthood, they increase in frequency with age and peak at approximately 70 years.[128,129,130] The ratio of females to males is approximately 3:1 after the age of 40, with an equal incidence before 40 years of age.[129]

Seventy-two different causes of leg ulcers have been recognized and grouped into three categories.[131] Seventy-five percent to 90% are of venous etiology,[3,132,133] 40% to 60% of which are associated with varicose veins,[132-134] and 35% to 90% are associated with a history of DVT.[3,36,132-135] Nonvenous causes of leg ulceration include arterial disease (8%) and ulcers caused by trauma or those that have bacteriologic, mycotic, hematologic, neoplastic, neurologic, or systemic origins (2%).[131]

The cost for treating leg ulcers in the United States was estimated in 1991 to be between $775 million and $1 billion, based on the annual cost of ulcer care in Sweden.[136] In addition to this cost, there is an estimated loss of 2,000,000 work days annually in the United States because of leg ulcers.[137] Therefore, optimizing treatment or, better yet, prevention is important. Curiously, despite its importance, very little government funding is allocated toward ulcer treatment. The longest diagnosis-related group time allowed for leg ulcer admission in the United States is 12.1 days.[138] Because leg ulcers frequently take much longer to heal with bed rest and ancillary care, this form of therapy is impractical and not properly reimbursable.

Twenty percent to 25% of ulcerations have either superficial venous insufficiency alone with perforating vein incompetence or as a significant component combined with deep venous insufficiency.[139,92,96,97,140] In one practice of more than 20,000 lifetime patients, it was estimated that nearly 15% of patients with major varicose veins developed ulcerations.[6] Although ulcerations are more common in patients with DVT, 13% of all venous ulcerations are observed in limbs with superficial venous insufficiency alone.

Cutaneous ulceration usually occurs 10 to 35 years (mean 24 years) after the onset of varicose veins[141] and is commonly assumed to be specifically associated

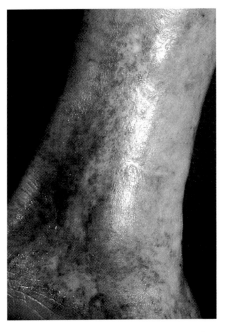

Fig. 2-17 Middle-aged woman with venous insufficiency and atrophie blanche of the medial malleolar area. (Courtesy Kim Butterwick, M.D.)

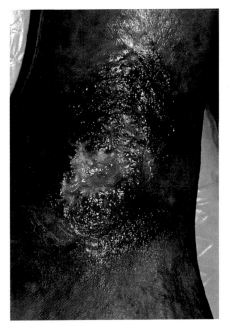

Fig. 2-18 Chronic venous insufficiency with cutaneous ulceration in a 68-year-old man before treatment.

with incompetent calf perforating veins (see Chapter 9).[15,142,143,144] Dodd and Cockett[15] surgically explored 135 limbs with ankle ulceration and found that the most severe lesions always were associated with an incompetent perforating vein. Lawrence, Fish, and Kakkar[143] studied patients with varicosities, both with and without associated ulceration, with Doppler ultrasound. They found sustained retrograde flow in incompetent veins in eight of nine ulcer patients, but found it in only one of seven patients with varicose veins without ulceration. However, a recent study using duplex sonography showed no direct correlation between incompetent perforators and venous ulceration. Plethysmographic examination indicated that venous hypertension in superficial veins was the more important factor.[145] One study of 213 consecutive patients with venous ulceration demonstrated that 90% of patients will have sustained ulcer healing with a mean follow-up period of 3.4 years when treated with saphenous ligation alone, without perforating vein treatment, even when incompetence of the perforating veins can be demonstrated.[146] Thus any operative procedure on varicose ulcers must correct the underlying abnormal communicating superficial or perforating veins. Interestingly, no evidence or history of DVT was reported in up to 24% of patients with chronic venous leg ulcers.[134,147] Therefore, the etiology may be multifactorial, with the majority of patients having a similar initiating event: superficial venous hypertension. This may arise from incompetent perforating veins alone, associated with an abnormal deep venous system, or with an incompetent superficial venous system.

Stasis ulcerations, unlike most other causes of cutaneous ulcerations, appear in the gaiter area.[37,134] The ulcers appear cyanotic, edematous, and friable. The base usually is covered with thick granulation tissue that rarely penetrates the deep fascia. The skin edges are painless, thickened, and bleed easily. Adjacent skin is edematous and inflamed, with associated dilated venules, eczematous changes, and pigmentation.[36,148] Calcification of the subcutaneous tissue, often not even adjacent to the ulceration, occurs in a significant number of patients,[113,149,150] up to 25% in one study (Fig. 2-19).[151] The calcium, acting as a foreign body, may perpetuate the ulceration or may actually be an essential cause of the lesion. Calcification is probably caused by venous insufficiency and represents the last stage of the inflammatory response. It almost always precedes the ulceration.[113]

In contrast to venous/stasis ulceration, ischemic ulcers occur most commonly on the anterior and/or lateral leg and ankle. The base of an ischemic ulcer is often obscured by a pale yellow, purulent exudate. Often, the borders are poorly epithelialized, with a "punched-out" appearance, and are necrotic with islands of gangrenous skin. Deep fascia and tendon may be exposed at the base, with little or no spontaneous granulation tissue.

Malignant Degeneration

A potentially fatal, but fortunately rare, secondary change in venous ulcers is malignant degeneration (Fig. 2-20). There have been more than 100 case reports of malignant degeneration of a stasis ulcer in the world literature.[144, 152-159] The most common cancers reported are carcinomas (squamous and basal cell) and sarcomas (fibrosarcoma, osteosarcoma, and angiosarcoma). The incidence of malignant degeneration of venous stasis ulcerations is 0.4% to 1%.[159,160] The average duration of the ulcer before tumor growth is 21 years, with a reported span of 10 to 40 years.[161] The onset of malignant change usually appears as a rapid growth of exuberant cauliflower-like masses, an increase in pain, or, in a smaller number of cases, a rapid extension of the ulcer crater.[161] An increase in induration of the ulcer borders and surrounding tissue and a failure of the ulcer to respond to prolonged conservative treatment are also suspect.[162] Transition into a

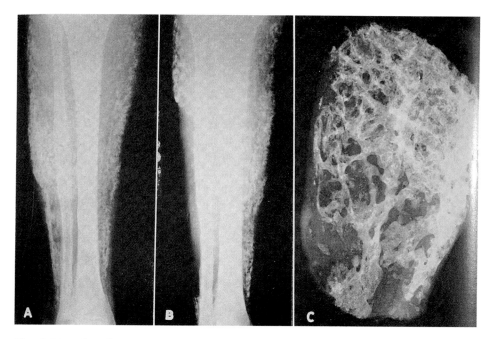

Fig. 2-19   Sixty-five-year-old woman with varicose veins, stasis dermatitis, and medial malleolar ulcerations bilaterally. **A,** Right leg; **B,** left leg; **C,** close-up view of left medial calf demonstrating extensive subcutaneous calcium deposits.

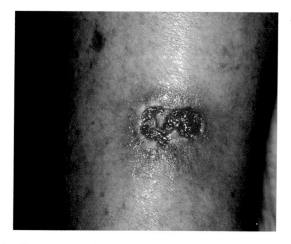

Fig. 2-20   Basal cell carcinoma (keratinizing type) arising in an ulcer in the setting of chronic venous insufficiency in a 77-year-old woman. The ulceration has been present for at least 6 years. An incompetent perforating vein was found at the base of the ulceration.

malignant growth is thought to be stimulated by many factors, including chronic dermatitis, irritation, and/or infection.[163,162] Implanted epithelial cells may produce a chronic foreign-body reaction with subsequent neoplasia.[164] Chronic scarring from the sequelae of ulceration mentioned above may obliterate lymphatic channels, leading to decreased immune surveillance of the scar by immunologically competent cells. This relative localized immune deficiency provides less protection against cellular mutation, which allows cellular progression into neoplasia.[165] Therefore, it seems prudent to biopsy the base and border areas of ulcers

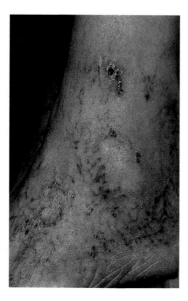

Fig. 2-21   Venulectasia in a 90-year-old male that bled profusely while the patient was standing. Sclerotherapy caused rapid healing.

with these characteristics or ulcers that persist for more than 4 months. This is particularly important when surgically correcting the ulceration with a skin graft. One patient developed a squamous cell carcinoma following split skin grafting and, in spite of amputation and radiotherapy, died from multiple metastasis.[144]

Although the appearance of malignant degeneration in a nonhealing leg ulcer is often characteristic, basal cell carcinoma in the ulcer may appear as either exuberant and translucent "granulation tissue" or may have no clinical features to suggest malignancy.[157,154]

Secondary Complications of Venous Hypertension/Stasis

In addition to the varicose ulcers and dermatologic abnormalities already discussed, external hemorrhage, superficial thrombophlebitis, and DVT are the three most severe and acute complications of varicose veins.

Hemorrhage

Hemorrhage from varicose veins may not be a rare event. Tretbar[166] has reported treating 12 patients in 3 years for 18 episodes of hemorrhagic varicose veins. All but two of his patients had varicose veins for more than 20 years. The bleeding area typically consisted of a mat of "blue blebs" 1 to 2 mm in diameter on the medial ankle. Doppler examination usually disclosed an underlying incompetent communicating vein. None of Tretbar's patients developed serious sequelae from the bleeding episodes, and all were treated successfully with compression sclerotherapy of the affected veins. However, bleeding can be profuse and, if unnoticed or improperly treated, can be fatal.[167-169,15] Hemorrhage is usually spontaneous but may also occur when the skin overlying a varicose vein becomes traumatized or eroded. Most cases described in the literature occur in patients with ulcers overlying varices, but profuse bleeding may occur also from varicosities 1 to 2 mm in diameter (Fig. 2-21). Twenty-three fatal cases of hemorrhage were reported in England and Wales in 1971.[167] The patients most at risk are solitary elderly patients with long-standing varicose veins. These patients usually live alone and are unable to apply pressure to the bleeding varix or get help because of physical disabilities. Rarely, patients may have no history of long-standing varices or overlying ulcers. Hemorrhage in this setting usually is attributable to the rapid development of venous hypertension that occurs from DVT.[170]

If the varicose vein is under high pressure from venous insufficiency, as it usually is, the acute hemorrhage may appear to be arterial in origin. This may result in the inappropriate application of a tourniquet, which only increases venous hypertension. Properly recognized, bleeding of venous origin is easily controlled by raising the affected area above the level of the heart and applying localized pressure to the bleeding vein. Sclerotherapy or ligation of the affected vein is curative but may not prevent further episodes of hemorrhage from other varices.

Superficial Thrombophlebitis

Superficial thrombophlebitis (ST) is a painful condition that fortunately seldom results in serious embolic complications. In the absence of malignancy, thrombophlebitis of the leg is almost invariably associated with varicose veins.[4,171,172,173] Patients with varicose vein ST are younger and have a decreased incidence of coexistent DVT (9.75% versus 43.75%).[172] ST results from the development of a clot in a varicose vein caused by one or more of the following factors: trauma to the varicosity, stasis of blood flow, or occlusion of blood flow. Fifty percent of cases may occur spontaneously.[171,174] The greater saphenous system is the usual site of ascending ST. Clinically, one notes a painful, tender, hot, erythematous swelling along the course of the vein with a variable amount of perivascular edema. The pain associated with ST is often severe, probably resulting from inflammation of the dense network of somatic nerve fibers in the associated subcutaneous tissue.[4]

ST increases in incidence with advancing age and inactivity and with bed rest as the result of surgery, childbirth, or cardiac disease.[175,176] In patients in whom the incidence of varicose veins is not stated, ST has been estimated to occur in 0.7% of women in their fourth decade of life, increasing to 2.6% of women in the seventh decade.[56] The actual number of patients with ST in the United States was estimated in 1973 to occur in 123,000 persons yearly. In men, the incidence of ST has been estimated to be 0.4% in the fourth decade, increasing to 1.7% in the seventh decade.[56]

The incidence of ST is substantially higher when related to the presence of varicose veins.[4] A review of the lifetime work of one physician with more than 20,000 patients notes an incidence of ST in as many as 20% of patients with prominent major varicosities.[6] Older papers have estimated a 50% lifetime incidence of thrombophlebitis in patients with varicose veins.[177] Fegan estimates that the incidence of ST occurs in approximately 4% of those with varicose veins.[80]

Although the condition is usually treated as a benign complication of varicose veins, the development of DVT, venous hypertension, and pulmonary emboli may occur in a significant percentage of patients.[171,174,178-180,181,182] A review of 340 cases of ST in a university hospital disclosed a 10% incidence of pulmonary emboli with 5 deaths.[174] This risk has been confirmed by others.[183] The development of pulmonary emboli may also be related in some cases to a coexistent DVT.[4,184,185] One study of 44 consecutive patients with ST found coexistent DVT in 23%. All of these cases were clinically occult with the site of ST not predictive of DVT.[173] Thus noninvasive deep venous studies are recommended for all patients with ST.

DVT and pulmonary emboli, by definition, do not complicate ST unless the thrombus progresses into the deep venous system. This may occur because of either progression into a perforating vein or ascending involvement of the common femoral vein at the saphenofemoral junction (Fig. 2-22). When either of these events occurs, superficial or deep venous hypertension develops as a result of valvular destruction.[176] Propagation of the thrombotic process into the deep system has been reported to occur in 6%[186] to 32%[178] of all cases of ST. In an 11-year retrospective series, 17% of 133 patients were noted to have extension of the clot into the deep system.[187] Surgical exploration of the saphenofemoral junction, followed by ligation, thrombectomy, and limited vein stripping, has been advocated, particularly if clinical signs of thrombophlebitis reach the midthigh. Alternatively, full anticoagulation is advocated by some.[188] Surgical removal of the thrombosed vein segments and associated varicosities shortens the convalescence and mitigates recurrences.[186,189] Unfortunately, this latter form of treatment usually results in extensive scarring. Finally, because DVT may manifest partly in the appearance of ST, patients should be examined carefully.

Deep Venous Thrombosis

Varicose veins, by virtue of their low blood flow, are considered a high risk factor for DVT.[4] Without other predisposing factors, patients with varicose veins have an incidence of DVT ninefold that of the normal population.[190] Platelet aggregation is thought to occur behind valve cusps, especially when the valves are in-

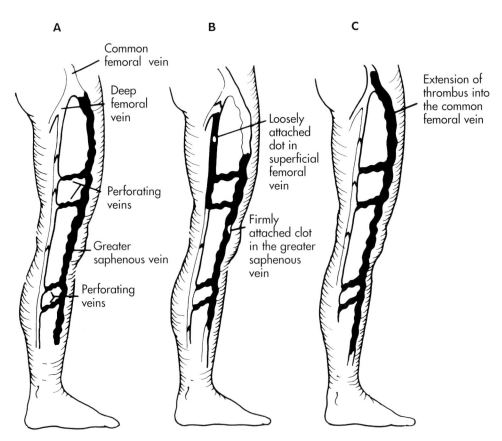

Fig. 2-22 Diagrammatic representation of three methods of propagation of superficial thrombophlebitis. **A,** Thrombophlebitis limited to the superficial system with blockage by the perforating vein valves and at the saphenofemoral junction. **B,** Extension of the thrombus into the deep system via destruction and incompetence of perforating veins. **C,** Direct extension of the thrombus into the femoral vein at the saphenofemoral junction. (Redrawn from Totten HP: Angiology, the journal of vascular diseases, Fig 2, vol 16:37, 1965. Reproduced with permission of the copyright owner, Westminster Publications, Inc, Roslyn, New York. All rights reserved.)

competent in varicose veins.[191,192] Thrombosis on the valve cusps then triggers the coagulation cascade and results in clot propagation.

Stasis of blood flow may cause activation of factors XII, XI, and IX, which initiates thrombin activity to propagate thrombus formation through fibrin formation and platelet aggregation.[193] Stasis may also result in a significant amount of endothelial sloughing with exposure of subendothelial collagen and subsequent activation of platelets.[194] An additional reason for the propensity for DVT in patients with chronic venous insufficiency (which commonly is associated with the presence of varicose veins) may be related to a faulty fibrinolytic system, correlated with pericapillary deposition of fibrin.[195] This hypothesis has been questioned because up to 70% of patients with idiopathic DVT have a decreased tissue plasminogen activator that probably reflects endothelial dysfunction and a decreased clearance of clotting factors.[195,196,197,198]

An increased incidence of DVT is also found in the postoperative period.[199-203] This may be related to the increased incidence of thrombophlebitis in varicose veins in the postoperative period, with an incidence estimated at 6%, versus the normal 0.5% to 0.7% incidence.[204] This is of particular significance in patients less than 60 years of age. With fibrinogen scanning, DVT occurs in 56% of patients over 60 with varicose veins versus 41% in patients over 60 without varicose veins, compared to 56% in patients younger than 60 years with varicose veins versus 19% in patients less than 60 without varicose veins.[205] Therefore, all patients with varicose veins who are about to undergo surgery, or who are bedridden or pregnant, should receive thrombosis prophylaxis, such as wearing a graduated support stocking, to prevent this potentially fatal, albeit rare, complication of varicose veins.

In summary, varicose veins are associated with a number of serious medical problems and are not just of cosmetic concern. Basle Study III[5] found that the incidence of the major complications of varicose veins—chronic venous insufficiency, phlebitis, and pulmonary embolism—increases with the severity of the varicosity (Fig. 2-23). Even patients with minor telangiectasias and reticular veins

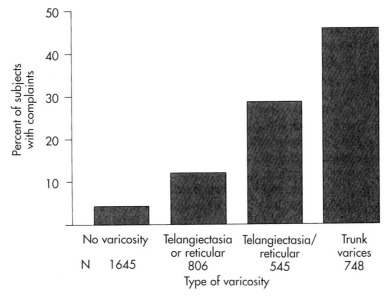

Fig. 2-23 Complications according to the type of varicose vein; *N* represents the number of persons in the defined group; *hyphenweb* refers to telangiectatic veins; * refers to the group composed of both telangiectasia and reticular veins. (Redrawn from Widmer L: Peripheral venous disorders: prevalence and socio-medical importance observations in 4529 apparently healthy persons. Basle Study III. Bern, Switzerland, 1978, Hans Huber.)

Table 2-1 Classification of varicosities of the lower extremities

Group	Varicosities	Saphenous system
1	Spider bursts; telangiectatic veins	Competent
2	Mild or moderate varicosities	Competent
3	Mild, moderate, or marked varicosities	Incompetent

From Heyerdale WW and Stalker LK: The management of varicose veins of the lower extremities, Ann Surg 114:1042, 1941.

ADVANTAGES OF LIGATION OF INCOMPETENT GREAT SAPHENOUS VEIN

1. Continuity of the vein is interrupted at the most proximal point
2. Possibility of cannulization is reduced to a minimum
3. Number of local injections necessary for obliteration is decreased
4. Period of treatment is shortened
5. Adequate complete thrombosis is obtained with greater ease
6. Pulmonary showers are less likely to occur

From Heyerdale WW and Stalker LK: The management of varicose veins of the lower extremities, Ann Surg 114:1042, 1941.

---

in combination demonstrated a significant increase of these serious medical complications when compared to patients without these types of veins.

CLASSIFICATION

A classification of varicose veins should be based on anatomic and/or subsequent therapeutic considerations. The first anatomic classification was proposed by Heyerdale and Stalker[206] in 1941 (Table 2-1). This classification is useful in determining when surgical ligation of the great saphenous vein is advantageous before performing sclerotherapy. The list of advantages presented by Heyerdale and Stalker still holds true today (see box above). The Basle study[207] classified varicose veins into three groups:

1. Dilated saphenous veins (stem veins)
2. Dilated superficial branches (reticular veins)
3. Dilated venules (hyphenwebs)

Duffy[208] proposed a more complete classification of "unwanted leg veins." Since one purpose of a classification is to provide a mechanism for evaluating pathophysiology and treatment, a modification of the Duffy classification appears useful. It provides comprehensive clinical and therapeutic criteria in an effort to optimize treatment (see box on p. 73) (Figs. 2-24 to 2-29).

Varicose veins can also be classified into four developmental stages. The first stage appears as a somewhat dilated blue vein in association with normal greater and lesser saphenous veins. This stage usually occurs in teenagers with a family history of varicose veins. It is asymptomatic.

The second stage appears as a palpable, bulging, moderately dilated vein, usually in association with a larger saphenous vein. Venous Doppler examination is normal. Duplex scanning may show a dilated but competent saphenofemoral and/or saphenopopliteal junction. These veins may be symptomatic after prolonged immobilization or standing.

VESSEL CLASSIFICATION

TYPE 1-TELANGIECTASIA, "SPIDER VEINS"
0.1-1.0 mm diameter
Red to cyanotic

TYPE 1A-TELANGIECTATIC MATTING
<0.2 mm diameter
Red

TYPE 1B-COMMUNICATING TELANGIECTASIA
Type 1 veins in direct communication with varicose veins of the saphenous system

TYPE 2-MIXED TELANGIECTATIC/VARICOSE VEINS (NO DIRECT COMMUNICATION WITH THE SAPHENOUS SYSTEM)
1.0-6.0 mm diameter
Cyanotic to blue

TYPE 3-NONSAPHENOUS VARICOSE VEINS (RETICULAR VEINS)
2-8 mm diameter
Blue to blue-green

TYPE 4-SAPHENOUS VARICOSE VEINS
Usually over 8 mm in diameter
Blue to blue-green

Modified from Duffy DM: Small vessel sclerotherapy: an overview. In Callen et al, editors: Advances in dermatology, vol 3, Chicago, 1988, Year Book.

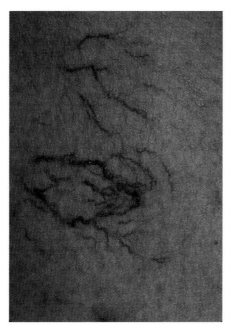

Fig. 2-24 Duffy type 1 (telangiectasia) on the inner thigh of a 58-year-old woman.

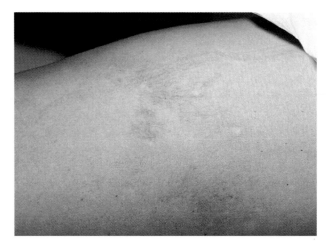

Fig. 2-25 Duffy type 1A (telangiectatic matting) 6 weeks after sclerotherapy treatment on the lateral calf. Note associated reticular veins, postsclerotherapy hyperpigmentation, and bruising.

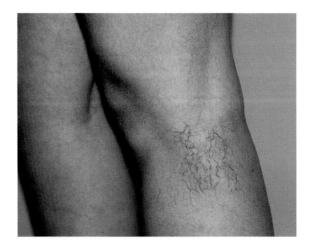

Fig. 2-26 Duffy type 1B (communicating telangiectasia) in a 20-year-old woman.

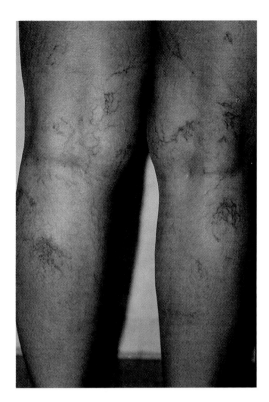

Fig. 2-27   Duffy type 2 (mixed telangiectasia and varicose veins with no direct communication with the saphenous system) in a 54-year-old woman. There was no evidence (venous Doppler) of incompetence of the saphenofemoral or saphenopopliteal junctions or of perforating veins.

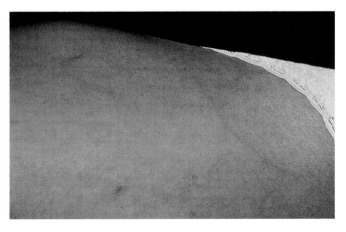

Fig. 2-28   Duffy type 3 (nonsaphenous varicose [reticular] veins) located over the proximal anterolateral thigh of a 24-year-old woman.

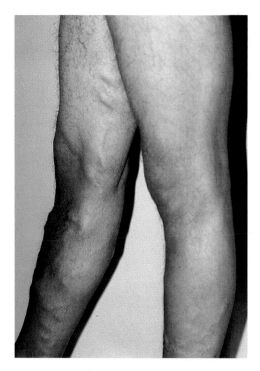

Fig. 2-29 Duffy type 4 (saphenous varicose veins). Varicose GSV with incompetent valvular function throughout its length and a grossly incompetent saphenofemoral junction in a 32-year-old man.

The third stage represents established varicose vein disease. The greater and/or lessor saphenous veins are dilated over all or part of their length. There are associated varicose veins over the thigh and lower leg with accompanying venules and spider veins. The varicose veins themselves may or may not be incompetent, but gross incompetence is present at the saphenofemoral and/or saphenopopliteal junctions.

The final, or fourth, stage consists of complications arising from chronic venous insufficiency and varicose veins. Perforating vein incompetence is present along with cutaneous manifestations of venous stasis disease, including ulcerations.

The development of varicose vein disease is generally progressive. Six different patterns of greater saphenous vein varicosity have been described.[102] These relate to the duration of varicose vein disease (Fig. 2-30). Certain patients may experience spontaneous stabilization of the disease in the early stages. Treatment of early-stage disease may prevent the progression and cause regression of the disease process. A complete understanding of the anatomy and pathophysiology of the venous system with regard to varicose veins allows the development of a rational treatment plan.

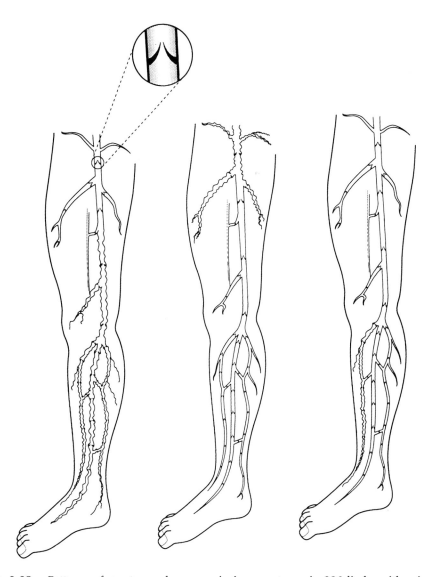

Fig. 2-30   Patterns of greater saphenous vein incompetence in 296 limbs with primary varicose veins. (Modified from Almgren B and Eriksson I: Valvular incompetence in superficial, deep and perforator veins of the limbs with varicose veins, Acta Chir Scand 156:69, 1990.)   *Continued*

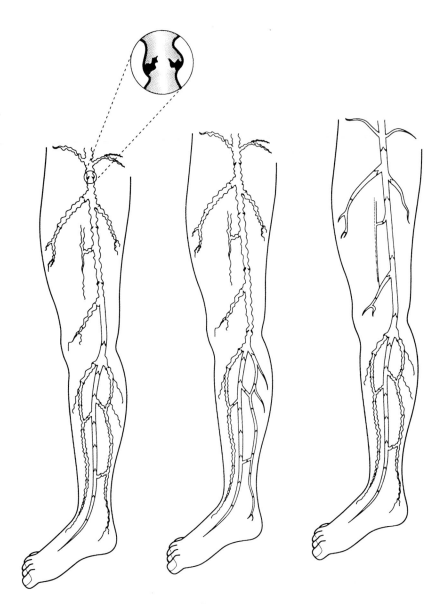

Fig. 2-30, cont'd For legend see opposite page.

REFERENCES

1. Baron HC: Varicose veins, Consultant, May:108, 1983.
2. Hobbs JT: The problem of the post-thrombotic syndrome, Postgrad Med J (Aug supp):48, 1973.
3. Beninson J and Livingood CS: Stasis dermatitis in clinical dermatology. In Demis DJ, editor: Clinical dermatology, vol 2, Philadelphia, 1985, Harper & Row.
4. Strandness DE Jr and Thiele BL: Selected topics in venous disorders, Mt Kisco, NY, 1981, Futura.
5. Widmer LK: Peripheral venous disorders: prevalence and socio-medical importance observations in 4529 apparently healthy persons, Basle Study III, Bern, Switzerland, 1978, Hans Huber.
6. Gallagher PG: Major contributing role of sclerotherapy in the treatment of varicose veins, J Vasc Surg 20:139, 1986.
7. Homans J: The operative treatment of varicose veins and ulcers, based upon a classification of these lesions, Surg Gynecol Obstet 22:143, 1916.
8. Haeger KHM and Bergman L: Skin temperature of normal and varicose veins and some reflections on the etiology of varicose veins, Angiology 14:473, 1963.
9. Linton R: The post-thrombotic ulceration of the lower extremities: its etiology and surgical treatment, Ann Surg 138:415, 1953.
10. Burnand KG et al: The relative importance of incompetent communicating veins in the production of varicose veins and venous ulcers, Surgery 82:9, 1977.
11. Warren R, White EA, and Belcher CB: Venous pressure in the saphenous system in normal, varicose, and post-phlebitic extremities, Surgery 26:435, 1949.
12. Farber EM and Batts EE: Pathologic physiology of stasis dermatitis, Arch Dermatol 70:653, 1954.
13. Smith HG: Complicating factors in the surgical management of varicose veins, Surgery 17:590, 1945.
14. Cockett FB and Jones BE: The ankle blow-out syndrome: a new approach to the varicose ulcer problem, Lancet 1:17, 1953.
15. Dodd H and Cockett FB: The pathology and surgery of the veins of the lower limbs, ed 2, London, 1976, Churchill Livingstone.
16. Landis EM: Factors controlling the movement of fluid through the human capillary wall, Yale J Biol Med 5:201, 1933.
17. Burnand KG et al: The effects of sustained venous hypertension of the skin capillaries of the canine hind limb, Br J Surg 69:41, 1982.
18. Ryan TJ and Wilkinson DS: Diseases of the veins: venous leg ulcers. In Rook A, Wilkinson DS, and Ebling FTG, editors: Textbook of dermatology, ed 3, London, 1979, Blackwell Scientific.
19. Ryan TJ: Diseases of the skin: management of varicose ulcers and eczema, Br Med J 1:192, 1974.
20. Whimster I. Cited in Dodd H and Cockett FP: The pathology and surgery of the veins of the lower limb, Edinburgh & London, 1956, Churchill Livingstone.
21. van Bremmelen SP et al: A study of valve incompetence that developed in an experimental model of venous hypertension, Arch Surg 121:1048, 1986.
22. Nicoaides AN, Hussein MK, Szendro G: The Relation of venous ulceration with ambulatory venous pressure measurements, J Vasc Surg 17:414, 1993.
23. Christopoulos DG et al: Air-plethysmography and the effect of elastic compression on hemodynamics of the leg, J Vasc Surg 5:148, 1987.
24. Calman JS et al: Venous obstruction in the aetiology of lymphoedema praecox, Br J Med 2:221, 1964.
25. Farber EM and Barnes VR: The stasis syndrome, Arch Dermatol Syph 73:277, 1956.
26. Lofgren KA: Varicose veins: their symptoms, complications, and management, Postgrad Med 65:131, 1979.
27. Veal JR and Hossey H: The pathologic physiology of the circulation in the post-thrombotic syndrome, Am Heart J 23:390, 1942.
28. Drinker CK, Field ME, and Homans J: Experimental production of edema and elephantiasis as a result of lymphatic obstruction, Am J Physiol 108:509, 1934.
29. Isenring G, Franzeck UK, and Bollinger A: Lymphatische Mikroangiopathie bei Chronisch-Venoeser Insuffizienz (CVI), Vasa 11:104, 1982.
30. Bull RH et al: Abnormal lymph drainage in patients with chronic venous leg ulcers, J Am Acad Dermatol 28:585, 1993.
31. McMaster PD: Changes in the cutaneous lymphatics of human beings and in the lymph flow under normal and pathological conditions, J Exp Med 65:345, 1937.
32. Campbell RT: Chronic varicose ulcer with pseudoepitheliomatous hyperplasia, Proc R Soc Med 44:923, 1951.

33. Nemeth AJ et al: Ulcerated edematous limbs: effect of edema removal on transcutaneous oxygen measurements, J Am Acad Dermatol 20:191, 1989.
34. Mortimer PS: Investigation and treatment of lymphedema, Vasc Med Rev 1:1, 1990.
35. Myers MB et al: The effect of edema and external pressure on wound healing, Arch Surg 94:218, 1967.
36. Dodd H and Cockett FB: The pathology and surgery of the veins of the lower limbs, Edinburgh & London, 1956, ES Livingstone.
37. Falanga V et al: Dermal pericapillary fibrin in venous disease and venous ulceration, Arch Dermatol 123:620, 1987.
38. Browse NL and Burnand KG: The cause of venous ulceration, Lancet 2:243, 1982.
39. Coleridge Smith PD et al: Causes of wound ulceration: a new hypothesis, Br Med J 296:1726, 1988.
40. Michel CC: Oxygen diffusion in oedematous tissue and through pericapillary cuffs, Phlebology 5:223, 1990.
41. Cheatle TR et al: Skin damage in chronic venous insufficiency: does an oxygen diffuson barrier really exist? Roy Soc Med 83:493, 1990.
42. Stibe E et al: Liposclerotic skin: a diffusion block or a perfusion problem? Phlebology 5:231, 1990.
43. Bollinger A et al: Fluorescence microlymphography in chronic venous incompetence, Int Angiol 8:23, 1989.
44. Thomas PRS, Nash GB, and Dormandy JA: White cell accumulation in dependent legs of patients with venous hypertension: a possible mechanism for trophic changes in the skin, Br Med J 296:1693, 1988.
45. Nash GB, Thomas PRS, and Dormandy JA: Abnormal flow properties of white blood cells in patients with severe ischemia of the leg, Br Med J 296:1699, 1988.
46. Scott HJ et al: Venous ulceration: the role of the white blood cell, Phlebology 4:153, 1989.
47. Veraart JCJM et al: Adhesion molecule expression in venous leg ulcers, Vasa 22:213, 1993.
48. Sullivan GW et al: Inhibition of the inflammatory action of interleukin-1 and tumor necrosis factor (alpha) on neutrophil function by pentoxyfylline, Infest Immunol 56:1722, 1988.
49. Colgan M-P et al: Oxpentifylline treatment of venous ulcers of the leg, Br Med J 300:972, 1990.
50. Allen JC: The micro-circulation of the skin of the normal leg in varicose veins and in the post-thrombotic syndrome, S Afr J Surg 10:29, 1972.
51. Wilkinson LS et al: Leukocytes: their role in the etiopathogenesis of skin damage in venous disease, J Vasc Surg 17:669, 1993.
52. Jorizzo JL et al: Sclerosing panniculitis: a clinopathologic assessment, Arch Dermatol 127:554, 1991.
53. Fagrell B: Local microcirculation in chronic venous incompetence and leg ulcers, Vasc Surg 13:217, 1979.
54. Speiser DE and Bollinger A: Microangiopathy in mild chronic venous incompetence (CVI): morphological alterations and increased transcapillary diffusion detected by fluorescence video-microscopy, Int J Microcirc Clin Exp 10:55, 1991.
55. Strandness DE Jr: Varicose veins. In Dermis DJ, editor: Clinical dermatology, Philadelphia, 1985, Harper & Row.
56. Coon WW, Willis PW III, and Keller JB: Venous thromboembolism and other venous disease in the Tecumseh community health study, Circulation 48:839, 1973.
57. Engel A, Johnson ML, and Haynes SG: Health effects of sunlight exposure in the United States: results from the first national health and nutrition examination survey, 1971-1974, Arch Dermatol 124:72, 1988.
58. Dinn A and Henry M: Value of lightweight elastic tights in standing occupations, Phlebology 4:45, 1989.
59. Lake M, Pratt GH, and Wright IS: Arteriosclerosis and varicose veins: occupational activities and other factors, JAMA 119:696, 1942.
60. Tianco EAV, Buendia-Teodosio G, and Alberto NL: Survey of skin lesions in the Filipino elderly, Int J Dermatol 31:196, 1992.
61. Brand FN et al: The epidemiology of varicose veins: the Framingham study, Am J Prev Med 4:96, 1988.
62. Oster J and Nielsen A: Nuchal naevi and intrascapular telangiectasies, Acta Paediat Scand 59:416, 1970.
63. Heede G: Prevaricose epidemiological symptoms in 8 to 18 aged pupils. In Davy A and Stemmer R, editors: Phlebologie '89, Montrouge, France, 1989, John Libbey Eurotext.
64. Strejcek J: The first experience with using digital photoplethysmography in epidemiological study of children (Bohemian Study I), Prakticka Flebologie 2:5, 1992.

65. Schultz-Ehrenburg U et al: Prospective epidemiological investigations on early and preclinical stages of varicosis. In Davy A and Stemmer R, editors: Phlebologie '89, Montrouge, France, 1989, John Libbey Eurotext.

66. Schultz-Ehrenburg U et al: New epidemiological findings with regard to initial stages of varicose veins (Bochum Study I-III). In Raymond-Martimbeau P, Prescott R, and Zummo M, editors: Phlebologie '92, Paris, 1992, John Libbey, Eurotext.

67. Fischer H: Socio-epidemiological study on distribution of venous disorders among a residential population, Int Angiol 3:89, 1984.

68. Galen: Galen on the affected parts. Translated by Rudolph E. Siegel, Basel, 1976, S. Karger.

69. Delater G and Hugel R: Apercu de pathologie veineuse le systeme veineux peripherique superficiel, Rev Gen Clin Ther 41:166, 1927.

70. Neumann HAM and van den Broek MJTB: Evaluation of O-(B-hydroxyethyl)-rutosides in chronic venous insufficiency by means of non-invasive techniques, Phlebology 5(suppl 1):13, 1990.

71. de Jongste AB et al: A double-blind trial on the short-term efficacy of HR in patients with the post-thrombotic syndrome, Phlebology 5(suppl 1):21, 1990.

72. Nocker W, Diebschlag W, and Lehmacher W: Clinical trials of the dose-related effects of O-(B hydroxyethyl)-rutosides in patients with chronic venous insufficiency, Phlebology 5(suppl 1):23, 1990.

73. Conrad P: Painful legs: the GP's dilemma, Aust Fam Physician 9:691, 1980.

74. Negus D: Calf pain in the post-thrombotic syndrome, Br Med J 2:156, 1968.

75. Cocket FB and Lea Thomas M: The iliac compression syndrome, Br J Surg 52:816, 1965.

76. Qvarfordt P, Eklof B, and Ohlin P: Intramuscular pressure in the lower extremity in deep venous thrombosis and phlegmasia cerulea dolens, Ann Surg 197:450, 1983.

77. Qvarfordt P et al: Intra-muscular pressure, blood flow and skeletal muscle metabolism in patients with venous claudication, Surgery 95:191, 1984.

78. Kistner RL: Primary venous valve incompetence of the leg, Am J Surg 140:218, 1980.

79. McPheeters HO: The value of estrogen therapy in the treatment of varicose veins complicating pregnancy, Lancet 69:2, 1949.

80. Fegan G: Varicose veins, London, 1967, William Heinemann.

81. Summer DS: Hemodynamics and pathophysiology of venous disease. In Rutherford RB, editor: Vascular surgery, Philadelphia, 1984, WB Saunders.

82. Sumner DS: Venous dynamics-varicosities, Clin Obstet Gynecol 24:743, 1981.

83. Burnand KG: Management of varicose veins of the legs, Nursing Mirror 144:45, 1977.

84. Weiss R and Weiss M: Resolution of pain associated with varicose and telangiectatic leg veins after compression sclerotherapy, J Dermatol Surg Oncol, 16:333, 1990.

85. Murray RY: A retrospective analysis of varying symptoms in patients presenting for sclerotherapy of telangiectasia, J Dermatol Surg Oncol (ABST) 1994.

86. Wilder CS: Prevalence of selected chronic circulatory conditions, Vital Health Stat 94:1, 1974.

87. Fegan WG, Lambe R, and Henry M: Steroid hormones and varicose veins, Lancet 1:1070, 1967.

88. MacCausland AM: Varicose veins in pregnancy, Ca West Med 50:258, 1939.

89. Browse NL, Burnand KG, and Thomas ML: Diseases of the veins: pathology, diagnosis, and treatment, London, 1988, Edward Arnold.

90. Gay J: On varicose disease of the lower extremities, London, 1868, J Churchill & Sons.

91. Pleuss J: Contribution a letude etiopathogenique des ulceres de jambe, Bull Soc Franc Phlebologie 4:137, 1952.

92. McEnroe CS, O'Donnell TF Jr, and Mackey WC: Correlation of clinical findings with venous hemodynamics in 386 patients with chronic venous insufficiency, Am J Surg 156:148, 1988.

93. Morano JU and Raju S: Chronic venous insufficiency: assessment with descending venography, Radiology 174:441, 1990.

94. Train JS et al: Radiological evaluation of the chronic venous stasis syndrome, JAMA 258:941, 1987.

95. Darke SG and Andress MR: The value of venography in the management of chronic venous disorders of the lower limb. In Greenhalgh RM, editor: Diagnostic techniques and assessment procedures in vascular surgery, London, 1985, Grune & Stratton.

96. Moore DJ, Himmel PD, and Sumner DS: Distribution of venous valvular incompetence in patients with postphlebotic syndrome, J Vasc Surg 3:49, 1986.

97. Mastroroberto M, Chello M, and Marchese AR: Distribution of valvular incompetence in patients with venous stasis ulceration, J Vasc Surg 14:307, 1992.

98. Hanrahan LM et al: Patterns of venous insufficiency in patients with varicose veins, Arch Surg 126:687, 1991.

99. Schanzer H and Converse Peirce E II: A rational approach to surgery of the chronic venous stasis syndrome, Ann Surg 195:25, 1982.

100. Raju S and Fredericks R: Evaluation of methods for detecting venous reflux, Arch Surg 125:1463, 1990.

101. Walsh JC et al: Femoral venous reflux is abolished by greater saphenous vein stripping, J Dermatol Surg Oncol 20:65, 1994.
102. Almgren B and Eriksson I: Valvular incompetence in superficial, deep and perforator veins of the limbs with varicose veins, Acta Chir Scand 156:69, 1990.
103. Allen EV, Barker NW, and Hines EA Jr: Peripheral vascular diseases, Philadelphia, 1946, WB Saunders.
104. Hojensgard IC and Sturup H: On the function of the venous pump and the venous return from the lower limbs, Acta Derm Venerol Stockn 29(Suppl):169, 1952.
105. Ryan TJ: Microvascular injury: vasculitis, stasis, and ischemia, London, 1976, WB Saunders.
106. Fagrell B: Vital microscopy in the pathophysiology of deep venous insufficiency. In Eklof B et al, editors: Controversies in the management of venous disorders, London, 1989, Butterworths.
107. Burnand KG et al: Pericapillary fibrin in the ulcer-bearing skin of the leg: the cause of lipodermatosclerosis and venous ulcerations, Br Med J 285:1071, 1982.
108. Fagrell B: Microcirculatory disturbances: the final cause for venous leg ulcers? Vasa 11:101, 1982.
109. Browse NL et al: The treatment of liposclerosis of the leg by fibrinolytic enhancement: a preliminary report, Br Med J 2:434, 1977.
110. Wenner A et al: Ultrastructural changes of capillaries in chronic venous insufficiency, Exp Cell Biol 48:1, 1980.
111. Hobbs JT: The post-thrombotic syndrome. In Hobbs JT, editor: The treatment of venous disorders, Philadelphia, 1977, JB Lippincott.
112. Shelley WB, Swaminathan R, and Shelley ED: Lichen aureus: a hemosiderin tattoo associated with perforator vein incompetence, J Am Acad Dermatol 11:260, 1984.
113. Gravatational eczema. In Rook A et al, editors: Textbook of dermatology, ed 4, Melbourne, 1986, Blackwell Scientific.
114. McPheeters HO and Anderson JK: Injection treatment of varicose veins and hemorrhoids, Philadelphia, 1943, FA Davis.
115. Zimmerman LM and Rattner H: Infra-red photography of subcutaneous veins, Am J Surg 27:502, 1935.
116. Droller H: Dermatologic findings in a random sample of old persons, Geriatrics 10:421, 1955.
117. Weismann K, Krakauer R, and Wanscher B: Prevalence of skin disease in old age, Acta Derm Venereol 60:352, 1980.
118. Beauregard S and Gilchrest BA: A survey of skin problems and skin care in the elderly, Arch Dermatol 123:1638, 1987.
119. Larsen WG and Maibach HI: Dermatitis and eczema. In Mosschella SL and Hurley HJ, editors: Dermatology, ed 2, Philadelphia, 1985, WB Saunders.
120. Biegeleisen HI: Varicose veins, related diseases, and sclerotherapy: a guide for practitioners, London, 1984, Eden.
121. Jeghers H and Edelstein L: Skin color in health and disease. In MacBryde CM and Blackslow RS, editors: Signs and symptoms, ed 6, Philadelphia, 1983, JB Lippincott.
122. Kulwin MH and Hines EA Jr: Blood vessels of the skin in chronic venous insufficiency: clinical pathologic studies, Arch Dermatol Syph 62:293, 1950.
123. Milian G: Les atrophies cutanees syphilitiques, Bull Soc Franc Dermatol Syph 36:865, 1929.
124. Bollinger A: Transcapillary and interstitial diffusion of Na-fluroscein in chronic venous insufficiency with white atrophy, Int J Microcirc Clin Exp 1:5, 1982.
125. Anning ST: Leg ulcers: their causes and treatment, London, 1954, J & A Churchill.
126. Wiseman R: Severall chirurgical treatises, London, 1676, Royston and Took.
127. Dale WA and Foster J: Leg ulcers: comprehensive plan of diagnosis and management, Med Sci 15:56, 1964.
128. Callam MJ et al: Chronic ulceration of the leg: extent of the problem and provision of care, Br Med J 290:1855, 1985.
129. Baker SR et al: Epidemiology of chronic venous ulcers, Br J Surg 78:864, 1991.
130. Nelzen O et al: Chronic leg ulcers: an underestimated problem in primary health care among elderly patients, J Epidemiol Community Health 45:184, 1991.
131. Haeger K, editor: Venous and lymphatic disorders of the leg, Lund, Sweden, 1966, Bokforlaget Universitet och Skola.
132. Sicard JA, Forestier J, and Gaugier L: Treatment of varicose ulcers, Proc R Soc Med 21:1837, 1929.
133. Sigg K: Varizen, ulcus cruris, und Thrombose, Berlin, 1958, Springer-Verlag.
134. Ruckley CV et al: Causes of chronic leg ulcer, Lancet 2:615, 1982.
135. Bauer G: Heparin as a therapeutic against thrombosis: results of a one-year treatment at Mariestal Hospital, Acta Chir Scand 86:217, 1942.
136. Gjores JE: Symposium on venous ulcers: opening comments, Acta Chir Scand 544(suppl):7, 1988.

137. Browse NL and Burnand KG: The postphlebetic syndrome: a new look. In Bergan JJ and Yao JST, editors: Venous problems, Chicago, 1978, Yearbook.
138. Neldner KH: The management of venous leg ulcers, Curr Concepts Skin Disorders 8:5, 1987.
139. Gooley NA and Sumner DS: Relationship of venous reflux to the site of venous valvular incompetence: implications for venous reconstructive surgery, J Vasc Surg 7:50, 1988.
140. Hanraham LM et al: Distribution of valvular incompetence in patients with venous stasis ulceration, J Vasc Surg 13:805, 1991.
141. Hoare MC et al: The role of primary varicose veins in venous ulceration, Surgery 92:450, 1982.
142. Editorial: Venous ulcers, Lancet 1:522, 1977.
143. Lawrence D, Fish PJ, and Kakkar VV: Blood-flow in incompetent perforating veins, Lancet 1:117, 1977.
144. Negus D: Prevention and treatment of venous ulceration, Ann R Coll Surg Engl 67:144, 1985.
145. Koyano K and Sakaguchi S: Ultrasonographic detection and the role of the perforating veins in primary varicose veins. In Raymond-Martimbeau P, Prescott R, and Zummo M, editors: Phlebologie '92, Paris, 1992, John Libbey Eurotext.
146. Darke SG and Penfold C: Venous ulceration and saphenous ligation, Eur J Vasc Surg 6:4, 1992.
147. Burnand K et al: Relationship between postphlebitic changes in the deep veins and results of surgical treatment of venous ulcers, Lancet 1:936, 1976.
148. Lofgren EP: Leg ulcers: symptoms of an underlying disorder, Postgrad Med 76:51, 1984.
149. Lippman HI: Subcutaneous ossification in chronic venous insufficiency, presentation of 23 cases: preliminary report, Angiology 8:378, 1957.
150. Ward WH: Leg ulcers, Australas J Dermatol 5:145, 1960.
151. Lippman HI and Goldin RR: Subcutaneous ossification of the legs in chronic venous insufficiency, Radiology 74:279, 1960.
152. Michael: Uber der primaren Krebs der Extremitaten, Tübingen, Germany, 1890, Inaug Diss.
153. Balestrino E et al: Malignant degeneration of chronic venous ulcer (Marjolin's ulcer), Min Chir 38:211, 1983.
154. Phillips TJ, Salman SM, and Rogers GS: Nonhealing leg ulcers: a manifestation of basal cell carcinoma, J Am Acad Dermatol 25:47, 1991.
155. Kaufmann R, Klein CE, and Sterry W: Neoplastic diseases associated with leg ulcers. In Raymond-Martimbeau P, Prescott R, and Zummo M, editors: Phlebologie '92, Paris, 1992, John Libbey Eurotext.
156. Igarzabal C and Feisilberg D: Secondary malignant degeneration of chronic leg ulcers. In Raymond-Martimbeau P, Prescott R, and Zummo M, editors: Phlebologie '92, Paris, 1992, John Libbey Eurotext.
157. Harris B, Eaglstein WH, and Falanga V: Basal cell carcinoma arising in venous ulcers and mimicking granulation tissue, J Dermatol Surg Oncol 19:150, 1993.
158. Kofler H et al: Hemangiosarcoma in chronic leg ulcer, Arch Dermatol 124:1080, 1988.
159. Hassan SA, Cheatle TR, and Fox JA: Marjolin's ulcer: a report of three cases and review of the literature, Phlebology 8:34, 1993.
160. Tenopyr J and Silverman T: The relation of chronic varicose ulcer to epithelioma, Ann Surg 95:754, 1932.
161. Knox LC: Epithelioma and the chronic varicose ulcer, JAMA 85:1046, 1925.
162. Pannell TC and Hightower F: Malignant changes in post-phlebitic ulcers, S Med J 58:779, 1965.
163. Grusser M: Cancer of leg, Arch f Klin f Klin Chir 127:529, 1923; abstr JAMA 81:2156, 1923.
164. Neumann Z, Ben-Hur N, and Shulman J: Trauma and skin cancer: implantation of epidermal elements and possible causes, Plast Reconstr Surg 32:649, 1963.
165. Bostwick J, Prendergast WJ, and Vasconez LO: Marjolin's ulcer: an immunologically privileged tumour, Plast Reconstr Surg 57:66, 1975.
166. Tretbar LI: Bleeding from varicose veins, treatment with injection sclerotherapy. In Davy A and Stemmer R, editors: Phlebologie '89, Montrouge, France, 1989, John Libbey Eurotext.
167. Evans GA et al: Spontaneous fatal hemorrhage caused by varicose veins, Lancet 2:1359, 1973.
168. Harman RRM: Haemorrhage from varicose veins, Lancet 1:363, 1974.
169. Du Toit DF, Knott-Craig C, and Laker L: Bleeding from varicose veins—still potentially fatal, S Afr Med J 67:303, 1985.
170. Teitelbaum GP and Davis PS: Spontaneous rupture of a lower extremity varix: case report, Cardiovasc Intervent Radiol 12:101, 1989.
171. Husni EA and Williams WA: Superficial thrombophlebitis of the lower limbs, Surgery 91:70, 1982.
172. Prountjos P et al: Superficial venous thrombosis of the lower extremities co-existing with deep venous thrombosis, Int Angiol 10:63, 1991.
173. Jorgensen JO et al: The incidence of deep venous thrombosis in patients with superficial thrombophlebitis of the lower limbs, J Vasc Surg 18:70, 1993.

174. Zollinger RW, Williams RD, and Briggs DO: Problems in the diagnosis and treatment of thrombophlebitis, Arch Surg 85:18, 1962.

175. Raso AM et al: Studio su 357 casi di flebite degli arti inferiori su due campioni interregionali, Minerva Chir 34:553, 1979.

176. Totten HP: Superficial thrombophlebitis: observations on diagnosis and treatment, Geriatrics 22:151, 1967.

177. Edwards EA: Thrombophlebitis of varicose veins, Gynecol Obstet 60:236, 1938.

178. Gjores JE: Surgical therapy of ascending thrombophlebitis in the saphenous system, Angiology 13:241, 1962.

179. Husni EA, Pena LI, and Lenhert AE: Thrombophlebitis in pregnancy, Am J Obstet Gynecol 97:901, 1967.

180. Osius EA: Discussion of Hermann's paper, AMA Arch Surg 64:685, 1952.

181. Bergqvist D and Jaroszewski H: Deep vein thrombosis in patients with superficial thrombophlebitis of the leg, Br Med J 292:658, 1986.

182. Galloway JMD, Karmody AM, and Mavor GE: Thrombophlebitis of the long saphenous vein complicated by pulmonary embolism, Br J Surg 56:360, 1969.

183. Guilmot J-L, Wolman F, and Lasfargues G: Thromboses veineuses superficielles, Rev Prat 38:2062, 1988.

184. Plate G et al: Deep venous thrombosis, pulmonary embolism and acute surgery in thrombophlebitis of the long saphenous vein, Acta Chir Scand 151:241, 1985.

185. Skillman JJ et al: Simultaneous occurrence of superficial and deep thrombophlebitis in the lower extremity, J Vasc Surg 11:818, 1990.

186. Zollinger RW: Superficial thrombophlebitis, Surg Gynecol Obstet 124:1077, 1967.

187. Hafner CD et al: A method of managing superficial thrombophlebitis, Surgery 55:201, 1964.

188. Bergan J: Personal communication, 1989.

189. Lofgren EP and Lofgren KA: The surgical treatment of superficial thrombophlebitis, Surgery 90:49, 1981.

190. Widmer LK et al: Venen, Arterien-Krankheiten, koronare Herzkrankheit bei Beruistatigen, Bern Stuttgart, Wien, 1981, Hans Huber.

191. Stead RB: The hypercoagulable state. In Goldhaber SZ, editor: Pulmonary embolism and deep venous thrombosis, Philadelphia, 1985, WB Saunders.

192. Siegel B, Ipsen J, and Felix WR: Epidemiology of lower extremity deep venous thrombosis in surgical patients, Ann Surg 179:278, 1974.

193. Hume M, Sevitt S, and Thomas DP: Venous thrombosis and pulmonary embolism, Cambridge, Mass, 1970, Harvard University.

194. Bick RL: Disseminated intravascular coagulation. In Bick RL, editor: Disseminated intravascular coagulation and related syndromes, Boca Raton, Fl, 1983, CRC.

195. Falanga V, Bontempo FA, and Eaglstein WH: Protein C and protein S plasma levels in patients with lipodermatosclerosis and venous ulceration, Arch Dermatol 126:1195, 1990.

196. Samlaska CP: Protein C and protein S plasma levels in patients with lipodermatosclerosis and venous ulceration, Arch Dermatol 127:908, 1991.

197. Samlaska CP and James WD: Superficial thrombophlebitis I. Primary hypercoagulable states, J Am Acad Dermatol 22:975, 1990.

198. Samlaska CP and James WD: Superficial thrombophlebitis II. Secondary hypercoagulable states, J Am Acad Dermatol 23:1, 1990.

199. Barrow DW: The clinical management of varicose veins, ed 2, New York, 1957, Paul H. Hoeber.

200. Foote RR: Varicose veins, St Louis, 1949, CV Mosby.

201. Clayton JK, Anderson JA, and McNicol GP: Preoperative prediction of post-operative deep vein thrombosis, Br Med J 2:910, 1976.

202. Lowe GD et al: Prediction and selective prophylaxis of venous thrombosis in elective gastrointestinal surgery, Lancet 1:409, 1982.

203. Rakoczi I et al: Prediction of post-operative leg-vein thrombosis in gynecological patients, Lancet 1:509, 1978.

204. Matyas M: The clinical management of varicose veins, ed 2, New York, 1957, Paul H Hoeber.

205. Kakkar VV et al: Deep vein thrombosis of the leg. Is there a "high risk" group? Am J Surg 120:527, 1970.

206. Heyerdale WW and Stalker LK: The management of varicose veins of the lower extremities, Ann Surg 114:1042, 1941.

207. Widmer LK: Peripheral venous disorders: prevalence and socio-medical importance observations in 4529 apparently healthy persons. Basle Study III, Bern, Switzerland, 1978, Hans Huber.

208. Duffy DM: Small vessel sclerotherapy: an overview. In Callen et al, editors: Advances in dermatology, vol 3, Chicago, 1988, Year Book.

3 Pathophysiology of Varicose Veins

There are essentially three components of the venous system of the leg that act in concert: deep veins, superficial veins, and perforating/communicating veins. Dysfunction in any of these three systems results in dysfunction of the other two. When the superficial veins are placed under high pressure, they dilate and elongate to accommodate the increased blood volume. The tortuous appearance thus produced is termed *varicose*, derived from the Greek term for "grape-like." This term applies to both the large protruding veins within the superficial subcutaneous fascia and the smaller venectasia "spider veins" that occur just beneath the epidermis.

The World Health Organization[1] defines varicose veins as "Saccular dilatation of the veins which are often tortuous." Further, this definition specifically excludes any tortuous veins associated with previous thrombophlebitis or an arteriovenous fistula or with venectasia.

HISTOCHEMICAL PHYSIOLOGY OF VARICOSE VEINS

Varicose veins differ from nonvaricose veins in physiologic function. This may occur in one or all of the histologic layers. Endothelial damage has been noted to occur in parts of a varicose vein.[2] This has been noted both ultrastructurally and physiologically by a reduction in endothelial-mediated enhancement of norepinephrine-induced vasoconstriction (Fig. 3-1).[3,4]

The muscular layer has been found in most investigations to be altered. Varicose veins have been noted to have a considerable degree of smooth muscle hypertrophy and a 15% increase in muscle content compared with normal veins.[5] This is thought to be a secondary response to venous hypertension. Other investigators have found that smooth muscle cells are capable of phagocytosis and decomposition of collagen fibers.[6] Thus these cells may be part of the cellular basis for collagen breakdown. However, other investigators note a decrease in lactate dehydrogenase (LDH) and creatine kinase (CK) activity in varicose versus normal veins and postulate that varicose vein weakness is due to a thinning or damaged muscular layer.[7] This has been confirmed in a study of aging canine and human veins where a decrease in sympathetic innervation has been correlated to muscular layer thinning.[8] In addition, the protein content of varicose veins (which is predominantly smooth muscle) is reduced.[4] However, one research group has found no significant difference in the quantity of smooth muscle between normal and varicose veins.[9]

The adventitial layer has also been noted to be altered in varicose veins. Some investigators have found that varicose veins have an extremely dense and compact fibrosis between the intima and adventitia, with a diminished and atrophied elastic network and a disorganized muscular layer (Fig. 3-2).[10-12,13] Thickening and fibrillation of individual collagen fibers has also been noted.[2,11,14,15] This translates to a reduced compliance that may lead to poor coaptation of venous valves and increased varicose vein wall stiffness. An in vivo measurement of venous elasticity in patients with normal, "high-risk," and varicose veins confirmed both a reduced elasticity in varicose veins as well as in high-risk veins.[16] In this

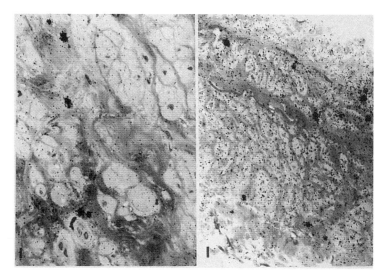

Fig. 3-1 Light microscope autoradiographies of human saphenous vein strips incubated with ^{3}H-nor-adrenaline. In the control vein *(right)*, clusters of silver grains indicative of adrenergic varicosities are seen throughout the media. Smooth muscle cells exhibit a high density of silver grains. In the varicose vein *(left)*, nerve varicosities are less abundant, and smooth muscle cells are larger and have a much lower density of silver grains. Collagen is more abundant. Bars = 10 μm. (Reproduced with permission from Azevedo I, Albino Teixeira A, and Osswald W: Changes induced by ageing and denervation in the canine saphenous vein: a comparison with the human varicose vein. In Vanhoutte PM, editor: Return circulation and norepinephrine: an update, Paris, 1991, John Libbey Eurotext.)

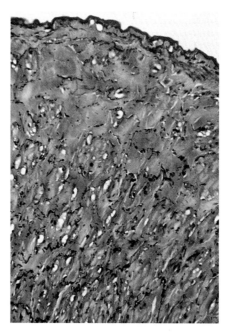

Fig. 3-2 Cross section of a tributary to the GSV in a 46-year-old man, stained with Verhoeff-van Gieson (×150). Note extensive fragmentation of elastin fibers interspersed between irregularly oriented muscle bundles with marked hypertrophy of collagen fibers. Elastic fibers stain *black;* collagen, *red;* muscle, *brown-yellow.*

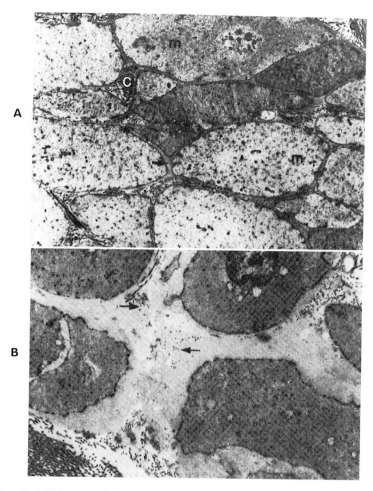

Fig. 3-3 **A,** Middle muscle layer of a saphenous vein of a young subject. Smooth muscle cells, *(m)*; narrow perimyocytic spaces containing collagen fibers, *(c)*. The basilar membrane of smooth muscle is clearly visible, *(arrow)*, (Uranyl acetate–lead citrate; ×4000.) **B,** Muscle fibers in an aged subject showing the wide separation of dystrophic muscle cells. A few collagen fibers are visible, *(arrows)*. (Uranyl acetate–lead citrate; ×5000.) (From Bouissou H et al: Phlebologie 3[suppl 1]:1, 1988.)

study, individuals with "high-risk" veins were defined as having a family history of varicose veins, standing occupations, symptoms of venous disease, and Doppler ultrasound reflux.

The loss of tonicity of varicose veins is primarily the result of the loss of coordinated communication between vein wall smooth muscle cells as previously described. Electron microscopic studies of nonvaricose veins demonstrate the close approximation of smooth muscle cells. When veins become varicose, smooth muscle cells become vacuolated and are separated by collagen.[10,11] With increasing varicose changes, intercellular collagen deposition accumulates and separates the smooth muscle cells, which then atrophy (Fig. 3-3). It is suggested that the resulting separation of smooth muscle cell hemidesmosomes results in inefficient smooth muscle contraction and increased venous distensibility.[9,11,17] However, at least some varicose veins are capable of constricting in response to an infusion of dihydroergotamine. This venoconstriction is even more pronounced than that which occurs in normal veins.[18] The reason for this paradoxical effect is unknown. Therefore, the varicose vein appears to be a dysplastic vein characterized by malformations. Whether this is the result of continual high venous pressure or whether it is the primary etiologic event in the development of valvular incompetence is unknown.

Although collagen accumulation is thought to separate smooth muscle cells within the varicose vein wall, the collagen content of varicose veins is less than that in normal tissues.[5,19] The bulk of the varicose vein wall is made up of mucopolysaccharides and other ground substances. Varicose veins contain 67% more hexosamine (which comprises about 0.3% of normal vein dry material) as compared with normal veins.

Dysplasticity of the varicose vein wall may explain why varicose veins have an even greater susceptibility to pressure-induced distention than nonvaricose veins. This anatomico-pathophysiologic correlation has been demonstrated by pharmacologic studies that show reduced maximal contraction of varicose veins as compared with control veins.[2,17] They have also been investigated with in vitro techniques measuring distensibility as a function of infused volumes of saline.[20] However, some investigations have failed to disclose a significant difference in the degree of intimal fibrosis between varicose and nonvaricose veins.[21] Therefore, fibrosis of the vein wall alone is not totally responsible for the development of varicose veins.

Finally, a decrease in tocopherol concentration has been noted in varicose veins.[22] There also appears to be a significant correlation between the inhibition of vessel wall tissues on lipoperoxidation and their tocopherol concentration, independent of serum concentrations. This may be the result of the protective effect of blocking peroxidation of membrane-associated fatty acids by tocopherol and other antioxidants to prevent vein wall damage.[23] It is clear that the dysplasticity of varicose veins correlates with the changes in their pharmacodynamics and histochemistry. Varicose veins have a demonstrated loss of contractility.[24]

Varicose veins are often complicated by local inflammation and thrombosis. This may be due to venous hypertension or to an inherent histochemical abnormality in the varicose vein/endothelial wall. The formation of arachidonic acid-derived prostanoids was investigated in segments of varicose and nonvaricose veins. Venous production of prostacyclin was decreased with an increase in thromboxane A_2 and prostaglandin E_2 in the varicose vein segments regardless of whether it was macroscopically affected.[25] It is unknown whether this change in the cyclooxygenase pathway in the varicose vein wall is the cause or effect of its dysplasticity. In addition, histochemical examination discloses a marked increase in the activity of lysosomal enzymes,[26] acid phosphatase, β-glucuronidase, and anaerobic isoenzymes (lactodehydrogenase) in primary varicose veins.[27-29] These enzyme patterns suggest a decline in energy metabolism and an increase in cellular damage in the varicose veins. It has also been found that varicose veins accumulate and metabolize norepinephrine less efficiently than normal veins.[30] Therefore, both anatomic and biochemical abnormalities in the varicose vein wall contribute to its increased distensibility.

PATHOPHYSIOLOGY

Approximately 75% of the body's total blood volume is contained within the peripheral venous system.[31] The quantity of blood within the legs is a function of body position. When erect, 300 to 800 ml of extracellular and vascular fluids (the quantity varies according to the experimental method and the size of the subject measured) collect in the legs.[32-34] This includes a 15% increase of blood volume.[32] Thus the venous system, especially in the legs, is an important component of the cardiovascular system's circulatory reservoir. However, the arterial system plays an equally important role in cardiovascular adaptation to postural changes by virtue of changes in arterial resistance. In fact, studies have demonstrated that reflex changes in venous tone are not essential for this fluid shift.[35]

Venous blood pressure is determined by several factors. Among these are pressure generated by the heart, the energy lost in the peripheral resistance of arterioles, hydrostatic gravitational forces, blood volume, anatomic composition of the venous wall, efficiency of one-way valves, vein wall distensibility (determined by hormonal, systemic alcohol, and other factors), and the contraction of venous smooth muscle as influenced by ambient temperature and sympathetic and parasympathetic nerve tone (Fig. 3-4).

Although arterial pressure comprises one factor in the development of venous pressure, arterial hypertension has been noted to be associated with the development of varicose veins in some epidemiologic studies[36] but not others.[37] Curiously, atherosclerotic disease has been linked epidemiologically to varicose veins.[38,39] It is postulated that this coincidence is probably related to an atherogenic risk profile, owing primarily to coexistent inactivity, obesity, and hypertension.[39] At rest, in the erect position, pressure in the saphenous vein is determined primarily by the height of the column of blood from the right atrium to the site of measurement (90 to 120 mm Hg at the ankle) (Fig. 3-5).[40,41] Contraction of calf muscles generates pressures between 200 and 300 mm Hg.[42-44]

Pressure generated deep to the fascia, outside of muscles, is between 100 and 150 mm Hg.[44,45] However, with muscular activity, pressure in the normal saphenous vein at the level of the malleoli falls 45 to 68 mm Hg below the resting level.[46] It is reduced from 80 to 40 mm Hg in the posterior tibial vein.[47] Because of the one-way valves, blood flow is directed from the superficial venous system to the deep venous system via perforating vessels. This has been visually demonstrated by serial phlebography of the normal lower leg (see Fig. 1-6).[48] The venous blood then flows toward the heart.

The venous pump in the foot is an important portion of the muscle pump of the lower leg. Weight bearing is usually necessary to propel blood up the leg. Bidirectional ultrasound velocity detector tracings of venous blood flow through the popliteal vein have demonstrated the importance of dorsiflexion of the foot when there is no weight bearing.[49] Therefore, full flexion of the foot is important after sclerotherapy to maximize the efficacy of the lower extremity muscle pump.

THEORETICAL CAUSES OF VARICOSE VEINS

Heredity	Primary valvular incompetence
Race	Decreased number
Gender	Aging
Posture	Incompetent perforating veins
Weight	Arteriovenous communication
Height	Vein wall weakness
Occupation	Secondary valvular incompetence
Hormones	Phlebitis
Estrogen	Deep vein thrombosis
Progesterone	
Pregnancy	

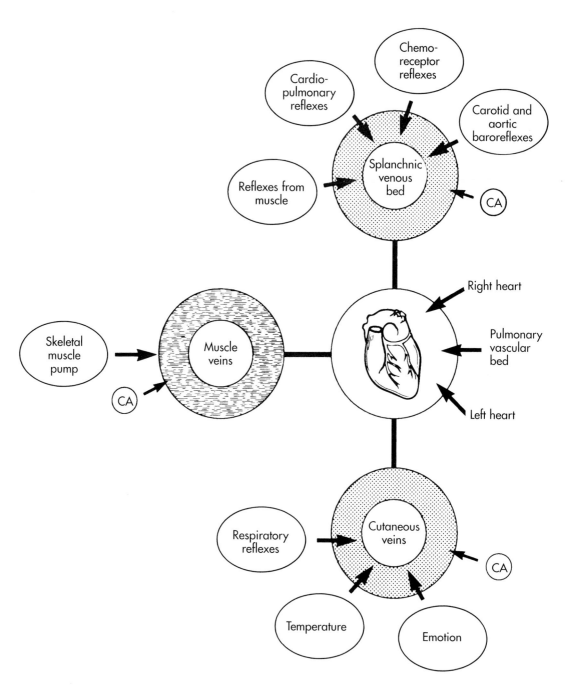

Fig. 3-4 Multiple environmental and internal factors act on the venous system to influence its dilation and constriction. (*CA* = catecholamines.)

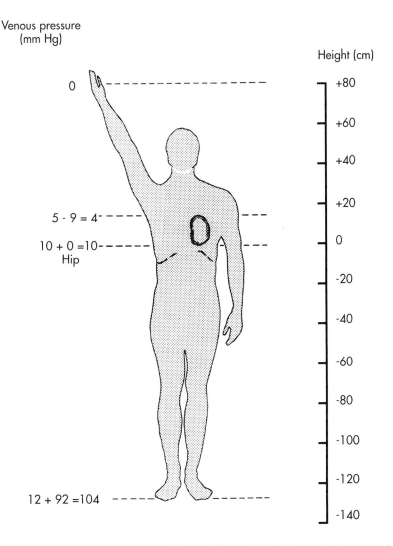

Fig. 3-5 Venous pressure is that exerted by a collum of blood from the heart to the location of measurement.

Respiration produces alterations in intraabdominal venous pressure. This "abdominal venous pump" contributes to the flow of blood even when an individual is erect.[34,50] Inspiration produces a rise in venous pressure in the external iliac vein, common iliac vein, and inferior vena cava when measured in both the horizontal and erect positions, 6.3 mm Hg and 8.7 mm Hg respectively.[50]

In the supine position, blood flows evenly along all superficial and deep vessels toward the heart. It is propelled by the relatively small vis-à-tergo (force from behind) from the capillaries[47] and the respiration-induced aspiration of blood into the abdominal and thoracic veins. In contrast to deep veins, superficial veins have smooth muscle in their walls. This allows contraction of these vessels in response to cold and to drugs such as dihydroergotamine[51,52] and allows dilation in response to topical and systemic alcohol, estrogen, and light physical trauma.[47] As previously described, part of the pathophysiology of varicose veins may be a diminished response of such smooth muscle contraction.

Regardless of its etiology, chronic venous hypertension in the lower extremities causes an increase in venous diameter. This may lead to valvular insufficiency, which usually causes a reversal of blood flow from the deep veins into the superficial veins through incompetent perforating veins. This "private circulation" may account for as much as 20% to 25% of the total femoral flow to be involved in a circular retrograde flow (Fig. 3-6).[53,54]

Direction of venous flow in varicose veins has been examined by McPheeters and Rice[55] using fluoroscopy. Reversal of flow caused by incompetent perforator valves is beneficial during sclerotherapy. When a superficial varicosity is injected, its venous flow is forced distally to the smaller branching veins, where it is arrested (see Chapter 8).[55] Thromboembolic disease is thereby prevented.

Superficial veins respond to increased pressure by dilating. Valvular incompetence occurs and varicosities appear.[56] Additionally, in muscular contraction, high compartmental pressure that normally occurs within the calf muscle pump is transmitted directly to the superficial veins and subcutaneous tissues drained by perforating veins.[57,58] When this occurs, venous pressure in the cuticular venules may reach 100 mm Hg in the erect position.[47] This causes venular dilation over a broad area and may cause capillary dilation, increased permeability,[59-62] and a subsequent increase in the subcutaneous capillary bed through angiogenesis.[60,63] This is expressed clinically as telangiectasia (venous blemishes). Histologically, cutaneous and subcutaneous hemosiderin deposition may also occur. This, in time, results in cutaneous pigmentation (see Chapter 2). However, some patients with chronic venous insufficiency are able to increase their venous blood flow through exercise.[64] It is postulated that various factors (such as sympathetic tone, temperature, tissue metabolites) compensate venous hypertension to normalize cuticular blood flow. This finding demonstrates the complexity of the superficial venous system.

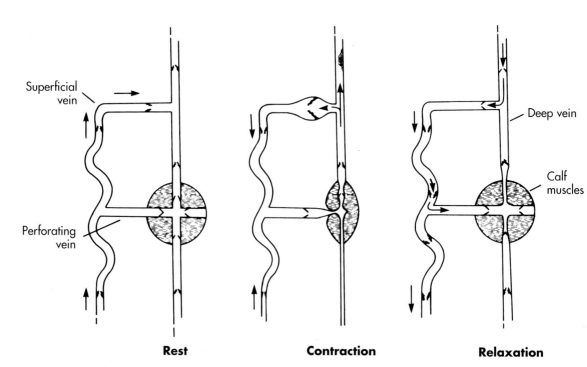

Fig. 3-6 Private circulation of blood flow in primary varicose veins demonstrating a retrograde circuitous blood flow with muscle contraction and relaxation.

A special situation develops in the area of the medial malleolus. In this area perforating veins are not surrounded by deep or superficial fascia. Therefore, any increase in deep venous pressure is transmitted directly through perforating veins to superficial connecting veins. This causes high cutaneous venous pressures and a transudation of extracellular fluid. This, in turn, leads to perivascular fibrin deposition, which may play a role in decreased oxygenation of cutaneous and supporting tissues, and this contributes to cutaneous ulceration (see Chapter 2).[60,65,66]

The effect of temperature variations on the venous system is well studied.[67,68] The cutaneous vasculature is intimately involved in thermoregulation. An increase in body core temperature results in cutaneous vasodilation. This does not occur as a result of relaxation of venous smooth muscle, but because of the reduction in the vasoconstrictor impulses to the vein wall. Such vasodilation also occurs in varicose veins. Recently strain gauge venous occlusion plethysmography has shown an increase in venous distensibility associated with temperature elevation.[69] Similarly, alcohol ingestion may influence the development of varicose veins. Alcohol intake, like increased environmental temperature, causes cutaneous vasodilation. In an examination of 136 men with primary varicose veins greater than 4 mm in diameter, it was found that a significantly increased incidence of varicose veins occurred among men who consumed 4 oz of alcohol a day.[70] Unfortunately, further experimental evaluations of this association have not been performed.

In summary, pathologic development of varicose veins can be divided into four broad categories. These may overlap. Increased deep venous pressure, primary valvular incompetence, secondary valvular incompetence, and hereditary factors such as vein wall weakness all coexist and are influenced by temperature, alcohol, and hormonal and other vasodilatory stimuli (see box, below).

PATHOPHYSIOLOGY OF VARICOSE VEINS

- Increased Deep Venous Pressure

  PROXIMAL
  Pelvic obstruction (indirect)
  Intraabdominal pressure secondary to Valsalva, leg crossing, constrictive clothing, squatting, obesity
  Saphenofemoral incompetence
  Venous obstruction

  DISTAL
  Perforator valvular incompetence
  Venous obstruction

- Arteriovenous Anastomoses
- Primary Valvular Incompetence
  Venous obstruction (thrombosis)
  Destruction of venous valves (thrombophlebitis)
  Congenital absence of venous valves
  Decreased number of venous valves
  Vein wall weakness
- Secondary Valvular Incompetence
  Deep venous obstruction
  Increased venous distensibility
  Hormonally induced through pregnancy, systemic estrogens, and progesterones (concentration and ratio-dependent)

Increased Deep Venous Pressure

An increase in the deep venous pressure may be of proximal or distal origin. Proximal causes include pelvic obstruction (resulting in indirect venous obstruction); increased intraabdominal pressure caused by straining during defecation or micturition, wearing constrictive clothing, sitting in chairs, obesity, and running; saphenofemoral incompetence; and intraluminal venous obstruction. Distal causes include perforating vein valvular incompetence, arteriovenous anastomoses, and intraluminal venous obstruction.

Proximal

Pelvic obstruction. Pelvic obstruction is an uncommon cause of varicose veins. Iliac vein compression syndrome is the phenomenon of compression of the right iliac vein by the right iliac artery overlying the fifth lumbar vertebra. This usually occurs in women, in whom it may be a cause of vulvar varicosities, but it has also been noted in men (see Chapter 5). Extravascular abdominal tumors, such as ovarian and uterine carcinoma or teratoma, may be causes of obstruction. More commonly, however, it is relative pelvic obstruction that provides a mechanism for impedance of return blood flow. Relative obstruction may occur in the third trimester of pregnancy, particularly during recumbency when the gravid uterus compresses the inferior vena cava against the lumbar spine and/or psoas muscles. Phlebographic studies have shown complete obstruction of the inferior vena cava at the confluence of the iliac veins in third-trimester pregnancies.[71] Partial obstruction has been shown in earlier months of pregnancy. Some degree of compression is evident using phlebography, even in the left lateral decubitus position.

Increased intraabdominal pressure. One popular hypothesis for the development of varicose veins is Western dietary and defecation habits that cause an increase in intraabdominal pressure. A distended cecum or sigmoid colon, the result of constipation, may drag on the iliac veins and obstruct venous return from the legs.[72] Population studies have demonstrated that a high-fiber diet is evacuated within an average of 35 hours.[73] In contrast, a low-fiber diet has an average transit time of 77 hours. An intermediate diet has a stool transit time of 47 hours.

It is possible that the small increase in abdominal intravenous pressure caused by less than optimal bowel habits, when transmitted intravenously distally, gradually breaks down venous valves of leg veins.[74,75] Evidence in support of this hypothesis is seen in populations of people who eat unprocessed high-fiber food. These persons are free of constipation and varicose veins.[76,77] However, if this population's diet is changed to low fiber, the incidence of varicose veins increases.[72,78-81] When a diet that is intermediate between Western low-fiber and high-fiber diets is consumed, the prevalence of varicose veins is also found to be in an intermediate range.[82]

Defecatory straining induced by Western-style toilet seats has also been cited as a cause of varicose veins, in contrast to the African custom of squatting during defecation.[79] However, venous pressures of subjects measured in both the sitting and squatting positions during defecation have not shown a significant difference.[83] Venous flow has not been accurately examined in constipated and nonconstipated populations.

Finally, there are other dietary factors besides fiber content that may explain the differences in prevalence of varicose veins. An increased incidence of varicose veins is found in populations of people who consume diets high in long-chain fatty acids, as opposed to diets high in short-chain fatty acids.[84] Long-chain fatty acids have been shown in experimental systems to enhance blood coagulation and stimulate the development of blood clots.[85-87] Clot lysis times were lower in the population group that consumed long-chain fatty acids.[84] Accordingly, the *type* of dietary fatty acids consumed also may predispose one to the development of varicose veins. In addition, the Western diet has been found to be relatively deficient in vitamin E.[88] It is hypothesized that the slight vitamin E deficiency, when aggravated by pregnancy, may predispose the vein wall to coagulation and fibrinolysis, thus causing the veins to become more sensitive to venous stasis and venous hypertension. Therefore, although it would seem prudent to recommend a high-fiber diet for several medical reasons, it remains an unproven treatment for the prevention of varicose veins.

An association between prostatic hypertrophy, inguinal hernia, and varicose veins also may be caused by straining at micturition with a resultant increase in intraabdominal pressure.[89]

Another mechanism for increasing distal venous pressure by proximal obstruction is the practice of wearing girdles or tight-fitting clothing. A statistically significant excess of varicose veins is noted in women who wear corsets compared with women who wear less constrictive garments.[90] This finding was not confirmed by a subsequent study.[91] A similar increased incidence was noted in women who stand at work compared with those whose jobs entail more walking and sitting.[37,40,90-95] However, this has not been confirmed universally.[96,97]

Leg crossing and sitting on chairs are two other potential mechanisms for producing a relative impedance in venous return. Habitual leg crossing is commonly thought to result in extravenous compression, but this has never been scientifically verified. A decreased incidence of varicose veins has been noted in population groups that do not sit in chairs.[98,99] It is thought that sitting may produce some compression on the posterior thigh that produces a relative impedance to blood flow. Wright and Osborn[100] have shown that the linear velocity of venous flow in the lower limbs in the recumbent position is reduced by half in the standing position and by two thirds when sitting. Alexander[99] found that the circumferential stress on the saphenous vein at the ankle was 2.54 times greater with chair sitting than with ground sitting. This may explain the increased incidence of varicose veins in men versus women in population groups where only men sit on chairs and women sit on the floor. In this population study,[98] varicose veins were present in 5.1% of men and only 0.1% of women. Finally, the practical implications regarding chair sitting concerns those who travel for long periods in airplanes. Pulmonary thromboembolism has occurred in many people after prolonged air travel and has been termed *economy class syndrome*.[101] Although preexisting venous disease, dehydration, and immobility are all contributing factors, chair sitting adds another insult to the venous system.

Most,[*] but not all,[91,104,105] studies have found that obesity is associated with the development of varicose veins. Careful examination of some of these epidemiologic studies shows that when the patient's age is correlated with obesity, the statistical significance is eliminated.[105] Obesity was especially correlated with the development of varicose veins in women when the varicosities occurred in unison with cutaneous changes indicative of venous stasis (see Chapter 2).[107,108]

Running has been demonstrated to raise the intraabdominal pressure by 22 mm Hg.[109] This increase in abdominal pressure occurs because of a reflex tightening of abdominal muscles during running, which prevents the pelvis from tipping forward during thigh flexion induced by contraction of the iliopsoas muscle group.[110] Therefore, during strenuous leg exercise, elevated abdominal pressures

---

*See references 36-38,94,95,102-104.

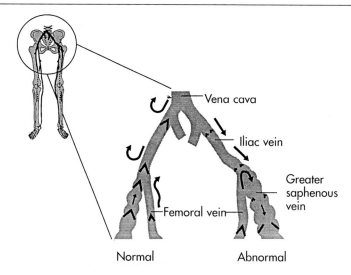

Fig. 3-7   Reflux of blood from the iliac vein into the greater saphenous vein occurs when the valves in the iliac vein and/or at the saphenofemoral junction are incompetent. With normal valvular function, blood flow from a Valsalva maneuver is prevented from going into the femoral and greater saphenous veins. (Reproduced with permission from Goldman MP: 7-31 varicose and telangiectatic leg veins. In Demis DJ, editor: Clinical dermatology, ed 19, Philadelphia, 1992, JB Lippincott.)

may impede venous return. By way of comparison, a Valsalva maneuver was shown to elevate the intraabdominal pressure by 50 mm Hg or more.[109] Strenuous exercise, particularly long-distance running, is often associated with prolonged increases in limb blood flow, which could theoretically overload the venous system and lead to progressive dilation.[56] Usually, dilated veins that occur in this situation are normal and do not require treatment.

Finally, it is commonly noted that occupations that require standing for prolonged periods have an increased incidence of varicose veins.[111] This may be exacerbated by tall height, although this factor has not been supported by other studies.[106]

Saphenofemoral incompetence. Saphenofemoral impedance rarely occurs because of anatomic abnormalities in the saphenofemoral triangle. When it does, pelvic tributary veins or accessory saphenous veins may converge in such a manner that flow to the femoral vein is impeded.[112] Likewise, iliac venous incompetence caused by congenital absence of or acquired damage to venous valves via thrombosis may cause distal venous hypertension.

Distal

Valvular incompetence. Unlike the foregoing, incompetence of the saphenofemoral junction clearly produces distal retrograde flow into the GSV and thus produces distal venous hypertension (Fig. 3-7). The GSV then dilates, producing further distal valvular incompetence sequentially. Retrograde flow thus produced is channeled via the perforator veins back into the deep venous system. This produces a private circuit of blood flow from the femoral vein to the saphenous vein and back to the femoral vein via perforating veins (see Fig. 3-5).[53] It has been estimated that the total volume of flow in this circuitous route may be 20% to 25% of the total limb blood flow during exercise.[54] This paradoxical circulation can be maintained for a long time, but eventually the quantity of blood channeled by the perforator veins increases. As this happens, there is hypertrophy and dilation of the veins, producing valvular incompetence and localized varicose veins.

In addition to increasing superficial venous volume through perforator incompetence, retrograde flow produces an increase in acidity and potassium concentration with a decrease in venous oxygen concentration. These three factors promote vasodilatation to exacerbate venous stasis.[113]

Perforator incompetence in the lower part of the leg may occur from localized thrombosis in the vein following trauma. It is believed that localized thrombosis usually is masked by the local tissue injury. The valve cusps become involved by the thrombus and, after recanalization, remain functionless.[114] Dodd and Cockett[47] found on examination of 54 legs with perforator incompetence that the lower leg incompetent perforators were in communication with the soleal plexus of veins and, as such, were the channels most likely to be damaged as a result of thrombotic episodes in this region. In support of this concept, Fegan,[115] Hobbs,[116] Lofgren,[117] and Beninson and Livingood[118] all have pointed out that the treatment of varicosities may have no effect on superficial venous pressure. These investigators hold that treatment of perforating veins draining the ankle and lower calf area is important.[57,90,116,119-121] The vessels may be either surgically ligated[57,119-121] or sclerosed (see Chapter 9).[116] Only then will retrograde flow under high pressure via the calf muscle pump be diverted upstream away from the skin. When this is done, a lowering of cuticular venous pressure and a decrease in dermal capillary pressure is accomplished. The excess transudation of fluid-producing edema and the associated decrease in tissue oxygenation and nutrition is halted. Quill and Fegan[122] have clearly demonstrated the narrowing of the proximal LSV after obliteration of incompetent distal perforating veins in 9 of 11 cases. This suggests that dilation and incompetence of the saphenous vein may be caused by distal reflux, as well as primary or irreversible abnormalities of the proximal venous wall. The finding has been confirmed through duplex examination of patients presenting for cosmetic veins or with primary varicose veins. In a study of 500 lower limbs in "cosmetic" patients, incompetence from below the knee extending upward was found in 63.3%. However, only 9% were found to have perforator incompetence.[123] An additional study of 167 consecutive patients with primary varicose veins demonstrated 31% with incompetence of the GSV without evidence for saphenofemoral junction incompetence, and 24% of limbs with incompetence of the LSV without incompetence of the saphenopopliteal junction.[124] Thus, perforator incompetence, although important as an etiologic factor, is not solely responsible for varicose vein development in all patients.

Direct ambulatory venous pressure measurements and duplex examination both have shown bidirectional flow through perforator veins. Exercise has been found to result in inward flow from the dilated superficial system and perforating veins into deep veins.[125] The perforator vein here functions as a drainage pipe to limit cuticular venous hypertension. Compression distal to perforator veins in patients with venous disease demonstrated inward flow in 55 of 56 perforator veins examined with duplex scanning.[126] Thus, venous hypertension is related to both perforator incompetence and to valvular dysfunction.

Venous obstruction. Venous obstruction may occur proximally or distally to varicose veins. An obstruction is produced typically by thrombus that may extend proximally and distally from its origin. The thrombus also may extend into communicating or perforating veins. Depending on the extent of thrombus, venous blood may be forced into the superficial veins in either a retrograde or lateral direction (see Fig. 1-11).

Finally, it is interesting to speculate that the wearing of high-heeled shoes may lead to distal compression of the vein walls by leg muscles that are strained as a result of these shoes. When high-heeled shoes are worn, calf muscles are compressed and the gluteal muscles are used for walking. This secondary, logical factor has been proposed previously but awaits experimental confirmation.[127] At least one study has been unable to substantiate an effect of walking barefoot versus wearing high heels on leg volume.[128]

Arteriovenous anastomosis. Another important factor that may lead to increased venous pressure in cutaneous veins is the opening of arteriovenous communications. Arteriovenous anastomoses (AVAs) were suggested to be a component in the pathogenesis of varicose veins in 1949 by Pratt[129] and by Piulachs, Vidal-Barraquer, and Biel[130] in 1952. Pratt hypothesized that AVAs represented the failure of closure of femoral artery branches to the saphenous system.

A clue to the presence of AVAs is often provided by the presence of varicostities in an unusual anatomic location in the absence of detectable abnormalities of the deep venous system.[56] Physical examination often shows a lack of complete emptying of the varicose veins when the limb is elevated, during very rapid refilling of the varicose vein or venules with diascopy, during warmth over affected varicose veins, and in the rare presence of a bruit or thrill over these vessels.[129] Arterial Doppler sounds are often demonstrated over varices, especially when they are associated with bright red venectasia. Between 60% and 80% of patients with congenital AVAs on the legs have associated varicose veins.[131,132]

AVAs have also been demonstrated by direct operative microscopic dissection by Schalin[133] and Gius.[134] Indirect support of this theory has been provided by evaluating the oxygen content of varicose blood and skin temperature over varicose veins.[134-138] These studies estimate that AVAs occur in 64% to 100% of patients with varicose veins. However, at least one study has found no difference in varicose vein blood oxygen levels.[139] These authors postulate that oxygenation of venous blood is also related to metabolic activity, blood flow, blood volume in the varicosity, body position, and intravenous pressure. This was confirmed indirectly by measuring skin oxygen levels in patients with and without varicose veins. In this study no significant difference could be appreciated.[140] Finally, Pratt[129] estimated that AVAs occur in 24% of varicose veins and in 50% of patients with recurrent varicose veins after surgical ligation and stripping.

Schalin has demonstrated AVAs with thermography (Fig. 3-8). Schalin[141] recently reviewed the role of arteriovenous shunting in the development of varicose veins and concluded that the recurrent and varying flow of arterial blood transmitted to veins over years causes the venous wall to distend. He observed that this occurs by operative microscopy, demonstrating that AVAs connect to varicose veins at the convex curves. Although AVAs are difficult to detect radiographically in association with varicose veins,[142] rapid venous filling is commonly seen in arteriograms of limbs with severe venous stasis.

Opening of the AVA may occur through developmental or functional abnormalities of vasa vasorum of the venous wall. In one scenario, an association of excessive alcohol consumption in male patients with varicose veins was proposed to cause arteriolar dilation and new capillary formation, which may act like multiple AVAs.[70] Alternatively, opening of the AVA may be caused by proximal venous hypertension that breaks down the capillary barrier.[142] Once dysfunction of the

AVA is established, shunting of arterial blood directly into the venous system further increases venous dilation. It is still uncertain whether AVAs are the cause or the result of varicosities. Despite this, there are common observations that tend to support the concept of AVA-induced varicosities. Varicose veins may recur after anatomically correct sclerotherapy that obliterates all perforating veins. This may result from an AVA distal to the point of injection. Also, the bright red color of some leg telangiectasias may be caused by underlying AVA. Finally, cutaneous ulceration after sclerotherapy treatment also may be related to injection of venules and their associated AVAs (see Chapter 8). Therefore, the AVA is important either as an etiologic or associated factor in the cause and treatment of varicose veins, but it is not the primary cause of all varicose veins.

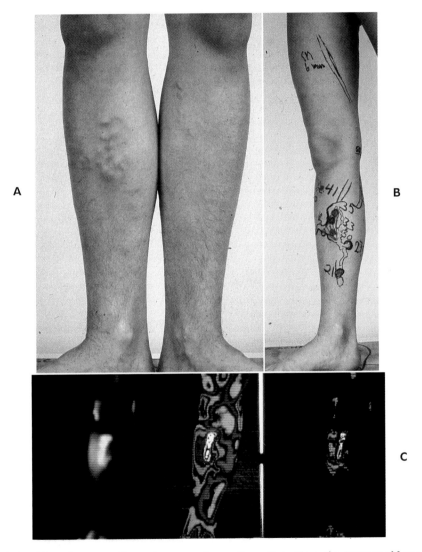

Fig. 3-8   Use of an operation microscope in cautious dissection of a 27-year-old woman identified two small pulsating vessels at the medial calf, **A**, 33 to 35 cm above the floor, **B**, corresponding to a thermographically hot (35° centigrade) varicosity, **C**.

Continued.

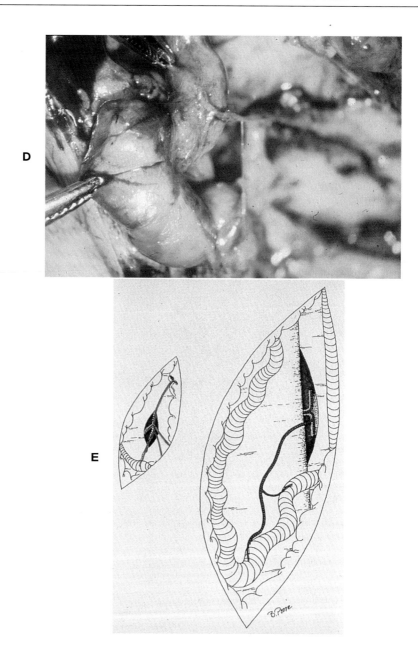

Fig. 3-8, cont'd   **D**, These arteries joined the meandering (tortuous) vein at the convex bends. No alternative arterial runoff was identified. The drawing, **E**, illustrates the connection of the arteries with the varicose vein. (Courtesy Lars Schalin, M.D.)

Primary Valvular Incompetence

Primary valvular incompetence is a serious precursor of varicose veins because, by definition, such valves are permanently damaged, absent, or incompetent. Thus, as originally suggested by William Harvey,[143] an incompetent valve causes distention of the distal vein by gravitational back pressure and may produce a varicosity. Many factors may be responsible for the development of valvular incompetence, including developmental abnormalities and destruction of the venous valves. Direct venoscopic evaluation in 25 patients with varicose veins disclosed that the GSV was valveless from the SFJ to the upper calf where the first normal valve appeared.[144] Thus, regional differences occur in varicosities.

Congenital valvular agenesis is a very rare cause of varicose veins.[145-149] Multiple case reports and a series of 14 patients have been described.[145,150] Such patients have partial or complete absence of deep vein valves in the lower extremities. Familial occurrence in two pedigrees suggests a simple dominant mode of inheritance. Clinically, such patients are detected by development of venous insufficiency at an early age. Interestingly, signs and symptoms invariably occurred only after puberty. The most serious physical finding was cutaneous ulceration in the typical medial malleolar area. The most notable physical finding was ankle edema occurring during the day with complete resolution at night or during rest. Another common sign was marked orthostatic hypotension from venous pooling in the legs. In these patients, wide variations in the number of valves was seen. This ranged from complete agenesis in both lower extremities to agenesis in only one leg or even partial agenesis. Therefore, although rarely reported, valvular agenesis in some degree may be found on careful examination of some patients. Its diagnosis is critical before performing injection sclerotherapy because a major complication of injecting veins without valves is a possible progression of venous fibrosis and thrombosis to the deep venous system. This could worsen venous insufficiency, even to the extent of jeopardizing the viability of the limb.

Scientific evaluation of the relative significance of valvular deficiency in relation to the development of varicose veins is not as clear. An autopsy study of 44 limbs disclosed 4 limbs with varicose veins that had normal valves in the femoral vein and the saphenofemoral junction (SFJ). Valves were absent proximal to the SFJ in 3 of the 4 varicose vein limbs. This was statistically significant when compared with nonvaricose vein limbs.[151]

Another autopsy study demonstrated a decreased number of venous valves in the left internal iliac vein compared with the right iliac vein. This could explain the relative increased incidence in left-sided varicose veins; the relative obstruction caused by the right iliac artery may be unimportant.[152] Anatomic studies do not define functional significance of venous valves. In a radiographic functional study of external iliac and femoral valves performed on 12 male volunteers with and without varicose veins, it was found that subjects with a family history of varicose veins did not have femoral or external iliac valves.[153] Conversely, those men without a family history of varicose veins did have such valves. Another study of 54 normal adults and 19 children of patients with varicose veins confirmed these findings. Using venous Doppler examination, incompetent iliofemoral valves were present in 16% of the normal adults and 32% of the children of patients with varicose veins.[154] These studies lend support to the theory of descending sequential valvular incompetence as a pathogenic mechanism for the development of varicose veins. Interestingly, a Nigerian study found that Caucasians show a relative deficiency of venous valves relative to Africans.[155] However, this cannot explain the lack of difference in the incidence of varicose veins between American Blacks and Caucasians.

Unfortunately, other studies have failed to show a convincing association between the absence of iliofemoral valves and the presence of LSV incompetence.[156] In addition, veins that have been reversed, rendering their valves incompetent, and used as arterial grafts fail to elongate or dilate. They certainly do not develop into varicose veins.[157] Therefore, primary valvular deficiency, with or without

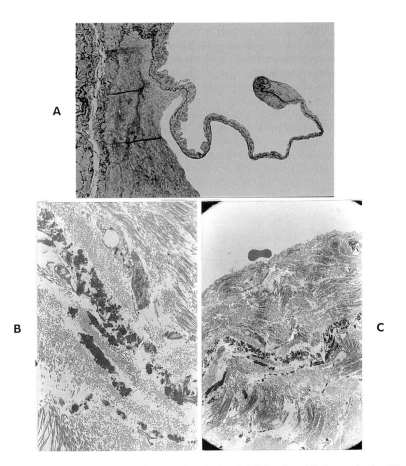

Fig. 3-9 **A,** Valve cusp in a varicose vein. Intimal thickening (*) is marked with thinning of the tunica media. (Elastic von Gieson ×20.) **B,** Protofibrils are proliferative with a complect course in a varicose vein. (Electron microscope stained with silicotangstic acid uranyl acetate.) **C,** Elastic fibers are torn with an aberrant course. (Electron microscope stained with silicotangstic acid uranyl acetate.) (Reproduced with permission from Obitsu Y et al: Histopathological studies of the valves of varicose veins, Phlebology 5:245, 21990.

increased transmural pressure, is best thought of as a contributory factor and not as an absolute etiologic factor in all patients with varicose veins.

Light microscopic findings of the venous valve in varicose veins consist of multiple dystrophic changes. There is a proliferation of collagen fibers and smooth muscle cells, as well as distortion and tearing of elastic fibers in the cusp. This translates to intimal thickening and tortuosity[158] (Fig. 3-9).

Common mechanisms for the destruction of these valves are deep venous thrombosis (DVT) and thrombophlebitis. DVT is estimated to precede the development of varicose veins in as many as 25% of patients.[159] Incompetence of the veins may also occur because of destruction of the valves by the inflammatory process of thrombophlebitis.[160-162] In addition to spontaneous DVT, thrombophlebitis may occur as a result of chemical or mechanical trauma or inflammatory bowel disease. Also, it may occur postsurgically in association with various malignancies or as a result of hormonal elevations in conjunction with birth control pills, postpartum, or even as a result of smoking.[162]

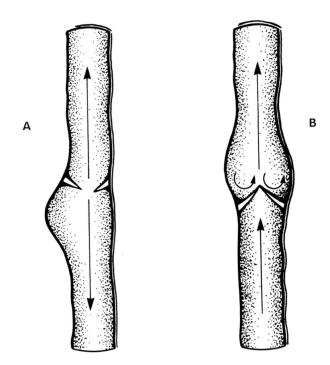

Fig. 3-10 A, Diagram of eccentric dilation beneath the valve cusps in a varicose vein. B, A normal valve is shown for comparison. (From Cotton L: Br J Surg 48:589, 1961.)

Finally, chronic venous dilation may in itself result in valvular fibrosis. Venous dilation increases tension on the cusps of the valves, which causes them to project into the lumen of the vein as rigid flanges (Fig. 3-10; see also Figs. 1-8A & B and 1-9). The resultant turbulence of blood flow is thought to cause sclerosis and contraction of the valve, and its eventual disappearance. This has been noted on histologic examination of varicose veins removed at surgery or postmortem.[163]

Secondary Valvular Incompetence

Secondary valvular incompetence is a common cause of varicose veins. In this situation the valves are normal but become incompetent because of dilation of the vein wall. Secondary valvular incompetence may occur as a result of destruction of the valvular system after DVT or because of the expansion in the diameter of the vein. This later process may occur via an increase in venous volume, obstruction in venous return, or a hormonally induced increase in venous distensibility. Thrombotic destruction of venous valves usually begins in the venous sinuses, such as in the soleal sinuses. Here the thrombus may spread to the posterior tibial vein and subsequently into the ankle communicating veins.[47] Organization and recanalization of the thrombus destroys the valves.[47] An even more dangerous event occurs when the thrombus spreads proximally as a precursor to the development of pulmonary embolism.

Pregnancy is typically associated with secondary valvular incompetence. Many epidemiologic studies have found a significantly increased incidence of varicose veins in women who have been pregnant.[39,94-96,164] However, some epidemiologic studies have failed to confirm this association when the effect of age

Fig. 3-11 Woman, 33 years old. **A,** Before pregnancy. **B,** 20 weeks into pregnancy with a 15-lb weight gain. Note the dramatic increase in the size and number of varicose veins. (Courtesy Anton Butie, M.D.)

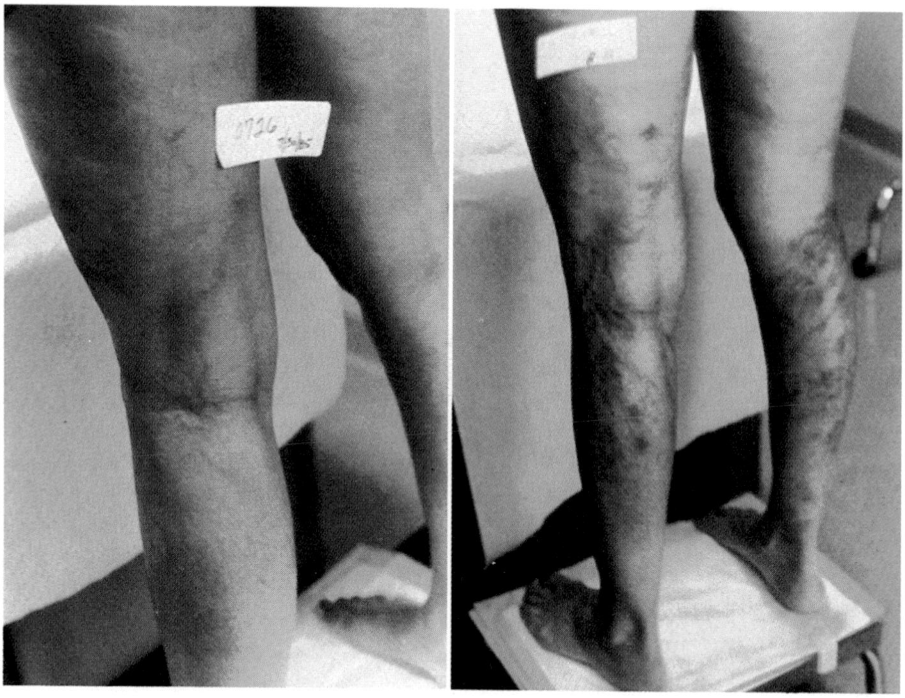

is controlled.[37,91] Varices are often first noted during pregnancy and are exceedingly rare before puberty.[165] Indeed, population studies have found that only 12% of women with varicose veins have never been pregnant.[166] It has been suggested that, in addition to hormonal effects (discussed below), increased total blood flow in the iliac veins from the uterine and ovarian veins may explain the occurrence of varicose veins in early pregnancy.[167] Pregnancy is accompanied by an increase in plasma volume to 149% of normal shortly before parturition.[168] Blood flow through the uterine veins is increased 4 to 16 times in the first 2 months of pregnancy and doubles again during the third month.[169] Although uterine obstruction to venous flow and an increase in iliac blood volume and flow are measurable physiologic factors in pregnancy, it is obvious that factors other than venous congestion are important in the development of varicose veins.

Femoral vein obstruction by the gravid uterus also may lead to secondary valvular incompetence through an increase in proximal venous pressures. The obstructive effects of the uterus do not develop during pregnancy until the second and third trimesters.[170] A sequential study of 50 gravid women through the first, second, and third trimesters using Doppler ultrasound demonstrated that femoral venous flow was obstructed in 72% of erect patients in the second trimester and 86% of patients in the third trimester.[171] An additional study of femoral blood flow in 61 pregnant patients demonstrated that the most significant decrease in femoral blood flow occurred when the head of the fetus became engaged during the latter part of the third trimester.[172] However, a study of venous capacitance and outflow in pregnant women at term, 1 week, 6 weeks, and 3 months after delivery demonstrated a decrease that persisted until 3 months postpartum.[173] Thus, other factors affect venous function in pregnancy.

The effect of the gravid uterus on the impedance of femoral blood flow may be influenced by hereditary factors. Although some investigators have not found a consistent relationship between the presence or absence of varicose veins and obstruction to venous flow,[171] others[174] have measured venous pressure in the popliteal vein in pregnant patients in the third trimester and found a marked increase in venous pressure only in those women with varicose veins. Therefore, both an increase in blood volume and an obstruction of venous return are responsible for the development of varicose veins in pregnancy. However, these two factors do not account for the development of smaller telangiectasias and venectasias; nor do these factors account for the development of varicose veins in the first trimester.

In pregnancy, hormonal factors are primarily responsible for venous dilation. As many as 70% to 80% of patients develop varicose veins during the first trimester when the uterus is only slightly enlarged (Fig. 3-11). In the second trimester, 20% to 25% of patients develop varicose veins, and 1% to 5% of patients develop them in the third trimester.[175-177]

Varicose veins of the legs are first apparent as early as 6 weeks into gestation, a time when the uterus is not yet large enough to significantly impede venous return from the leg veins. In contrast, vulvar varices usually develop in the third trimester but may appear late in the first trimester.[167,178] Furthermore, Mullane[177] notes that symptoms of varicose veins may be the first sign of pregnancy and can occur even before the first missed menstrual period. This confirms observations of many multiparous women and argues for a profound influence of progesterone on venous dilation and valvular insufficiency. Siegler[179] states that 40% of all pregnant patients are affected and maintains that all women will develop varicosities if they have a sufficient number of pregnancies. Berg estimates that 30% of primigravidas and 60% of multigravidas suffer varicose changes in the veins during pregnancy.[180] In support of this theory is Mullane's patient, who developed varicose veins for the first time in her eleventh pregnancy.[177] However, an evaluation of venous refilling times in primiparae and multiparae patients with varicose veins demonstrated no difference between the two groups.[181,182] Therefore, the first pregnancy most likely represents the most important injurious factor, with each subsequent pregnancy producing minor deterioration of venous function.

Venous distensibility has been found to increase in both forearm and calf veins with the progression of pregnancy, particularly after the thirteenth week.[183] The increase in distensibility was greater in the calf than in the forearm and returned to normal by the eighth postpartum week.[183]

Incompetence of the saphenous veins may occur because of excessive dilation of the vein when there is sufficient separation of the valve cusps.[161] Interestingly, retrospective studies have shown that 40% to 78% of patients note the development of varicosities during the second pregnancy rather than during the first.[11,176,177] Rose and Ahmed[11] postulate that veins that become subclinically varicose after the first pregnancy become clinically obvious after the second. As previously mentioned, this impression has been confirmed with photoplethysmography evaluation of venous refilling times.[181]

The pregnant state is associated with elevations of multiple hormones. Estrogen produces a relaxation of smooth muscle and softening of collagen fibers in general, which may explain the increased distensibility of veins.[184,185] The increased distensibility of vein walls has been reported to occur as a result of estrogen therapy.[186,187] McCausland[176] believes that the progesterone level, and, more importantly, the estrogen/progesterone ratio are primarily responsible for increased venous distensibility. Supporting this theory is the marked venous distensibility demonstrated in women who are given a synthetic progesterone.[188] Furthermore, a study in 1946 reported that the administration of an estrogenic substance, diovocylin (CIBA Pharmaceutical Company), to 27 pregnant patients with either varicose or telangiectatic veins in weekly doses throughout pregnancy actually produced an amelioration of the smaller and larger types of veins, and a reduction of peripheral edema and subjective complaints in the majority of patients.[189] This was confirmed in a subsequent study of 34 patients treated with oral ethinyl estradiol 0.05 mg 2 to 4 times daily.[190] Presumably, administration of this substance altered the progesterone/estrogen ratio. (No mention was made of feminization of male babies on follow-up examination.) An additional study has demonstrated a complete relief of symptoms in 13 of 15 patients with angiectids (small, intradermal, raised, bluish mats of blood vessels) in pregnancy with diethylstilbestrol (E. R. Squibb & Sons, Inc.) in doses ranging from 50 to 150 mg daily.[191] In this regard, the degree of pain and disability caused by the "angiectid" was frequently related to the level of subnormal estrogen. Symptomless angiectids were correlated with low normal amounts of estrogen and progesterone. Therefore, the hormonal factor responsible for the development or exacerbation of varicosities in pregnancy may very well be related to estrogen-progesterone balance. Hormonal influences may also explain why varicose veins that develop in pregnancy resolve postpartum (Fig. 3-12).

One additional hypothesis to explain the development of varicose veins in pregnancy is the development of arteriovenous anastamoses (AVA). Venous volume with correction for capillary filtration was found to be larger in pregnant

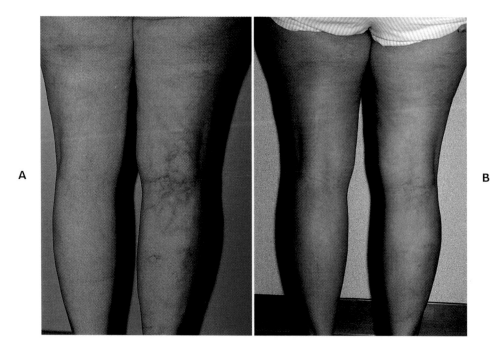

Fig. 3-12 **A,** Twenty-eight-year-old woman in her sixth month of pregnancy. Note prominent varicose, reticular, and telangiectatic veins on the right posterior thigh and calf. **B,** Six months postpartum. Note near complete resolution of all new veins without treatment.

women with varices than in pregnant women without varices or in nonpregnant women. This may indicate the presence of AVM.[192]

In pregnancy, two factors operate to dilate leg veins: increased venous distensibility from hormonal stimulation and increased venous pressure from obstruction by the gravid uterus and an increased blood volume. Sumner[193] has estimated that 80% to 90% of varicose veins tend to regress during the puerperium. He advises physicians to wait 6 to 12 weeks postpartum before performing surgery or sclerotherapy to allow time for the varices to regress. This will not only enhance treatment efficacy, but it also allows the physician to make a more accurate assessment of the true extent and severity of the disease.

The hormonal influence on the venous system extends beyond pregnancy. Studies have demonstrated that the increase in venous distensibility is different for different oral contraceptive agents. Oral contraceptives with a high progestogen component appear to increase venous capacitance and may induce venous stasis, whereas coagulability is partially enhanced by estrogen-dominant contraceptives.[194] The effect of systemic estrogen and progesterone can be demonstrated with photoplethysmography, venous Doppler tensiometry, and biomicroscopy. With these evaluations, women taking a low-dose oral contraceptive agent (0.020 mg ethinyl estradiol plus 0.150 mg desogestrel) undergo observable microcirculatory changes without clinical evidence of varicose or telangiectatic vein development. When women take a higher estrogen oral contraceptive (0.030 mg ethinyl estradiol plus 0.075 mg gestodene), significant capillaroscopic changes and a significant impairment of photoplethysmography occur associated with clinical signs and symptoms such as orthostatic edema, itching, heaviness, and slight pain in the lower limbs.[195] A retrospective evaluation of 2295 patients who took various concentrations and types of oral contraceptives determined the existence of a significant relationship between the intensity and functional symptomatology and the dosage of estrogen and progesterone.[196] However, epidemiologic evaluations concerning the use of oral contraceptives demonstrate a trend but do not prove a statistically significant risk for their use in the development of varicose veins.[95,197] In addition, alterations in leg vein distensibility were not found in the first half of pregnancy or during oral contraceptive therapy with estrogen-dominant ethyl-adrianol (10 mg) by means of ascending phlebography.[198]

Finally, it has been noted by Gallagher[199] in his practice of 20,000 patients that the incidence of minor asymptomatic varices decreases after menopause. This is correlated with a fall in estradiol production and plasma concentration. Therefore, estrogen or progesterone does not seem to be an independent factor influencing venous capacitance; their proportional concentrations may be more important.

A change in venous distensibility also occurs during the menstrual cycle.[188,194] Venous distensibility is higher during the luteal phase than during the follicular phase of the menstrual cycle.[194] This increase in distensibility correlates most closely with progesterone levels.[188] However, studies on vein distensibility do not distinguish between relaxation of smooth muscle and alteration in the visoelastic properties of the venous wall. Also, these studies do not exclude the possibility that the increased distensibility may result from the release of vasoconstrictor tone. Therefore, it is difficult to make recommendations regarding the timing of sclerotherapy with the menstrual cycle or the necessity to discontinue oral contraceptives during sclerotherapy.

Of more clinical concern is postpartum thrombophlebitis and its attendant dangers of pulmonary embolism and eventual development of the postphlebitic syndrome.[200] The reported incidence of thrombophlebitis in pregnancy ranges from 0.35%, with a 0.085% incidence antepartum and 0.27% postpartum,[201] up to 3.6% when mild cases are included in statistical analysis.[202] There are multiple factors responsible for the increased incidence of thrombophlebitis in this group of patients. In late pregnancy, blood volume is increased, the uterus impedes venous return, and elevated hormonal levels produce an increased distensibility of veins with resulting valvular incompetence. In addition, multiple factors are present at childbirth, including increased clotting factors and a hormonal environment conducive to clotting, that appear to predispose this physiologic milieu to the development of thrombophlebitis.[203,204] Therefore, graduated elastic support hosiery should be worn before, during, and immediately after delivery.[200]

Heredity

Although development of varicose veins can usually be ascribed to one of the above-mentioned pathologic states, postmortem examination may not disclose the apparent source of the high-pressure leak from the deep to the superficial system.[205] Therefore, other inherent factors such as vein wall weakness, increased primary valvular dysfunction or agenesis, and other genetic factors may enhance the development of varicose veins.

A familial tendency toward the development of varicose veins has been described in many population groups.[93-95,106,206-209] This may also be demonstrated by the development over time of varicose veins bilaterally when patients with unilateral varicose and telangiectatic veins are followed for 10 years.[209] A limited study of 50 patients with varicose veins in Great Britain disclosed a simple dominant type of inheritance.[210] Only 28% of patients had no family history of varicose veins. In Scandinavia, questionnaires completed by 124 women with varicose veins disclosed a 72% prevalence of varicose veins of an autosomal type in the women's siblings.[207] Of these cases, 28% were of a recessive pattern. Troisier and Le Bayon[211] examined 154 families with 514 descendants. They found that if both parents had varicose veins, 85% of children had evidence of varicose veins, whereas 27% of the children were affected if neither parent had varicose veins, and 41% of the children were affected if one parent had varicosities. These authors conclude that the inheritance of varicose disease is recessive. However, some studies have not found a significant familial tendency.[97,212]

A single study on unselected twins found that 75% of 12 monozygotic pairs were concordant with regard to varicose veins. Of 25 dizygotic, same-sexed pairs, 52% had varicose veins.[213]

Other studies have found more of a multifactorial inheritance. In a detailed study from Sweden of 250 probands of patients with varicose veins presenting for treatment, the overall frequency of varicose veins in female relatives was 43%, compared with 19% in male relatives.[214]

The absence of venous valves in the external iliac and femoral veins has been shown to be a marker of varicose veins in a limited radiographic study of 12 male volunteers, some with and some without varicose veins,[153] and in a venous Doppler study of 54 patients with varicose veins.[215] In addition, a simple dominant mode of inheritance has been reported in 14 patients with congenital partial or total absence of venous valves of the leg.[145,216] Thus this genetic predisposition may be the result of multiple factors, and the subsequent development of varicose veins may depend on one or more occupational or hormonal factors.

Congenitally weak or nonfunctioning venous valves may be an initiating factor in the altered venous hemodynamics that lead to the formation of varicose veins.[217] The argument against this theory is that valvular cusps consist of a fibrous tissue core covered by endothelium. This structure has been demonstrated to be extremely strong in experimental models.[218] In fact, it has been estimated experimentally that valves will not rupture at the physiologic pressures to which a valve might be subjected during life. Therefore, it is most likely that alterations in the vein wall, and not valve strength, are responsible for the development of incompetence.

Rose and Ahmed[11] postulated that an inherited alteration in vein wall collagen and/or elastin, or an increase in vein wall collagen deposition with separation of smooth muscle cells (as previously described), is a major etiologic precursor to the development of varicose veins. They reason that increased venous pressure should lead to hypertrophy of the vein wall as demonstrated in arterialized venous bypass coronary grafts[218-222] and not the dilation associated with varicose veins. Accordingly, dilation of varicose veins, at times only in certain areas of the vein, must be caused by a vein wall defect—not merely by the presence of high venous pressure. A generalized increase in venous distensibility was found in superficial forearm and hand veins in patients with a saphenous varicosity compared with patients without varicosities.[223,224] Abnormal distensibility curves were found to be similar regardless of the age and sex of the patient. This may be related to a reported decrease in collagen content in the saphenous veins of patients with varicosities, which occurs even in vein segments that are not varicose.[19,28] The decrease in venous distensibility may also be related to a constitutional decrease in venous α-adrenergic receptor responsiveness in patients with varicosities. Patients with varicose veins require significantly higher doses of noradrenaline for vasoconstriction than do control subjects. This finding applies to both varicose and normal veins in the same individual.[225] The neural regulatory network in the saphenous vein also consists of acetylcholinergic and peptidergic neurons, as well as both circulating and endothelium-derived vasoactive substances.[226] Thus, neural as well as hormonal factors are important regulators of venous distensibility.

The decreased collagen content in varicose vein walls has been physically related to its visoelastic properties with varicose veins breaking at lower pressures than normal veins.[227] This may occur in certain patients from a genetic defect affecting the biosynthesis of certain collagen types. One example is type 4 Ehlers-Danlos syndrome, in which patients have a deficiency in collagen 3 normally present in the skin, arteries, and gut. These patients also frequently have varicose veins.[228] However, this theory does not explain why correction of proximal valvular dysfunction with a tourniquet can correct abnormal venous pressures distally if, indeed, it is the vein wall that is abnormally distensible.[229]

Generalized dystrophic changes in the vein wall were confirmed histologically through biopsy of normal dorsal foot veins in 97.3% of patients with varicose veins.[230] The generalization of venous wall changes from superficial to deep veins was also demonstrated.[19] The authors speculate that this generalized trend may allow improvement of sclerotherapy techniques by choosing a stronger sclerosing agent when a peripheral venous biopsy demonstrates severe dystrophy (see Chapter 9).

Another interesting relationship is the recently described association of varicose veins with the ABO blood group system. Numerous studies have demonstrated a relationship between blood groups of the ABO system and DVT of the lower limbs.[231-234] These studies indicate an increased incidence of DVT in patients with blood type O, particularly when associated with pregnancy or the use of oral contraceptive agents.[234] However, one study found an increased incidence of thromboembolism in people with blood group A.[235] A study of 569 French men and women showed the risk of varicose veins in patients with type A blood to be double that for patients of all other blood groups.[236] Varicose veins were defined

Table 3-1 Development of varicose veins (% of study population)

Age	10-12	14-16	18-20
Tel	0	3.7	12.9
Retic	10.2	30.3	35.3
Perf	0	4.1	5.2
Trib	0	0.8	5.0
Trunk	0	1.7	3.3
SFJ RF	0	12.3	19.8

Bochum Study I-III abstracted from Schultz-Ehrenberg U et al: New epidemiological findings with regard to initial stages of varicose veins (Bochum Study I-III). In Raymond-Martimbeau P, Prescott R, and Zummo M, editors: Phlebologie '92, Paris, 1992, John Libbey Eurotext.
(Tel, telangiectasia; Retic, reticular vein; Perf, perforating vein; Trib, tributary varicose vein: Trunk, truncal varicose vein; SFJ RF, saphenofemoral junction reflux.)

as the presence in the standing position of a permanent dilation of at least one leg vein with a diameter of 3 mm or more with reflux. The risk of varicose veins persisted after adjustment for age, sex, paternal or maternal history, and a personal history of DVT. No association was found between rhesus factor and varicose veins. Therefore, a patient's blood group may be taken into account when assessing the need for prophylactic treatment of varicose veins or assessing the risk of postoperative venous thrombosis.

Aging

The incidence of varicose veins increases with age (Table 3-1); therefore, vein wall damage also should be more pronounced in the veins of older patients. An autopsy study of the popliteal vein in 127 persons demonstrated diffuse changes with an increase in connective tissue in the media that becomes most pronounced in the fifth decade and is progressive thereafter. This is associated with the loss of muscle cells in the media.[237] The finding correlated with an abnormality in the physical property of axial tension testing in 93 specimens of saphenous veins from 22 patients harvested during coronary bypass surgery.[238] However, one study of 31 normal veins and 41 varicose veins in patients and autopsy samples ranging in age from 25 to 92 failed to disclose an age-related difference.[239] The latter study concluded that varicose veins were a predetermined disease unrelated to aging effects.

In conclusion, multiple studies of population groups have documented a significant relationship between heredity and the development of varicose veins.[240-242] There also appears to be a significant difference in the incidence of varicose veins among different cultures, with a rarity of varicose veins in non-Westernized populations.[243] Therefore, multiple factors—pathologic, intrinsic, and extrinsic—contribute to the development of varicose veins.

REFERENCES

1. Prerovsky I: Disease of the veins, internal communication, MHO-PA 10964, World Health Organization.
2. Thulesius O et al: The varicose saphenous vein: functional and ultrastructural studies with special reference to smooth muscle, Phlebology 3:89, 1988.
3. Thulesius O et al: Endothelial mediated enhancement of noradrenaline-induced vasoconstriction in normal and varicose veins, Clin Physiol 11:153, 1991.
4. Lowell RC, Gloviczki P, and Miller VM: In vitro evaluation of endothelial and smooth muscle function of primary varicose veins, J Vasc Surg 16:679, 1992.

5. Svjcar J et al: Biochemical differences in the composition of primary varicose veins, Am Heart J 67:572, 1964.
6. Jurukova Z and Milenkov C: Ultrastructural evidence for collagen degradation in the walls of varicose veins, Exp Mol Path 37:37, 1982.
7. Garcia-Rospide V, et al: Enzymatic and isoenzymatic study of varicose veins, Phlebology 6:187, 1991.
8. Azevedo I, Albino Teixeira A, and Osswald W: Changes induced by ageing and denervation in the canine saphenous vein: a comparison with the human varicose vein. In Vanhoutte PM, editor: Return circulation and norepinephrine: an update, Paris, 1991, John Libbey Eurotext.
9. Lees TA, Mantle D, and Lambert D: Analysis of the smooth muscle content of the normal and varicose vein wall via analytical electrophoresis. In Raymond-Martimbeau P, Prescott R, and Zummo M, editors: Phlebologie '92, Paris, 1992, John Libbey Eurotext.
10. Bouissou H et al: Vein morphology, Phlebology 3(Suppl 1):1, 1988.
11. Rose SS and Ahmed A: Some thoughts on the aetiology of varicose veins, Cardiovasc Surg 27:534, 1986.
12. Acsady G and Lengyel I: Modifications between histomorphological and pathobiochemical changes leading to primary varicosis. In Davy A and Stemmer R, editors: Phlebologie 89, Montrouge, France, 1989, John Libbey Eurotext.
13. Andreotti L and Cammelli D: Connective tissue in varicose veins, Angiology 30:798, 1979.
14. Zwillenberg LO, Laszt L, and Willenberg H: Die Feinstruktur der Venenwand bei Varikose, Angiologica 8:318, 1971.
15. Gandhi RH et al: Analysis of the connective tissue matrix and proteolytic activity of primary varicose veins, J Vasc Surg 18:814, 1993.
16. Clarke H et al: Role of venous elasticity in the development of varicose veins, Br J Surg 76:577, 1989.
17. Merlen JF et al: Le devenir histologique d'une veine sclerosee, Phlebologie 31:17, 1978.
18. Partsch H and Mostbeck A: Constriction of varicose veins and improvement of venous pumping by dihydroergotamine, Vasa 14:74, 1985.
19. Fuchs U and Petter O: Phlebosclerosis of the stem veins in varicosis, Phlebo Proktol 19:120, 1990.
20. Zsoter T, Moore S, and Keon W: Venous distensibility in patients with varicosities: in vitro studies, J Appl Physiol 22:505, 1967.
21. Leu HJ, Vogt M, and Pfrunder H: Morphological alterations of nonvaricose and varicose veins, Basic Res Cardiol 74:435, 1979.
22. Deby C et al: Decreased tocopherol concentration of varicose veins associated with a decrease in antilipoperoxidant activity without similar changes in plasma, Phlebology 4:113, 1989.
23. Kontos HA and Hess ML: Oxygen radicals and vascular damage, Adv Exp Med Biol 161:365, 1983.
24. Felix W: Pharmakologische Beeinflußbarkeit kapazitativer Venen. In Schneider KW, editor: Die venose Insuffizienz, Wittstock, East Germany, 1972, Baden-Baden.
25. Biagi G et al: Prostanoid production in varicose veins: evidence for decreased prostacyclin with increased thromboxane A_2 and prostaglandin E_2 formation, Angiology 39:1036, 1989.
26. Kreysel HW, Nissen HP, and Enghofer E: A possible role of lysosomal enzymes in the pathogenesis of varicosis and the reduction in their serum activity by venostasis, Vasa 12:377, 1983.
27. Haardt B: Histological comparison of the enzyme profiles of healthy veins and varicose veins, Phlebology 39:921, 1986.
28. Svejcar J et al: Content of collagen, elastine, and hexosamine in primary varicose veins, Clin Sci 24:325, 1963.
29. Niebes P: Biochemical studies of varicosis, Monogr Stand Cardioangeiological Methods 4:233, 1977.
30. Branco D and Osswald W: The influence of Ruscus extract on the uptake and metabolism of noradrenaline in the normal and varicose vein, Phlebology 3(suppl 1):33, 1988.
31. Mellander S: Operative studies on the adrenergic neuro-hormonal control of resistance and capacitance blood vessels in the cat, Acta Physiol Scand 50:5, 1960.
32. Waterfield RL: The effect of posture on the volume of the leg, J Physiol 72:121, 1931.
33. Ludbrook J and Loughlin J: Regulation of volume in postarteriolar vessels of the lower limb, Am Heart J 67:493, 1964.
34. Rushmer RF: Effects of posture. In Rushmer RF: Cardiovascular dynamics, ed 4, Philadelphia, 1976, WB Saunders.
35. Samueloff SL, Browse NL, and Shepherd JT: Response of capacity vessels in human limbs to head-up tilt and suction on lower body, J Appl Physiol 21:47, 1966.
36. Reinis Z et al: Incidence of diseases of veins of the lower extremities in the population, Vnitr Lek 29:105, 1983.

37. Abramson JH, Hopp C, and Epstein LM: The epidemiology of varicose veins: a survey in Western Jerusalem, J Epidemiol Community Health 35:213, 1981.

38. Ducimetiere P et al: Varicose veins: a risk factor for atherosclerotic disease in middle-aged men? Int J Epidemiol 10:329, 1981.

39. Brand FN et al: The epidemiology of varicose veins: the Framingham study, Am J Prev Med 4:96,1988.

40. Pollack AA et al: The effect of exercise and body position on the venous pressure at the ankle in patients having venous valvular defects, J Clin Invest 28:559, 1949.

41. Pollack AA and Wood EH: Venous pressure in the saphenous vein at the ankle in man during exercise and changes in posture, J Appl Physiol 1:649, 1949.

42. Barcroft H and Dornhorst AC: The blood flow through the human calf during rhythmic exercise, J Physiol (Lond) 107:402, 1949.

43. Wells HS, Youmans JB, and Miller DG: Tissue pressure, intracutaneous, subcutaneous, and intramuscular, as related to venous pressure, capillary filtration, and other factors, J Clin Invest 17:489, 1938.

44. Ludbrook J: The musculo-venous pumps of the human lower limb, Am Heart J 71:635, 1966.

45. Hojensgard IC and Sturup H: Static and dynamic pressures in superficial and deep veins of the lower extremity in man, Acta Physiol Scand 27:49, 1953.

46. Arnoldi CC: Venous pressure in the leg of healthy human subjects at rest and during muscular exercise in the nearly erect position, Acta Chir Scand 130:570, 1965.

47. Dodd H and Cockett FB, editors: The pathology and surgery of the veins of the lower limb, ed 2, Edinburgh, 1976, Churchill Livingstone.

48. Almen T and Nylander G: Serial phlebography of the normal lower leg during muscular contraction and relaxation, Acta Radiol 57:264, 1962.

49. Dicker Jr JW: A study of venous return from the leg during exercise, Phlebology 4:185, 1989.

50. Fegan WG, Milliken JC, and Fitzgerald DE: Abdominal venous pump, Arch Surg 92:44, 1966.

51. Lange L and Echt M: Comparative studies on drugs which increase venous tone using nor-adrenaline, ethyl-andrianol, dihydroergotamine, and horsechestnut extract, Fortschr Med 90:1161, 1972.

52. Mellander S and Nordenfelt L: Comparative effects of dihydroergotamine and noradrenaline on resistance, exchange, and capacitance functions in the peripheral circulation, Clin Sci 39:183, 1970.

53. Bjordal R: Simultaneous pressure and flow recordings in varicose veins of the lower extremities, Acta Chir Scand 136:309, 1970.

54. Strandness DE Jr and Thiele BL: Selected topics in venous disorders, New York, 1981, Futura.

55. McPheeters HO and Rice CO: Varicose veins: the circulation and direction of venous flow, Surg Gynecol Obstet 49:29, 1929.

56. Farber EM and Bates EE: Pathologic physiology of stasis dermatitis, Arch Dermatol 70:653, 1954.

57. Negus D and Friedgood A: The effective management of venous ulceration, Br J Surg 70:623, 1983.

58. Cockett FB and Jones BE: The ankle blow-out syndrome: a new approach to the varicose ulcer problem, Lancet 1:17, 1953.

59. Landis EM: Factors controlling the movement of fluid through the human capillary wall, Yale J Biol Med 5:201, 1933.

60. Burnand KG et al: The effect of sustained venous hypertension on the skin capillaries of the canine hind limb, Br J Surg 69:41, 1982.

61. Ryan TJ and Wilkinson DS: Diseases of the veins: venous ulcers. In Rook A, Wilkinson DS, and Ebling FJG, editors: Textbook of dermatology, ed 3, London, 1979, Blackwell Scientific Publications.

62. Ryan TJ: Diseases of the skin: management of varicose ulcers and eczema, Br Med J 1:192, 1974.

63. Whimster I. Cited in Dodd H and Cockett FB, editors: The pathology and surgery of the veins of the lower limb, ed 2, Edinburgh, 1976, Churchill Livingstone.

64. Peters K et al: Lower leg subcutaneous blood flow during walking and passive dependency in chronic venous insufficiency, Br J Dermatol 124:177, 1991.

65. Falanga V et al: Dermal pericapillary fibrin in venous disease and venous ulceration, Arch Dermatol 123:620, 1987.

66. Lotti T, Fabbri P, and Panconesi E: The pathogenesis of venous ulcers, J Am Acad Dermatol 16:877, 1987.

67. Ludbrook J and Loughlin J: Regulation of volume in postarteriolar vessels of the lower limb, Am Heart J 67:493, 1964.

68. Shepherd JT and Vanhoutte PM: Role of the venous system in circulatory control, Mayo Clin Proc 53:247, 1978.

69. Boccalon H and Ginestet MC: Influence of temperature variations on venous return: clinical observations, Phlebology 3(suppl 1):47, 1988.

70. Tanyol H and Menduke H: Alcohol as a possible etiologic agent in varicose veins: a study of drinking habits in 136 patients with varicose veins and in 70 control patients, Angiology 12:382, 1961.

71. Kerr MG, Scott DB, and Samuel E: Studies of the inferior vena cava in late pregnancy, Br Med J 1:532, 1964.

72. Cleave TL: On the causation of varicose veins and their prevention and arrest by natural means, Bristol, 1960, Wright & Sons.

73. Cambell GC and Cleave TL: Diverticular disease of colon, Br Med J 3:741, 1968.

74. Beaglehole R: Epidemiology of varicose veins, World J Surg 10:898, 1986.

75. Burkitt DP: Varicose veins: facts and fantasy, Arch Surg 111:1327, 1976.

76. Foote RR: Varicose veins, St Louis, 1949, CV Mosby.

77. Pirner F: Der varikose Symptomen-komplex mit seien Folgen und Nachkrakheiten un ter besoneren Bereichsichtigung der Fehlerquellen. In Diagnostik und Therapie, Stuttgart, 1957, ENKE.

78. Dodd H: The cause, prevention, and arrest of varicose veins, Lancet 2:809, 1964.

79. Burkitt DP: Varicose veins, deep vein thrombosis, and haemorrhoids: epidemiology and suggested etiology, Br Med J 2:556, 1972.

80. Stamler J: Epidemiology as an investigative method for study of human arteriosclerosis, J Natl Med Assoc, Tuskegee, Ala, 50:161, 1958.

81. Brodribb AJM and Humphreys DM: Diverticular disease: three studies. Part I—relation to other disorders of fibre intake, Br Med J 6:424, 1976.

82. Richardson JB and Dixon M: Varicose veins in tropical Africa, Lancet 1:791, 1977.

83. Martin A and Odling-Smee A: Pressure changes in varicose veins, Lancet 1:768, 1976.

84. Malhotra SL: An epidemiological study of varicose veins in Indian railroad workers from the south and north of India, with special reference to the causation and prevention of varicose veins, Int J Epidemiol 1:117, 1982.

85. Connor WE, Hoak JG, and Warner EA: Massive thrombosis produced by fatty acid infusion, J Clin Invest 42:860, 1963.

86. Connor WE and Poole JCF: The effect of fatty acids on the formation of thrombi, Q J Exp Physiol 46:1, 1961.

87. Poole JCF: Effective diet and lipidemia on coagulation and thrombosis, Fed Proc 21(4), pt 2:20, 1962.

88. Melet JJ: La place de l'alimentation parmi les facteurs de rísque des maladies veineuses, Phlebologie 34:469, 1981.

89. Abramson JH et al: The epidemiology of inguinal hernia: a survey in Western Jerusalem, J Epidemiol Community Health 32:59, 1978.

90. Schilling RSF and Walford J: Varicose veins in women cotton workers: an epidemiological study in England and Egypt, Br Med J 2:591, 1969.

91. Guberan E et al: Causative factors of varicose veins: myths and facts, Vasa 2:115, 1973.

92. Askar O and Emara A: Varicose veins and occupation, J Egypt Med Assoc 53:341, 1970.

93. Stvrtinova V, Kolesar J, and Wimmer G: Prevalence of varicose veins of the lower limbs in the women working at a department store, Int Angiol 10:2, 1991.

94. Reinis Z et al: Incidence of diseases of the veins of the lower extremities in the population, Vnitrni Lek (Prague) 29:105, 1983.

95. Sadick NS: Predisposing factors of varicose and telangiectatic leg veins, J Dermatol Surg Oncol 18:883, 1992.

96. Maffei FHA et al: Varicose veins and chronic venous insufficiency in Brazil: prevalence among 1755 inhabitants of a country town, Int J Epidemiol 15:210, 1986.

97. Weddell JM: Varicose veins pilot survey, 1966, Br J Prev Soc Med 23:179, 1969.

98. Stanhope JM: Varicose veins in a population of lowland New Guinea, Int J Epidemiol 4:221, 1975.

99. Alexander CJ: Chair-sitting and varicose veins, Lancet 1:822, 1972.

100. Wright HP and Osborn SB: Effect of posture on venous velocity, Br Heart J 14:325, 1952.

101. Symington IS and Stack BH: Pulmonary thromboembolism after travel, Br J Dis Chest 71:138, 1977.

102. Myers TT: Varicose veins. In Barker and Hines, editors: Barker and Hines's peripheral vascular diseases, ed 3, Philadelphia, 1962, WB Saunders.

103. Leipnitz G et al: Prevalence of venous disease in the population: first results from a prospective study carried out in greater Aachen. In Davy A and Stemmer R, editors: Phlebologie '89, Montrouge, France, 1989, John Libbey Eurotext.

104. Beaglehole R, Almond CE, and Prior IAM: Varicose veins in New Zealand: prevalence and severity, NZ Med J 84:396, 1976.

105. Widmer LK: Peripheral venous disorders: prevalence and socio-medical importance: observations in 4529 apparently healthy persons, Basle Study III, Berne, Switzerland, 1978, Huber.

106. Hirai M and Nakayama R: Prevalence and risk factors of varicose veins in Japanese women, Angiolology 3:228, 1990.

107. Ludbrook J: Obesity and varicose veins, Surg Gynecol Obstet 118:843, 1964.

108. Seidell JC et al: Fat distribution of overweight persons in relation to morbidity and subjective health, Int J Obes 9:363, 1985.

109. Stegall HF: Muscle pumping in the dependent leg, Circ Res 19:180, 1966.

110. Floyd WF and Silver PHS: Electromyographic study of patterns of activity of the anterior abdominal muscles in man, J Anat 84:132, 1950.

111. Stewart AM, Webb JW, and Hewitt D: Social medicine studies based on civilian medical board records. II. Physical and occupational characteristics of men with varicose conditions, Br J Prev Med 9:26, 1955.

112. Kriessmann A: Klinische Pathophysiologie des venosen Ruckstroms. In Ay RE and Kriessmann A, editors: Periphere Venendruckmessung, Stuttgart, 1978, Thieme.

113. Haddy FJ and Scott JB: Metabolic factors in peripheral circulatory regulation, Fed Proc 34:2006, 1975.

114. Fegan G: Varicose veins: compression sclerotherapy, London, 1967, William Heinemann.

115. Fegan WG: Continuous uninterrupted compression technique of injecting varicose veins, Proc R Soc Med 53:837, 1960.

116. Hobbs JT: The problem of the post-thrombotic syndrome, Postgrad Med J (Aug supp):48, 1973.

117. Lofgren EP: Leg ulcers: symptoms of an underlying disorder, Postgrad Med 76:51, 1984.

118. Beninson J and Livingood CS: Stasis dermatitis. In Demis DJ, editor: Clinical dermatology, vol 2, Philadelphia, 1985, Harper & Row.

119. Cockett FB and Thomas ML: The iliac compression syndrome, Br J Surg 52:816, 1965.

120. Kwaan JHM, Jones RN, and Connolly JE: Simplified technique for the management of refractory varicose ulcers, Surgery 80:743, 1976.

121. Lim LT, Michoda M, and Bergan JJ: Therapy of peripheral vascular ulcers: surgical management, Angiology 29:654, 1978.

122. Quill RD and Fegan WG: Reversibility of femorosaphenous reflux, Br J Surg 55:389, 1971.

123. Thibault P et al: Cosmetic leg veins: evaluation using duplex venous imaging, J Dermatol Surg Oncol 16:612, 1990.

124. Abu-Own A, Scurr JH, and Coleridge Smith PD: Saphenous vein reflux without sapheno-femoral or sapheno-popliteal junction incompetence. Presented at the sixth Annual Meeting of the American Venous Forum, Maui, 1994.

125. Bjordal RI: Circulation patterns in incompetent perforating veins of the calf in venous dysfunction. In May R, Partsch H, and Staubesand J, editors: Perforating Veins, Munich, 1981, Urban & Schwarzenberg.

126. McMullin GM, Coleridge Smith PD, and Scurr JH: Which way does blood flow in the perforating veins of the leg? Phlebology 6:127, 1991.

127. Lake M, Pratt GH, and Wright IS: Arteriosclerosis and varicose veins: occupational activities and other factors, JAMA 119:696, 1942.

128. Lindemayr H and Santler R: Der einfluss der Schuhabasastzhohe auf den Venendruk des Beines, Winer med Wochenschr 14:496, 1979.

129. Pratt GH: Arterial varices: a syndrome, Am J Surg 77:456, 1949.

130. Piulachs P, Vidal-Barraquer F, and Biel JM: Considerations pathogeniques sur les varices de la grossesse, Lyon Chir 47:263, 1952.

131. Szilagyi DE et al: Congenital arteriovenous anomalies of the limbs, Arch Surg 111:423, 1976.

132. Coursley G, Ivins JC, and Barker NW: Congenital arteriovenous fistulas in the extremities: an analysis of sixty-nine cases, Angiology 7:201, 1956.

133. Schalin L: Reevaluation of incompetent perforating veins: a review of all the facts and observations interpreted on account of a controversial opinion and our own results. In Tese M and Dormandy JA: Superficial and deep venous diseases of the lower limbs, Torino, Italy, 1984, Edizioni Panminerva Medica.

134. Gius JA: Arteriovenous anastomoses and varicose veins, Arch Surg 81:299, 1960.

135. Schroth R: Venose Sauerstoffsattigung bei varicen, Arch Klin Chir 300:419, 1962.
136. Haeger KHM and Bergman L: Skin temperature of normal and varicose legs and some reflections on the etiology of varicose veins, Angiology 14:473, 1963.
137. Piulachs P and Vidal-Barraquer F: Pathogenic study of varicose veins, Angiology 4:59, 1953.
138. Baron HC and Cassaro S: The role of arteriovenous shunts in the pathogenesis of varicose veins, J Vasc Surg 4:124, 1986.
139. McEwan AJ and McArdle CS: Effect of hydroxyethylrutosides on blood oxygen levels and venous insufficiency symptoms in varicose veins, Br Med J 2:138, 1971.
140. Clyne CAC et al: Oxygen tension of the skin of the gaiter area of limbs with venous disease, Br J Surg 72:644, 1985.
141. Schalin L: Role of arteriovenous shunting in the development of varicose veins. In Etilof B et al, editors: Controversies in the management of venous disorders, England, 1989, Butterworth.
142. Haimovici H, Steinman C, and Caplan LH: Role of arteriovenous anastomoses in vascular diseases of the lower extremity, Ann Surg 164:990, 1966.
143. Bylebyl JJ: Harvey on the valves in the veins, Bull Hist Med 3:351, 1983.
144. Gradman WS, Segalowitz J, and Grandfest W: Venoscopy in varicose vein surgery: initial experience, Phlebology 8:145, 1993.
145. Lindvall N and Lodin A: Congenital absence of venous valves, Acta Chir Scand 124:310, 1962.
146. Luke JC: The diagnosis of chronic enlargement of the leg: with description of a new syndrome, Surg Gynecol Obstet 73:472, 1941.
147. Norman AG: The significance of a venous cough impulse in the short saphenous vein, Angiology 7:523, 1956.
148. Ludin A: Congenital absence of valves in the veins. In van der Molen HR, editor: Progres cliniques et therapeutiques dans le domaine de la phlebologie, Apeldoorn, Netherlands, 1970, Stenvert.
149. Lodin A: Congenital absence of valves in the deep veins of the leg: a factor in venous insufficiency, Acta Derm Venerol 62(41):1, 1961.
150. Lodin A, Lindvall N, and Gentele H: Congenital absence of venous valves as a cause of leg ulcers, Acta Chir Scand 116:256, 1958-1959.
151. Chadwick SJD, Clowes T, and Dudley HAF: The relationship of varicose veins to the absence of venous valves, Br J Surg 71:222, 1984.
152. Villavicencio JL: Personal communication, 1989.
153. Ludbrook J and Beale G: Femoral vein valves in relation to varicose veins, Lancet 1:79, 1962.
154. Reagan B and Folse R: Lower limb venous dynamics in normal persons and children of patients with varicose veins, Surg Gynecol Obstet 132:15, 1971.
155. Geelhoed GW and Burkitt DP: Varicose veins: a reappraisal from a global perspective, South Med J 84:1131, 1991.
156. Basmajian JV: The distribution of valves in the femoral, external iliac, and common iliac veins and their relationship to varicose veins, Surg Gynecol Obstet 95:537, 1952.
157. LiCalzi LK and Stansel HC Jr: Failure of autogenous reversed vein femoropopliteal grafting: pathophysiology, Surgery 91:352, 1982.
158. Obitsu Y et al: Histopathological studies of the valves of varicose veins, Phlebology 5:245, 1990.
159. Gjores JE: The incidence of venous thrombosis and its sequelae in certain districts of Sweden, Acta Chir Scand (suppl)206:11, 1956.
160. Miller RP and Sparrow TD: The pathogenesis diagnosis and treatment of varicose veins and varicose ulcers, NC Med J 9:574, 1948.
161. Lofgren KA: Varicose veins: their symptoms, complications, and management, Postgrad Med 65:131, 1979.
162. Beninson J: Thrombophlebitis. In Demis DJ, editor: Clinical dermatology, Philadelphia, 1986, Harper & Row.
163. Cotton LT: Varicose veins: gross anatomy and development, Br J Surg 48:589, 1961.
164. Forconi S, Guerrim M, and DiPerri T: Vasa 6:282, 1977.
165. Tolins SH: Treatment of varicose veins, an update, Am J Surg 145:248, 1983.
166. Henry M and Corless C: The incidence of varicose veins in Ireland, Phlebology 4:133, 1989.
167. Nabatoff RA: Varicose veins of pregnancy, JAMA 174:1712, 1960.
168. Documenta Geigy: Scientific Tables. In Diem K, editor: Macclesfield, 1962, Geigy Switzerland.
169. Barrow DW: Clinical management of varicose veins, ed 2, New York, 1957, Paul B. Hoeber.
170. McLennan CE: Antecubital and femoral venous pressures in normal and toxemic pregnancy, Am J Obstet Gynecol 45:568, 1943.
171. Ikard RW, Ueland K, and Folse R: Lower limb venous dynamics in pregnant women, Surg Gynecol Obstet 132:483, 1971.
172. Wright HP, Osborn SB, and Edmonds DG: Changes in the rate of flow of venous blood in the leg during pregnancy, measured with radioactive sodium, Surg Gynecol Obstet 90:481, 1950.

173. Skudder Jr PA et al: Venous dysfunction of late pregnancy persists after delivery, J Cardiovasc Surg 31:748, 1990.

174. Veal JR and Hussey HH: Venous circulation in lower extremities during pregnancy, Surg Gynecol Obstet 72:841, 1941.

175. Tournay R and Wallois P: Les varices de la grossesse et leur traitment principalement par les injections sclerosantes, expansion, Paris, 1948, Scient Franc.

176. McCausland AM: Varicose veins in pregnancy, Cal West Med 50:258, 1939.

177. Mullane DJ: Varicose veins in pregnancy, Am J Obstet Gynecol 63:620, 1952.

178. Dodd H and Wright HP: Vulval varicose veins in pregnancy, Br Med J 1:831, 1959.

179. Siegler J: The treatment of varicose veins in pregnancy, Am J Surg 44:403, 1939.

180. Berg D: First results with Ruscus extract in the treatment of pregnancy-related varicose veins. In Vanhoutte PM, editor: Return circulation and norepinephrine: an update, Paris, 1991, John Libbey Eurotext.

181. Sohn CH, Karl C, and Zelihic N: Untersuchungen zum Einfluß der Schwangerschaftsanzahl auf das Venensystem, Phlebologie 20:41, 1991.

182. Struckmann JR et al: Venous muscle pump function during pregnancy: assessment of ambulatory strain-gauge plethysmography, Acta Obstet Gynecol Scand 69:209, 1990.

183. Barwin BN and Roddie IC: Venous distensibility during pregnancy determined by graded venous congestion, Am J Obstet Gynecol 125:921, 1976.

184. Wahl LM: Hormonal regulation of macrophage collagenase activity, Biochem Biophys Res Commun 74:838, 1977.

185. Woolley DE: On the sequential changes in levels of oestradiol and progesterone during pregnancy and parturition and collagenolytic activity. In Piez KA and Eddi AH, editors: Extracellular matrix biochemistry, New York, 1984, Elsevier Science Publishing.

186. Reynolds RM and Foster I: Peripheral vascular action of estrogen, observed in the ear of the rabbit, J Pharmacol Exp Ther 68:173, 1940.

187. Goodrich SM and Wood JE: Peripheral venous distensibility and velocity of venous blood flow during pregnancy or during oral contraceptive therapy, Am J Obstet Gynecol 90:740, 1964.

188. McCausland AM, Holmes F, and Trotter AD Jr: Venous distensibility during the menstrual cycle, Am J Obstet Gynecol 86:640, 1963.

189. Marazita AJD: The action of hormones on varicose veins in pregnancy, Med Rec 159:422, 1946.

190. McPheeters HO: The value of estrogen therapy in the treatment of varicose veins complicating pregnancy, Lancet 69:2, 1949.

191. Fried PH, Perilstein PK, and Wagner FB: Saphenous varicosities vs angiectids consideration of so-called varicose veins of the lower extremities complicating pregnancy, Obstet Gynecol 2:418, 1953.

192. Sandstrom B and Bjerle P: Calf blood flow and venous capacity during late pregnancy in women with varices, Acta Obstet Gynecol Scand 53:355, 1974.

193. Sumner DS: Venous dynamics—varicosities, Clin Obstet Gynecol 24:743, 1981.

194. Fawer R et al: Effect of menstrual cycle, oral contraception, and pregnancy on forearm blood flow, venous distensibility, and clotting factors, Eur J Clin Pharmacol 13:251, 1978.

195. Allegra C, Carlizza A, and Mari A: Estroprogestins and microcirculation. In Raymond-Martimbeau P, Prescott R, and Zummo M, editors: Phlebologie '92. Paris, 1992, John Libbey Eurotext.

196. Vin F, Allaert FA, and Levardon M: Influence of estrogens and progesterone on the venous system of the lower limbs in women, J Dermatol Surg Oncol 18:888, 1992.

197. Durand JL and Bressler R: Clinical pharmacology of the steroidal oral contraceptives, Adv Intern Med 24:97, 1979.

198. Dandstrom B and Lowegren L: Phlebographic studies of the leg veins in the first half of pregnancy, Acta Obstet Gynecol Scand 49:375, 1970.

199. Gallagher PG: Major contributing role of sclerotherapy in the treatment of varicose veins, Vasc Surg 20:139, 1986.

200. Harridge WH: The treatment of primary varicose veins, Surg Clin North Am 40:191, 1960.

201. Husni EA, Pena LI, and Lenhert AE: Thrombophlebitis in pregnancy, Am J Obstet Gynecol 97:901, 1967.

202. Quattlebaum FW and Hodgson JF: The surgical treatment of varicose veins in pregnancy, Surg Gynecol Obstet 95:336, 1952.

203. Pechet L and Alexander B: Increased clotting factors in pregnancy, N Engl J Med 265:1093, 1961.

204. Wood JE: Oral contraceptives, pregnancy, and the veins, Circulation 38:627, 1968.

205. Thompson H: The surgical anatomy of the superficial and perforating veins of the lower limb, Ann R Coll Surg Engl 61:198, 1979.

206. von Curtius F: Untersuchungen uber das menschliche Venensystem, Deutsches Arch Klin Med 162:194, 1928.

207. Arnoldi C: The heredity of venous insufficiency, Dan Med Bull 5:169, 1958.

208. Almgren B and Eriksson I: Primary deep venous incompetence in limbs with varicose veins, Acta Chir Scand 155:455, 1989.
209. Arenander E and Lindhagen A: The evolution of varicose veins studied in a material of initially unilateral varices, Vasa 7:180, 1978.
210. Ottley C: Heredity and varicose veins, Br Med J 1:528, 1934.
211. Troisier J and Le Bayon: Etude génétique des varices, Ann de Med (Fr) 41:30, 1937.
212. King ESJ: The genesis of varicose veins, Aust NZ J Surg 20:126, 1950.
213. Niermann H: Zwillingsdermatologie, Berlin, 1964, Springer-Verlag.
214. Gundersen J and Hauge M: Hereditary factors in venous insufficiency, Angiology 20:346, 1969.
215. Folse R: The influence of femoral vein dynamics on the development of varicose veins, Surgery 68:974, 1970.
216. Almgren B: Non-thrombotic deep venous incompetence with special reference to anatomic, haemodynamic and therapeutic aspects, Phlebology 5:255, 1990.
217. Baron HC: Varicose veins, Consultant, p 108, May 1983.
218. Ackroyd JS, Pattison M, and Browse NL: A study of the mechanical properties of fresh and preserved human femoral vein wall and valve cusps, Br J Surg 72:117, 1985.
219. Campbell PA, McGeachie JK, and Prendergast FJ: Vein grafts for arterial repair: their success and reasons for failure, Ann R Coll Surg Engl 4:257, 1981.
220. Szilagyi DE et al: Biological fate of autologous vein implants as arterial substitutes, Ann Surg 178:232, 1973.
221. Fuchs JCA, Michener JS, and Hagen PO: Postoperative changes in autologous vein grafts, Ann Surg 188:1, 1978.
222. Brody WR, Kosek JC, and Angell WW: Changes in vein grafts following aorto-coronary bypass induced by pressure and ischaemia, J Thorac Cardiovasc Surg 64:847, 1972.
223. Zsoter T and Cronin RFP: Venous distensibility in patients with varicose veins, Can Med Assoc J 4:1293, 1966.
224. Eiriksson E and Dahn I: Plethysmographic studies of venous distensibility in patients with varicose veins, Acta Chir Scand Suppl 398:19, 1968.
225. Blochl-Daum B et al: Primary defect in alpha-adrenergic responsiveness in patients with varicose veins, Clin Pharmacol Ther 49:49, 1991.
226. Herbst WM et al: The innervation of the great saphenous vein: an immunohistological study with special regard to regulatory peptides, Vasa 21:253, 1992.
227. Psaila JV and Melhuish J: Visoelastic properties and collagen content of the long saphenous vein in normal and varicose veins, Br J Surg 76:37, 1989.
228. Gertsch P et al: Changing patterns in the vascular form of Ehlers-Danlos syndrome, Arch Surg 121:1061, 1986.
229. Ludbrook J: Valvular defect in primary varicose veins: cause or effect? Lancet 2:1289, 1963.
230. Corcos L et al: Peripheral venous biopsy: significance, limitations, indications and clinical applications, Phlebology 4:271, 1989.
231. Jick H and Porter J: Thrombophlebitis of the lower extremities and the ABO type, Arch Intern Med 138:1566, 1978.
232. Robinson WN and Roisenberg I: Venous thromboembolism and the ABO blood groups in a Brazilian population, Hum Genet 55:129, 1980.
233. Talbot S et al: ABO blood groups and venous thromboembolic disease, Lancet 1:1257, 1970.
234. Jick H et al: Venous thromboembolic disease and the ABO blood type, Lancet 1:539, 1969.
235. Vessay MP and Mann JI: Female sex hormones and thrombosis, Br Med Bull 34:157, 1978.
236. Cornu-Thenard A et al: Relationship between blood groups (ABO) and varicose veins of the lower limbs: a case-control study, Phlebology 4:37, 1989.
237. Lev M and Saphir O: Endophlebohypertrophy and phlebosclerosis, Arch Pathol Lab Med 154, 1951.
238. Donovan DL et al: Material and structural characterization of human saphenous veins, J Vasc Surg 12:531, 1990.
239. Bouissou H et al: Structure of healthy and varicose veins. In Vanhoutte PM, editor: Return circulation and norepinephrine: an update, Paris, 1991, John Libbey Eurotext.
240. Cepelak V et al: Genetic backgrounds of varicosity. In van der Molen HR, van Limborgh J, and Boersma W, editors: Progres cliniques et therapeutiques dans le domanie de la phlebologie, Apeldoorn, Netherlands, 1970, Stenvert.
241. Niermann H: Genetische Problematik des varikosen Symptomenkomplexes, Ergebn Angiol 4:25, 1970.
242. Gundersen J: Hereditare Faktoren bei der Entstehung der Varikosis. In Schneider KW, editor: Die venose Insuffizienz, Wittstock, East Germany, 1972, Baden-Baden.
243. Alexander CJ: The epidemiology of varicose veins, Med J Aust 1:215, 1972.

4 PATHOPHYSIOLOGY OF TELANGIECTASIAS

The term *telangiectasia* was first coined in 1807 by Von Graf to describe a superficial vessel of the skin visible to the human eye.[1] Individually, the vessels measure 0.1 to 1 mm in diameter and represent an expanded venule, a capillary, or an arteriole. Telangiectasias that originate from arterioles on the arterial side of a capillary loop tend to be small, bright red, and do not protrude above the skin surface. Telangiectasias that originate from venules on the venous side of a capillary loop are blue, wider, and often protrude above the skin surface. Sometimes telangiectasias, especially those arising at the capillary loop, are red at first, but with time become blue, probably because of an increasing hydrostatic pressure and backflow from the venous side.[2]

CLASSIFICATION

Redisch and Pelzer[3] classified telangiectasias into 4 types based on clinical appearance: (1) sinus or simple (linear), (2) arborizing, (3) spider or star, and (4) puntiform (papular) (Fig. 4-1). Papular telangiectasias are frequently present in patients with collagen vascular disease. Spider telangiectasias are red and arise from a central filling vessel of arteriolar origin. Red linear telangiectasias occur on the face (especially the nose) or legs. Blue linear or anastomosing telangiectasias are found most often on the legs. This chapter discusses the pathophysiology and anatomy of telangiectasias that occur on the lower extremities.

PATTERNS

Two common patterns of telangiectasias on the legs of women, besides red or blue streaks, are the parallel linear pattern, usually found on the medial thigh (Fig. 4-2), and the arborizing or radiating cartwheel pattern, seen most often on the lateral thigh (Fig. 4-3).[4] These two subsets of telangiectasias seem to run in families and may form anastomosing complexes as large as 15 cm in diameter. The arborizing type on the lateral thigh usually appears with "feeding" reticular veins, (4-3) (see Chapter 1, Fig. 1-17). These complexes have been termed *venous stars, sunburst venous blemishes,* and *spider leg veins* by various authors.

PATHOGENESIS

The pathogenesis of each of the various types of telangiectasias is somewhat different. Many factors may play a role in the development of new blood vessels or the dilation of existing blood vessels (see Chapters 2 and 8). Also, acquired telangiectasias are thought to occur as a result of the release or activation of vasoactive substances, such as hormones and chemicals, under a multitude of conditions, including anoxia, infection, and the presence of certain physical factors, which results in capillary or venular neogenesis.[3,5,6] The box on p. 121 (which is an extension of the observations of Shelley[7] and Anderson and Smith[8]) lists the major causes and diseases associated with telangiectasias that may appear on the lower extremities.

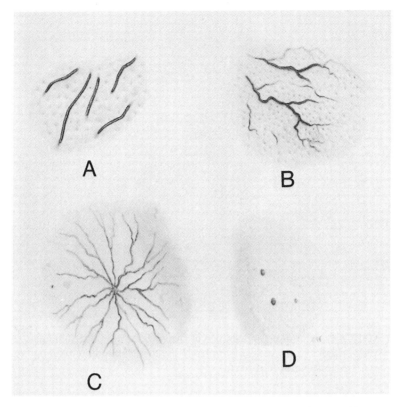

Fig. 4-1 Four types of telangiectasias. **A,** Simple. **B,** Arborized. **C,** Spider. **D,** Papular. (Adapted from Reddish W and Peltzer RH: Am Heart J 37:106, 1949.)

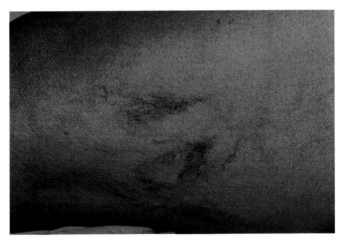

Fig. 4-2 Typical appearance of telangiectasia located at the medial thigh in a 54-year-old woman. Note the feeding reticular vein proximal to the telangiectasia.

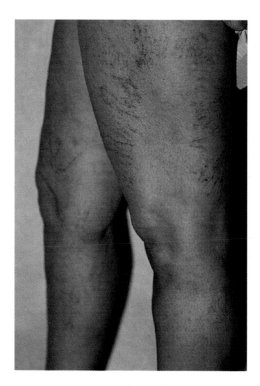

Fig. 4-3   Common appearance of cartwheel or radiating telangiectasia pattern on the lateral thigh of a 42-year-old woman. Note the feeding blue reticular vein at the distal aspect of the telangiectatic pattern.

INCIDENCE

The incidence of varicose and telangiectatic leg veins in the general population is presented in Chapter 2. The relationship between varicose veins and spider leg veins (telangiectasias) is intimate, so much of the anatomy and pathophysiology of telangiectasia is presented in Chapters 1 and 3.

Telangiectasia increase in incidence with advancing age.[9] The prevalence of telangiectasia in the neonate is 3.8%, with 26% occurring on the legs.[10]

Two recent surveys have detailed the characteristics of patients seeking treatment of these unwanted spider leg veins. Duffy,[11] in a nonrandomized survey of his patients, reported a 90% family history of varicose or telangiectatic leg veins. The patients included three sets of identical twins with similar appearances of leg telangiectasia. Sadick,[12] in a nonrandomized survey of 100 patients seeking treatment, found a 43% family history of varicose or telangiectatic leg veins. Both surveys found that one third of the patients first noted the development of these veins during pregnancy. Duffy notes that the veins became most severe after the third pregnancy. Between 20% and 30% of patients developed these veins before pregnancy, and 18% of women noted the onset of the veins when they were taking oral contraceptives. Both authors conclude that the development of leg telangiectasia is probably a partially sex-linked, autosomal, dominant condition with incomplete penetrance and variable expressivity.

PATHOPHYSIOLOGY

Many conditions—inherited, acquired, and iatrogenic—are known to be involved in the formation of telangiectasias.

CAUSES OF CUTANEOUS TELANGIECTASIA OF THE LOWER EXTREMITIES

GENETIC/CONGENITAL FACTORS
Vascular nevi
  Nevus flammeus
    Klippel-Trenaunay syndrome
  Nevus araneus
  Angioma serpiginosum
  Bockenheimer's syndrome
Congenital neuroangiopathies
  Maffucci's syndrome
Congenital poikiloderma
  (Rothmund-Thomson syndrome)
Essential progressive telangiectasia
Cutis marmorata telangiectatica congenita
Diffuse neonatal hemangiomatosis

**ACQUIRED DISEASE WITH A SECONDARY
  CUTANEOUS COMPONENT**
Collagen vascular diseases
  Lupus erythematosus
  Dermatomyositis
  Progressive systemic sclerosis
  Cryoglobulinemia
Other
  Telangiectasia macularis eruptiva perstans
    (mastocytosis)
  Human immunodeficiency virus
    (HTLV-III)

**COMPONENT OF A PRIMARY CUTANEOUS
  DISEASE**
Varicose veins
Keratosis lichenoides chronica
Other acquired/primary cutaneous diseases
  Necrobiosis lipoidica diabeticorum
  Capillaritis (purpura annularis telangi-
    ectodes)
  Malignant atrophic papulosis (Degos'
    disease)

HORMONAL FACTORS
Pregnancy
Estrogen therapy
Topical corticosteroid preparations

PHYSICAL FACTORS
Actinic neovascularization and/or vascular
  dilation
Trauma
  Contusion
  Surgical incision/laceration
Infection
  Generalized essential telangiectasia
  Progressive ascending telangiectasia
  Human immunodeficiency virus
    (HTLV-III)
Radiodermatitis
Erythema ab igne (heat/infrared radiation)

Modified from Goldman MP and Bennett RG: Treatment of telangiectasia: a review, J Am Acad Dermatol 17:167, 1987.

Genetic/Congenital Factors

Numerous genetic or congenital conditions (listed in the box above) display cutaneous telangiectasia. The pathogenesis for the development of telangiectasia in these syndromes is unknown. Genetic syndromes that may produce telangiectasias on the legs include nevus flammeus (alone or as a component of Klippel-Trenaunay syndrome), nevus araneus, angioma serpiginosum, congenital neuroangiopathies (especially Maffucci's syndrome), congenital poikiloderma, essential progressive or generalized telangiectasia, cutis marmorata telangiectatica congenita, and diffuse neonatal hemangiomatosis.

Nevus flammeus

Nevus flammeus (port-wine stain) affects 0.3% to 1% of the population.[13,14] Women are affected twice as often as men.[15,16] The occurrence is usually sporadic, but a 10% familial incidence,[15] and an autosomal dominant inheritance have been described.[17-20] The lesions occur in various shapes and sizes on any part of the body. They most commonly occur on the face but may cover large areas of the skin, in-

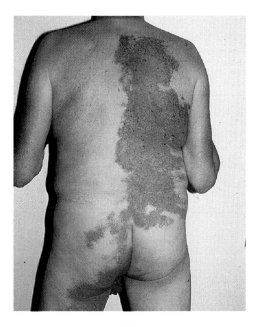

Fig. 4-4 Nevus flammeus in a 68-year-old man without any associated soft tissue abnormalities. Note that the lesion extends down the posterior thigh.

cluding an entire arm, leg, or trunk (Fig. 4-4). Lesions often overlay the distribution of peripheral nerves. Nevus flammeus is usually macular and varies in color depending on the extent and depth of vascular involvement. Lesions become progressively nodular and darker with time and may ulcerate and bleed from minor trauma.

Histologic examination shows a collection of thin-walled capillary and cavernous vessels arranged in a loose fashion throughout the superficial and deep dermis (Fig. 4-5). These vessels represent dilations of the postcapillary venules of the superficial dermis with a mean vessel depth of 0.46 mm.[21] In infancy, histopathologic changes of the cutaneous vasculature are minimal. With advancing age, these lesions usually undergo a progressive ectasia and erythrocyte stasis.[21] Rarely, cavernous hemangiomas arising from arteriovenous malformations may occur within the lesions.[22] There also may be evidence of neovascularization or other vascular malformation.[21] Further, some lesions may be associated with prominent telangiectasias and reticular varicose veins when present over the lower limbs.

Nevus flammeus can also be a component of other congenital vascular diseases. The most commonly associated disease involving the leg is Klippel-Trenaunay syndrome (KTS) (Fig. 4-6). With this latter entity, the cutaneous vascular abnormality is associated with underlying varicose and telangiectatic veins with or without significant abnormalities of the deep and superficial system or arteriovenous anastomoses. In addition, hypertrophy of soft tissue and bone may occur with overgrowth of the involved extremity (Figs. 4-7 and 4-8).

The cause of KTS is unknown. Its prevalence in newborns is estimated to be 1:25,000.[23] There is no apparent hereditary factor.[24] Some authors speculate that

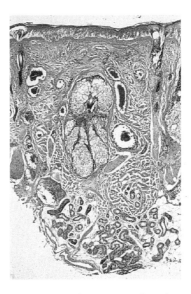

Fig. 4-5 Histologic section of a nevus flammeus taken from the forehead of a 66-year-old man immediately after treatment with the argon laser. Note the location of the enlarged blood vessels within the middle and deep dermis. Because this lesion has just been treated, the overlying epidermis demonstrates thermal changes, and the vessels are thrombosed. (Hematoxylin-eosin, ×80) (Courtesy Richard Fitzpatrick, M.D.)

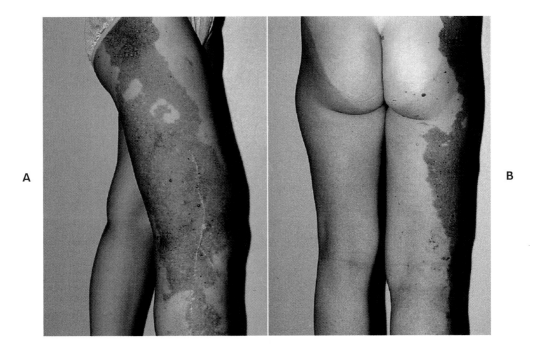

Fig. 4-6 **A** and **B**, Woman, 16 years old, with Klippel-Trenaunay syndrome and associated varicose veins and nevus flammeus of the right lower extremity from the toes to buttock.

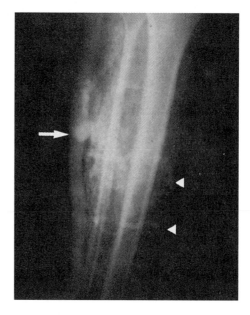

Fig. 4-7 Venogram film of the right calf (anteroposterior projection) of patient shown in Fig. 4-6. There are multiple dilated collateral dermal venules *(arrowheads)* and a grossly enlarged lateral accessory saphenous vein along the posterolateral aspect of the calf *(arrow)*, which is avalvular. The deep venous system is absent. (Courtesy Christopher Sebrechts, M.D.)

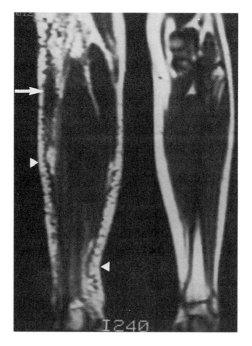

Fig. 4-8 Magnetic resonance image, coronal T1-weighted, of the calves (TR500, TE 20) of patient in Fig. 4-6. There are multiple small collateral vessels in the subcutaneous fat of the right calf seen as a spaghetti-like accumulation of dermal venulectases *(arrowheads)*. Note the enlarged lateral accessory vein present along the posterolateral aspect of the right calf *(arrow)*.

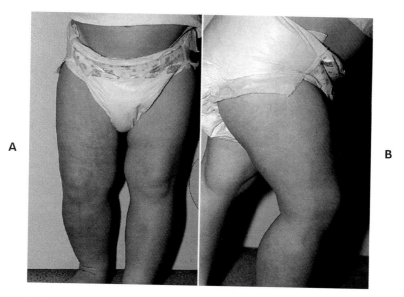

Fig. 4-9 A, One-year-old girl with KTS on the right leg manifesting as cutaneous port-wine stain vascular malformation of the medial calf and thigh, elongation of the affected limb (note bent knee to compensate for the 1 cm increased length), and soft tissue hypertrophy of the affected limb noted in an increased diameter. B, Lateral view demonstrating a prominent lateral varicosity 6 mm in diameter that was incompetent through its entire length with Valsalva positive incompetence.

an atresia, agenesis, or compression of the deep venous system by fibrous tissue is the cause.[25] Other authors suggest that a congenital weakness of the venous wall in combination with vascular hypertension from an abnormal venous system leads to the development of KTS.[26] Baskerville et al.[27] found that 68% of 49 patients with KTS had a superficial, embryologic venous channel on the lateral aspect of the thigh (Fig. 4-9). Because these veins are usually present at birth and are avalvular, histologic and venous flow studies suggest that KTS is caused by a mesodermal abnormality during fetal development, leading to persistence of arteriovenous communications that result in the triad of nevus flammeus, soft tissue hypertrophy, and varicosities.[28] This entire patient population had clinical varicose veins, and 88% had pain and limb swelling. Twenty-two percent had severe hemorrhage from varicose vein rupture, and 6% had a history of superficial thrombophlebitis. Baskerville et al. recommended sugical excision/avulsion of symptomatic *superficial* varices. Villavilacencio recently reported his experience with 14 patients and also recommends surgical excision followed by sclerotherapy to treat patients with intractable symptoms.[29]

Servelle unquestionably has the largest experience with KTS, reporting on 786 patients.[30] He found venographic evidence for obstruction in most of his patients and postulates that changes seen in this syndrome are manifestations of this process. In addition to the cutaneous and soft tissue findings described above, he notes a 36% incidence of varicose veins in his patient population. Concomitant malformations of the deep venous system (avalvulia, aneurysmata, aplasia, lateral marginal veins) have been found in up to 94% of all patients.[31] He recommends surgical intervention to the *deep* venous system and cautions against treating superficial varicosities because of the possibility of increasing outflow obstruction.

Proteus syndrome is a congenital hamartomatous condition that may have overlapping features with KTS.[32] Wiedemann et al. in 1983 described the syndrome as consisting of partial gigantism of the hands and/or feet, hemihypertrophy, pigmented nevi, soft tissue tumors, macrocephaly, and other hamartomatous changes.[33] Prominent capillary hemangiomas, telangiectasia, and varicosities also have been noted in these patients.[34-37] These clinical findings are evident usually at or shortly after birth. This condition may represent a somatic mutation that influences the local regulation or production of tissue growth factors.[38]

When associated with KTS, cutaneous telangiectasias, venulectases, and varicose veins occur in the distribution of the underlying vascular malformation of soft tissue and bone. Some patients may have a persistence of an embryologic lateral limb bud vein. The large drainage capacity of this vein may limit venous hypertension. In this instance, microcirculatory change, rather than large vessel change, may account for limb hypertrophy.[39]

Therefore, because KTS can be composed of a variable venous system, sclerotherapy treatment must be performed only after a thorough vascular evaluation. A complete discussion of the surgical management of KTS or the vascular component of Proteus syndrome is beyond the scope of this text. In short, if an incompetent feeding varicose vein is found along with an intact deep venous system, it can be avulsed safely. This is often combined with sclerotherapy to distal varices. Care must be taken to ensure adequate venous return from remaining vessels. Treating perforating veins is usually quite difficult because there may be hundreds of connections between the superficial and deep venous systems.[40]

Sclerotherapy to nontruncal varicose and telangiectatic veins can restore some degree of venous competency and relieve symptoms. In addition to a heavy, tired feeling of the affected limb, patients may be bothered by recurrent bleeding from cutaneous vascular blebs. These vessels are easily traumatized, and trauma may lead to cutaneous and soft-tissue infections. Sclerosing these vessels is helpful and has been practiced for more than 60 years.[41]

Laser or photocoagulation is reserved for cutaneous ectasia, which usually occurs within the nevus flammeus. These manifestations are not treated for cosmetic reasons but to prevent bleeding and infection (Fig. 4-10) (see Chapter 12).

Nevus araneus

Nevus araneus (spider telangiectasia) may occur as a component of a number of congenital and acquired diseases. They are found in up to 15% of the normal population and increase in number during pregnancy, liver disease, and many other conditions.[42] Ninety-nine percent occur above the umbilicus.[42,43]

The lesions appear as bright red macules composed of a central red dot, with fine blood vessels radiating from the center (Fig. 4-11). The central vessel may pulsate, indicating its arteriolar origin. Point compression of the central dot blanches the radiating vessels. One genetic disease with this form of telangiectasia distributed on the lower extremities is ataxia telangiectasia, which may have lesions in the popliteal fossae.[44,45]

Vascular spiders arise from the terminal arteriole (see Fig. 4-11).[3] The pressure of blood within the spider telangiectasia is lower than systolic pressure and higher than venous pressure. One measurement demonstrated its pressure to be 85 mm Hg when systolic pressure was 120 mm Hg.[46] The vessels arise within the deep dermis and push their way up into the superficial dermis as a space-occupying lesion. The central arteriole connects to dilated venous saccules with radiating venous legs in the papillary dermis.[42] Detailed histologic studies have provided little understanding of the factors responsible for the initial growth.[47]

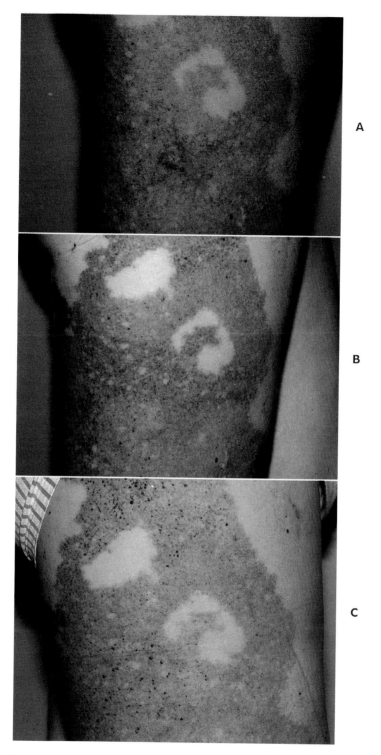

Fig. 4-10 Before (A) and after (B) treatment of a section of the nevus flammeus and associated superficial varicosity of the patient shown in Fig. 4-6. The reticular veins were treated with polidocanol 0.75% (6 ml total) followed by multiple impacts with the Candela SPTL-I pulsed-dye laser at 8J/cm². **C,** Clinical appearance 5 years after last sclerotherapy/laser treatment. Note the recurrence of venules and vascular ectasia.

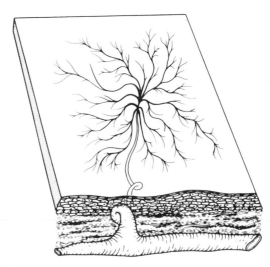

Fig. 4-11 Schematic diagram of a nevus araneus (arteriolar spider) showing the origin at a dermal arteriole with coiled extension to the superficial dermis and branching horizontal "arms."

Because the spider telangiectasia is composed of a central arteriole, sclerotherapy of these lesions usually produces cutaneous ulcerations (see Chapter 8). Therefore, treatment with the pulsed-dye laser at 577 to 585 nm, continuous wave lasers at 511 to 577 nm, Photoderm™ thermal coagulation or electrodesiccation to fibrose the central feeding arteriole is recommended (see Chapter 12).

Angioma serpiginosum

Angioma serpiginosum is a rare nevoid disorder of the upper dermal vasculature. The disease usually occurs on the lower extremities in women, and has its onset in childhood. Although occurrence of most cases is sporadic, one family study suggests an autosomal dominant inheritance.[48] Lesions appear as small erythematous puncta occurring in groups that enlarge by forming new puncta at the periphery while those at the center fade. This results in a reticular or serpiginous pattern. A dilation of the subpapillary venous plexus may lead to telangiectasia. Histologic examination shows a number of ectatic capillaries in the superficial dermis. Endothelial cells appear hyperplastic and have an increased number of interendothelial junctions and vacuolization. Capillary walls are thickened with multiple basal laminae and a "heavy" precipitation of fine fibrillar material. The deeper dermis is unremarkable.[49] Therefore, angioma serpiginosum may represent a type of capillary nevus.

Bockenheimer's syndrome (diffuse genuine phlebectasia)

Diffuse genuine phlebectasia was first described by Bockenheimer in 1907.[50] A recent review has documented 40 cases in the literature.[51] This rare syndrome represents a deep venous malformation that begins in childhood (rarely present at birth). Large multiple venous sinusoids or cavernous hemangiomas develop, usually on an extremity. These frequently thrombose, hemorrhage, and ulcerate, and they may ultimately progress to gangrenous infection. Unilateral localization is common. Secondary cutaneous telangiectasia develops in response to venous hypertension. Late manifestations are soft tissue and/or bone hypotrophy or hypertrophy.

Compression therapy is generally beneficial to prevent the manifestations of both venous hypertension and thrombosis. Surgical excision and phlebectomy have produced varying results, generally with recurrence.[52,53] Sclerotherapy has been successful in one of two cases.[54,55]

Maffucci's syndrome

Maffucci's syndrome is a congenital, nonfamilial dysplasia consisting of a constellation of vascular malformation and dyschondroplasia. Patients have single or multiple hemangiomas, varicosities, and telangiectasia of the legs. Dyschondroplasia and endochondromas occur as bony nodules on the fingers, toes, and extremities, and patients have unequal bone growth and slow union of easily sustained fractures. The distribution of vascular lesions often does not correspond to that of the skeletal lesions. In addition to the hemangioma, lymphangiomas and lymphectasis may be present.

The syndrome affects all races, affects men and women equally, and has no evidence of a familial tendency.[56] Twenty-five percent of patients have symptoms within the first year of life, and 78% manifest symptoms before puberty.[56] From 25% to 30% of patients develop malignancies including chondrosarcoma, angiosarcoma, lymphangiosarcoma, glioma, fibrosarcoma, pancreatic carcinoma, and ovarian teratoma.[56-59] Surgical excision or sclerotherapy treatment to symptomatic vascular lesions is helpful.[29]

Congenital poikiloderma

Congenital poikiloderma (Rothmund-Thomson syndrome) is a rare neurocutaneous syndrome that has its onset in the first year of life. There appears to be a female predominance. Although an autosomal dominant inheritance has been demonstrated, 70% of cases show a familial recessive inheritance.[60] A fine telangiectatic network first appears on the cheeks and progresses within a year to the head, arms, buttocks, and legs. There may be associated scaling of the skin and lichenoid papules. The hair is often sparse, and the skin is soft and translucent. Dwarfism, cataracts, dental abnormalities, mental retardation, hypogenitalism, and diabetes mellitus may occur.[60]

Essential progressive telangiectasia

Essential progressive telangiectasia (EPT) is a rare entity that has been reported in association with bronchogenic carcinoma,[61] angiokeratomas,[62] chronic sinusitis,[63] and an autoimmune setting.[64] It most commonly is essential in nature. EPT has been reported to be associated with small varicose veins that occur many years after disease onset.[65] Histochemical examination establishes the vessels in EPT to be venular in origin.[66] Lesions appear as blue to bright-red telangiectasias 0.1 to 0.4 mm in diameter. There may be an associated peritelangiectatic atrophy of the subcutaneous tissues. Lesions most commonly appear on the feet and distal leg but rarely involve the entire leg.

The treatment of these lesions is often fraught with complications because many of the telangiectasias are intimately associated with arterioles. This leads to frequent recurrence of previously treated vessels. However, cautious treatment with sclerotherapy, pulsed-dye laser, or Photoderm™ thermal coagulation may be successful[65] (see Chapter 12).

Cutis marmorata telangiectatica congenita

Cutis marmorata telangiectatica congenita is a rare congenital cutaneous vascular anomaly consisting of a sharply demarcated, reticulated vascular network of blue-violet venules associated with telangiectasia, with or without varicose veins. The cutis marmorata component is neither transient nor related to temperature. Telangiectasias may not appear in the first 2 years.[67-69] Lesions are most prominent on the lower extremities but may involve any cutaneous surface. Involvement may be unilateral or bilateral. Atrophy and ulcerations of the overlying skin may occur over time.[70] There may be an associated nevus flammeus. Lesions have also been reported to spontaneously improve in up to three-fourths of patients within the first 2 years.[69]

Most cases of this disease occur sporadically, and two thirds of the approximately 80 reported cases occurred in women.[67-69,71] The pathogenesis is most likely multifactorial; genetic (autosomal dominant inheritance[72,73]) and teratogenic factors are most commonly cited.

Histologic examination demonstrates an abnormal dilation of capillaries and veins.[74] Associated congenital abnormalities have been reported in up to 50% of patients. These include structural defects of the musculoskeletal system, ocular and dental malformations, and arteriovenous malformations.[75] Cutaneous atrophy, nevus telangiectaticus, and hypertrophy or atrophy of the affected limbs are also reported.[76]

Diffuse neonatal hemangiomatosis

Diffuse neonatal hemangiomatosis is a rare congenital disorder of vascular development, occurring in infancy with multiple visceral hemangiomas. The combination of hepatic and cutaneous hemangiomas occurs twice as often in girls as in boys.[77] Hemangiomas are usually present on the skin and may be associated with large areas involved with telangiectasias and venulectases (Fig. 4-12).

Infants with this disorder often die of high-output cardiac failure as a result of arteriovenous shunting of blood flow through the hemangiomas. Recognition of the cutaneous component, which may be minimal in some infants, will help to prevent confusion of the cardiac failure with a congenital heart disease.[78] Therapy consists of systemic steroids, selective embolization, and/or surgical excision.[56] Selective sclerotherapy of the telangiectasias may be performed for cosmetic improvement.

Acquired Disease with a Secondary Cutaneous Component

Telangiectasias that occur as a component of an acquired or primary cutaneous disease evolve from multiple factors. When associated with collagen vascular diseases, relative tissue anoxia may result in the appearance of telangiectasias, especially in connection with an acral distribution. Alternatively, circulating cryoglobulins may lead to acral telangiectasia. Periungual telangiectasia is particularly common in lupus erythematosus and progressive systemic sclerosis. In addition, various vasculitic factors or other immunologic factors associated with these diseases may lead to the appearance of telangiectasias, particularly in areas where other physical factors (such as actinic damage) are prominent.

In some conditions (for example, mastocytosis), a component of the disease itself, such as the release of various mast cell vasoactive factors, especially histamine or heparin, may lead to the development of telangiectasias.[79,80] Histologic studies in a patient with unilateral facial telangiectasia macularis eruptiva perstans demonstrated an accumulation of mast cells.[81]

Component of a Primary Cutaneous Disease
Varicose veins

Varicose veins lead to the development of telangiectasia most likely through associated venous hypertension with resulting angiogenesis or vascular dilation,[42]

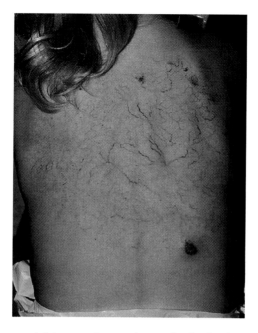

Fig. 4-12 Diffuse neonatal hemangiomatosis on the back of a $2\frac{1}{2}$-year-old girl. The telangiectatic component was present at birth. Within the first few months cutaneous hemangiomas began to appear. A large mediastinal hemangioma was also noted surrounding the esophagus. Systemic treatment with corticosteroids did not result in any notable decrease in the size of the internal or cutaneous hemangiomas. The patient remains well now at age 13.

or through an associated increased distensibility of the telangiectatic vein wall (see Chapter 3). Although telangiectasias associated with varicose veins may appear at first as erythematous streaks, with time they turn blue. Often they are directly associated with underlying varicose veins, so the distinction between telangiectasias and varicose veins becomes blurred.[42] Telangiectasias have been shown by multiple investigators with various techniques to be associated with underlying reticular veins. Tretbar[82] studied 100 patients with telangiectasias (<1 mm diameter) with the venous Doppler and found that they are connected with associated "feeding" reticular veins. These veins were separate from any truncal varicosities that may have been present. All blue reticular veins demonstrated reflux that did not appear to originate from the greater or lessor saphenous veins. In patients with blue reticular veins, 50% demonstrated reflux from incompetent calf perforating veins. Weiss and Weiss confirmed these findings with Doppler examination of 700 patients. They noted audible reflux in 88% of patients whose telangiectasias were associated with a "feeding" reticular vein.[83] In addition, they confirmed that enhanced therapeutic efficacy with decreased postsclerotherapy hyperpigmentation occurred when the reticular veins were treated prior to treating distal telangiectasia.[84] Duplex scanning also has demonstrated telangiectasia to be associated with "feeding" reticular veins.[85,86] Somjen et al. found that 89% of telangiectasia had closely situated incompetent reticular veins.[86] Finally, direct radiographic imaging has shown connections between telangiectasia and both the deep and superficial venous systems.[87] Importantly, 2 of 15 telangiectasias examined were found to connect directly to the deep venous system without any obvious cutaneous sign. This emphasizes the importance of postsclerotherapy compression when treating telangiectasia (see Chapters 6, 8, and 11). Therefore, it is clear that treatment of the feeding varicosity results in treatment of the distal telangiectasia (see Chapters 9 and 11). If no apparent connection exists between deep collecting or reticular vessels, the telangiectasia may arise from a terminal arteriole or arteriovenous anastomosis.[88]

Telangiectasias may be associated with underlying venous disease even when there are no clinical abnormalities. Thibault and Bray[89] have evaluated 83 patients with spider leg veins with duplex and Doppler examinations. They found that 23% of these patients without clinically apparent varicose veins had incompetence of the superficial venous system. In addition, 1.2% had incompetence of a perforator vein. Nineteen patients, each with one clinically abnormal leg and one clinically normal leg, were also evaluated. Interestingly, 37% of clinically normal legs demonstrated incompetence of the superficial system. The abnormal legs in this group had a 74% incidence of incompetence of the superficial system, and 21% had saphenofemoral incompetence. This study demonstrates the need for both a clinical and noninvasive diagnostic work-up in patients who have spider veins and reinforces the view that spider veins arise from underlying varicose veins via venous hypertension.

A proposed mechanism for the development of leg telangiectasia associated with underlying venous disease is that preexisting vascular anastomotic channels open in response to venous stasis.[90] Venous stasis with resulting venous hypertension leads to a reversal of flow from venules back to capillaries. The resulting capillary hypertension leads to opening and dilation of normally closed vessels. Consequently, relative anoxia, as a result of reversed venous flow, leads to angiogenesis. Merlen[88] states that capillaries and venules have an enhanced neogenic potential and a remarkable tendency toward neogenesis in a hypoxic atmosphere.

In addition, Braverman has distinguished between the arterial and venous sides of the microcirculation based on the ultrastructural characteristic of the vascular basement membrane, which appears homogeneous in arterial vessels and multilaminated in venous vessels.[91] With this finding, he has demonstrated changes from arterial to venous vessels in various cutaneous disorders, such as psoriasis, within 48 to 72 hours. It is postulated that this change occurs secondary to changes in circulation pressure. Thus, the development of venulectases and telangiectasias in venous hypertension may respresent the conversion of preexisting capillaries into venules.

Keratosis lichenoides chronica

Prominent telangiectasia of the feet and legs has been described in patients with keratosis lichenoides chronica.[92] This condition is usually not associated with telangiectasia.[93] However, severe pruritus was also present in these patients, and, although the authors ascribed the development of the telangiectasia and lichenoid papules to the same process, it appears to be equally likely that both physical manifestations could be caused by chronic rubbing and scratching. Thus it is difficult to separate the development of telangiectasia into primary and secondary processes in this disease.

Other acquired primary cutaneous diseases

As with telangiectasia of acquired cutaneous disease, telangiectasia of primary cutaneous disease rarely affects the legs, with the obvious exception of varicose veins. Other cutaneous diseases with associated telangiectasia are necrobiosis lipoidica diabeticorum, capillaritis (purpura annularis telangiectodes [Majocchi's disease]) and malignant atrophic papulosis (Degos' disease).

The pigmented purpuric eruptions (progressive pigmentary dermatitis (Schamberg's disease), pigmented purpuric lichenoid dermatosis (Gougerot-Blum syndrome), lichen aureus, and purpura annularis telangiectodes (Majocchi's disease) share the common pathogenic denominator of dilatation of the superficial papillary dermal capillaries with occasional endothelial proliferation. These conditions are manifested by punctate purpuric lesions and telangiectasia predominately located on the lower legs. Most patients do not have manifestations of venous hypertension. Capillary microscopy in 12 patients disclosed ectatic dilated venules in the subpapillary plexus.[94] Iwatsuki et al. have found fibrinoid degeneration and occlusive damage with swollen endothelia in 3 of 8 patients with this condition. Eight of 8 had evidence of direct immunofluorescence with C3, C1q, and fibrin in papillary vessels.[95] These findings suggest an immunologic process for the pathogenesis.

Treatment of telangiectasias caused by an acquired or primary cutaneous disease usually is best accomplished by treatment of the acquired disease itself. The telangiectatic component of these lesions is usually asymptomatic and requires no treatment except for cosmesis. In that case, electrodesiccation or the tunable continuous dye, pulsed-dye lasers, or Photoderm™ thermal coagulation may be the treatment of choice (see Chapter 12).

Hormonal Factors

Pregnancy and estrogen therapy

The hormonal influence in the development of telangiectasia is well known. Pregnancy is perhaps the most common physiologic condition that leads to the development of telangiectasia. This was first suggested by Corbett in 1914.[46] Bean[42] has estimated that almost 70% of women develop telangiectasia during pregnancy, the majority of which disappear between 3 and 6 weeks postpartum (Fig. 4-13). Pregnant women often develop telangiectasia on the legs within a few

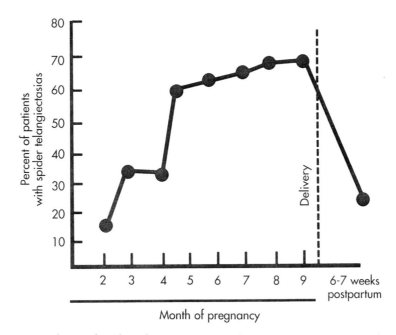

Fig. 4-13   Incidence of spider telangiectasias in white pregnant women as a function of the duration of pregnancy. (From Bean WB: Vascular spiders and related lesions of the skin, Springfield, Ill, 1958, Charles C Thomas.)

weeks of conception, even before the uterus has enlarged to compress venous return to the pelvis.[96,97] Also, pregnant women and those taking birth control pills have been shown to have an increase in the distensibility of vein walls.[98] This increase in distensibility has also been noted to fluctuate with the normal menstrual cycle.[99] It was found that leg volume was greatest just before ovulation and during menses. The increased distensibility did not fully correlate with one specific hormone but was related to both estrogen and progesterone levels or ratios.

Hormonal stimulation may also lead to the development of telangiectasia, independent of the effect on venous distensibility. Paradoxically, estrogen has been found to be beneficial in controlling symptoms of venous distensibility during pregnancy (see Chapter 3).[100] Thus some hormonal influence is involved in the development of varicose veins and their associated telangiectasias in women (see Chapter 2), but the exact hormonal mechanism for telangiectasia development is unknown.

Davis and Duffy[101] reported an apparent association of estrogen excess states with the development of telangiectatic matting after sclerotherapy of spider leg veins. In their selected patient population of 160, 29% of women who developed "new" telangiectasias were taking systemic estrogens or became pregnant, compared with 19% of patients on hormones who did not develop telangiectatic matting. One additional patient noted the disappearance of both spider veins and telangiectatic matting after taking the antiestrogen tamoxifen citrate (Nolvadex). Biopsies of these patients were not performed.

Estrogen acts by entering its target cell and associating with an extranuclear receptor protein. This complex then enters the nucleus and modulates ribonucleic acid (RNA) synthesis.[102] Because endothelial cells have been found to possess estrogen receptors, they may be potential target cells.[103] Sadick and Neidt[104] assayed 20 patients with leg telangiectasias for estrogen receptors. Interestingly, they failed to find any evidence of such receptors in their patient population. They postulated that either estrogen receptors are not present in increased numbers in leg telangiectasia, or estrogen acts on endothelium through an indirect pathway. This pathway may be a stimulation of angiogenic factors (see Chapter 8) or an increase in vascular distensibility.

The hormonal influence in telangiectasia neogenesis has been noted in 17 of 46, and 10 of 15, reported cases of unilateral nevoid telangiectasia syndrome respectively.[105,106] In these female patients, the telangiectasias did not occur until triggered by pregnancy or puberty and correlated with high serum estrogen levels. Four of the remaining 5 cases were associated with alcoholic cirrhosis, and 1 was congenital. There was no association with the development of varicose veins. Progesterone receptors have also been reported in 2 patients with unilateral nevoid telangiectasia; one developed following metastases from a carcinoid tumor of the stomach.[107,108]

Topical corticosteroid preparations

The development of telangiectatic blood vessels may also occur from self-induced hormonal manipulation. A common form of iatrogenic telangiectasia may occur from the use of high-potency topical steroid preparations. Leyden[109] first reported the development of rosacea associated with telangiectasia in 10 patients who regularly used topical fluorinated steroids on the face. Katz and Prawer[110] demonstrated clinical cutaneous vascular dilation and network development within 2 weeks of treatment with superpotent topical steroids (betamethasone dipropionate in an optimized vehicle and clobetasol ointment). This type of steroid-induced telangiectasia probably reflects the loss of perivascular ground substance, allowing distention of existing vessels, or the capillary elongation and distortion generated to meet the requirement of the hyperplastic epidermis.[111] In support of this theory, covert vascular visualization has been shown to represent the early changes of cutaneous atrophy that occur as a result of steroid use.[112] Facial telangiectasia has been reported to develop in association with long-term application of a topical corticosteroid to the scalp.[113] In this report the long-term use of betamethasone valerate lotion allowed percutaneous absorption of a sufficient amount to spread locally from the scalp to the face via the dermal vasculature. Therefore, topical application of corticosteroid preparations can induce the development or appearance of telangiectasia.

Physical Factors

Actinic neovascularization and vascular dilation

Physical factors are commonly responsible for acquired telangiectasia. Telangiectasias are noted to appear after many types of physical trauma. The most common form of physical damage to the skin is that caused from sun exposure.[114,115] Telangiectasia of the face is probably a manifestation of persistent active arteriolar vasodilation caused by weakness in the vessel wall, resulting from degenerative elastic changes or weakness in the surrounding connective tissue caused by chronic sun exposure. Alternatively, Ultraviolet B (UVB) exposure has been shown to elevate epidermal tumor necrosis factor (TNF).[116] TNF has been demonstrated to promote angiogenesis by various mechanisms that may also lead to the development of new vessels, in addition to dilation of existing vessels.[117] Finally, the aging process itself may lead to vessel dilation. Perivascular veil cells and adventitial cells are believed to be responsible for the synthesis and maintenance of the peripheral portion of the vascular wall of dermal blood vessels.[91] These cells are decreased in number with aging, which correlates with a histologic thinning of vascular walls.[118] Thus, direct or indirect ultraviolet light and the aging process contribute to the development of telangiectasia.

Ultraviolet-induced telangiectasias most often arise from arterioles and are seen frequently in individuals with fair complexions, often on the nose, especially on the ala and nasolabial crease. A similar mechanism for the pathogenesis of type I telangiectasias may also apply to their occurrence on the legs. An examination of more than 20,000 Americans[119] demonstrated the presence of fine telangiectasias in 17.3% of men and 11.6% of women with low sun exposure, compared with 30.1% of men and 26.2% of women who report high sun exposure. More significant, 15.5% of men and 40.9% of women with actinic skin damage were shown to have spider leg veins, compared with 6% of men and 28.9% of women without actinic skin damage. Sun exposure with resulting damage to subcutaneous and cutaneous tissues is a significant etiologic factor in the appearance of telangiectasias.

Trauma

Contusion

Various forms of physical trauma may lead to the development of new blood vessel growth. Contusion injuries are a common mechanism for the development of a localized growth of telangiectasias (Fig. 4-14). Neovascularization in this case is probably the result of epidermal and endothelial damage with the release of angiogenic factors, including fibrin.[120] Trauma also causes a rapid change in the permeability of cutaneous blood vessels through the release of various mediators.[80] The increased permeability of endothelium may lead to angiogenesis through multiple mechanisms.[121]

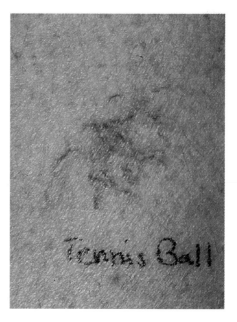

Fig. 4-14   Posterior thigh of a 35-year-old woman hit with a tennis ball 1 year previously. The resulting telangiectatic mass developed shortly after resolution of the bruise.

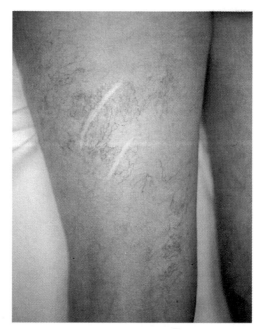

Fig. 4-15   At 18 years of age this woman underwent an extensive ligation and stripping of her varicose veins. She developed extensive telangiectasia around all of the surgical sites within weeks of the surgical procedure. This photograph was taken 22 years after the surgical procedure. (Courtesy John Bergan, M.D.)

A solitary giant spider angioma with an overlying pyogenic granuloma was described recently.[122] This spider angioma was associated with alcoholic liver cirrhosis. The authors postulated that local mechanical irritation led to a reactive proliferation of the endothelial cells. When the central pyogenic granuloma was removed, the surrounding spider telangiectasia disappeared.

Surgical incision/lacerations

Surgical incision or cutaneous laceration are common events that require physiologic neovascularization. Here angiogenesis is a prerequisite for the development of wound healing.[120] Fibrin deposition appears to play a prominent role in wound healing by stimulating new blood vessel growth.[120,123] The resulting formation of blood vessels has been demonstrated to represent a dilation and extension of existing blood vessels.[80] Unfortunately, some postsurgical patients develop an exaggerated angiogenic response with resulting cutaneous telangiectasia. Although this may occur at sites of ligation for vein stripping (Fig. 4-15), the most common surgical event that leads to the development of telangiectasia is the skin flap procedure. When a skin flap is under excessive tension, telangiectasias may develop at the edge of the flap. This excessive blood vessel growth may result from the influence of mechanical forces on the wound. Histologic examination demonstrates the orientation of vascular fiber networks along lines of tension. This orientation may be related to the activation of cell growth through stretching.[124] Thus the vascularization of skin flaps and grafts supports the concept of an epidermal stimulus for vasculogenesis.[125,126]

Infection

Generalized essential telangiectasia

Generalized essential telangiectasia is a benign form of telangiectasia of unknown etiology. It often begins in late childhood as extensive linear telangiectasia of the legs. It is more common in girls, but estrogen and progesterone receptors in the vascular lesions have not been found to be elevated.

Various infections have been associated with the development of this form of telangiectasia. Bacterium may stimulate endothelial proliferation in vitro.[127] Becker,[128] in 1926, first noted the association of generalized telangiectasia with syphilitic infection in a review of patients with generalized telangiectasia. Of those patients, 16 had evidence of syphilis, and 4% had evidence of a focal infection. Ayres Jr., Burrows, and Anderson[129] later described a patient with generalized telangiectasia and sinus infection. Resolution of the sinusitis with antibiotic treatment resulted in the disappearance of the telangiectasia.

Progressive ascending telangiectasia

Shelley[130] and Shelley and Fierer[131] described two cases of essential progressive telangiectasia that resolved after empiric treatment with tetracycline and ketoconazole respectively. Electron microscopic studies in one patient[131] demonstrated focal fibrin clots in some of the dilated vessels, which disappeared within a month of ketoconazole therapy. They postulated a microbial-induced focal intravascular coagulation as the etiologic factor in the pathogenesis of this rare form of acquired telangiectasia.

Human immunodeficiency virus

Immunosupressed populations are frequently infected with a wide variety of bacteria, fungal, and yeast species. The first report of neovascularization in immunosupressed patients was an HIV-positive hemophiliac man with numerous telangiectasias on the shins, which resolved after treatment with tetracycline.[132] Unfortunately, the specific infection involved is usually difficult to identify because a myriad of infections occur in this immunosuppressed population. Also, a recent survey of homosexual men with and without lymphadenopathy demonstrated that 47% had focal telangiectasias in a broad distribution across the anterior chest.[133] The presence of telangiectasias was significantly, although not exclusively, associated with HIV seropositivity. Telangiectasias in this group did not appear to be related to underlying bacterial or fungal infection or to sun exposure. The authors postulated that this clinical finding may have been a direct manifestation of HIV infectivity.

Although not telangiectatic, bacillary angiomatosis (also called epithelioid angiomatosis) is a newly recognized disease most often characterized by multiple cutaneous reddish papules. Tissue sections of these lesions have demonstrated a weakly reactive gram-negative bacillus. The cutaneous lesions resolve with antibiotic therapy. Thus, this new entity confirms an infectious etiology for the stimulation of vascular proliferation.[134]

In summary, circumstantial evidence exists that indicates a systemic or localized infection promotes the development of neovascularization. Because this association is so rare, when one considers the ubiquitous occurrence of infections in humans, the pathophysiology of this clinical association is obscure.

Radiodermatitis

Therapeutic radiation therapy may lead to the development of telangiectasia (Fig. 4-16). Chronic radiodermatitis has been noticeably decreased with the advent of mega-voltage equipment and better technique. Mega-voltage radiation beams are more penetrating than the older, lower-energy beams; this minimizes the radiation dose to the skin. However, at least 5% of patients irradiated during therapeutic radiation therapy develop cutaneous telangiectasia.[135] The fundamental pathology of chronic radiodermatitis is fibrosis of the vessels with occlusion and varying degrees of homogenization of the connective tissue. Residual superficial blood vessels are usually dilated.[136]

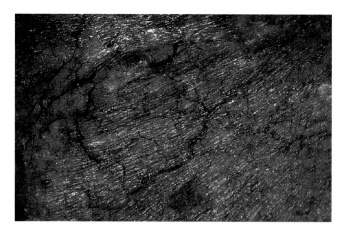

Fig. 4-16   Appearance of telangiectasia occurring as a result of radiation treatment on the lateral neck for laryngeal carcinoma 20 years previously.

Erythema ab igne

Infrared radiation/heat exposure can lead to the appearance of telangiectasia. Erythema ab igne is a localized dermatosis that occurs as reticular pigmentation and telangiectasia produced by repeated exposures to heat. It is commonly seen on the legs of women who sit close to heating units in countries without central heating. Histologic findings include epidermal atrophy, vasodilation, a dermal mixed-cellular infiltrate, and an increase in melanophages and free-lying melanin granules.[137]

REFERENCES

1. Merlen JF: Red telangiectasia, blue telangiectasias, Soc Franc Phlebol 22:167,1970.
2. Goldman MP and Bennett RG: Treatment of telangiectasia: a review, J Am Acad Dermatol 17:167, 1987.
3. Redisch W and Pelzer RH: Localized vascular dilatations of the human skin: capillary microscopy and related studies, Am Heart J 37:106, 1949.
4. Kaplan I and Peled I: The carbon dioxide laser in the treatment of superficial telangiectasias, Br J Plast Surg 28:214, 1975.
5. Ayres S Jr, Burrows LA, and Anderson NP: Generalized telangiectasias and sinus infection: report of a case with cure by treatment of chronic sinusitis, Arch Derm Syph 26:56, 1931.
6. Noe JM et al: Post rhinoplasty "red nose": differential diagnosis and treatment by laser, Plast Reconstr Surg 67:661, 1981.
7. Shelley WB: Essential progressive telangiectasia, JAMA 210:1343, 1971.
8. Anderson RL and Smith JG Jr: Unilateral nevoid telangiectasia with gastric involvement, Arch Dermatol 111:617, 1975.
9. Widmer LK: Peripheral venous disorders: prevalence and socio-medical importance: observations in 4529 apparently healthy persons. Basle Study III, Berne, Switzerland. 1978, Hans Huber.
10. Rivers JK, Frederiksen PC, and Dibdin C: A prevalence survey of dermatoses in the Australian neonate, J Am Acad Dermatol 23:77, 1990.
11. Duffy DM: Small vessel sclerotherapy: an overview, Adv Dermatol 3:221, 1988.
12. Sadick N: Treatment of varicose and telangiectatic leg veins with hypertonic saline: a comparative study of heparin and saline, J Dermatol Surg Oncol 16:24, 1990.
13. Pratt AG: Birthmarks in infants, Arch Dermat Syph 67:302, 1953.
14. Jacobs AH and Walton RG: The incidence of birthmarks in the neonate, Pediatrics 58:218, 1970.
15. Cosman B: Clinical experience in the laser therapy of port-wine stains, Lasers Surg Med 1:133, 1980.
16. Hobby LW: Treatment of port-wine stains and other cutaneous lesions, Contemp Surg 18:21, 1981.
17. Shelley WB and Livingood CS: Familial multiple nevi flammei, Arch Dermat Syph 59:343, 1949.
18. Kaplan P, Hollenberg RD, and Fraser FC: A spinal arteriovenous malformation in hereditary cutaneous hemangiomas, Am J Dis Child 130:1329, 1976.
19. Nova HR: Familial communicating hydrocephalus, posterior cerebellar agenesis, mega cisterna magna, and port-wine nevi, J Neurosurg 51:862, 1979.
20. Zaremba J et al: Hereditary neurocutaneous angioma: a new genetic entity? J Med Genet 6:443, 1979.
21. Barsky SH et al: The nature and evolution of port-wine stains: a computer-assisted study, J Invest Dermatol 74:154, 1980.
22. Finley JL et al: Port-wine stains: morphologic variations and developmental lesions, Arch Dermatol 120:1453, 1984.
23. Higurashi M et al: Live birth prevalence and follow-up of malformation syndromes in 27,472 newborns, Brain Dev 12:770, 1990.
24. Glovicki P et al: Surgical implications of Klippel-Trenaunay syndrome, Ann Surg 19:353, 1983.
25. Servelle M et al: Haematuria and rectal bleeding in the child with Klippel-Trenaunay syndrome, Ann Surg 183:410, 1976.
26. Vollmar JF et al: Aneurysmatische Transformation des Venensystems bei venosen Angiodysplasien der Gliedmassen, Vasa 18:96, 1989.
27. Baskerville PA et al: The Klippel-Trenaunay syndrome: clinical, radiological and haemodynamic features and management, Br J Surg 72:232, 1985.
28. Baskerville PA, Ackroyd JS, and Browse NL: The etiology of the Klippel-Trenaunay syndrome, Ann Surg 202:624, 1985.

29. Villavilacencio L: Treatment of varicose veins associated with congenital vascular malformations. In Bergan JB and Goldman MP, editors: Varicose and telangiectatic leg veins: diagnosis and treatment, St. Louis, 1993, Quality Medical Publishers.

30. Servelle M: Klippel and Trenaunay's syndrome, Ann Surg 197:365, 1985.

31. Paes E and Vollmar J: Diagnosis and surgical aspects of congenital venous angiodysplasia in lower extremities, sixth Annual Meeting of the American Venous Forum, Maui, February 23-35, 1994.

32. Hulsmans R-FHJ et al: "Chimp's" feet and "Tarzan's" chest constitute clinical hallmarks in many pediatric patients with Proteus syndrome, Scripta Phlebologica 2:7, 1994.

33. Wiedemann HR et al: The Proteus syndrome: partial gigantism of the hands and/or feet, nevi, hemihypertrophy, subcutaneous tumors, macrocephaly or other skull anomalies and possible accelerated growth and other visceral afflictions, Eur J Pediatr 140:5, 1983.

34. Mayatepek R et al: Expanding the phenotype of the Proteus syndrome: a severely affected patient with new findings, Am J Med Genet 32:402, 1989.

35. Cohen MM Jr and Hayden PW: A newly recognized hamartomatous syndrome. In Bergsma D, editor: Penetrance and variability in malformation syndromes, New York, 1979, Alan R. Liss, Inc., for the National Foundation-March of Dimes.

36. Fay JT and Schow SR: A possible cause of Maffucci's syndrome: report of a case, J Oral Surg 26:739, 1968.

37. Kontras SB: Case report 19, Synd Indent 2:1, 1974.

38. Clark RD et al: Proteus syndrome: an expanded phenotype, Am J Med Genet 27:99, 1987.

39. Colver GB: The clinical relevance of abnormal cutaneous vascular patterns and related pathologies. In Ryan J and Cherry GW, editors: Vascular birthmarks: pathogenesis and management, New York, 1987, Oxford University.

40. Myers TT and Janes JM: Comprehensive surgical management of cavernous hemangioma of the lower extremity with special reference to stripping, Surgery 37:184, 1955.

41. de Takats G: Vascular anomalies of the extremities, Surg Gynecol Obstet 55:227, 1932.

42. Bean WB: Vascular spiders and related lesions of the skin, Springfield, Ill, 1958, Charles C Thomas.

43. Pasyk KA: Classification and clinical and histopathological features of haemangiomas and other vascular malformations. In Ryan J and Cherry GW, editors: Vascular birthmarks: pathogenesis and management, New York, 1987, Oxford University.

44. Reed WB et al: Cutaneous manifestations of ataxia-telangiectasia, JAMA 195:126, 1966.

45. Patek AJ, Post J, and Victor JC: The vascular "spider" associated with cirrhosis of the liver, Am J Med Sci 200:341, 1946.

46. Corbett D: Discussion, Br J Dermatol 26:200, 1914.

47. Martini GA and Staubesand J: Zur morphologie der gefäcbspinnen ("vascular spider") in der Hatu Leverknankev, Virchows Archiv 324:147, 1953.

48. Marriott P, Munro D, and Ryan TJ: Angioma serpiginosum—familial incidence, Br J Dermatol 93:701, 1975.

49. Kumakiri M: Angioma serpiginosum, J Cutan Pathol 7:410, 1980.

50. Bockenheimer Ph: Uber die genuine diffuse Phlebektasie deroberen Extremitat. In Festschrift fur Georg Eduard von Rindfleisch Leipzig, 1907.

51. Hulsmans R-FHJ, Woltil HA, and Groeneweg DA: Genuine diffuse phlebectasia (Bockenheimer's syndrome) report of 5 cases and a review of the literature, Scripta Phlebologica 1:4, 1993.

52. Sonntag E: Das Rankenagion, sowie die genuine diffuse Phlebarteriektasie und Phlebektasie, Ergebn Chir Orthop 11:99, 1919.

53. Malan E and Puglionisi A: Congenital angiodysplasias of the extremities, J Cardiovasc Surg 5:87, 1964.

54. Thompson AW and Shafer JC: Congenital vascular anomalies, JAMA 145:869, 1951.

55. Kluken N and Heller W: Die genuine diffuse Phlebektasie, Folia Angiol 20(2):66, 1972.

56. Young AE, Ackroyd AE, and Baskerville P: Combined vascular malformations. In Mulliken JB and Young AE, editors: Vascular birthmarks, Philadelphia, 1988, WB Saunders.

57. Lewis RJ and Ketcham AS: Maffucci's syndrome: functional and neoplastic significance, J Bone Joint Surg 55:1465, 1973.

58. Cremer H, Gullotta F, and Wolf L: Maffucci-Kast syndrome, J Cancer Res Clin Oncol 101:231, 1981.

59. Cheng FC: Maffucci's syndrome with fibroadenomas of the breasts, J R Coll Surg Edinb 26:181, 1981.

60. Silver HK: Rothmund-Thomson syndrome: an oculocutaneous disorder, Am J Dis Child 111:182, 1966.

61. Ochshorn M, Ilie B, and Blum I: Multiple telangiectasias preceding the appearance of undifferentiated bronchiogenic carcinoma, Dermatologica 165:620, 1982.

62. Draelos ZK, Hansen RC, and Hays SB: Symmetric progressive telangiectatic nevi with hemorrhagic angiokeratomas, Pediatr Dermatol 3:212, 1986.

63. Ayers S Jr, Burrows LA, and Anderson NP: Generalized telangiectasia and sinus infection: report of a case with cure by treatment of chronic sinusitus, Arch Dermat Syph 26:56, 1932.

64. Shelley WB and Shelley ED: Essential progressive telangiectasia in an autoimmune setting: successful treatment with acyclovir, J Am Acad Dermatol 21:1094, 1989.

65. Girbig P and Voigtlander V: Besenreiservarizen in Rahmen progressiver essentieller Telangiektasien, Phlebol und Proctol 17:116, 1988.

66. McGrae JD and Winkelmann RK: Generalized essential telangiectasia: report of a clinical and histologic study of 13 patients with acquired cutaneous lesions, JAMA 185:909, 1963.

67. Paller AS: Vascular disorders, Dermatol Clin 5:239, 1987.

68. Way BH et al: Cutis marmorata telangiectatic congenita, J Cutan Pathol 1:10, 1974.

69. Powell ST and Su WPD: Cutis marmorata telangiectatica congenita: report of nine cases and review of the literature, Cutis 34:305, 1984.

70. Picascia DD and Esterly NB: Cutis marmorata telangiectatica congenita: report of 22 cases, J Am Acad Dermatol 20:1098, 1989.

71. South DA and Jacobs AH: Cutis marmorata telangiectatica congenita (congenital generalized phlebectasia), J Pediatr 93:944, 1978.

72. Andreev VC and Pramatarov K: Cutis marmorata telangiectatic congenita in two sisters, Br J Dermatol 101:345, 1979.

73. Kurczynski TW: Hereditary cutis marmorata telangiectatic congenita, Pediatrics 70:52, 1982.

74. Van Lohuizen CHJ: Uber eine seltene angeborene Hautanomalie (Cutis marmorata telangiectatica congenita), Acta Derm Venerol (Stockh) 3:202, 1922.

75. Cohen PR and Zalar GL: Cutis marmorata telangiectatica congenita: cliniopathologic characteristics and differential diagnosis, Cutis 42:518, 1988.

76. Kennedy C, Oranje A, and Keizer K: Cutis marmorata telangiectatica congenita, Int J Dermatol 31:349, 1992.

77. de Lorimier AA: Hepatic tumors of infancy and childhood, Surg Clin North Am 57:443, 1977.

78. Hurwitz S: Clinical pediatric dermatology: a textbook of skin disorders of childhood and adolescence, Philadelphia, 1981, WB Saunders.

79. Azizkhan G et al: Mast cell heparin stimulates migration of capillary endothelial cells in vitro, J Exp Med 152:931, 1980.

80. Ryan TJ and Kurban AK: New vessel growth in the adult skin, Br J Derm 82(suppl):92, 1970.

81. Fried SZ and Lynfield L: Unilateral facial telangiectasia macularis eruptiva perstans, J Am Acad Dermatol 16:250, 1987.

82. Tretbar LL: The origin of reflux in incompetent blue reticular/telangiectasia veins. In Davy A and Stemmer R, editors: Phlebologie '89, Montrouge, France, 1989, John Libbey Eurotext.

83. Weiss RA and Weiss MA: Doppler ultrasound findings in reticular veins of the thigh subdermic lateral venous system and implications for sclerotherapy, J Dermatol Surg Oncol 19:947, 1993.

84. Goldman MP: Commentary: rational sclerotherapy techniques for leg telangiectasia, J Dermatol Surg Oncol 19:933, 1993.

85. Salles-Cunha SX: Telangiectasias: classification of feeder vessels with color flow, Radiology 186:615, 1993.

86. Somjen GM et al: Anatomical examination of leg telangiectases with duplex scanning, J Dermatol Surg Oncol 19:940, 1993.

87. Bohler-Sommeregger K et al: Do telangiectases communicate with the deep venous system? J Dermatol Surg Oncol 18:403, 1992.

88. Merlen JF: Telangiectasies rouges, telangiectasies bleues, Phlebologie 23:167, 1970.

89. Thibault P and Bray A: Cosmetic leg veins: evaluation using duplex venous imaging, J Dermatol Surg Oncol, 1990 (in press).

90. Curri GB and Lo Brutto ME: Influenza dei mucopolisaccaridi e dei loro costituenti sulla neoformazione vascolare, Riv Pat Clin Sper 8:379, 1967.

91. Braverman IM: Microcirculation in psoriasis. In Roenigk HH Jr and Maibach HA, editors: Psoriasis, New York, 1985, Marcel Dekker.

92. David M et al: Keratosis lichenoides chronica with prominent telangiectasia: response to etretinate, J Am Acad Dermatol 21:1112, 1989.

93. Margolis MH, Cooper GA, and Johnson SAM: Keratosis lichenoides chronica, Arch Dermatol 105:739, 1972.

94. Davis MJ and Lawler JC: Capillary alterations in pigmented purpuric disease of the skin, Arch Dermatol 78:723, 1958.

95. Iwatsuki K et al: Immunofluorescence study in purpura pigmentosa chronica, Acta Dermatovener (Stockholm) 60:341, 1980.

96. Miller SS: Investigation and management of varicose veins, Ann R Coll Surg Engl 55:245, 1974.

97. Mullane DJ: Varicose veins of pregnancy, Am J Obstet Gynecol 63:620, 1952.
98. Goodrich SM and Wood JE: Peripheral venous distensibility and velocity of venous blood flow during pregnancy or during oral contraceptive therapy, Am J Obstet Gynecol 90:740, 1964.
99. Keates JS and Fitzgerald DE: An interim report on lower limb volume and blood flow changes during a normal menstrual cycle, 5th Europ Conf Microcirculation, Gothenburg, 1968, Bibl Anat 10:189, Basle, Switzerland, 1969, Karger.
100. McPheeters HO: The value of estrogen therapy in the treatment of varicose veins complicating pregnancy, J Lancet 69:2, 1949.
101. Davis LT and Duffy DM: Determination of incidence and risk factors for post-sclerotherapy telangiectatic matting of the lower extremity: a retrospective analysis, J Dermatol Surg Oncol 16:327, 1990.
102. Jensen EV et al: Receptors reconsidered: a 20-year perspective, Rec Prog Horm Res 38:1, 1982.
103. Colburn P and Buonossisi: Estrogen binding sites in endothelial cell cultures, Science 201:817, 1978.
104. Sadick NS and Niedt G: A study of estrogen receptors in spider telangiectasia of the lower extremities, J Dermatol Surg Oncol 16:620, 1990.
105. Wilkin JK et al: Unilateral dermatomal superficial telangiectasia, J Am Acad Dermatol 8:468, 1983.
106. Wilkin JK: Unilateral nevoid telangiectasias, Arch Dermatol 113:486, 1977.
107. Beacham BE and Kurgansky D: Unilateral naevoid telangiectasia syndrome associated with metastatic carcinoma tumour, Br J Dermatol 124:86, 1991.
108. Uhlin SR and McCarty KS: Unilateral naevoid telangiectatic syndrome. The role of estrogen and progesterone receptors, Arch Dermatol 119:226, 1983.
109. Leyden JJ, Thew M, and Kligman AM: Steroid rosacea, Arch Dermatol 110:619, 1974.
110. Katz HI and Prawer SE: Morphologic diagnosis of pre-atrophy of the skin. Scientific exhibit presented at the American Academy of Dermatology, New Orleans, December 6-11, 1986.
111. Zheng P et al: Morphologic investigations on the rebound phenomenon after corticosteroid-induced atrophy in human skin, J Invest Dermatol 82:345, 1984.
112. Katz HI et al: Preatrophy: covert sign of thinned skin, J Am Acad Dermatol 20:731, 1989.
113. Hogan DJ and Rooney ME: Facial telangiectasia associated with long-term application of a topical corticosteroid to the scalp, J Am Acad Dermatol 20:1129, 1989.
114. O'Brian JP: Solar and radiant damage to elastic tissue as a cause of internal vascular disease, Aust J Dermatol 21:1, 1980.
115. Kumakari M, Hashimoto K, and Willis I: Biologic changes due to long wave ultraviolet irradiation on human skin, J Invest Dermatol 69:392, 1977.
116. Oxholm A et al: Immunohistochemical detection of interleukin I-like molecules and tumour necrosis factor in human epidermis before and after UVB-irraditation in vivo, Br J Dermatol 118:369, 1988.
117. Braverman IM and Fonferko E: Studies in cutaneous aging: II. The microvasculature, J Invest Dermatol 78:444, 1982.
118. Piquet PF, Grau GE, and Vassali P: Subcutaneous perfusion of tumor necrosis factor induces local proliferation of fibroblasts, capillaries, and epidermal cells, or massive tissue necrosis, Am J Pathol 136:103, 1990.
119. Engel A, Johnson M-L, and Haynes SG: Health effects of sunlight exposure in the United States: results from the first national health and nutrition examination survey, 1971-1974, Arch Dermatol 124:72, 1988.
120. Dvorak HF: Tumors: wounds that do not heal: similarities between tumor stroma generation and wound healing, New Engl J Med 26:1650, 1986.
121. Ryan TJ: Factors influencing the growth of vascular endothelium in the skin, Br J Derm (suppl 5)82:99, 1970.
122. Okada N: Solitary giant spider angioma with an overlying pyogenic granuloma, J Am Acad Dermatol 5:1053, 1987.
123. Folkman J and Klagsbrun M: Angiogenic factors, Science 235:442, 1987.
124. Ryan TJ and Barnhill RL: Physical factors and angiogenesis. In Nugent J and O'Connor M, editors: Development of the vascular system, Ciba Foundation Symposium. London, 1983, Pitman.
125. Smahel J: The healing of skin grafts, Clin Plast Surg 4:409, 1977.
126. Myers MB: Attempts to augment survival in skin flaps—mechanism of the delay phenomenon. In Grabb WC and Myers MB, editors: Skin flaps, Boston, 1975, Little, Brown.
127. Garcia FN, Ojta T, and Hoover RL: Stimulation of human umbilical vein endothelial cells (HUVEC) by Bartonella bacilliformis (BB), FASEB J A1189, 1988.
128. Becker SW: Generalized telangiectasia, Arch Dermatol Syph 14:387, 1926.
129. Ayers S Jr, Burrows A, and Anderson NP: Generalized telangiectasia and sinus infection: report of a case with cure by treatment of chronic sinusitis, Arch Dermat Syph 26:56, 1932.

130. Shelley WB: Essential progressive telangiectasia: successful treatment with tetracycline, JAMA 216:1343, 1971.
131. Shelley WB and Fierer JA: Focal intravascular coagulation in progressive ascending telangiectasia: ultrastructural studies of ketoconazole-induced involution of vessels, J Am Acad Dermatol 10:876, 1984.
132. Jimenez-Acosta F, Fonseca E, and Magallon M: Response to tetracycline of telangiectasias in a male hemophiliac with human immunodeficiency virus infection, J Am Acad Dermatol 19:369, 1988.
133. Fallon T Jr et al: Telangiectasias of the anterior chest in homosexual men, Ann Intern Med 105:679, 1986.
134. Cockerell CJ and LeBoit PE: Bacillary angiomatosis: a newly characterized, pseudoneoplastic infectious, cutaneous vascular disorder, J Am Acad Dermatol 22:501, 1990.
135. Clarke D, Martinez A, and Cox RS: Analysis of cosmetic results and complications in patients with stage I and II breast cancer treated by biopsy and irradiation, Int J Radiat Oncol Biol Phys 9:1807, 1983.
136. Goldschmidt H and Sherwin WK: Reactions to ionizing radiation, J Am Acad Dermatol 3:551, 1980.
137. Dover JS, Phillips TJ, and Arndt KA: Cutaneous effects and therapeutic uses of heat with emphasis on infrared radiation, J Am Acad Dermatol 20:278, 1989.

NONINVASIVE EXAMINATION OF THE PATIENT BEFORE SCLEROTHERAPY

Helane S. Fronek

The simplicity of sclerotherapy treatment of varicose vein disease invites certain problems. Physicians unfamiliar with the anatomy and pathophysiology of the venous system can easily feel otherwise well-prepared to simply "inject veins" and are thus lured into treating patients who may actually have very complicated conditions. Unfortunately, evidence of venous disease on examination is subtle. For this reason, it is quite possible, and frequently the case, that an asymptomatic patient with no grossly visible varicose veins actually has significant venous disease that will lead either to treatment failure with a rapid recurrence of symptoms or to serious complications or worsened venous function if it goes unrecognized. Imaging of 83 limbs with clinical evidence of only telangiectatic vessels demonstrated that nearly 25% had insufficiency of the greater or lessor saphenous veins, which was not apparent on physical examination.[1] Incomplete appreciation of the actual condition of the patient's venous system can thus subject the patient to avoidable risks and unnecessary treatment. As with any medical procedure, a great deal of thought, examination, and treatment planning is essential to achieve success. Therefore, a screening evaluation of the venous system should be performed before undertaking sclerotherapy. More involved examinations may also be necessary based on the initial findings.

MEDICAL HISTORY

The approach to the patient who seeks treatment is to begin with a directed medical history. The duration of the known venous disease and the course of its evolution are important factors to consider in understanding both the severity of the disease and in planning treatment. Patients who noted the onset of large varicose veins by their early 20s, especially those with a strong family history of varicose vein disease, will undoubtedly have an aggressive disease. These patients require a thorough examination of their venous system since long-standing varicose veins may be not only the result of, but also the cause of, venous valvular insufficiency in both the superficial and perforating veins and may be the sole cause of serious problems, including venous ulceration.[2-6]

Worsening of varicose veins or the symptoms attributed to them following a period of immobilization, travel, or an operation suggests the occurrence of a clinically unrecognized deep vein thrombosis (DVT). These patients should be examined for calf muscle pump function, perforator vein valvular insufficiency, and deep venous valvular insufficiency. Persons with a confirmed history of DVT or even superficial thrombophlebitis may also be at risk for these complications because the thrombus or the inflammatory reaction may spread to perforating and deep veins, leading to valvular damage at these sites. A rapid or simply progressive increase in the size of the varicose veins or the recent onset of edema may be indicative of an abdominal or pelvic tumor compressing the inferior vena cava, interfering with venous outflow; therefore, abdominal and pelvic physical exam-

SYMPTOMS ATTRIBUTABLE TO VARICOSE VEINS

Aching	Itching
Heaviness, tiredness	Cramping
Pain (throbbing, burning, sharp, tingling)	

ination, supplemented with radiologic studies such as ultrasound, computerized axial tomography, or magnetic resonance imaging should be considered.

Prior Treatment

It is important that prior treatment for venous disease be discussed. However, the physician must realize that although proper ligation, with or without stripping of the main saphenous trunks, implies that reflux through the saphenofemoral (SFJ) and saphenopopliteal (SPJ) junctions has been prevented, this is not always the case. In up to 27% of people there is a duplication of the greater saphenous vein (GSV),[7-9] thus the removal of the GSV may be followed by the development of varicosity in the remaining GSV. In 20% to 40%, the lessor saphenous vein (LSV) has an aberrant termination[10-12] that is not in the popliteal vein or that is in the popliteal vein above the popliteal fossa. Therefore, the actual SPJ may easily be missed, leading to an apparent rapid recurrence with varicose changes occurring in the remaining segment of the LSV and its tributaries. Finally, in a number of patients, a recurrence of varicose veins in the upper thigh may be the result of incomplete ligation and division of the other tributaries arising at the level of the SFJ or failure to accomplish the ligation flush with the femoral vein. In fact, in a review of 341 extremities that underwent repeat operations for varicose veins, Lofgren, Myers, and Webb[13] found that 61% had inadequate ligation. These facts make it imperative that, even in the patient with a history of ligation, division, and stripping, an examination for reflux through the SFJ and SPJ be performed.

Responses to and complications from all treatment modalities (sclerotherapy, laser, etc.) also should be discussed. Certain complications, such as ischemic ulceration due to injection into an arteriovenous malformation, can be avoided more easily if one is aware of their prior occurrence. Given the predilection for these to occur in a particular anatomic distribution(s), one might avoid treating that area or use greater caution in the previously affected region. A history of prior hyperpigmentation, blushing, or poor response to a particular sclerosing agent may support a variety of changes in treatment protocol, such as altering the sclerosant concentration, increasing the strength or duration of compression, and paying greater attention to posttreatment thrombectomy.

Symptoms

It is well known that the presence and severity of symptoms does not correlate with the size or severity of the varicose veins present. Symptoms usually attributable to varicose veins include feelings of heaviness, tiredness, aching, burning, throbbing, itching, and cramping in the legs (see box above). These symptoms are generally worse with prolonged sitting or standing and are improved with leg elevation or walking. A premenstrual exacerbation of symptoms is also common. Generally, patients find relief with the use of compression, in the form of either support hose or an elastic bandage. Weight loss may also be accompanied by a diminution in the severity of varicose vein symptoms, as may the commencement of a regular program of lower extremity exercise. Clearly, these symptoms are not specific, as they may also be indicative of a variety of rheumatologic or orthopedic problems. However, their relationship to lower extremity movement and compression is usually helpful in establishing a venous origin for the symptoms. Significant symptoms suggestive of venous disease should prompt further evaluation for valvular insufficiency and calf muscle pump dysfunction. If a venous etiology is suspected but all examinations are negative, repeat examination during a symptomatic period is warranted and often fruitful.

The recent development of an extremely painful area on the lower leg associated with an overlying area of erythema and warmth may be indicative of lipodermatosclerosis, which may be associated with insufficiency of an underlying perforator vein, and examination for this lesion should be performed. Lipodermatosclerosis may precede ulceration and has been shown to be improved by certain pharmacologic interventions.[14]

Patients with a history of iliofemoral thrombophlebitis who describe "bursting" pain with walking may be suffering from venous claudication. In these patients, an evaluation for persistent hemodynamically significant obstruction, possibly treatable with venous bypass surgery, is in order.[15]

Complications of Varicose Vein Disease

Complications such as ulceration and hemorrhage should be discussed with the patient, because this provides additional insight into both the severity and the probable locations of abnormality within the venous system. A history of ulceration of the medial aspect of the lower leg should prompt further examination of the GSV trunk,[2] whereas involvement of the lateral aspect of the lower leg suggests an abnormality in the LSV, in addition to the deep and perforating vein systems. A history of hemorrhage from telangiectasia in a particular area suggests further examination for underlying incompetent perforators and is an indication to treat all suspicious telangiectasias.[16]

PURPOSE OF VENOUS EVALUATION

More extensive evaluation can provide essential information regarding both venous anatomy and function. Abnormalities of the superficial, perforating, or deep systems can be diagnosed, and the exact sites of valvular insufficiency within the various systems (and therefore the sites where treatment must be directed) can be determined. The hemodynamic significance of each of these abnormalities may be defined, and the effect of correcting each site of reflux may be assessed. Insufficiency at a particular site within the venous system may be found to have no importance in the patient's pathologic venous hypertension or symptoms and, therefore, may be ignored in the treatment plan, preventing unnecessary treatment. Using the following examination techniques, the result of sclerotherapy may be documented in a more accurate and sensitive manner than with simple observation and palpation. Therefore, treatment success may be enhanced significantly because treatment can be continued until its endpoint, sclerosis and restoration of normal venous flow, is evident. Finally, the presence of DVT and deep venous valvular insufficiency, absolute and relative contraindications to sclerotherapy, respectively, may be diagnosed, thus allowing improved patient selection and avoidance of serious complications.

PHYSICAL EXAMINATION

The best way to approach the examination of the venous system before sclerotherapy is a matter of personal preference because many methods are available. Each has something to contribute, and each has limitations.

Using no special equipment, one can obtain a degree of information regarding overall venous outflow from the leg, the sites of valvular insufficiency, the presence of primary versus secondary varicose veins, and the presence of DVT.

The screening physical examination consists of careful observation of the legs. Any patient with large varicose veins; bulges in the thigh, calf, or the inguinal region representative of incompetent perforating veins or a saphena varix;[17] signs of superficial venous hypertension such as an accumulation of telangiectasias in the ankle region; or any of the findings suggestive of venous dermatitis (pigmentation, induration, eczema) should be examined more fully. This includes patients with obvious cutaneous signs of venous disease such as venous ulceration, atrophie blanche, or lipodermatosclerosis. An obvious but often forgotten point is the necessity of observing the entire leg and not confining the examination simply to the area that the patient feels is abnormal. The importance of this is demonstrated in Fig. 5-1. This patient came for treatment of an obviously dilated anterior thigh vein, but further inspection revealed a saphena varix, indicative of incompetence at the level of the SFJ, thus defining the first step in her treatment. Similarly, patients often seek treatment of specific clusters of telangiectasia and do not notice the underlying reticular veins that should be treated before or at the same time as the telangiectasia (see Chapter 11).

Finally, because the veins of the leg empty into the pelvic and abdominal veins, inspection of the abdomen is very important since dilation of veins on the abdominal wall or across the pubic region suggests an old iliofemoral thrombus[18] or, rarely, a developmental anomaly of the venous system.[19] Dilated veins along the medial or posterior aspect of the proximal thigh or buttocks most often arise from varicosities involving the pudendal or other pelvic vessels. These can be associated with vulvar varices that may remain symptomatic after the completion

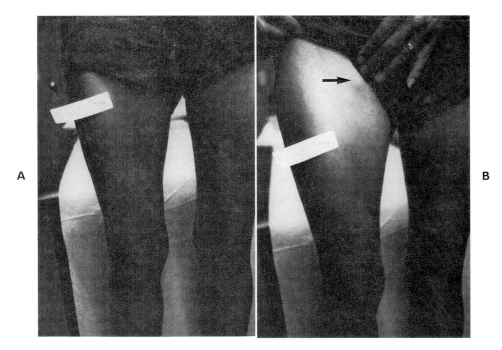

Fig. 5-1   A, This patient sought treatment because of an obviously enlarged vein in her thigh. **B,** Further inspection revealed a saphena varix *(arrow)* indicative of SFJ insufficiency. (Courtesy Anton Butie, M.D.)

of the pregnancy during which they formed. The enlarged veins in the thigh or buttocks may also be quite symptomatic and respond well to treatment.

A tourniquet may be placed around the patient's proximal thigh while the patient is standing. The patient then assumes the supine position with the affected leg elevated 45 degrees. The tourniquet is removed and the time required for the leg veins to empty, which is indicative of the adequacy of venous drainage, is recorded.

When compared with the contralateral leg, this method may demonstrate a degree of venous obstructive disease. Another approach is to elevate the leg while the patient is supine and observe the height of the heel in relation to the level of the heart that is required for the prominent veins to collapse (Fig. 5-2). Unfortunately, neither procedure is sufficiently sensitive nor accurate, and does not differentiate acute from chronic obstruction, thus being of minimal assistance in current-day medical practice. However, there are several physical examination maneuvers that can provide information on the competence of the venous valves.

Cough Test

One hand is placed gently over the GSV or the SFJ, and the patient is asked to cough or perform a Valsalva maneuver (Fig. 5-3). Simply palpating an impulse over the vein being examined may be indicative of insufficiency of the valve at the saphenofemoral junction and below to the level of the palpating hand. This test is not, however, applicable to the examination of the LSV and SPJ (see below).[10] Palpation of a thrill during this maneuver is generally more diagnostic.

Percussion/Schwartz Test

One hand is placed over the SFJ or SPJ while the other hand is used to tap very lightly on a distal segment of the GSV or LSV (Fig. 5-4). The production of an im-

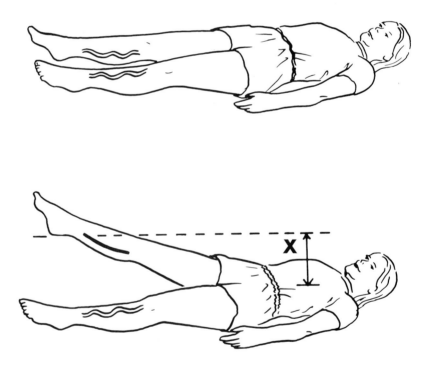

Fig. 5-2 Venous outflow may also be assessed by elevating the leg until the superficial veins collapse and then measuring the distance *(X)* from the heart to the heel and comparing this measurement with the other leg.

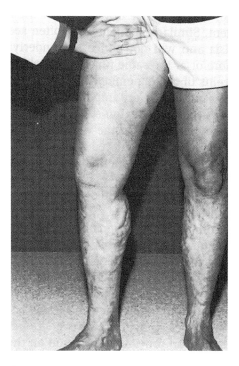

Fig. 5-3 Cough test. The SFJ is palpated while the patient coughs. Palpation of an impulse is indicative of SFJ insufficiency.

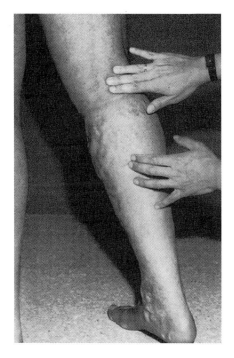

Fig. 5-4 Percussion test. The SPJ is palpated while the LSV is gently percussed. Palpation of an impulse is indicative of SPJ insufficiency.

pulse in this manner implies insufficiency of the valves in the segment between the two hands. Confirmation of the valvular insufficiency can be achieved by tapping proximally while palpating distally. This test can also be used to detect whether an enlarged tributary is in direct connection with the GSV or LSV by palpating over the main trunk and tapping lightly on the dilated tributary, or vice versa. The presence of a direct connection results in a palpable impulse being transmitted from the percussing to the palpating hand. As might be expected, these tests are far from infallible. In a study of 105 limbs, Chan, Chisholm, and Royle[20] found that these clinical examination techniques correctly identified SFJ incompetence in only 82%. False negatives were felt to be caused primarily by previous groin surgery with resultant scarring and by obesity, whereas false positives were the result of variations in ve-

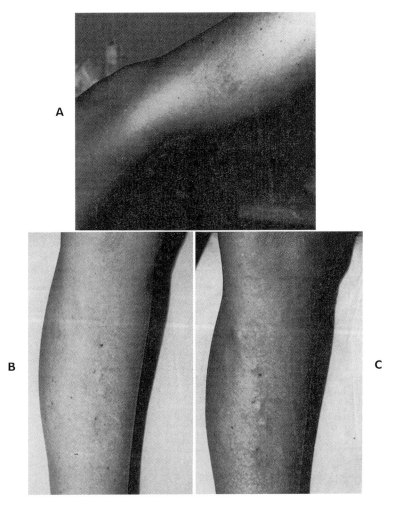

Fig. 5-5   Brodie-Trendelenburg test. **A,** The proximal portion of the GSV is obstructed after the veins have emptied with the leg elevated. **B,** The distal veins are then observed after the patient stands. **C,** The veins are further inspected after the tourniquet is released. In this case, filling of the veins on standing and additional filling after tourniquet removal constitutes a double-positive test.

nous anatomy, such as a dilated tributary emptying into the common femoral vein adjacent to the GSV or the absence of valves in the otherwise normal common femoral vein and the external iliac vein (seen in 5% to 30% of persons).[21,22] Another source of error with the cough test is simply a misinterpretation of the muscle contraction that occurs with coughing as a reflux impulse.

Brodie-Trendelenburg Test

The well-known Brodie-Trendelenburg test traditionally involves the manual obstruction of the proximal end of the GSV (or LSV) while the patient lies supine with the leg elevated, after stroking the vein in a cephalad direction to empty it of blood.[18,23-26] The patient then assumes the standing position, and the leg is observed for 30 seconds (Fig. 5-5). In "nil" test, there is slow filling of the veins from below and the release of the compression does not result in rapid filling from above, indicating competence of valves in deep and perforating veins, as well as at the SFJ (Fig. 5-6, A). Rapid filling of the GSV or more distal tributaries that occurs only after release of the compression constitutes a "positive" test, indicating the presence of an insufficient valve at the SFJ (Fig. 5-6, B). In the "double-positive" test, there is some distension of the veins within the initial 30 seconds while the compression is maintained, as well as additional filling once the compression is released (Fig. 5-6, C). This is taken as evidence of incompetent deep and perforating veins as well as reflux through the SFJ. A "negative" test occurs when the veins fill within the initial 30 seconds with no increased filling after the compression is released, implying

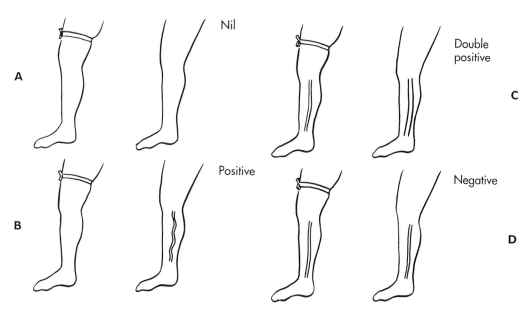

Fig. 5-6 Interpreting the Brodie-Trendelenburg test. **A,** Nil—no distention of the veins for 30 seconds both while the tourniquet remains on and after it is removed implies a lack of reflux. **B,** Positive—distention of the veins only after the tourniquet is released implies reflux only through the SFJ. **C,** Double positive—distention of the veins while the tourniquet remains on and further distention after it is removed implies reflux through perforating veins as well as the SFJ. **D,** Negative—distention of the veins while the tourniquet remains on and no additional distention once it is removed implies reflux only through perforating veins.

only deep and perforating valvular insufficiency (Fig. 5-6, *D*). The reverse may not be true; that is, filling in greater than 30 seconds does not imply competence of perforating veins. In a study of 901 extremities, Sherman[27] found that 95% had a nil Trendelenburg test, but surgical exploration later showed incompetent perforators in 90% of these patients. The Brodie-Trendelenburg test can thus be an important method of localizing the most proximal site of reflux in most dilated superficial veins by obstructing the GSV, LSV, or whichever vein is suspected of refluxing into a more distal vein. Also, by placing the examining finger over palpable fascial defects in the leg while the patient is supine and then releasing the obstructions one by one after the patient is standing, the sites of insufficient perforators, or "points of control" (considered so crucial in Fegan's technique of sclerotherapy) may be defined because the superficial veins distal to the insufficient perforator fill rapidly once the obstructing fingers are removed (see Chapter 9).[28,29]

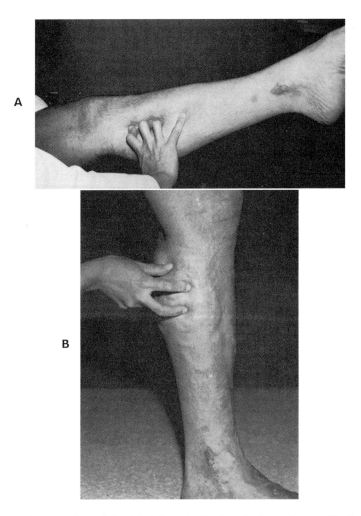

Fig. 5-7 **A,** Compression of fascial defects indicating "points of control" of an incompetent perforating vein with the leg elevated. **B,** When the patient stands, the varicose vein remains collapsed while pressure is maintained over control points and distends when the control point is released.

With this technique, described well in many papers,[17,28-31] one first marks on the leg the sites of all dilated varicosities in the leg. The patient then assumes the supine position with the leg elevated to approximately 60 degrees to empty the veins. After at least 20 seconds, or when the distended veins are flattened, the leg is gently and rapidly palpated to detect any defects in the fascia. With experience these can be detected easily as places that allow the entrance of the examining finger without the use of any pressure. Fascial defects can be caused by many abnormalities other than perforating veins, thus one continues the examination by compressing the individual fascial defects with one's fingers and then having the patient stand. The fingers are then released one by one, starting with the most distal defect, and rapid filling of more distal varicosities is noted (Fig. 5-7). Those defects that result in distal filling when released are assumed to correspond to sites of incompetent perforating veins. In the presence of a dilated GSV or LSV, these points of reflux must first be controlled with either digital compression or a tourniquet to evaluate the lower volume reflux through the perforators. Compression of the defects must first result in sustained flattening of the varicosities when the patient initially stands for the evaluation to be helpful. If the veins fill before any of the fingers are released, the test must be restarted and other sites compressed until the sites responsible for the reflux are located. This examination is associated with a 50% to 70% accuracy[30-33] compared with findings at surgical exploration. Repeated examination at different times and improvement of edema allows the detection of increased numbers of perforators.

Bracey variation. A clever variation of the Brodie-Trendelenburg technique was proposed by Bracey[34] in 1958 (Fig. 5-8). He used a flat rubber tourniquet 3.8 cm wide and two rubber rings covered with latex, with inside diameters of 7 cm and 8.2 cm. The small ring is used between the ankle and knee and may also be used for the thigh if the patient is thin. If not, the larger ring is used for the thigh. With the patient standing, the small ring is rolled over the foot to just above the ankle, and the rubber tourniquet is then placed below the ring to obstruct any upward flow of blood through the superficial veins. The small ring is then slowly

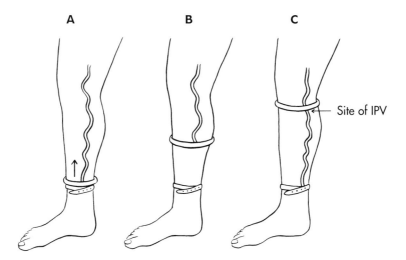

Fig. 5-8 Device for the detection of incompetent perforating veins (IPV). **A,** Two rubber rings are placed around the ankle, and, **B,** the more proximally placed ring is slowly rolled upward. **C,** As it rolls above an IPV the reflux of blood through the IPV results in an immediate distention of a superficial varix or the formation of a large bulge at the site of the IPV.

rolled upward, emptying the superficial veins as it moves. As soon as it passes an incompetent perforating vein, the blood enters the superficial vein that connects with it, causing a dilation of the vein. The exit site of the perforating vein may then be marked. This reflux of blood can be accentuated by asking the patient to repetitively dorsiflex the foot. When the ring reaches the knee, the tourniquet is moved up to the knee, just below the ring. Either the small or larger ring is then used similarly to examine the thigh.

Perthes' Test

The Perthes' test[18,26,35] has several uses, including distinguishing between venous valvular insufficiency in the deep, perforator, and superficial systems and screening for DVT (Table 5-1). To localize the site of valvular disease, one places a tourniquet around the proximal thigh with the patient standing. When the patient ambulates, a decrease in the distention of varicose veins suggests a primary process without underlying deep venous disease because the calf muscle pump

Table 5-1   Perthes' test

Finding	Interpretation
Decreased diameter of varicose veins	Primary varicose veins
No change in diameter of varicose veins	Secondary varicose veins
	Impairment of calf muscle pump
	Deep venous patency
Increased diameter of varicose veins	Deep venous obstruction

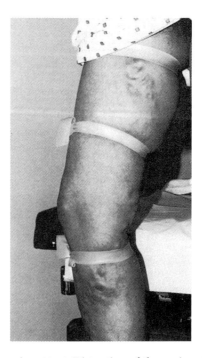

Fig. 5-9   Comparative tourniquet test. Distention of the varices in each segment of the leg when the patient ambulates implies the presence of IPVs in each segment.

effectively removes blood from the leg and the varicose veins empty. Secondary varicose veins do not change caliber (if there is patency of the deep venous system) because of the inability to empty blood out of the veins as a result of impairment of the calf muscle pump. In the setting of a current DVT, they may increase in size. If there is significant chronic or acute obstructive disease in the iliofemoral segment, the patient may note pain (venous claudication)[36-38] as a result of the obstruction to outflow through both the deep and superficial systems. Information regarding the presence of deep venous valvular insufficiency and thrombosis is important to note in patient selection to avoid causing catastrophic complications, such as pulmonary embolism resulting from an undiagnosed and worsened DVT or venous claudication caused by further impairment of venous return. Indeed, these two complications are serious enough to warrant the use of a much more sensitive and accurate method, and therefore the Perthes' test is now of more historical than actual clinical importance.

To test for perforator valvular defects, one may embellish the traditional Perthes' test by placing a tourniquet around the calf just below the popliteal fossa.[28] If the dilated superficial veins in the calf and ankle become less prominent as the patient ambulates, this implies that the blood is being drawn into the deep system through competent perforating veins. However, if the veins become increasingly dilated, the perforating veins must be incompetent. A more involved test, the Mahorner-Ochsner comparative tourniquet test,[26] similarly localizes the site(s) of reflux by observing the leg while the patient walks with the tourniquet placed at various levels on the leg (upper, middle, and lower thigh) (Fig. 5-9).

NONINVASIVE DIAGNOSTIC TECHNIQUES

The preceding three decades have been very fruitful and have provided us with a wealth of noninvasive technology that has revolutionized vascular diagnosis. A thorough description of all these techniques is certainly beyond the scope of this book, but those not presented here may be found in several excellent texts.[9,39,40] Some of the new technologies have real utility in the everyday performance of sclerotherapy, and the following discussion attempts to acquaint you with their uses and limitations.

Doppler Ultrasound

Probably the most useful, practical instrument for evaluating patients with venous disease is the Doppler ultrasound. Its first vascular application came in 1960 when Satomura and Kaneko[41] described a method of studying changes in blood flow in peripheral arteries using an ultrasonic blood rheograph. Its use in the field of venous disease was promoted by many groups, including Sumner, Baker, and Strandness,[42] Strandness et al.,[43] Felix and Sigel,[44] and Sigel et al.[45-49] The instrument is based on the principle of the Doppler effect and consists of an emitting crystal and a receiving crystal. Sound waves are directed into the limb and reflected off of the blood cells traveling through the vessel being examined (Fig. 5-10). The input picked up by the receiving crystal may be connected to a variety of audio or graphic recording systems. Dopplers come with either continuous or pulsed-wave ultrasound beams; the continuous-wave Doppler is adequate for venous examination even though the signal represents a composite of the flow in all vessels in the path of the ultrasound beam. Thus selective examination of one particular vessel may not always be possible. Pulsed Dopplers are used in sonar systems, as well as in medical ultrasound imaging, and are required when the intent is to focus the beam at a particular depth. Dopplers are also available in either directional or nondirectional forms. The directional type is capable of determining the direction of blood flow and depicts the direction on the tracing as either a positive (toward the probe)

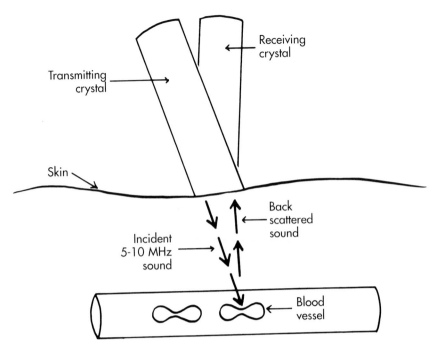

Fig. 5-10 Doppler ultrasound. Sound waves are emitted from the transmitting crystal, reflected by moving particles (blood cells) within the vessel being examined, and picked up by the sensing crystal.

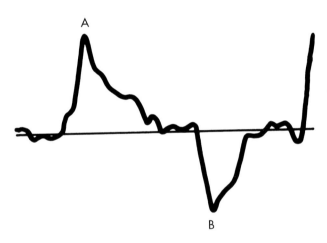

Fig. 5-11 Bidirectional Doppler tracing. *A,* Positive deflection indicates flow toward the probe; *B,* negative deflection indicates flow away from the probe.

or negative (away from the probe) deflection (Fig. 5-11). Although the directionality greatly simplifies the interpretation of the tracing, experience with a nondirectional Doppler allows one to make this determination easily based on certain augmentation maneuvers.

The transmission frequency of the ultrasound beam may range from 2 to 10 MHz; the depth of penetration varies inversely with the frequency. Therefore, a frequency of 4 MHz produces a broad beam with deep penetration, especially useful for examining the deep veins in the pelvis and abdomen. A frequency of 8 MHz is much better suited to the examination of more superficial veins, includ-

---

VENOUS DOPPLER CHARACTERISTICS

Spontaneous   Nonpulsatile
Unidirectional   Augmentation
Phasic with respiratory cycle

---

ing superficial segments of the deep veins of the legs, since it produces a narrower beam with relatively less penetration. Dopplers used for evaluation of the venous system generally permit detection of flow rates as low as 6 cm/sec.[46]

Characteristics of Doppler waveform. Venous Doppler signals display five characteristics (see box above). In a normal patient, there should be a *spontaneous* signal over any vessel not otherwise vasoconstricted, and the flow should be only *unidirectional.* This signal diminishes in intensity with inspiration as descension of the diaphragm results in a rise in intraabdominal pressure, thus decreasing venous outflow from the leg. It will be augmented similarly with exhalation. This waxing and waning of the intensity of the signal with the respiratory cycle is a phenomenon known as *phasicity.* Venous signals are continuous except for their respiratory variation and are *not pulsatile,* except in the setting of elevated right heart pressure such as congestive heart failure or tricuspid insufficiency[50] or in the normal common femoral vein (CFV).[51] Finally, and most important to their usefulness in the evaluation of patients with varicose veins, venous signals may be *augmented* with certain compression maneuvers. It is the response to these maneuvers that provides information regarding the sites of valvular insufficiency and obstruction of the venous system.

By compressing the limb distal to the Doppler probe (Fig. 5-12), one increases the flow through the vein, and an immediate increase in the signal intensity should be heard if there is no proximal obstruction. In the presence of a hemodynamically significant DVT, the augmented response is weaker and delayed compared with the contralateral side. With the patient in the upright position, release of distal compression should be followed by silence as the valves close in response to the downward pressure of the blood being pulled by gravity. With the patient in the supine position, release of the compression normally should be followed by the return of the lower intensity spontaneous signal or by silence in the smaller veins. In the setting of valvular insufficiency at the level of the Doppler probe, a loud reflux flow signal can be heard on release of distal compression as blood is pulled in a caudad direction by gravity. To quantitate this reflux flow, the compression used may be standardized by using a pneumatic cuff inflated to a standard pressure (for example, 80 to 120 mm Hg), and the amplitude and duration of reflux may be read from the tracing obtained. In order to be considered true reflux and not merely delayed valve closure, the duration of reflux must be at least 0.5 second.[4,52]

The other method of augmentation is proximal compression and release (Fig. 5-13). Proximal compression produces a transient obstruction to outflow and thus causes an accumulation of blood distally, with an associated interruption of the Doppler signal. On its release, the large bolus of blood flowing past the Doppler probe results in a loud signal. This has also been found to be the more sensitive maneuver in diagnosing DVT, even that limited to calf veins, with a diminished or delayed signal indicative of a significant thrombosis.[53,54] Valvular insufficiency is discovered easily because proximal compression will, instead of resulting in silence, yield a loud reflux flow.

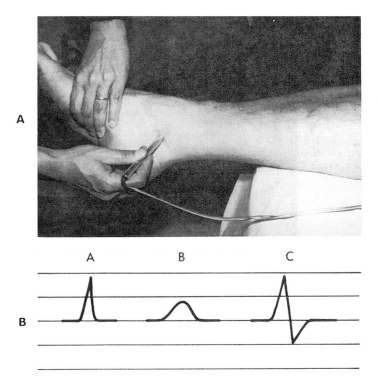

Fig. 5-12 **A,** Method of producing augmentation of flow in the posterior tibial vein by distal (foot) compression. **B,** Shows, *A,* normal flow; *B,* venous obstruction; *C,* valvular insufficiency.

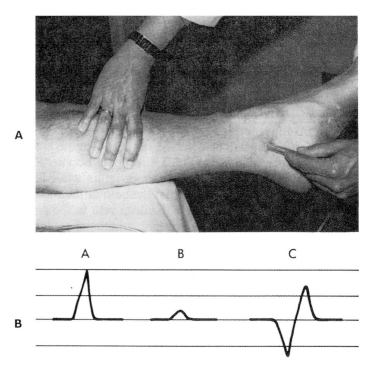

Fig. 5-13 **A,** Method of producing augmentation of flow in the posterior tibial vein by release of proximal (calf) compression. **B,** Shows, *A,* normal flow; *B,* venous obstruction; *C,* valvular insufficiency.

In early descriptions of the use of Doppler ultrasound for detection of venous disease, Sigel et al.[46] named the various sounds "S" for spontaneous and "A" for augmented. They further specified A sounds as *distal* (if the compression was distal to the probe) or *proximal* (if the compression was proximal to the probe) and *positive* if the A sound was heard directly with compression or *negative* if the A sound was heard on release of the compression. This notation thus makes it possible for four A sounds to be generated at each site being examined. Table 5-2 summarizes these sounds and their significance. This schema provides a useful method of categorizing these sounds, however, the "S" and "A" nomenclature has not found generalized acceptance. Instead, sounds are referred to as manifesting flux or reflux, antegrade or retrograde flow, patency or incompetence, etc.

Augmentation of the most proximal portion of the GSV and of the more proximal deep veins is accomplished either by compressing the abdomen or by using a variation of the proximal compression and release, the Valsalva maneuver (Fig. 5-14). The rise in intraabdominal pressure caused by descension of the diaphragm is accentuated by contraction of the intercostal muscles. In the normal patient an abrupt closure of the valves results in silence. However, more than 38% of normal persons have a brief period of reflux at the commencement of the Valsalva.[55] Also, with a weak effort by the patient, a slow retrograde flow may pass through the valve and produce a Doppler flow signal because sufficient force to cause valve closure has not been generated. Visualization of the valves using ultrasound

Table 5-2 Interpretation of A sounds

Type of A sound	Condition if present	Condition if absent
Distal positive	Normal	Venous obstruction
Distal negative	Valvular insufficiency	Normal
Proximal positive	Valvular insufficiency	Normal
Proximal negative	Normal	Venous obstruction or marked valvular insufficiency

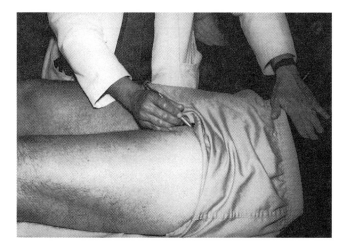

Fig. 5-14 Augmentation of flow in the common femoral vein or through the SFJ with intermittent compression of the abdomen or with Valsalva maneuver and release (not shown).

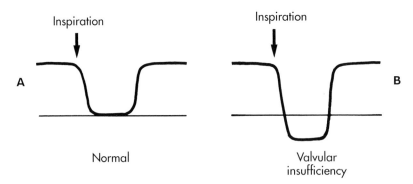

Fig. 5-15   Venous Doppler tracings. **A,** Normal phasic flow. **B,** Reflux with deep inspiration in the setting of valvular insufficiency.

demonstrates that these valves do eventually close, and that they are not actually insufficient.[56] Therefore, the continuation of reflux through at least half of the period of compression or at least 0.5 seconds (usually 1 to 4 seconds) is important in diagnosing pathologic valvular incompetence.[4,52] A less sensitive, but perhaps more specific, response may be elicited simply with deep breathing. With valvular insufficiency, instead of hearing the cessation of flow as the patient takes a deep breath, flow will be reversed and a continuous signal will be heard, which will show a reverse deflection on a directional Doppler tracing (Fig. 5-15). When using the Valsalva maneuver to produce reflux while listening over more distal veins, it is important to realize that the path of the reflux may be either straight down the superficial vein or via the deep vein to the perforating vein to the superficial vein (Fig. 5-16).[57] Therefore, additional testing is necessary to further delineate the exact site of abnormality. This is easily accomplished by manually obstructing the superficial vein, and, if reflux is still heard, the retrograde flow is assumed to be traveling through the deep and perforating systems.

Doppler examination technique. The Doppler examination of the patient is begun with the deep veins, several of which are easily accessible.

Femoral vein. With the patient supine and the hips slightly flexed and externally rotated, one first locates the pulsatile signal of the femoral artery in the groin. If desired, the examination can also be performed with the patient standing, which may provide a more physiologic evaluation, because most symptoms occur when the patient is upright and reflux is more easily elicited in this position. The Doppler probe is then gradually angled medially until the spontaneous, continuous sound of the femoral vein, suggestive of a windstorm, is heard. Clear phasicity with respiration should be detected easily. Patency can be further tested by manually compressing the thigh or the calf and listening for a strongly augmented signal. Valvular competence may be assessed by listening first for the phasic waxing and waning of the signal that, in severe cases of insufficiency, shows a decrease in intensity of the signal followed by a reversal of flow direction as inspiration progresses, rather than the expected silence. The patient is then asked to perform a Valsalva maneuver; alternatively, one may press on the abdomen. These latter maneuvers should result in an abrupt closure of the valve and silence, followed by a more intense antegrade flow on release if the valves are competent. A loud reflux flow heard through the Valsalva maneuver is pathognomonic of valvular insufficiency, which may be present in 5% to 30% of normal patients and, in one study, was found in 100% of patients with bilateral GSV vari-

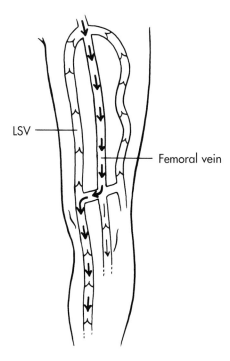

Fig. 5-16 Pathways of reflux are typically through the SFJ but may also be through atypical channels, such as via a deep vein through a perforating vein into a superficial vein (shown). Reflux may also travel via a superficial vein through a perforating vein into another superficial vein (not shown). (Redrawn from Schultz-Ehrenburg U and Hubner H-J: Reflux diagnosis with Doppler ultrasound. In Findings in angiology and phlebology, vol 35, New York, 1989, FK Schattauer Verlag.)

cosities.[48] The effort invested in the Valsalva maneuver may be standardized to ensure the proper force and reproducibility by asking the patient to blow into a tube connected to a mercury manometer so the mercury column rises to 30 mm.

Differentiation of femoral from saphenous veins. Because the SFJ is located in close proximity to the femoral artery pulsation, valvular incompetence at the junction can sometimes be mistaken for common femoral vein insufficiency. Several techniques can be used to aid in making this important differentiation. The saphenous vein is much easier to compress than the femoral vein, so manual compression using the Doppler probe may occlude the saphenous vein and allow the physician to listen selectively to the femoral vein. A separate occlusive device, such as the physician's other hand or a tourniquet, may be used to compress the GSV distal to the Doppler probe and thus prevent reflux through it. Any reflux still heard is then assumed to be through the femoral vein. Finally, moving or angling the Doppler probe in a cephalad direction may enable the physician to direct the ultrasound beam away from the saphenous vein to a more proximal segment of the femoral vein. Still, there are a small number of patients in whom differentiation of femoral from junctional signals may be impossible using only the continuous-wave Doppler, and an imaging procedure such as Duplex scanning, which uses a pulsed ultrasound beam, may be necessary.[59,60]

Popliteal vein. For the next site of examination, the popliteal vein, the patient may be in the supine, prone, or standing position. The most physiologic position is standing, and it is advisable to perform all presclerotherapy Doppler examinations in this position. It is important to have the knee slightly flexed, however, since full extension of the knee joint may cause a functional obstruction of the popliteal vein. Also, if the examination is performed while the patient is standing, the weight should be borne on the opposite foot (Fig. 5-17). The pulsatile arterial signal is located, generally, in the popliteal crease just lateral to the midline, and the Doppler probe may be angled medially to find a softer, though spontaneous, venous signal, or it may be left over the popliteal artery. Augmentation with either calf compression or thigh compression and release will, as described above, disclose both obstruction and valvular insufficiency. The Valsalva maneuver will only disclose reflux if the more proximal deep veins (common femoral vein) are also incompetent. As with reflux heard at the femoral level, reflux at the popliteal level may actually be caused by reflux through the SPJ. Therefore, in any patient who appears to have reflux through the popliteal vein, the test should be repeated while firm manual compression is applied to the LSV. Obliteration of the reflux in this manner will localize the site of reflux to the SPJ and not the popliteal vein itself. Another method consists of slightly compressing an uninvolved portion of the calf with one finger, which causes flow through the popliteal vein and not the lessor saphenous vein.[57] Popliteal vein reflux can be detected in this way with a sensitivity of 100% and a specificity of 92%, with most false-positives being the result of variations in the anatomy of the LSV (see Chapter 1).[4,11,61] The presence of popliteal valvular insufficiency is an important finding because it is associated with diminished calf muscle pump function and may be the most important prognostic factor in the development of venous ulceration.[4,62,63] This relationship is not, however, absolute; one study showed that popliteal incompetence was found in only 20% of patients with ulceration and 31.2% of postphlebitic legs.[55]

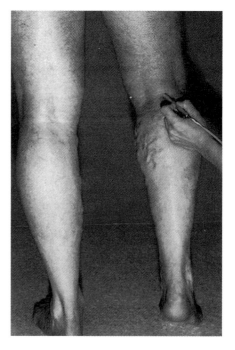

Fig. 5-17 The popliteal vein is examined with the knee flexed and the weight borne on the opposite foot.

Posterior tibial vein. The final deep vein that should be examined is the posterior tibial vein, located just posterior to the medial malleolus and beside the posterior tibial artery, whose pulsatile signal is easily located. This vein is frequently vasoconstricted, except if the patient is examined in a warm room, and therefore a spontaneous signal may not be noticeable. Augmentation maneuvers are the same as described for the other deep veins. Again, although the Doppler is generally not felt to be sufficiently sensitive in the diagnosis of DVT below the knee, the response of posterior tibial venous flow to release of calf compression has been found to allow an 87% accuracy in this diagnosis.[53,54]

Superficial veins. After the deep veins mentioned above are examined, attention is then turned to the superficial and perforating systems. The major saphenous trunks and their junctions with the deep veins should be examined with the patient in the standing position. Because of the lower flow rate in these vessels, a spontaneous signal may only rarely be audible. The presence of a saphena varix, or a visible bulge over the SFJ, is nearly pathognomonic of valvular incompetence. The junction is easily located with the Doppler approximately two fingerbreadths below the inguinal ligament, in the femoral triangle. Alternatively, one may first locate the LSV in the thigh and then gradually move the Doppler probe superiorly and laterally while repetitively compressing the GSV until its location is reached. A positive cough or percussion test may also help to localize the site of the SFJ. The presence of reflux on release of more distal compression is indicative of SFJ insufficiency. The magnitude of the compression can, again, be standardized for serial comparisons by using a pneumatic cuff inflated to a specific level. Also, the Valsalva maneuver may be employed to elicit reflux, although manual compression of the SFJ by the inguinal ligament may occur during a forceful Valsalva, and more proximal competent valves may impede the retrograde flow,[64] thus creating the false impression of a competent valve.

If no reflux is heard over the SFJ, it should not be assumed that the entire GSV is competent.[65-67] The perforator(s) in Hunter's canal may frequently be the first abnormality to develop, leading to dilation and incompetence beginning just below the level of the middle thigh (see Chapters 1 and 3).[27,68] Reflux may also originate in branches of the GSV, the "atypical refluxes" described by Schultz-Ehrenburg and Hubner.[57] Incompetence of the GSV that is limited to the calf suggests insufficiency of the geniculate or lower leg perforators. Therefore, it is important to test the GSV for reflux in the groin, at the level of the knee, and in the lower leg, not assuming that it is normal until all sites fail to demonstrate reflux. In addition, there is a growing consensus that dilation may occur due to biochemical abnormalities in the muscle of the varicose vein wall. Thus, valvular insufficiency may not necessarily be a descending process, as was once assumed. This underscores the need to evaluate the entire length of the GSV in determining which portions of the vein to treat.[65]

Examination of the LSV and the SPJ is best carried out with the patient standing and the knee slightly flexed, as previously described. The LSV is felt more easily with the knee flexed and the popliteal fossa relaxed.[10] When enlarged, the LSV generally is still not visible, but it is easily palpable as a spongy tubular structure leading inferiorly from the popliteal crease. By listening over the popliteal vein and tapping the leg very gently 5 to 10 cm below the probe, one will selectively compress and thus listen to the LSV and not the popliteal vein, which requires a much stronger force. Since the termination of the LSV is variable, the exact location of the probe cannot be known for certain; therefore, it is difficult to determine if any reflux heard is originating from the SPJ or is simply within a dilated LSV. The Valsalva maneuver or compression of the thigh aids in this differentiation because it results in reflux only if the SPJ is incompetent. Distinction between flow through the SPJ and popliteal vein can also be difficult but is facilitated by manually compressing the LSV below the probe while pressing on the calf as described previously. Abolition of the reflux is evidence that the source is the SPJ.[11] Another method is to listen over a more distal segment of the LSV, along the posterolateral calf, and to compress and release the LSV at the popliteal crease. Reflux or only augmentation after release will be detected easily.

Perforating veins. The examination of perforating veins is, at best, only 80% accurate using the Doppler,[69-71] and many believe that physical examination—that is, palpation of fascial defects where the incompetent perforator meets a dilated superficial vein at the depth of the superficial fascia—is perhaps even more helpful.[72] In fact, published studies document that palpation is accurate only 51%[31] to 69%[33] of the time. This technique, which is discussed more fully in Chapter 9, yields a large number of false-positive results, because a fascial defect may result merely from dilation of a superficial varicosity or even from a separate pathologic process, such as a muscle hernia. In these situations the Doppler will afford increased reliability. In fact, Doppler examination for incompetent perforating veins is advised after preliminary clinical localization of suspected sites, listening for the characteristic to and fro movement of blood over sites of palpable defects in the fascia. Some authors have advocated placing tourniquets at 4-inch increments along the course of the lower leg before listening for flux and reflux at the sites of fascial weakness while the calf or thigh is repetitively compressed.[69-71] A simpler approach is to place one tourniquet just below the level of the fascial defect and another just above it. While listening with the Doppler over each marked fascial defect, one compresses the foot. (Fig. 5-18) Any audible signal will thus represent flow proximally through the deep system and outward through an incompetent perforating vein. This provides greater specificity, because it interrupts the flow through the superficial veins, thus allowing selective examination of the perforating veins. Fig. 5-19 provides a rational method of recording the venous Doppler examination findings.

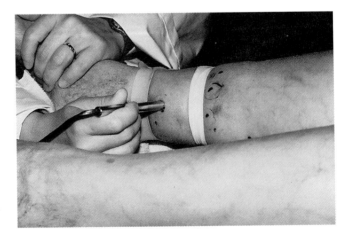

Fig. 5-18 After making fascial defects palpable with the leg elevated, the Doppler is used to detect outward flow at each site. Tourniquets are placed just proximal and distal to each potential incompetent perforating vein and the foot is compressed to produce flow upward through the deep veins.

PRESCLEROTHERAPY EXAMINATION

Deep veins		Right	Left
Common femoral	Phasicity		
	Reflux w/inspiration		
	Reflux w/Valsalva		
	Duration		
Popliteal	Reflux w/Valsalva		
	Reflux w/thigh compression		
	Reflux w/calf release		
Posterior tibial	Reflux w/calf compression		
	Reflux w/foot release		
SFJ	Reflux w/Valsalva		
	Reflux w/calf release		
	Duration		
	Trendelenburg test		
LSV distal thigh	Reflux		
	Diameter		
LSV calf	Reflux		
	Diameter		
SPJ	Reflux		
	Diameter		
SSV	Reflux		
	Diameter		

Tributary 1: Location _____ Diameter _____ LSV _____ SSV _____

Tributary 2: Location _____ Diameter _____ LSV _____ SSV _____

Tributary 3: Location _____ Diameter _____ LSV _____ SSV _____

Tributary 4: Location _____ Diameter _____ LSV _____ SSV _____

Fig. 5-19 Chart for recording venous Doppler examination.

Table 5-3 A comparison of Doppler ultrasound and Duplex scanning in the presclerotherapy evaluation

	Doppler	**Duplex**
Portability	Portable	Not easily portable "Luggable" units available
Ease of use	Requires short period of training and experience	Requires longer period of training
Cost (approx.)	Unidirectional—$300 Bidirectional—$2500	Grey scale—$40,000 and up Color—$150,000 and up
Information obtained	1. Patency, competence of venous valves 2. DVT in thigh (?calf)	1. Patency, competence of venous valves 2. DVT w/greater accuracy 3. Velocity of reflux 4. Anatomy and anomalies of venous system 5. Termination of SSV 6. Thrombosis vs. sclerosis
Reliability	Less reliable because of blind, nonpulsed sound beam	More reliable because of actual visualization of vein being examined

Posttreatment evaluation. Follow-up examinations of injected veins using the Doppler contribute more precise information regarding the response to treatment than physical examination because a vein that has been sclerosed loses both spontaneous and augmented flow signals. However, the Doppler detects flow through any vessel passing within the sound wave beam and thus does not allow the examiner to be certain that the signal is from a particular vessel. Also, the Doppler does not differentiate thrombus from fibrosis because both lead to an absence of a flow signal. These limitations illustrate the advantages of the Duplex scanner, another technological advance that is revolutionizing the practice of phlebology (Table 5-3).[73-76]

Duplex Scanners

Duplex scanners are ultrasound machines that generally use a 7.5- or 10-MHz imaging probe along with a 3-MHz pulsed Doppler to enable visualization of the superficial venous system as well as to determine the direction of blood flow within the examined veins. Anatomy, flow within the veins, and the movement of the valves may also be studied (Fig. 5-20). Newer scanners (sometimes termed *triplex*) employ a computer-generated color system in which antegrade and retrograde flow may be coded to appear as different colors (red or blue), with varying intensities (brighter with lower velocities, paler with higher velocities), thus allowing immediate integration of this information by the examiner (Fig. 5-21). Visual ultrasound images have found their greatest use within the field of venous disease in the diagnosis of DVT and have now all but replaced venography in centers where the instrumentation is available (Fig. 5-22).[77-82] More recent alterations in the frequency range of the probes have enabled clear resolution of superficial and deep veins, thus introducing an entirely new era in the treatment of varicose veins by sclerotherapy.

As an aid to sclerotherapy. If the Doppler is the "ears" of the phlebologist, the Duplex scanner may be considered both the ears and a pair of binoculars, because it allows the examiner to "see" much more than can be ascertained other-

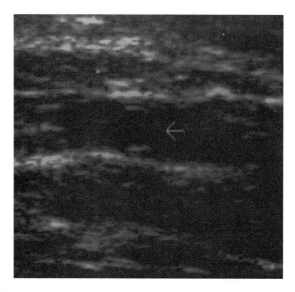

Fig. 5-20 Duplex scanners may provide clear images of anatomic structures such as the SFJ and venous valves *(arrow).*

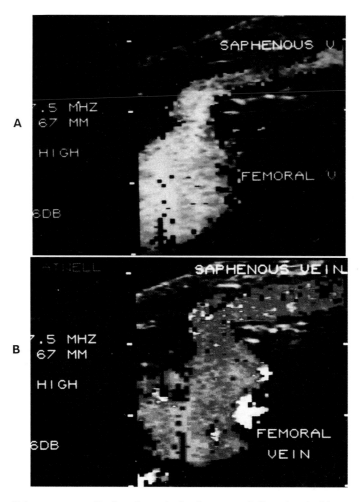

Fig. 5-21 Color scanners display flow, **A**, in the normal direction in blue and **B**, reflux flow in red.

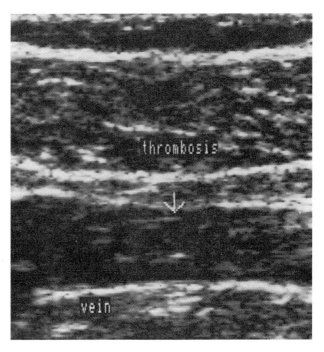

Fig. 5-22 Ultrasound provides clear images of DVT. Thrombus may appear as an echogenic mass or simply result in the vein being noncompressible.

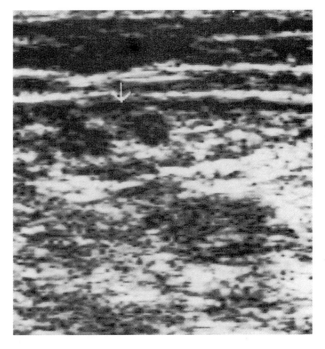

Fig. 5-23 Anomalies such as this duplication of the GSV *(arrow)* may be visualized with a Duplex scanner.

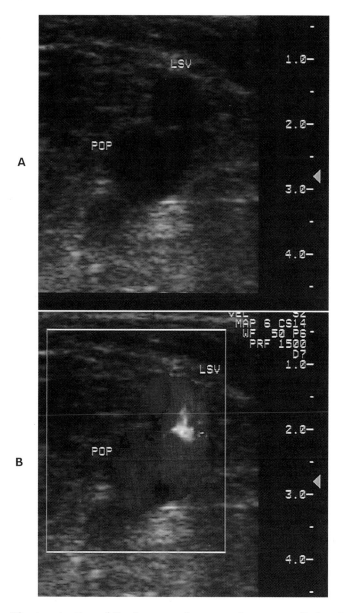

Fig. 5-24 The termination of the lessor saphenous vein can usually be visualized quite easily with Duplex scanning. **A,** Transverse image, grey scale. **B,** After release of the calf compression, showing reflux.

wise. The Duplex scanner allows for determination of the exact anatomy, including the important saphenofemoral and saphenopopliteal junctions. Although the anatomy of the SFJ is generally believed to be similar in all persons, there is actually significant variation. Duplication of the GSV can be found in up to 27% of persons[7-9] and is easily demonstrable with this technology (Fig. 5-23). Because the termination of the LSV is so variable, the exact location of the SPJ or the termination of the LSV in the GSV or its tributaries (the superficial or common femoral veins) or in tributaries of the internal iliac veins[82] can be seen on the Duplex scan (Fig 5-24). Before operating on the LSV, selective venography was once advised to determine the exact site of termination of the LSV.[83-85] Now the Duplex scanner may provide this piece of information noninvasively.[86,87] Injections into the SFJ or SPJ, if performed under ultrasonic guidance,[88,89] confer an added degree of accuracy and safety to this procedure (Fig. 5-25). Injections into incompetent perforating veins, particularly in areas of ulceration or lipodermatosclerosis, can be facilitated greatly by performing them under ultrasonic guidance.[90] This area may be particularly difficult to examine clinically or with a Doppler alone, and injections done blindly into this area can be quite risky due to the proximity of the posterior tibial vein and artery. Finally, the anatomic basis for proximal recurrences following GSV or LSV ligation may be found through Duplex scanning. If the recurrent varicosities are found to communicate directly with the common femoral or popliteal veins, repeat ligation at the junction may be indicated.

In addition, as McMullin and Appleberg have found, Duplex measurement of antegrade flow rates through the common femoral vein, superficial femoral vein, popliteal vein, and GSV may be used to determine the degree of resistance within the deep veins and thus the preferential flow up the superficial veins in patients with chronic venous insufficiency. If it is found that the flow rate upward through an incompetent GSV is quite high in a given patient with disease in more than one segment of their venous system, removal or closure of this vein might be contraindicated. The amount of flow generated by active dorsiflexion of the foot may also provide information on the efficacy of the musculovenous pump.[91]

Posttreatment evaluation. Another major use of the Duplex scanner with sclerotherapy is in the follow-up of patients. As mentioned above, the Doppler does not allow differentiation between thrombus and fibrosis, both of which yield abolition of flow through the involved vein segment. The Duplex scanner can differentiate these two situations more clearly. Depending on its age, thrombus may appear as a variably echogenic space associated with soft tissue swelling and inflammation, whereas fibrosis appears more often as a dense line with no associated inflammatory reaction (Fig. 5-26). Because patient response to treatment is so variable, one can now more accurately determine if the treatment rendered has been completely effective, producing fibrosis, or if the vessel is occluded by

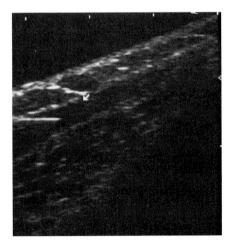

Fig. 5-25   Injection into the SFJ may be performed under ultrasonic guidance. The needle is seen inside of the SFJ. (Courtesy Robert M. Knight, M.D.) © 1989 R.M. Knight, M.D.

thrombus, thereby necessitating additional treatment. Many apparent treatment failures with early recurrence are likely to be found to be the result of inadequate treatment and not inadequate response. One might surmise, therefore, that exact assessment of the presence or absence of fibrosis will allow the technique of sclerotherapy to progress to a science instead of the art that now dominates this field.

Another important advantage of the Duplex scanner over the Doppler is its ability to quantitate venous reflux. This parameter has been found to have some prognostic potential. The flow in milliliters per second at peak reflux was measured in 47 limbs of patients who presented with chronic venous problems. It was found that dermatitis or ulceration did not develop if the sum of the peak refluxes in the GSV, LSV, and popliteal vein was less than 10 ml/sec. A sum of greater than 15 ml/sec was associated with a high incidence of these sequelae.[4,92] In addition, superficial venous reflux alone may result in ulceration if the peak flow is greater than 7 ml/sec.[93]

In summary, advantages provided by Duplex scanning include the ability to evaluate the anatomy of the main saphenous trunks and recurrences, inject

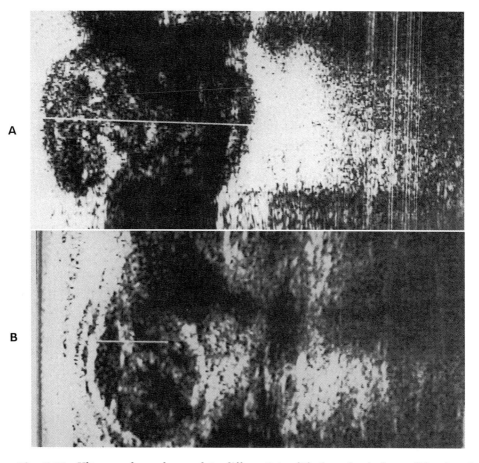

Fig. 5-26 Ultrasound can be used to differentiate, **(A)** thrombosis from, **(B)** sclerosis. (Horizontal white line indicates the diameter of the vessel.) (Courtesy Pauline Raymond-Martimbeau, M.D.)

difficult areas under ultrasonic guidance, determine the presence of fibrosis, and quantitate both reflux and forward flow. Unfortunately, both the Doppler and Duplex scanners are usually used to obtain only anatomic information and thus leave the actual hemodynamic effect of the various abnormalities unknown. Therefore, especially in the setting of deep as well as superficial venous insufficiency or when multiple segments of the superficial system are incompetent (for example, both the SFJ and lower leg perforators), a functional study is necessary.

Photoplethysmography

The most widely used functional evaluation for presclerotherapy purposes is photoplethysmography (PPG).[94-97] Various forms of plethysmography have been used to evaluate venous function since 1956,[98] and they have been shown to correlate well with venographic findings[99] and ambulatory venous pressure (AVP) measurements. In one study of 338 paired measurements of PPG and AVP, the correlation coefficient was 0.9.[94] The principle of PPG is quite simple, and the test is easy and quick to perform. An infrared light source and sensor are attached with adhesive to the medial aspect of the lower leg approximately 10 cm proximal to the medial malleolus. The infrared light is transmitted into the leg to a depth of approximately 0.5 to 1.5 mm, within the subdermal venous plexus, where it is absorbed by hemoglobin in red blood cells. Of the light that is not absorbed, a certain amount returns to the sensor. Therefore, the amount of infrared light reflected is inversely proportional to the volume of blood in the skin. Once a baseline level is reached, the patient is asked to actively dorsiflex the foot 5 to 10 times, resulting in activation of the calf muscle pump and producing venous outflow (Fig. 5-27). With a reduced volume of blood in the calf and the subdermal plexus, more light is reflected and the tracing shows a gradual deflection (the direction of the deflection depends on the electronics of the particular instrument). At the conclusion of exercise, the patient is asked to relax and the tracing then returns to either the original baseline value or levels off at a new value of light transmission. The time required for this value to be reached, the venous refilling time (VRT), provides information on the presence and degree of reflux of blood through either superficial or deep veins (Fig. 5-28).

Normally, refilling of blood occurs only through the arterial circuit and takes at least 20 to 25 seconds. A value less than 20 seconds is indicative of the presence of an abnormal refilling channel, namely retrograde flow through incompetent superficial or deep veins. Repeating the test while firmly compressing a particular vein allows one to assess the degree of hemodynamic disturbance contributed by that vein. Specifically, if the venous refilling time lengthens from 15 to 35 seconds when a vein is compressed, one can be assured that this vein is contributing significantly to the patient's problem. Similarly, in the setting of both superficial and deep venous incompetence, by compressing the superficial veins one can theoretically prevent reflux of blood through these veins and observe the effect of the deep venous system alone. If the VRT lengthens significantly when a tourniquet is placed around the thigh to occlude the superficial veins, this implies the dominance of the superficial system in the patient's pathology. If the VRT remains essentially unchanged, one can assume that the deep veins are the primary problem. A word of caution must be mentioned, however, relating to the method of compression of the vein(s). A simple tourniquet, such as that used in phlebotomy, is used frequently and has the advantage of compressing all of the superficial veins, even those that are not suspected of being enlarged and insufficient. However, it is important to be aware that this type of compression may not adequately compress all of the superficial veins, particularly large, thick-walled varicosities.

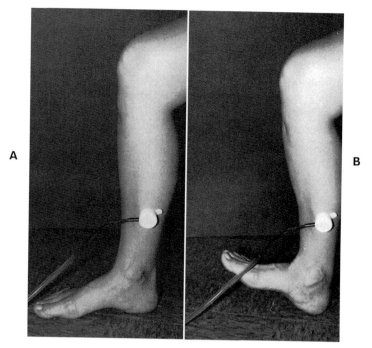

Fig. 5-27 **A,** Photoplethysmography measures venous emptying during and refilling after exercise of the calf and foot muscles. **B,** Emptying is accomplished with 5 to 10 dorsiflexions of the foot.

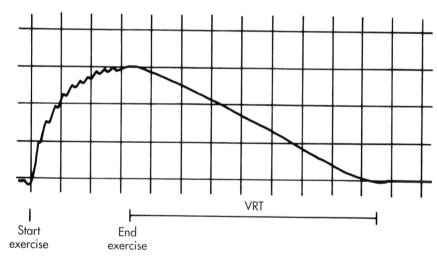

Fig. 5-28 Photoplethysmography. Light reflection is enhanced as the calf muscle is exercised and blood is pumped out of the leg. A reduction in light reflection is seen once the leg is allowed to rest. The venous refilling time *(VRT)* is indicative of the degree of reflux, although it is not quantitative.

The need for this awareness is especially important in obese patients, but it is also necessary in patients of normal weight. By using a Duplex scanner to visualize the flow through the GSV, McMullin, Coleridge Smith, and Scurr[100] found that the pressure within a 2.5-cm-wide tourniquet required to prevent reflux through the vein varied between 40 and 300 mm Hg in the 40 patients studied. Therefore, manual compression applied directly to the vein being considered is the preferred method because it is allows more reliable interruption of the flow and gives reproducibly accurate results.

VRT has been found to correlate well with AVP measurements that have long been considered the gold standard in the functional evaluation of venous hemodynamics. VRT may vary between 20 and 65 seconds when AVP is below 40 mm Hg, but a VRT less than 15 seconds is found only if the AVP is higher than 40 mm Hg.[101] AVP measurements show a linear relationship between their value and the incidence of venous ulceration.[4,102]

PPG may also be used to quantify the blood changes within the subdermal plexus, thus quantifying the degree of reflux. This involves performing an in vivo calibration maneuver that allows one to assign a numerical value to the deflections on the tracing.[103,104] The transducer is placed on the leg in its usual location while the patient rests in the supine position, and the tracing on the recorder is set to a zero baseline. The patient then stands, bearing weight on the opposite leg, and after the tracing levels off, the gain is adjusted so that the deflection reflects the calculated hydrostatic pressure in the superficial veins, measured by the distance from the right atrium to the site of the transducer on the leg. This maneuver is repeated until the zero baseline and standing levels of subdermal plexus blood content reproducibly reflect the hydrostatic pressures. The decrement in the tracing is then proportional to the degree of fall in AVP, as measured by invasive venous pressure recordings.

Light Reflection Rheography

Light reflection rheography (LRR), which is basically a form of photoplethysmography, was intended to improve upon the original PPG system.[105,106] Due to its incorporation of three light sources, the infrared light beam can be focused at a standardized depth of penetration (0.3 to 2.3 mm) to cover the subcutaneous venous plexus. Dermal pigment, such as that commonly found in patients with chronic venous insufficiency, is concentrated in the more superficial layers of the skin and interferes with light transmission, yielding inaccurate and variable values. It was hoped that by focusing its light beam on the deeper tissues, the LRR would not be as affected by the tissues containing the majority of the pigment. This did not prove to be the case, however, and it was felt that calibration of the system might neutralize the effect of the variables of skin thickness, skin pigment, and local blood volume on light absorption. This improvement is now available as D-PPG (Digital PPG) or C-PPG (calibratable PPG).[101]

The D-PPG contains a computer that permits changes in light intensity from the infrared light source according to the optical properties of the skin. The machine emits a standard light intensity and awaits reflection of the unabsorbed light. If it is below a certain level, the intensity of the emitted light is automatically increased until the intensity of reflected light reaches a level at which the machine can function accurately. This was demonstrated nicely by Kerner, Schultz-Ehrenburg, and Blazek, who recorded essentially the same response to dorsiflexion even after the leg was covered with a dark paint.[107,108]

The C-PPG is essentially the same except that the changes in light intensity are adjusted manually. This device was tested on normal subjects and on patients with venous disease. By comparing the time to 90% refilling, or by combining the results obtained during postural changes and dorsiflexion in order to obtain exercise drainage volume, it was possible to significantly differentiate patients with venous ulcers from those with varicose veins and from the normal controls.[101] Other parameters that can be calculated include venous filling volume and pump efficiency.

The usefulness of PPG in assessing venous valvular insufficiency is undisputed; however, the claims that it is accurate in diagnosing DVT are controversial. The general statement that a "picket fence" pattern (Fig. 5-29) produced by the 10 dorsiflexions with essentially no vertical movement off of the baseline is diagnostic of DVT certainly is incorrect, because there are many false positives using this criterion. In a study of 30 limbs, the correlation coefficient between venous emptying and AVP was only 0.73.[105] However, in a study performed at the University of Miami,[109] the slope of the deflection correlated well with the presence of acute DVT as documented by venography. As in Fig. 5-30, the finding of a slope (R/T) of less than 0.31 mm/sec predicts the presence of DVT with a 96% sensitivity. Still, at this time, LRR alone is not considered sufficient to make the diagnosis of DVT, and at least one other noninvasive test is required to confirm the diagnosis.

Air Plethysmography

Another technology, which is just as simple to use and potentially supplies a great deal of additional information compared with the conventional PPG, is the air plethysmograph (APG).[110] This device consists of a 14-inch long tubular polyvinylchloride air chamber that surrounds the leg from knee to ankle. This is inflated to 6 mm Hg and connected to a pressure transducer, an amplifier, and a recorder. A smaller bag placed between the air chamber and the leg is used for calibration by injecting a certain volume of air or water and measuring the change in the recording that is associated with that volume (Fig. 5-31). Parameters assessed include (a) functional venous volume (VV), the volume in the leg while the patient stands; (b) venous filling time 90 (VFT 90), the time required to achieve 90% of the VV; (c) venous filling index (VFI), 90% VV/VFT 90; (d) ejection volume (EV), the volume expelled from the leg with one tip-toe motion; (f) residual volume (RV), the volume at the end of 10 tip-toe motions; and (g) residual volume fraction (RVF), RV/VV 100 (Fig. 5-32). In a study of 22 patients with superficial venous insufficiency and 9 patients with deep venous disease,[111]

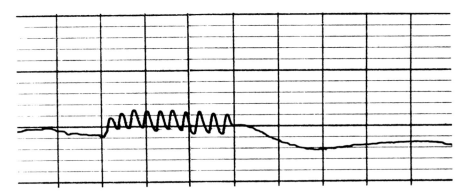

Fig. 5-29 A "picket fence" pattern may indicate DVT but may also be seen with chronic venous insufficiency without thrombosis.

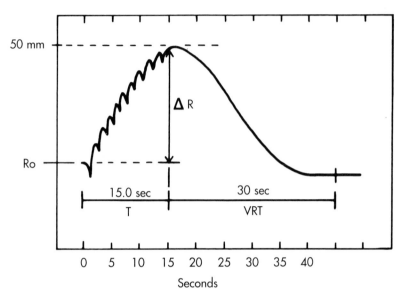

Fig. 5-30 Usefulness of PPG in the diagnosis of DVT may be improved by examination of the slope R/T; $< .31$ mm/sec predicts the presence of DVT with a 96% sensitivity.

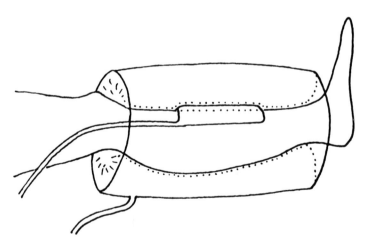

Fig. 5-31 The air plethysmograph consists of a long tubular polyvinyl chamber that surrounds the entire leg. This chamber is inflated to 6 mm Hg and is connected to a pressure transducer, an amplifier, and a recorder. A smaller bag is placed between the air chamber and the leg for calibration. (From Christopoulos DG et al: J Vasc Surg 5[1]:148, 1987.)

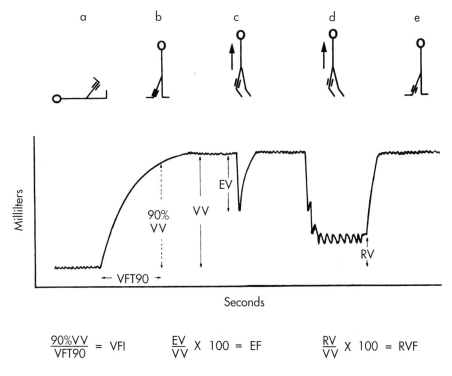

$$\frac{90\% VV}{VFT90} = VFI \qquad \frac{EV}{VV} \times 100 = EF \qquad \frac{RV}{VV} \times 100 = RVF$$

Fig. 5-32 Diagrammatic representation of typical recording of volume changes during standard sequence of postural changes and exercise using the air plethysmograph. Patient in supine position with leg elevated 45 degrees *(a)*; patient standing with weight on nonexamined leg *(b)*; single tip-toe movement *(c)*; ten tip-toe movements *(d)*; single tip-toe movement *(e)*. *VV* = functional venous volume; *VFT* = venous filling time; *VFI* = venous filling index; *EV* = ejected volume; *RV* = residual volume; *EF* = ejection fraction; *RVF* = residual volume fraction. (From Christopoulos DG et al: J Vasc Surg 5[1]:148, 1987.)

it was found that VV was elevated in 80% of patients. VFT 90 was greater than 70 seconds in normal limbs, 8 to 82 seconds in limbs with superficial venous insufficiency, and 9 to 19 seconds in limbs with deep venous disease. VFI was less than 1.7 ml/sec in normal limbs, 2 to 30 ml/sec in limbs with superficial venous insufficiency, and 7 to 28 ml/sec in limbs with deep venous disease. Ejection fraction (EF) appeared to show better discrimination than EV. The RVF was 20% in normal legs, 45% in legs with superficial venous insufficiency, and 60% in legs with deep venous disease (Fig. 5-33).

A linear correlation with r = 0.83 was present between RVF and AVP. In another study of 104 patients,[93,112] VFI was found to correlate with the incidence of sequelae of venous disease such as chronic swelling, skin changes, and ulceration, as seen in Table 5-4 on p. 179. In a third study of 205 limbs,[113] the same authors found an increasing incidence of ulceration in patients with diminished EF and elevated VFI (Table 5-5 on p. 179) and found that the RVF showed a good correlation (r = 0.81) with the incidence of ulceration and AVP measurements. The real advantages of this method are its ability to quantitate reflux with the VFI and thus determine prognosis, and its ability to measure calf muscle pump func-

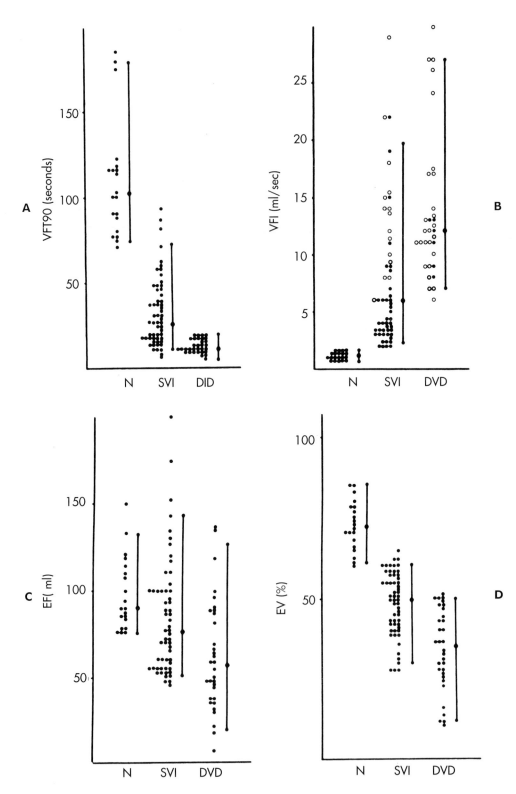

Fig. 5-33 Air plethysmography. Results of **A**, VFT/90; **B**, VFI; **C**, EV, **D**, EF. (*N* = normal limbs; *SVI* = limbs with superficial venous incompetence; *DVD* = limbs with deep venous disease.) (From Christopoulos DG et al: J Vasc Surg 5[1]:148, 1987.)

Table 5-4 Venous filling index and sequelae of venous disease

VFI (ml/sec)	Chronic swelling (%)	Ulceration (%)	Skin change (+/− ulcer)
<3	0	0	0
3-5	12	0	19
5-10	46	46	61
>10	76	58	76

Table 5-5 Effect of VFI and EF on incidence of venous ulceration

	EF >40%			EF <40%			
	Total no. of limbs	Limbs w/ulcers		Total no. of limbs	Limbs w/ulcers		
		No.	%		No.	%	p
VFI < 5	41	1	2	19	6	32	<0.01
5 < VFI < 10	37	11	30	19	12	63	<0.02
VFI > 10	32	13	41	27	19	70	<0.05

From Christopoulos DG et al: Surgery 106(5):829, 1989.

tion through the determination of the EF.[93,111-114] Still, APG measurements should not be used in a vacuum. They should be combined with Doppler or Duplex findings and clinical evaluation, since a great deal of overlap in values between normal and abnormal occur, decreasing the predictive value of abnormal APG measurements.[115] Neglen and Raju demonstrated quite well in their evaluation of 118 limbs that VFI alone had a positive predictive value of 66% in separating clinical severity class zero or class one from class two or class three. VFI combined with information gleaned from Duplex scanning had a positive predictive value of 83%.[116]

Foot Volumetry

Yet another method for evaluation of the functional state of the venous system is foot volumetry.[117-122] Introduced in the early 1970s, this technique has not earned a prominent place in phlebology, probably because of certain logistics of performing the test. The patient stands with the feet in an open water-filled plethysmograph (Fig. 5-34). The water level is monitored by a photoelectric sensor and changes in foot volume are continuously measured, first while the patient is standing still, then during the performance of 20 knee bends, and again while standing still. The parameters measured include the volume of blood expelled from the foot during exercise, the flow rate after exercise, and the time required for half and then full refilling to occur. Norgren et al.[120] have shown good correlation between foot volumetry and invasive venous pressure measurements in control subjects (r = 0.662) and in patients with varicose veins (r = 0.760), but poor correlation in patients with deep venous valvular insufficiency (r = 0.410). In their study, venous pressure measurements differed significantly in patients with varicose veins and controls, but were similar in patients with primary varicose veins and those with deep venous valvular insufficiency. However, using foot volumetry, there were significant differences between all three groups. Thus, although it is possible that foot volumetry is inaccurate in this important categorization, it is likely that this technique is more sensitive in distinguishing these groups than are venous pressure measurements.[121] It has been shown that both

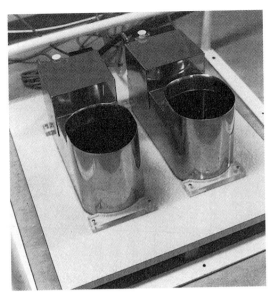

Fig. 5-34 The apparatus for foot volumetry consists of an open water-filled plethysmograph that allows continuous measurement of foot volume at rest and during exercise via monitoring of the water level by a photo-electric floatsensor. (Courtesy Lars Norgren, M.D.)

Table 5-6 Functional venous studies

	PPG	Foot volumetry	APG
Ease of use	Easy	Easy	Requires practice by patient
	Hygienic	Communal bath	Hygienic
	5 min test	5-10 min test	5-10 min test
Cost	$2500 and up		$7500
Information obtained	1. Presence of reflux	1. Presence and degree of reflux	1. Presence and degree of reflux
	2. Superficial vs deep	2. Calf muscle pump function	2. Superficial vs. deep
	3. ?DVT		3. Calf muscle pump function

the volume expelled with exercise and the refilling time increase after treatment of varicose veins.[122] Therefore, this test could be used to evaluate the success of a particular treatment, to follow the effect of different stages in treatment, and to monitor the severity of chronic venous insufficiency. It does not, however, allow localization of a particular site of reflux, thus limiting its usefulness for pre-sclerotherapy evaluation when compared with other methods (Table 5-6).

Venography

Venography is still felt by many clinicians to represent the "gold standard" in the evaluation of venous obstructive disease, and the results of all studies evaluating newer methods for the diagnosis of DVT are compared with those of venography. The most serious disadvantages of venography are its invasive method, the frequent development of superficial phlebitis as a result of the procedure, and a 5% to

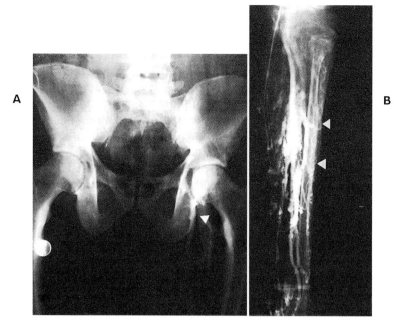

Fig. 5-35 Ascending venography demonstrating, (**A**) thrombus as a space-filling defect *(arrowhead)* and, (**B**) incompetent perforating vein *(arrowheads)*.

10% incidence of allergy to the contrast medium. The latter complications have been significantly reduced through the introduction of newer nonionic contrast media,[9] and venography continues to find frequent use in the diagnosis and treatment planning of venous disease. It also has great utility in the evaluation of groin and pelvic recurrences, including vulvar varicosities.[123] Four techniques have been described: ascending, descending, intraosseous venography, and varicography.

A variation of venography involving the injection of fluorescein into a vein on the dorsum of the foot has been used for the localization of incompetent ankle perforating veins.[124] This simple bedside test is performed by placing a 2.5-cm cuff, inflated to 80 mm Hg, just above the malleoli. The leg is elevated to 90 degrees, and the patient is asked to plantarflex the foot 10 times. A second 13-cm cuff is then inflated to 120 mm Hg just above the knee, and the leg is lowered. Aqueous fluorescein 5 ml is then injected into the distal portion of the foot, and an ultraviolet light is directed toward the leg in the darkened room. A second set of 10 plantarflexions is performed, drawing the solution into the deep veins and outward through any incompetent perforators. This is reflected on the skin surface as a circle of yellow-green fluorescence, 1 to 2 cm in diameter, within 30 seconds to 2 minutes. In 37 legs studied, this method had a 96% accuracy, identifying 50 of the 52 perforating veins later found to be incompetent at surgery, with two false negatives and four false positives.

Ascending venography. Ascending venography[9] is performed by injecting the contrast medium into a superficial vein on the dorsum of the foot after a 2.5-cm tourniquet is placed around the ankle to prevent flow through the superficial venous system. This forces the contrast to enter only the deep veins and allows clearer visualization of the deep system. Fluoroscopic imaging with the patient in various positions allows examination of the deep veins from the foot to the lower segment of the inferior vena cava for the presence of thrombi (Fig. 5-35, *A*). Passage of the contrast into the perforating veins is abnormal and diagnostic of valvular insufficiency (Fig. 5-35, *B*).[32] The addition of a Valsalva maneuver shows competent venous valves and defines bicuspid structures with a concentration of contrast media in their sinuses and may obviate the need for descending venography if this procedure was to be considered later. Ascending functional venography requires the patient to plantarflex the foot, thus forcing the contrast into the superficial veins through any incompetent perforating veins during muscle relaxation.[4]

Descending venography. Descending venography involves injection of the contrast into the femoral or the popliteal vein with the patient supine or tilted head up and performing a Valsalva maneuver. Valvular insufficiency is readily demonstrated because the contrast flows rapidly in a retrograde direction. Five grades of reflux have been described (Fig. 5-36).[55,125] One of the disadvantages of this technique is that the demonstration of reflux at a given level relies on the presence of reflux at the higher levels. Therefore, using descending venography alone, one might miss isolated incompetence of tibial veins or gastrocnemius veins, both of which have been shown to be responsible for the production of significant symptoms (see Chapters 3 and 4).[126,127]

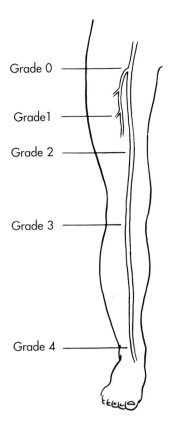

Fig. 5-36 Descending venography may demonstrate 5 grades of reflux: *Grade 0*—no reflux below the confluence of the superficial and profunda femoris veins; *Grade 1*—reflux into the superficial femoral vein but not below the middle of the thigh; *Grade 2*—reflux into the superficial femoral vein but not through the popliteal vein; *Grade 3*—reflux to just below the knee; *Grade 4*—reflux to the ankle level.

Intraosseus venography. Intraosseus venography is simply a variation of ascending venography in which the contrast is injected into bone rather than directly into a vein, with rapid distribution throughout the deep venous system. This technique may be significantly easier to perform in patients with edema[128] and may be especially helpful in diagnosing incompetent perforating veins,[32] yet it has not been found to have significant use recently.

Varicography. Varicography (Fig. 5-37) is a very helpful technique in which the contrast agent is injected directly into the dilated varix, showing the extent of the varicosities and their connection with other superficial, perforating, and deep veins.[9,123,129,130] The direction of blood flow and, therefore, the competence of valves is not discernible, although other criteria have been found to correlate with valvular insufficiency. For instance, if a perforator is greater than 3 mm in diameter and is seen to be tortuous, it is assumed to be incompetent.[9] When other methods, such as Duplex scanning, fail to demonstrate the proximal connections of a varicosity (due to obesity of the patient, masses of varicosities in the area, etc.), varicography provides a relatively simple way of clearly showing this anatomy (Fig. 5-38).

Thermography

Infrared thermography is based on the fact that infrared waves radiate from the skin surface in proportion to the temperature of that surface.[131,132] It is possible to scan the surface with an infrared detector and create an image where gradations of white and black or color reflect degrees of heat. Two identical symmetric skin areas of the body should be at the same temperature unless certain factors are present. These factors include structural abnormalities of vessels (dilation and incompetence), abnormalities of vascular control, local effects on vessels, changes

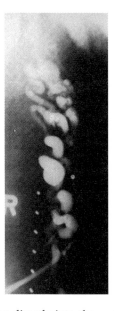

Fig. 5-37 Varicography. Injection directly into the varix may demonstrate the origin of a recurrence in the groin after vein stripping. (From Lea Thomas M and Mahraj RPM: Phlebology 3:155, 1988.)

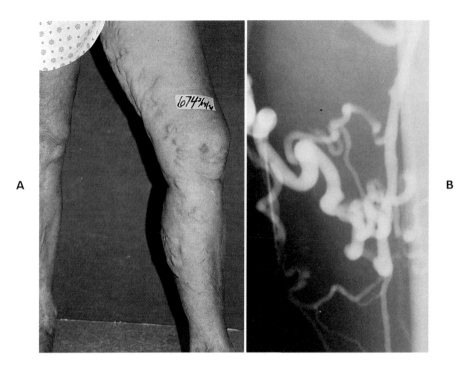

Fig. 5-38   This patient presented with a recurrent varicosity 25 years after GSV stripping (**A**). Duplex ultrasound showed no reflux at the level of the SFJ and no evidence of a GSV but was unable to demonstrate the connection of the varicosity to the deep venous system. Varicography clearly showed the proximal site of connection as well as sites of additional incompetent perforating veins (**B**).

in thermal conductivity of the tissues, or increased heat production of the tissues. When veins are dilated, such as with varicose veins or with an underlying arteriovenous communication, the overlying skin is warmer because of the accumulation of the extra volume of blood in the dilated vein. Similarly, when venous valves are incompetent, the reflux of blood from the more central common femoral vein down the GSV when the limb is lowered or outward from the warmer deep veins through a perforating vein when the calf muscle is activated produces a rise in skin temperature, and this may be visualized on the thermograph as a white, or "hot," spot (Fig. 5-39). In fact, this technique may be used to localize the site of an incompetent perforating vein (see Chapter 3).[33] After recording the general distribution of thermal patterns in the standing position, the leg is elevated for 1 minute to drain the veins, and the leg temperature is lowered with a cold, wet towel or a fan for 5 minutes. A tourniquet is placed around the proximal thigh to occlude the superficial veins, and the patient is asked to stand. Areas of rapid rewarming suggest possible sites of incompetent perforating veins. These areas are reexamined after placing tourniquets above and below each site. The segment in question is again cooled, and the appearance of a hot area within 60 seconds of standing (in the case of a thigh perforator) or of calf muscle action (in the case of a lower leg perforator) identifies the site of an incompetent perforator. Of 84 incompetent perforating veins later found at operation, thermography correctly identified 79 (94%). The five that were missed by thermography were found at surgery to be very small in diameter or in close proximity to a larger incompetent perforator that was correctly identified. Of the 12 false positives, 4

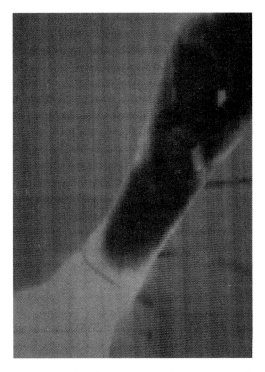

Fig. 5-39   Positive thermograph. The presence of an IPV may be indicated by a "hot" spot. (Courtesy K. Lloyd Williams, M.D., CHIR, FRCS.)

were caused by inadequate surgical exploration of the area, and the others were the result of heat changes from communicating sites of superficial veins or from the penetration of the GSV into the deep fascia of the thigh.

USE OF NONINVASIVE TECHNIQUES

Each of the above described techniques has advantages, limitations, and uses in specific situations. Prohibitive cost or limited access may preclude the use of the most sensitive and accurate method. Therefore, the following section discusses a reasonable use of various noninvasive techniques for a variety of situations commonly encountered in the everyday practice of sclerotherapy (Table 5-7).

Many practitioners have noted changes in the findings of flow and reflux depending on timing within the menstrual cycle, time of day, recent use of compression hosiery, and psychologic stress of the patient. Clearly, there is enough experimental data to support a physiologic cause for these fluctuations.[133] Therefore, an effort to examine patients in the most physiologic circumstances (for example, premenstrually, late in the day, etc.) may be rewarded by a more revealing study.

Examination of Deep Veins

One of the simplest techniques available for the detection of valvular competence in the deep venous system also happens to be quite sensitive and accurate. The Doppler ultrasound can be used to completely examine the common femoral, popliteal, and posterior tibial veins in less than 5 minutes, as described above, giving information on the presence and specific location of incompetent valves. Pitfalls occur in the differentiation of the femoral from the SFJ and the popliteal from the SPJ, yet these generally can be sorted out by compressing the superficial

Table 5-7 Preferred methods of evaluation

	Preferred method	Pitfalls	Additional methods
Deep veins	Doppler ultrasound	Differentiation SFJ vs CFV, SPJ vs popliteal vein	PPG/LRR Venography Duplex
Saphenous trunks	Doppler ultrasound	Same as above	Percussion Trendelenburg Venography Duplex
Tributaries of saphenous trunks	Doppler ultrasound		Percussion Duplex
Perforating veins	Clinical exam + Doppler	50%-80% accurate	Venography Duplex Thermography Fluorescein
Contribution of superficial vs deep reflux	PPG/LRR		AVP Duplex velocities
Functional evaluation	PPG/LRR		AVP Foot volumetry
Vulvar varices	Clinical exam for LSV reflux		Varicography

vein and repeating the test. If confusion still exists, a limited Duplex scan easily provides the answer. This examination should be carried out with the patient in the standing position. A reflux duration of at least 0.5 seconds after the release of calf compression will identify valvular insufficiency.[52] Descending venography will, similarly, provide accurate information on the state of the deep venous valves. Although its invasiveness, associated risks, and pain make it a much less attractive option for routine use, occasionally it will provide information unobtainable with other studies (Fig. 5-40). PPG will detect the presence of valvular insufficiency, and compression of the superficial veins (either manually or with a tourniquet) will allow differentiation between superficial and deep venous reflux; however, it cannot localize the reflux to the level within the deep system (femoral versus popliteal, etc.). When both superficial and deep venous reflux are present, the PPG will allow the determination of the relative importance of each segment. Although ascending venography was once considered the gold standard for the diagnosis of acute or chronic deep venous obstructive disease, most institutions now use B-mode ultrasound or color Duplex scanning in everyday clinical practice. Magnetic resonance venography may find a place in the diagnostic armamentarium as well, since it has been found to be as accurate as Duplex scanning in the diagnosis of DVT.[134]

Descending venography will detect deep venous valvular reflux but, again, the Duplex scanner offers the additional advantage of quantifying the reflux by determining flow velocities. The finding of deep venous valvular insufficiency is worrisome, because it may be associated with chronic venous obstructive disease that may give rise to venous claudication,[36-38] since there are a small number of patients who rely on their dilated superficial channels for venous return. This was determined using strain gauge plethysmography[135] and most likely may be assessed with PPG as well. Impairment of VRT with the tourniquet might caution one to avoid treatment. Alternatively, the simplest and most practical test is to

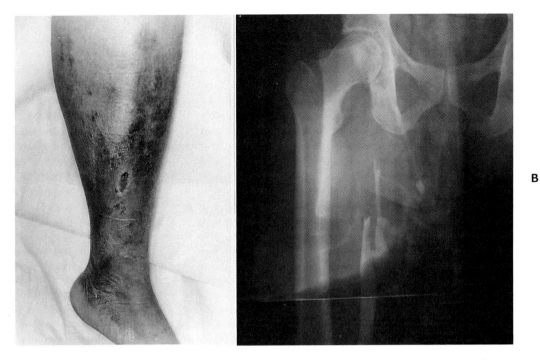

Fig. 5-40   This 36-year-old man with recurrent venous ulcers (**A**) was noted to have numerous large varices in the anteromedial thigh. A Duplex scan was complicated due to the large number of veins. Descending venography was successful in showing an absent/occluded segment of the common femoral and superficial femoral veins with a large number of collateral veins (**B**) around the obstruction.

place a 30- to 40-mm Hg compression stocking on the patient for 24 hours. The development of pain while walking contraindicates sclerotherapy and suggests the need for a venous bypass procedure. Using air plethysmography, Spence et al.[136] found that compression therapy in patients with venous claudication caused a deterioration in the ejection fraction and/or ambulatory venous pressure as measured by residual volume fraction. Noninvasive tests will not provide sufficient sensitivity if there is genuine concern about venous claudication. One must proceed with invasive pressure measurements such as the arm-foot vein pressure differential or the foot vein pressure elevation after reactive hyperemia, as described by Shami et al.[6] Deep venous valvular insufficiency has also been found to reduce the likelihood of successful long-term sclerosis of the main saphenous trunk.[57]

Examination of Saphenous Vein Trunks

Although many physicians use percussion and Trendelenburg tests as their first maneuver in assessing the competence of the saphenous trunks, Doppler ultrasound is assumed to be the most useful preliminary technique for this examination. In most cases it will provide an accurate evaluation of competence in the greater and lessor saphenous trunks as described previously. However, Lea Thomas and Bowles[137] found that it grossly overdiagnosed incompetence when compared with venography, and they recommended that all GSVs be examined with venography before ligation and stripping. One reason for this is the fact that Doppler examination is "blind," and thus dilated tributaries of the saphenous vein or pelvic varicosities may easily be mistaken for the GSV. This was addressed in two early studies[59,60] that compared the results of continuous wave Doppler examination with those obtained with Duplex scanning. The researchers found that in the examination of the GSV, Doppler was no better than 77% sensitive and 83% specific compared with the Duplex scan. In a more recent study using Duplex scanners with even greater sensitivities, DePalma et al.[138] found a sensitivity of 48%, specificity of 83%, positive predictive value of 83%, and negative predictive value of 44% in the determination of GSV reflux. By obtaining Duplex scans preoperatively, 10 limbs out of 80 were spared GSV stripping.

On the basis of this data, it might be argued that all patients with GSV varicosity should undergo Duplex scanning prior to treatment. However, the cost of this testing is high and the equipment is not readily available to many clinicians. Therefore, at this time Doppler examination affords the physician the most practical approach to this important segment of the venous system and, certainly, the Duplex scan may be obtained if there is any doubt about the diagnosis.

The Doppler examination of the junction of the saphenous trunks with the deep veins (SFJ and SPJ) and the distinction between reflux through these junctions versus reflux through the deep veins themselves is often difficult and a common source of error. In fact, studies using Doppler ultrasound have quoted an incidence of deep venous valvular reflux from 5% to 30%,[21,22,57] a range that is most likely partially determined by the difficulty of the examination and not solely by differences between the populations examined. The distinction between junctional and actual deep venous reflux is important for several reasons. First, Schultz-Ehrenburg[21,57] found that patients with deep venous valvular incompetence fared far better with a surgical approach to their disease than with treatment that was limited to sclerotherapy. Thus, the accuracy of this portion of the examination has a direct application to the treatment plan. In addition, patients with deep venous valvular insufficiency should be questioned regarding a history of iliofemoral thrombosis and possible chronic venous obstructive disease, which might contraindicate treatment of their GSV. Finally, it is possible to have only deep venous valvular insufficiency with a normally functioning saphenous vein. Thus, without this differentiation, a patient may be sent for treatment of a normal superficial vein. The technique of examination is quite simple. The Doppler probe may be placed over the site of the SFJ or over the femoral vein with the patient standing or supine, and the patient is asked to perform the Valsalva maneuver. The procedure is then repeated with the GSV firmly compressed below the Doppler probe. If reflux can still be heard after compression is applied, one assumes that the reflux is in the femoral vein. In contrast, if the reflux is obliterated with this maneuver, the retrograde flow is only through the SFJ and not through the femoral vein itself.

Examination of Tributaries of the Saphenous Trunks

The examination of the tributaries of the saphenous trunks focuses on two major questions: (1) to which saphenous trunk does the tributary belong, and (2) is there reflux of blood from the deep vein directly into the tributary? Both answers may be obtained by either physical examination maneuvers or with the Doppler. The origin of any tributary may be assessed with the percussion test, in which the palpating hand is placed gently over the tributary while the GSV or LSV is percussed with the other hand (or vice versa). The palpation of an impulse with percussion of a particular trunk localizes the origin of the tributary to that trunk. Alternatively, a modified Trendelenburg test supplies this information. The patient is asked to lie down with the leg elevated to nearly 90 degrees. The proximal GSV or LSV is then firmly compressed and the patient is asked to stand. If the varicose tributary remains empty and fills only when the compression is released from the GSV, the origin of the tributary is localized to that system. The presence of reflux from the deep system may then be discovered by using the cough test, in which the palpation of an impulse over the tributary when the patient coughs implies reflux of blood from the deep system through incompetent valves into the tributary.

As mentioned previously, although the Trendelenburg test is reasonably accurate, the cough and percussion tests are now considered confirmatory because the Doppler provides a more accurate answer to these questions. Placement of the Doppler probe over the tributary while intermittently compressing or percussing either the GSV or LSV allows determination of the origin of the tributary (Fig. 5-41). Listening for reflux while the patient coughs or performs the Valsalva maneuver uncovers connections to the deep system (since there should be no reflux unless there is a pathway directly to the deep vein that is unobstructed by competent valves). The applicability of the first piece of information is obvious. Careful evaluation must then be directed to that particular incompetent saphenous trunk to achieve sclerosis of the tributary as well. However, the connection of the tributary to the deep system must be explored further, because the exact route that the blood has taken from the deep to the superficial system must be defined. If the connection is simply through the SFJ or SPJ, again, the treatment directive is apparent. On the other hand, if the connection is actually through a perforating vein or another tributary,[57] treatment must be aimed at that particular vein and, perhaps, treatment of the saphenous trunk may be unnecessary. Manual

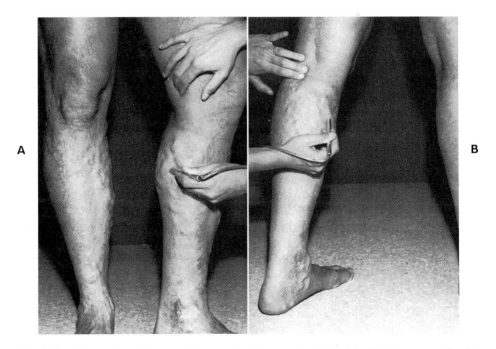

Fig. 5-41 The origin of a particular varicosity may be defined by listening over the dilated vein while alternately compressing the LSV (**A**) and, SSV trunks (**B**).

occlusion of the involved saphenous trunk at its proximal end followed by repeat examination will afford this important differentiation. If this occlusion results in the obliteration of reflux with the cough or Valsalva maneuver, then the blood must have flowed through the SFJ or SPJ. If, on the other hand, this maneuver does not change the result of the test, then the saphenous trunk is an important conduit, and the perforating vein must be the important route.

Examination of Perforating Veins

The perforator segment of the venous system is probably the most mysterious because of its variability, the difficulty of locating perforators even under direct visualization in the operating room, and the overwhelming importance ascribed to perforating veins in the development of varicose veins and the skin changes associated with chronic venous insufficiency.[139] It is no wonder, therefore, that there is no consensus about what constitutes the best method for examination of perforating veins and their valvular competence. Nearly every technique, including venography, Doppler, Duplex, thermography, fluorescein injection, and physical examination of fascial defects, has been employed with varying degrees of success. Complicating the evaluation of each method is the fact that all are compared with later surgical findings, which most likely also miss many incompetent perforating veins and which are impossible to standardize. Underscoring the current difficulties in this aspect of venous diagnosis are data that show that the number of incompetent perforating veins detected per limb in studies of the various diagnostic methods may be 1 to 4, whereas anatomic studies have shown a range of 1 to 14, with an average of 7.[26] Thus, it is still impossible to test the exact sensitivity and accuracy of each method. At best, one may miss a great deal of important pathology. In spite of the pitfalls and limitations of current diagnostic methods, examination for incompetent perforating veins is crucial and is usually productive. As mentioned previously, in a study of 901 limbs with varicose veins,[26] 90% were found to have incompetent perforators. Of interest, only 9% of the perforators were found in the thigh. Thigh perforators may be either single or multiple and may occur anywhere from just proximal to the patella to just below the SFJ, with most being single and located in the middle third of the thigh.[140] In evaluating patients with incompetent perforating veins in the lower leg, Dodd[141] found that 45% were associated with incompetence of the GSV, 15% with incompetence of the LSV, and 2% with an incompetent perforating vein in Hunter's canal. Therefore, any patient with significant truncal varicosities, as well as those with signs of chronic venous insufficiency, should undergo evaluation for perforator valvular insufficiency.

Historically, the most important and probably the most commonly employed technique for detection of outward flow through perforating veins was that of clinical examination. With its ability to detect 50% to 70% of incompetent perforating veins, clinical examination should be the first step in the evaluation. Other techniques have been studied extensively, such as thermography,[30,33,142,143] fluorescein injection,[144,145] and ascending[30,31,144] and intraosseus[33] venography, generally demonstrating accuracies in the range of 60% to 90%. Unfortunately, the instrumentation that is required makes these techniques impractical for most practitioners. The techniques can, however, be used when perforator disease is strongly suspected but has escaped localization by other methods.

Ultrasound technology can also be helpful and is associated with greater ease and lower risks than the other methods. Doppler evaluation of perforator incompetence provides a diagnostic accuracy of 60% to 90%[31,69-71,145] and definitely improves with experience. In one study of 39 legs,[31] its accuracy improved from 60%

to 87% when it was combined with clinical examination, thus making this combination of techniques well suited for routine clinical practice. Duplex scans are extremely useful in visualizing the site(s) of incompetent perforating veins (Fig. 5-42) and may be considered if one is otherwise unable to localize a vein in a suspected area and has the necessary equipment.

The clinical significance of outward flow through perforating veins has long been debated and the physiologic to and fro movement of blood through perforating veins in normal feet is well accepted. Thus the finding by Sarin, Scurr, and Coleridge-Smith[146] that the direction of blood flow within medial calf perforators

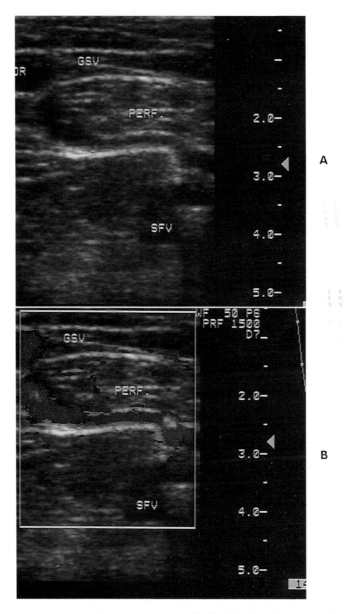

Fig. 5-42   Incompetent perforating veins can usually be discerned with Duplex scanning. **A,** Grey scale, longitudinal scan. **B,** Color image showing reflux.

can be both inward or outward in legs without venous disease is quite interesting. They observed outward blood flow in 21% of medial calf perforators in normal limbs during compression of the foot with a cuff inflated to 60 mm Hg. However, during the relaxation phase (distal cuff deflation) flow occurred in 33% to 44% of perforators in limbs with venous disease but in none of the perforators in limbs without venous disease. Thus, this criterion may allow the first true differentiation of pathologic flow within perforating veins.

Differentiation of the Relative Contribution of Deep and Superficial Reflux

The PPG, with and without compression, is especially useful in the setting of both deep and superficial venous disease; it is also simple and inexpensive to use. If the Doppler examination has disclosed that both the superficial (GSV or LSV) and deep veins (CFV or popliteal) are incompetent, this test will help to determine the relative importance of each segment of the venous system and whether correction of the superficial problem will afford the patient sufficient benefit, given the persistent deep vein reflux, to be worth the potential risks of treatment. This is exemplified by the case of a 40-year-old woman with congenital absence of valves within her femoral veins and a history of bilateral leg edema, lymphedema, and more recently the progressive enlargement of varicosities of her main long saphenous trunks. Although it was felt that her main problem was a deep venous defect, the application of this relatively simple examination scheme allowed a more precise understanding of her condition. By manually compressing the patient's GSV, her initial refilling time of 8 seconds lengthened to 19 seconds, indicating a significant contribution by her superficial system to her pathologic hemodynamics. To further test these findings, a Duplex scan was performed, showing that the peak velocity of reflux flow through the GSV was greater than 33 cm/sec, whereas that through her CFV was only 9.5 cm/sec. The patient underwent high ligation and division of her GSVs and postoperative sclerotherapy. Marked improvement in the discomfort and the edema in her legs resulted, and she was able to reduce the usage of her lymphapress and periodically wear hose with less compression without the disabling aching in her legs that she had experienced previously.

Other examples of the usefulness of the PPG are illustrated below:

J.S., a 59-year-old woman, sought treatment for dilated veins in her left calf. These connected with a minimally enlarged GSV in her thigh, and reflux was heard with the Doppler through her SFJ, whereas her deep veins all displayed valvular competence. The refilling time with PPG was found to be 15 seconds and lengthened to 25 seconds with obstruction of her GSV, thus indicating that obliteration of the flow through her SFJ would provide significantly improved hemodynamics.

R.S., on the other hand, a 72-year-old woman having a similar picture of dilated veins only in her right calf, had a different etiology. The Doppler examination revealed reflux through her SFJ and normal deep venous valvular function as well. However, her refilling time of 15 seconds did not improve with obstruction of her GSV, thus implicating her perforating veins as the origin of the problem. By further varying the location at which the GSV was obstructed, the exact location of the responsible perforator was found.

If obstruction of the GSV just above the knee results in improvement in the refilling time, the Hunterian perforator must be involved. If the refilling time is not improved until the GSV is obstructed just below the knee, the geniculate perforator must be responsible. If this fails to improve the refilling time, the Boyd or Cockett perforators may be implicated.

As mentioned previously, the method of compression of the superficial vein(s) is of extreme importance because one must assure that adequate pressure is achieved to prevent flow through the vein. When attempting to compress a particular vein, manual pressure directly over the vein is probably most effective. On the other hand, when there are multiple veins, placement of a tourniquet might be a more appropriate method.

Evaluation of the Origin of Recurrences after Ligation and Stripping

It is indeed disconcerting for both patient and physician to have to approach the treatment of varicosities that have developed in the groin or the popliteal fossa after previous ligation or ligation and stripping. Again, there are several noninvasive or minimally invasive methods that will provide information crucial to understanding the remaining connections and therefore the necessary sites of treatment. As found by Lofgren[13] in his study of 510 operations performed on patients with recurrence after ligation and stripping, most of the recurrences are found to be the result of inadequate surgery. Either treatment of a dilated tributary with the actual saphenous trunk left untouched or ligation distal to the SFJ/SPJ are the usual findings.

Lofgren felt strongly that all patients with recurrence should be explored surgically, thus obviating the need for an imaging procedure. Since many of these

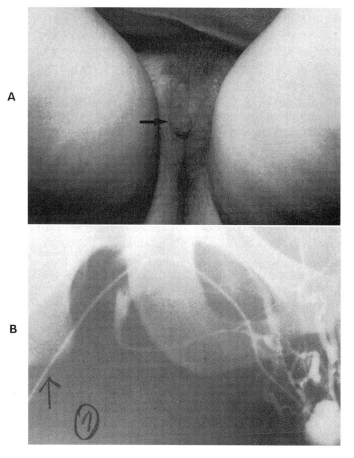

Fig. 5-43   A, Vulvar varix. **B,** Varicography may be used to define its origin. (Courtesy Jeffrey Weisfeld, D.O.)

patients will be found to have problems amenable to sclerotherapy alone, this is not a very satisfying approach, and one should first attempt to define the anatomy of the recurrence before proceeding with treatment decisions.

The approach to such a patient begins in the same way as the approach to any patient with involvement of the saphenous trunk. The palpation of the GSV or LSV is attempted, followed by the Doppler examination for reflux. It is always possible that the dilated vein noticed by the patient may, in fact, simply be a collateral that is functioning normally and does not need to be treated. Once reflux through the vein has been documented, a Valsalva maneuver will demonstrate whether this vein is still in connection with the deep venous system. If not, sclerotherapy may generally be employed successfully. If reflux is heard with a Valsalva maneuver, the patient may then be approached as if he or she were presenting de novo with SFJ or SPJ reflux. Historically, venography has been used in this situation and provides a good image of the exact connection of the recurrent varix. However, Duplex scanning provides excellent images, without the associated risks of the contrast media and radiation.

Evaluation of Vulvar Varices

Vulvar varices generally arise from the pudendal or iliac veins and require treatment only of the varices themselves. In some cases, however, they connect directly with the long saphenous system. Therefore, before treatment the presence of an incompetent SFJ should be sought, since long-term control of these varices requires control of the SFJ if blood is refluxing through it into the vulvar veins. The technique for this determination is as previously described. The exact connection may also be determined by varicography (Fig. 5-43).

REFERENCES

1. Thibault P, Bray A, and Wlodarczyk J: Cosmetic leg veins—evaluation using Duplex venous imaging, J Derm Surg Oncol, 1990 (in press).
2. Hoare MC et al: The role of primary varicose veins in venous ulceration, Surgery 92(3):450, 1982.
3. Sethia KK and Darke SG: Long saphenous incompetence as a cause of venous ulceration, Br J Surg 71:754, 1984.
4. Nicolaides A, Christopoulous D, and Vasdekis S: Progress in the investigation of chronic venous insufficiency, Ann Vasc Surg 3(3):278, 1989.
5. Hanrahan LM, Araki CT, and Rodriguez AA: Distribution of valvular incompetence in patients with venous stasis ulceration, J Vasc Surg 13:805, 1991.
6. Shami SK et al: Venous ulcers and the superficial venous system, J Vasc Surg, 17:487, 1993.
7. Haeger D: The anatomy of the veins of the leg. In Hobbs JT, editor: The treatment of venous disorders, Philadelphia, 1977, Lancaster MTP.
8. May R and Nissl R: Surgery of the veins of the leg and pelvis. In May R, editor: Anatomy, Stuttgart, 1979, Thieme.
9. Browse NL, Burnand KG, and Lea TM: Diseases of the veins: pathology, diagnosis, and treatment, London, 1988, Arnold.
10. Dodd H: The varicose tributaries of the popliteal vein, Br J Surg 52(5):350, 1965.
11. Hoare MC and Royle JP: Doppler ultrasound detection of saphenofemoral and saphenopopliteal incompetence and operative venography to ensure precise saphenopopliteal ligation, Aust N Z J Surg 54:49, 1984.
12. Sherman RS: Varicose veins: anatomy, reevaluation of Trendelenburg tests, and an operative procedure, Surg Clin North Am 44:13 69, 1964.
13. Lofgren KA, Myers TT, and Webb WD: Recurrent varicose veins, Surg Gynecol Obstet 102:729, 1956.
14. The Alexander House Group: Consensus paper on venous leg ulcer, J Dermatol Surg Oncol 18:592, 1992.
15. Neglen P and Raju S: Detection of outflow obstruction in chronic venous insufficiency, J Vasc Surg 17:583, 1993.

16. Tretbar LL: Bleeding from varicose veins: treatment with injection sclerotherapy. Presented at tenth World Congress of Phlebology, Abstract 3G 15, Strasbourg, September 25-29, 1989.
17. Nabatoff RA: Simple palpation to detect valvular incompetence in patients with varicose veins, JAMA 159:27, 1955.
18. Dodd H and Cockett FB: The pathology and surgery of the veins of the lower limb, ed 2, London, 1986, Churchill Livingstone.
19. Knudtzen J, Gudmundsen TE, and Svane S: Congenital absence of the entire inferior vena cava, Acta Chir Scand 152:541, 1986.
20. Chan A, Chisholm I, and Royle JP: The use of directional ultrasound in the assessment of saphenofemoral incompetence, Aust N Z J Surg 53:399, 1983.
21. Schultz-Ehrenburg U: Functional sclerotherapy. Presented at the second annual Congress of the North American Society of Phlebology, New Orleans, February 25-26, 1989.
22. Schadeck M: Personal communication, September, 1989.
23. Brodie B: Lecture illustrative of various subjects in pathology and surgery, London, 1846, Longman.
24. Trendelenburg F: Ueber die Unterbindung der Vena Saphena magna bei Unterschendelvaricen, Beitr Z Klin Chir 7:195, 1891.
25. Steiner CA and Palmer LH: A simplification of the diagnosis of varicose veins, Ann Surg 127(2):362, 1948.
26. Mahorner HR and Ochsner A: The modern treatment of varicose veins as indicated by the comparative tourniquet test, Ann Surg 10 7:927, 1938.
27. Sherman RS: Varicose veins: further findings based on anatomic and surgical dissections, Ann Surg 130(2):218, 1949.
28. Fegan WG: Compression sclerotherapy, Ann R Coll Surg Engl 41(4):364, 1967.
29. Fegan G: Varicose veins: compression sclerotherapy, London, 1967, Heinemann.
30. Beesley WH and Fegan WG: An investigation into the localization of incompetent perforating veins, Br J Surg 57(1):30, 1970.
31. O'Donnell TF Jr et al: Doppler examination vs clinical and phlebographic detection of the location of incompetent perforating veins, Arch Surg 112:31, 1977.
32. Townsend J, Jones H, and Williams JE: Detection of incompetent perforating veins by venography at operation, Br Med J 3:583, 1967.
33. Patil KD, Williams JR, and Williams KL: Thermographic localization of incompetent perforating veins in the leg, Br Med J 1:195, 1970.
34. Bracey DW: Simple device for location of perforating veins, Br Med J 2:101, 1958.
35. Perthes G: Über die Operation der Unterschenkelvaricen nach Trendelenburg, Deutsche Med Wehrschr 21:253, 1895.
36. Killewich LA et al: Pathophysiology of venous claudication, J Vasc Surg 1(4):507, 1984.
37. Anastasios JT: The physiology of venous claudication, Am J Surg 139:447, 1980.
38. Tripolitis AJ et al: The physiology of venous claudication, Am J Surg 139:447, 1980.
39. Fronek A: Noninvasive diagnostics in vascular disease, New York, 1989, McGraw-Hill.
40. Bernstein EF, editor: Noninvasive diagnostic techniques in vascular disease, ed 3, St Louis, 1985, CV Mosby.
41. Satomura S and Kaneko Z: Study of the flow patterns in peripheral arteries by ultrasonics, J Acoust Soc Japan 15:151, 1959.
42. Sumner DS, Baker DW, and Strandness DE Jr: The ultrasonic velocity detector in a clinical study of venous disease, Arch Surg 97:75, 1968.
43. Strandness DE Jr et al: Ultrasonic flow detection: a useful technique in the evaluation of peripheral vascular disease, Am J Surg 113:311, 1967.
44. Felix WR and Sigel B: Doppler ultrasound diagnosis in vascular disease, Penn Med 75:67, 1972.
45. Sigel B et al: A Doppler ultrasound method for diagnosing lower extremity venous disease, Surg Gynecol Obstet 127:339, 1968.
46. Sigel B et al: Augmentation flow sounds in the ultrasonic detection of venous abnormalities: a preliminary report, Invest Radiol 2:256, 1967.
47. Sigel B et al: Diagnosis of venous disease by ultrasonic detection, Surg Forum 18:185, 1967.
48. Sigel B et al: Comparison of clinical and Doppler ultrasound evaluation of confirmed lower extremity venous disease, Surgery 64(1):332, 1968.
49. Sigel B et al: Evaluation of Doppler ultrasound examination, Arch Surg 100(5):535, 1970.
50. Krahenbuhl B, Restellini A, and Frangos A: Peripheral venous pulsatility detected by Doppler method for diagnosis of right heart failure, Cardiology 71:173, 1984.
51. Folse R: The influence of femoral vein dynamics on the development of varicose veins, Surgery 68(6):974, 1970.

52. Araki CT et al: Refinements in the ultrasonographic detection of popliteal vein reflux, J Vasc Surg 17(2):425, 1993.

53. Barnes RW et al: Accuracy of Doppler ultrasound in clinically suspected venous thrombosis of the calf, Surg Gynecol Obstet 143:425, 1976.

54. Sumner DS and Lambeth A: Reliability of Doppler ultrasound in the diagnosis of acute venous thrombosis both above and below the knee, Am J Surg 130(2):218, 1979.

55. Ackroyd JS, Lea Thomas M, and Browse NL: Deep venous reflux: an assessment by descending venography, Br J Surg 73:31, 1986.

56. Bishop C: Personal communication, September, 1989.

57. Schultz-Ehrenburg U and Hubner H-J: Reflux diagnosis with Doppler ultrasound. In Findings in angiology and phlebology, vol 35, New York, 1989, FK Schattauer Verlag.

58. Barnes RW, Russell HE, and Wilson MR: Doppler ultrasonic evaluation of venous disease—a programmed audiovisual instruction, ed 2, Iowa City, 1975, University of Iowa.

59. Stonebridge PA et al: Comparison of Doppler and Duplex scanning for the evaluation of valvular reflux within the veins of the lower limb, Abstract 4S 09:20. Presented at the tenth World Congress of Phlebology, Strasbourg, September 25-29, 1989.

60. Bishop C et al: Real time color Duplex scanning following sclerotherapy of the greater saphenous vein. Submitted to the Society for Vascular Surgery, June 1990.

61. Vasdekis S et al: A comparison of Duplex scanning, Doppler ultrasound, and perioperative venography in assessing the termination of the short saphenous vein, Abstract 25 ii2. Presented at the fourth European-American Symposium on Venous Diseases, Washington DC, March 31-April 2, 1987.

62. Partsch H: Investigations on the pathogenesis of venous leg ulcers, Acta Chir Scand Suppl 544:25, 1988.

63. Shull KC et al: Significance of popliteal reflux in relation to ambulatory venous pressure and ulceration, Arch Surg 114:1304, 1979.

64. van Bemmelen PS et al: Quantitative segmental evaluation of venous valvular reflux with Duplex ultrasound scanning, J Vasc Surg 10:425, 1989.

65. Rose SR and Ahmed A: Some thoughts on the aetiology of varicose veins, J Cardiovasc Surg 27:534, 1986.

66. Goren G and Yellin AE: Primary varicose veins: topographic and hemodynamic correlations, J Cardiovasc Surg 31:672, 1990.

67. Abu-Own A, Scurr JH, and Coleridge-Smith PD: Saphenous vein reflux without sapheno-femoral or sapheno-popliteal junction incompetence, presented at the seventh annual Congress of the North American Society of Phlebology, Maui, February 21-23, 1994.

68. Rettori R: Recurrence of varicose veins due to the incompetence of the perforating veins at the medial aspect of the thigh, Abstract W51-18. Presented at the ninth World Congress of Phlebology, Kyoto, 1986.

69. Folse A and Alexander RH: Directional flow detection for localizing venous valvular incompetency, Surgery 67(1):114, 1970.

70. Miller SS and Foote AV: The ultrasonic detection of incompetent perforating veins, Br J Surg 61:653, 1974.

71. Foote AV and Miller SS: Ultrasonic flow probe detection of incompetent perforating veins, Scott Med J 14:96, 1969.

72. O'Donnell TF et al: Doppler examination vs clinical and phlebographic detection of the location of incompetent perforating veins, Arch Surg 112:31, 1977.

73. Zweibel WJ, editor: Introduction to vascular ultrasonography, ed 2, Philadelphia, 1986, WB Saunders.

74. Knight RM and Zygmunt JA: Ultrasonic detection of the efficacy of injection sclerotherapy of the saphenofemoral junction, Abstract 3G 15. Presented at the tenth World Congress of Phlebology, Strasbourg, September 25-29, 1989.

75. Schadeck M: Sclerotherapy of the long saphenous veins: methodology and results controlled by Echo-Doppler on 400 patients. Abstract 2S 15:30. Presented at the tenth World Congress of Phlebology, Strasbourg, September 25-29, 1989.

76. Raymond-Martimbeau P: Duplex ultrasonography, color flow Doppler and magnetic resonance imaging in phlebology, Abstract 1T 15:50. Presented at the tenth World Congress of Phlebology, Strasbourg, September 15-19, 1989.

77. Day TK, Rish PJ, and Kakkar VV: Detection of deep vein thrombosis by Doppler angiography, Br Med J 1:618, 1976.

78. Sullivan ED, Peter DJ, and Cranley JJ: Real-time B-mode venous ultrasound, J Vasc Surg 1:465, 1984.

79. Raghavendra BN et al: Deep venous thrombosis: detection by probe compression of veins, J Ultrasound Med 5:80, 1986.

80. Talbot SR: Use of real time imaging in identifying deep venous obstruction: a preliminary report, Bruit 1:41, 1982.

81. Hannan LJ et al: Venous imaging of the extremities: our first 2500 cases, Bruit 10:29, 1986.

82. Flanagan LD, Sullivan ED, and Cranley JJ: Venous imaging of the extremities using real-time B-mode ultrasound. In Bergan JJ and Yao JST, editors: Surgery of the veins, Orlando, 1984, Grune & Stratton.

83. Hobbs JT et al: Comparison of clinical examination, Doppler ultrasound, and color Duplex scanning with perioperative venography in the assessment of the short saphenous vein termination. Presented at the second annual Congress of the North American Society of Phlebology, New Orleans, February 25-26, 1989.

84. Hobbs JT: Perioperative venography to ensure accurate saphenopopliteal vein ligation, Br Med J 280:1578, 1980.

85. Corcos L et al: Intra-operative phlebography of the short saphenous vein, Phlebology 2:241, 1987.

86. Vasdekis SN et al: Evaluation of noninvasive and invasive methods in the assessment of short saphenous vein termination, Br J Surg 76:929, 1989.

87. Somjen GM et al: Venous reflux patterns in the popliteal fossa, J Cardiovasc Surg 33:85, 1992.

88. Knight RM, Vin F, and Zygmunt JA: Ultrasonic guidance of injections into the superficial venous system, Abstract 4S 14:50. Presented at the tenth World Congress of Phlebology, Strasbourg, September 25-29, 1989.

89. Kanter A Grondin L, Soriano J: Echosclerotherapy: a Canadian Study. In Phlebologie '92, Raymond-Martinbeau P, Prescott R, Zumme M (eds) p. 828, John Libbey Eurotext, Paris, 1992.

90. Thibault PK and Lewis WA: Recurrent varicose veins: injection of incompetent perforating veins using ultrasound guidance, J Dermatol Surg Oncol 18:895, 1992.

91. McMullin G and Appleberg M: Measurement of venous flow rates by Duplex Doppler ultrasound. Presented at the seventh Annual Congress of the North American Society of Phlebology, Maui, February 1994.

92. Vasdekis SN, Clarke GH, and Nicolaides AN: Quantification of venous reflux by means of Duplex scanning, J Vasc Surg 10:670, 1989.

93. Christopoulos D, Nicolaides AN, and Szendro G: Venous reflux: quantitation and correlation with the clinical severity of chronic venous disease, Br J Surg 75:352, 1988.

94. Abramowitz HB et al: The use of photoplethysmography in the assessment of venous insufficiency: a comparison to venous pressure measurements, Surgery 86(3):434, 1979.

95. Pearce WH et al: Hemodynamic assessment of venous problems, Surgery 93(5):715, 1983.

96. Barnes RW et al: Photoplethysmographic assessment of altered cutaneous circulation in the postphlebitic syndrome, Proc AAMI thirteenth annual meeting, Washington DC, March 28-Apr 1, 1978.

97. Killewich LA et al: An objective assessment of the physiologic changes in the postthrombotic syndrome, Arch Surg 120:424, 1985.

98. Dohn K: Plethysmography during functional states for investigation of the peripheral circulation, Copenhagen, 1957, Proc Second Int Congress Phys Med.

99. Bygdeman S, Aschberg S, and Hindmarsh T: Venous plethysmography in the diagnosis of chronic venous insufficiency, Acta Chir Scand 137:423, 1971.

100. McMullin G, Coleridge-Smith P, and Scurr J: An assessment of pneumatic tourniquets, Personal communication, 1990.

101. Fronek A: Recent developments in venous photoplethysmography. In Bernstein EF, editor, Vascular diagnosis, ed 4, St. Louis, 1993, Mosby.

102. Nicolaides AN et al: The relation of venous ulceration with ambulatory venous pressure measurements, J Vasc Surg 17:414, 1993.

103. Barnes RW and Yao JST: Photoplethysmography in chronic venous insufficiency. In Bernstein EF, editor: Noninvasive diagnostic techniques in vascular disease, ed 2, St Louis, 1982, CV Mosby.

104. Norris CS, Beyrau A, and Barnes RW: Quantitative photoplethysmography in chronic venous insufficiency: a new method of noninvasive estimation of ambulatory venous pressure, Surgery 94(5):758, 1983.

105. Shepard AD et al: Light reflection rheography (LRR): a new non-invasive test of venous function, Bruit 8:266, 1984.

106. Hubner K: Is the light reflection rheography (LRR) suitable as a diagnostic method for the phlebology practice? Phlebol Proctol 15:209, 1986.

107. Kerner J, Schultz-Ehrenburg U, and Blazek V: Digitale photoplethysmograph (D-PPG), Phlebologie Proktologie 18:98, 1989.
108. Kerner J, Schultz-Ehrenburg U, and Blazek V: First clinical experiences on two new plethysmographic measuring systems: digital-PPG and computer aided gravimetric plethysmography (CGP), Abstract 5T 08:40. Presented at the tenth World Congress of Phlebology, Strasbourg, September 25-29, 1989.
109. Hemodynamics Inc: Guidelines for measuring venous emptying with LRR as validated by the University of Miami. Personal communication, 1989.
110. Christopoulos D and Nicolaides AN: Air plethysmography in the assessment of the calf muscle pump in man, J Phys 374:11, 1986.
111. Christopoulos DG et al: Air-plethysmography and effect of elastic compression on venous hemodynamics of the leg, J Vasc Surg 5(1):148, 1987.
112. Nicolaides AN and Christopoulos D: Diagnosis and quantitation of venous reflux. In Baccolon H: Angiologie, Paris, 1988, John Libbey Eurotext.
113. Christopoulos D et al: Pathogenesis of venous ulceration in relation to calf muscle pump function, Surgery 106:829, 1989.
114. Christopoulos DG and Nicolaides AN: Noninvasive diagnosis and quantitation of popliteal reflux in the swollen and ulcerated leg, J Cardiovasc Surg 29:535, 1988.
115. Van Bemmelen PS et al: Does air plethysmography correlate with Duplex scanning in patients with chronic venous insufficiency? J Vasc Surg 18:798, 1993.
116. Neglen P and Raju S: A rational approach to detection of significant reflux with Duplex Doppler scanning and air plethysmography, J Vasc Surg 17:590, 1993.
117. Norgren L: Functional evaluation of chronic venous insufficiency by foot volumetry, Acta Chir Scand Suppl 444:1, 1974.
118. Kakkar VV and Lawrence DA: Venous pressure measurement and foot volumetry in venous disease, Int Angiol 1:87, 1982.
119. Thulesius O, Norgren L, and Gjores JE: Foot-volumetry, a new method for objective assessment of edema and venous function, Vasa 2(4):325, 1973.
120. Norgren L et al: Foot-volumetry and simultaneous venous pressure measurements for evaluation of venous insufficiency, Vasa 3(2):140, 1974.
121. Lawrence D and Kakkar VV: Post-phlebitic syndrome—a functional assessment, Br J Surg 67:686, 1980.
122. Norgren L: Foot-volumetry before and after surgical treatment of patients with varicose veins, Acta Chir Scand 141:129, 1975.
123. Lea Thomas M and Mahraj RPM: A comparison of varicography and descending phlebography in clinically suspected recurrent groin and upper thigh varicose veins, Phlebology 3:155, 1988.
124. Chilvers AS and Thomas MH: A method for the localization of incompetent ankle perforating veins, Br Med J 2:577, 1970.
125. Herman RJ, Neiman HL, and Yao JST: Descending venography: a method of evaluating lower extremity valvular function, Radiology 137:63, 1980.
126. Moore DF, Himmel PD, and Sumner DS: Distribution of venous valvular incompetence in patients with post phlebitic syndrome, J Vasc Surg 3(1):49, 1986.
127. Thiery L: Varicose veins as a result of gastrocnemial vein pathology: a 20-year survey. Presented at the second annual Congress of the North American Society of Phlebology, New Orleans, February 25-26, 1989.
128. Begg AC: Intraosseus venography of the lower limb and pelvis, Br J Radiol 27:318, 1954.
129. Lea Thomas M and Posniak HV: Varicography, Int Angiol 4:475, 1985.
130. Lea Thomas M and Keeling FP: Varicography in the management of recurrent varicose veins, Angiology 37:570, 1986.
131. Rosenberg N and Stefanides A: Thermography in the management of varicose veins and venous insufficiency, Ann NY Acad Sci 122:113, 1964.
132. Williams KL: Infrared thermography as a tool in medical research, Ann NY Acad Sci 121:99, 1964.
133. Camerota AJ, Datz ML, and Derr RP: Variability of venous valve function with daily activity, J Vasc Surg 17(2):440, 1993.
134. Carpenter JP et al: Magnetic resonance venography for the detection of deep venous thrombosis: comparison with contrast venography and Duplex Doppler ultrasonography, J Vasc Surg 17(2):425, 1993.
135. Barnes RW, Ross EA, and Strandness DE Jr: Differentiation of primary from secondary varicose veins by Doppler ultrasound and strain gauge plethysmography, Surg Gynecol Obstet 141:207, 1975.
136. Spence RK et al: Compression therapy fails to relieve venous claudication: a plethysmographic analysis of treatment failure and guidelines for surgical treatment, J Vasc Surg 17(2):432, 1993.

137. Lea Thomas M and Bowles JN: Descending phlebography in the assessment of long saphenous vein incompetence, Am J Radiol 145:1255, 1985.
138. DePalma RG et al: Physical examination, Doppler ultrasound, and colour flow Duplex scanning: guides to therapy for primary varicose veins, Phlebology 8:7, 1993.
139. Burnand KG et al: The relative importance of incompetent communicating veins in the production of varicose veins and venous ulcers, Surgery 82(1):9, 1977.
140. Papadakis K et al: Number and anatomical distribution of incompetent thigh perforating veins, Br J Surg 76(6):581, 1989.
141. Dodd H: The diagnosis and ligation of incompetent ankle perforating veins, Ann R Coll Surg Engl 34:186, 1964.
142. Noble J and Gunn AA: Varicose veins: comparative study of methods of detecting incompetent perforators, Lancet 1:1253, 1972.
143. Elem B, Shorey BA, and Williams KL: Comparison between thermography and fluorescein test in the detection of incompetent perforating veins, Br Med J 4:651, 1971.
144. Lea Thomas M et al: A simplified technique of phlebography for the localization of incompetent perforating veins of the legs, Clin Radiol 23:486, 1972.
145. Miller SS, Crossman JA, and Foote AV: The ultrasound detection of incompetent perforating veins, Br J Surg 58:872, 1971.
146. Sarin S, Scurr JH, and Coleridge-Smith PD: Medial calf perforators in venous disease: the significance of outward flow, J Vasc Surg 16:40, 1992.

6 COMPRESSION HOSIERY AND ELASTIC BANDAGES

*Their Use in the Prevention and Treatment of Varicose
and Telangiectatic Leg Veins*

HISTORICAL DEVELOPMENTS

Compression therapy of the leg is not a new procedure. Ancient Egyptians used paste bandages in the treatment of leg ulcers. Orbach[1] points out that the use of compression therapy for treatment of venous disease is mentioned in the Old Testament (book of Isaiah, Chapter 1, Verse 6), placing its use in the eight century BC. It was practiced by Hippocrates in the fourth century BC. Celcus discovered plaster and linen bandages. Virgo refers to compression treatment with circular bandages after application of caustic agents, white lead, and litharage.[2] Roman soldiers in 20 BC allegedly noted that leg fatigue could be reduced by applying tight strappings to the legs.[3]

The physicians of the Middle Ages used compression bandages, plaster dressings, and laced stockings made from dog leather. An early reference to compression treatment for varicose/stasis ulceration is found in the *Memoires D'Ambroise Paré, Voyage de Hedin,* published in 1553. Theden, one of Fredrick the Great's three surgeons in the late 1700s, used a modification of lace-up dog-leather stockings described by Fabrizio d'Aquapendente (1537-1619).[4] Theden reported in 1771 that he had cured a woman of varices in her eight month of pregnancy by enveloping her legs to the abdomen with 20 "ell-long" bandages.[2] In 1839, John Watson, M.D., reported on the usefulness of an elastic stocking in treating varicose veins in a 23-year-old woman with Klippel-Trenaunay syndrome in 1829. He remarked that the use of the elastic stocking resulted in "her thigh being reduced to its natural size . . . and the veins were also much diminished in size."[5]

The development of elastic medical compression bandages and stockings began in the middle 1800s with the discovery by Charles Goodyear in 1839 of a heating process for rubber that would increase its elasticity and durability. This, after much investigation, led to the manufacturing of rubber threads into stockings by William Brown in England in 1848. These stockings, made exclusively from rubber threads, were uncomfortable. It was not until Jonathan Sparks patented a method for winding cotton and silk around the rubber threads that elastic stockings became popular.[4]

During the late 1800s and early 1900s, technical advances in the manufacturing process led from the development of the frame-knitting to the flat-knitting method. Ultra-fine rounded latex yarns became available that permitted the construction of seamless stockings. Two-way-stretch stockings were then developed. Finally, the development of synthetic elastomers in the 1960s gave rise to rubberless compression stockings.

MECHANISM OF ACTION

External compression can benefit the patient with venous insufficiency by augmentation of the body's natural muscle pump through application of a graduation

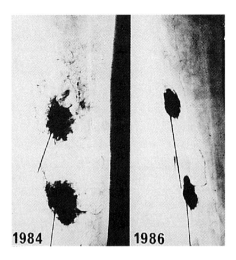

Fig. 6-1   Indirect lymphography by subdermal infusion of water-soluble contrast into lipodermatosclerotic skin above the inner malleolus. Before treatment (1984) irregular lymphatics with dermal back-flow and extravasation can be seen. After compression therapy, with removal of edema and normalization of the skin changes (1986), normal lymph drainage is obtained. (Reproduced with permission from Partsch H: Compression therapy of the legs: a review, J Dermatol Surg Oncol 17:799, 1991.)

of pressure in the leg, forcing blood toward the heart.[6-10] This effect has been demonstrated in patients with superficial venous insufficiency who wear a graduated compression stocking with an ankle pressure of as little as 18 mm Hg.[6] In addition, venous flow is improved by returning the distended veins to normal size, rendering incompetent nonfunctioning venous valves competent. This summarizes the present theory. However, other benefits of compression may be realized with future research. For example, vein diameter alone, irrespective of valvular function, may be important. This later effect is demonstrated in patients with postthrombotic venous stasis whose valves are destroyed, but who achieve an improvement in hemodynamic function with the use of external compression. Also, other as yet unknown effects may stimulate an improvement in microcirculation. One study demonstrated that elastic compression with 30 to 40 mm Hg or 40 to 50 mm Hg graduated compression stockings did not improve deep venous hemodynamics assessed by ambulatory venous pressure, venous refilling time, maximum venous pressure with exercise, or the amplitude of venous pressure excursion in patients with venous stasis disease.[11]

   Histologic examination of similar patients after 90 days of elastic compression with a 30-to-40 mm Hg graduated compression stocking showed remarkable changes in the structural pattern of dermal connective tissue. New capillaries are formed with a reduction in the diameter of existing capillaries and efferent venular systems.[12] In addition, correction of edema places the skin and dermal tissues in direct contact with the superficial capillary network, which is otherwise separated by a pericapillary halo of protein-rich edema fluid (see Chapter 2).[13] This leads to normalized nutritional exchange. Finally, external compression counterbalances the lost elasticity of the tissues to help lymph flow by "graduated" compression. Lymphatic flow is also augmented through an increase in hydrostatic pressure that discourages reaccumulation of edema (Fig. 6-1).[14]

   The adaptation of compression in the treatment of varicose veins has been used with sclerosing treatment for more than 50 years. Postsclerosis compression initially described by Brunstein in 1941,[15] Sigg[16] and Orbach[17] in the 1950s, and Fegan in the 1960s[18] is perhaps the most important advance in sclerotherapy treatment of varicose veins since the introduction of relatively safe synthetic sclerosing agents in the 1940s.

PHARMACOLOGIC VENOUS CONSTRICTION

As an addition to graduated compression stockings that produce a mechanical constriction of superficial veins via external pressure, venous constriction can also be induced pharmacologically. Dihydroergotamine (DHE), when given intravenously to patients with varicose veins, has been shown to produce venous constriction and changes in local venous hemodynamics comparable to that caused by compression bandages and stockings.[19] DHE exerts a relatively selective effect on smooth muscle stimulation of capacitance vessels in the peripheral circulation.[20] This effect can be demonstrated experimentally and visualized clinically when 1 mg of DHE is given intravenously, producing a mean reduction of 20.4% in the volume of blood in the legs.[19] This dose of DHE has been estimated to equal the compressive effect of a 25-mm Hg graduated compression stocking. The vasoconstrictive effect also occurs in the arms and the abdomen with a simultaneous increase in thoracic blood volume. Unfortunately, the frequency of side effects, especially headaches, limits its practical use. An oral preparation of DHE is being evaluated that would increase the efficiency of the calf muscle pump.[21]

This chapter examines the rationale for the use of compression in both the prevention and treatment of varicose and telangiectatic veins. An evaluation of the various compression stockings available, including an in-depth discussion regarding their production and composition, follows.

THE USE OF COMPRESSION ALONE IN PREVENTING VARICOSE AND TELANGIECTATIC LEG VEINS

Varicose and telangiectatic leg veins progress when the volume and subsequent pressure of blood within the vessel lumen exceeds the vessel's capacity to enclose that volume. The deep venous system, by virtue of its position within a musculofibrous sheath, can accommodate such changes by pumping more blood toward the heart. The superficial venous system is not enclosed in a rigid sheath. Thus, to accommodate the increase in flow, the vessel lumen increases in diameter. When this increase in diameter is supraphysiologic, the one-way valve cusps no longer meet, and they become incompetent. This causes excessive pressure with blood volume routed into smaller branching vessels, producing an abnormal dilation. This hemodynamical explanation of varicose vein development is best regarded as a vicious cycle (Fig. 6-2).

The primary method of reversing these changes is to first normalize the pressure and quantity of blood within the vessel lumen. This can be accomplished by sealing off incompetent perforator veins or junctions between the deep and su-

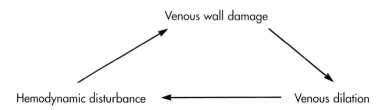

Fig. 6-2 Vicious cycle of varicose veins.

perficial systems through surgical ligation or sclerotherapy-induced endofibrosis. When this is not possible, blood must be pushed from the superficial venous system to the heart. This is accomplished by restoring the competency of valves within the vessel lumen or by establishing a sheath around the vessel so that blood flow will be propelled upward toward the heart instead of laterally against the vein wall. Bandages and graduated compression stockings provide the external support needed to produce this effect.

External Pressure Provided by Medical Support Stockings

The principle governing the magnitude of the applied pressure to the external leg is Laplace's law:

$$\text{Pressure} = \frac{\text{Tension (force of the bandage)}}{\text{Radius (of the leg)}}$$

In general, pressure is calculated for the circumference of the limb at a specific level. Because the leg is oval and not circular (in cross section), the applied point pressures vary at different locations around the leg. Using this formula, it is evident that the effective pressure is greatest at the point of maximum radius and least at the point of minimum radius in inverse proportions. Thus, when a stocking is applied, the anterior and posterior aspects of the leg receive the greatest amount of pressure, and the lateral and medial sides of the leg receive the least compression pressure. Therefore, to achieve uniform pressure around the leg circumference, the lateral and medial aspects should be padded to make the contour more circular (Figs. 6-3 and 6-4). This is especially important in the malleolar area, where the greatest degree of compression occurs, because the medial and lateral surfaces are flat or hollow (Fig. 6-5). Also, as is obvious from Laplace's law, a very thick leg requires more tension to achieve the optimum cutaneous and subcutaneous pressures. This factor should be considered when treating large-legged people.

Regarding large-legged people, one must also consider skin and subcutaneous tissue displacement when calculating the effective pressure over a given point. In 15 varicose veins from 12 subjects, skin displacement ranged from 6.3 to 1.2 mm, which decreased the effective compression of the elastic hosiery.[22]

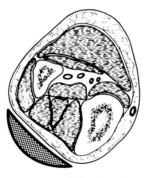 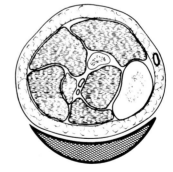

Midcalf level   Midthigh level

Fig. 6-3 Schematized cross section at the midcalf and midthigh levels after application of compression pads and stocking. The pads are placed to create both increased compression over the treated vein and rounding out of the otherwise oval calf or thigh to more uniformly distribute the graduated compression from the stocking.

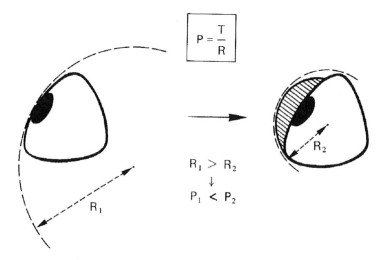

Fig. 6-4   According to Laplace's law, the pressure exerted by a bandage is in direct proportion to the radius of the leg. To increase local pressure on flat parts of the lower leg circumference, rubber pads are attached over the area (black oval) to decrease the radius. (Reproduced with permission from Partsch H: Compression therapy of the legs: a review, J Dermatol Surg Oncol 17:799, 1991.)

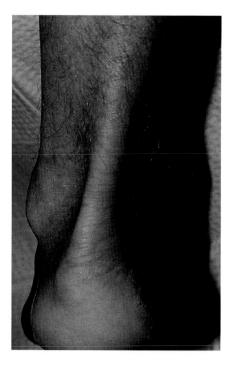

Fig. 6-5   Typical appearance of an ankle in posterior orientation. Note the bulging malleoli and the resulting concavity produced on the lateral and medial aspects.

Thus one disadvantage in treating obese patients is the difficulty in providing optimal compression to the treated varicose vein.

Not all elastic compression stockings reduce ambulatory superficial venous pressure. This is because of the lack of *graduated* compression, which is caused by ankle-calf disproportion—narrow ankles and wide calves.[23] Therefore, a graduated compression stocking is effective only if it has been properly measured and fitted to a patient's limb (customized). When properly fitted, graduated compression stockings have been demonstrated to reduce ambulatory venous pressures by as much as 20 to 30 mm Hg.[23] Even in recumbency, a graduation in pressure produced by stockings (18 mm Hg at the ankle falling to 8 mm Hg at the thigh) results in a significantly increased deep femoral vein flow velocity when uniform compression (11 mm Hg) is applied.[24] In the future, pressure-sensing devices used at the time of fitting the stocking may allow for a more accurate graduation of pressure to be obtained.[25]

Fegan has demonstrated that incompetent venous valves can become competent with the application of external pressure. However, if the valves are allowed to remain incompetent for prolonged periods, fibrosis of the cusps may occur and cause irreversible damage.[26] This effect is noted commonly in multiparous women who first note the temporary development of varicose veins during their first or second pregnancy. When the factors responsible for dilation of pregnancy-induced varicose veins (excessive blood volume, hormonally induced relaxation of the vein wall, etc.) resolve, the veins return to normal. However, after repeated pregnancies, varicose veins may become permanent. This progression is probably related to recurrent insult on the valves, resulting in fibrosis and permanent incompetence. Therefore, the use of graduated compression stockings for pregnancy-induced varicose veins should be considered preventative medicine, the goal being to maintain valvular competence and to prevent sustained valvular damage.

At the first indication of pregnancy, patients should be fitted with a 10- to 30-mm Hg graduated panty hose. In multiparous women, or in those with a history of varicose veins, a stronger 30- to 40-mm Hg panty hose should be worn. In women with large legs, or in patients who are too uncomfortable with a 30- to 40-mm Hg panty hose, a calf length 20- to 30-mm Hg compression stocking can be worn over a 20- to 30-mm Hg panty hose. Even for women in their 35th week of pregnancy, graduated compression stockings are able to increase expelled venous volume, while the refilling rate is influenced to a lesser degree, thus minimizing venous congestion in the leg.[27] This has been demonstrated to decrease postural changes in heart rate, negating uterovascular syndrome.[28] Using these guidelines, compression stockings worn during pregnancy can prevent or lessen the development of venous insufficiency. At the very least, the use of 25 mm Hg graduated compression stockings decreased subjective discomfort from 82% to 13% in pregnant women between 30 and 40 weeks gestation and decreased edema from 75% to 14% in these pregnant women.[28]

The above rationale also applies to most other forms of venous stasis disease. External pressure restores the calf muscle pump, thereby alleviating the increase in superficial venous pressure and thus preventing the sequelae of venous hypertension. In addition to increasing deep venous flow and decreasing the caliber of superficial veins, compression stockings counteract the lateral expansion and dilation of superficial veins during muscle contraction (venous systole) by encasing the veins in a semirigid elastic envelope.[29]

In addition to restoring the calf muscle pump function, graduated compression stockings or bandages correct venous hypertension by increasing the interstitial fluid pressure that both assists in transporting excess fluid back into circulation and prevents the leakage of fluid into the interstitium. Unfortunately, this effect is not always beneficial. Increasing the interstitial pressure forces the arterial circulation to increase its pressure to effect the release of interstitial fluid. When this occurs, the syndrome of intermittent claudication (pain in a limb, caused by exercise relieved by rest) is produced. Therefore, if pain worsens when walking during compression therapy, the stocking should be removed, and an evaluation for arterial disease should be undertaken.

Compression Bandaging Versus Graduated Compression Stockings

For most patients, there is no such thing as an attractive or comfortable compression stocking; there are only degrees of ugliness and discomfort. This is not true for compression bandages. Patients note that a bandage is worn only for a short time and is perceived as a sign of illness. It is therefore regarded by others with sympathy. A stockinged leg, however, is seen as an infirmity or a defect and arouses pity. This perception must be discussed with every patient if one is to ensure compliance with medical instruction.

One study compared the efficacy of sclerotherapy followed by compression with a 35 to 40 mm Hg graduated compression stocking versus compression with three four-inch Elastocrepe bandages (Smith and Nephew, UK) applied evenly from toe to groin for 18 or 16 days respectively.[30] Patients had varicose veins without evidence of saphenofemoral incompetence or incompetent high thigh perforating veins. All patients were assessed at 3 weeks postinjection. In the stockinged leg, 144 of 156 injections were successful versus 117 of 147 injections in the bandaged leg group (P < 0.001). In addition, there was significantly less pigmentation and superficial thrombophlebitis in the stockinged legs. Finally, patient tolerance and acceptability was greater in the stockinged group. However, some patients cannot be treated with graduated stockings because of irregular leg diameters or edema. In these patients compression bandages are mandatory.

Compression bandages. The primary difference between bandages and stockings is that the effect of bandages can be modified by bandaging technique. Pressure can be altered by varying the strength of wrapping. The elasticity of bandages, although limited, changes somewhat according to the type used and functions as a fixed support. Stockings, however, with elastic properties and graduated pressures fixed at the time of manufacture, undergo no change until the stocking is worn out and no longer usable. In fact, stockings must be made of highly elastic materials to enable them to be pulled over the heel of the foot.

Bandages are therefore best indicated when temporary compression is required, such as with edema or inflammatory conditions associated with a predisposing condition. Another benefit of bandages is that they can be reapplied as necessary as the edema in the affected limb is reduced. In this way, the optimum compression needed for efficient therapy is obtainable. Bandages, by providing a limited stretch, also reduce peripheral mean ambulatory venous pressure. This forces the deep system to increase its working pressure with muscular contraction; however, it also exerts a lower pressure during muscular relaxation, thus allowing a more intense retrograde refilling of superficial veins to occur. This explains the relative increase in upward flow of blood.[31]

In short, there are three basic types of bandages: nonelastic, short-stretch, and long-stretch (Fig. 6-6). Nonelastic bandages must be applied with great skill and

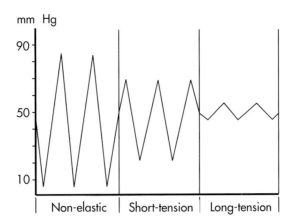

Fig. 6-6 Schematic illustration of the compression curves of bandages when walking (measurement performed at the calf). (Adapted from Stemmer R, Marescaux J, and Furderer C: Compression treatment of the lower extremities particularly with compression stockings, Der Hautarzt 31:355, 1980.)

without tension to avoid arterial ischemia and/or increased compartmental pressure. These bandages do not lengthen with stretching. An example is an Unna boot.

Short-stretch bandages are the most suitable for postsclerotherapy compression. They have similar properties to nonelastic bandages but minimize potential arterial ischemia. They can be extended 30% to 90%. They have a low to slight resting pressure and a very high working pressure. These bandages exert their effect mainly within the deep venous system. They exert little pressure when the calf muscles are relaxed and prevent expansion in calf diameter when the muscles are contracting ("working"). They are, therefore, comfortable when patients are recumbent and act to decrease superficial venous pressure mainly with ambulation.

Long-stretch bandages can be extended 130% to 200% and thus have a high resting pressure; that is, they exert pressure on the superficial venous system when the limb is at rest with a slightly decreased working pressure as compared with short-stretch bandages. They are therefore useful in maintaining compression of superficial veins at all times and are useful for postsclerotherapy compression, but they are very difficult to properly apply in a *graduated* manner. Because of their intrinsic high resting pressure, they can damage arterial, lymphatic, and venous flow if not applied carefully, so they are best used while patients are ambulatory.

A major drawback of bandages is their nonuniform application. A comparison of the range in pressures measured during application of a long-stretch elastic bandage by skilled persons versus nursing students demonstrated that skilled personnel applied the bandages with a pressure of 34 mm Hg $+/-$ 4.7 versus 36.6 mm Hg $+/-$ 15.6 of nursing students.[32] The skilled bandagers' pressure ranged from 25 to 50 mm Hg and the unskilled bandagers' pressure ranged from 15 to 70 mm Hg. In addition, even when bandages are applied by physicians who are experts in their use, a true graduation in pressure may not always be obtained. If graduated compression does not occur, thrombosis of normal veins may occur because of stagnation of blood flow caused by a tourniquet effect (Fig. 6-7).[33] Intra-

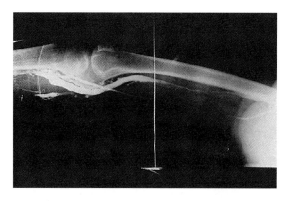

Fig. 6-7 Phlebolgram showing narrowing of veins under compression bandages on the lower leg and thigh (inelastic bandage, Porelast 50 mm Hg, no compression at knee level). The diameter of the deep femoral vein is compressed to a thin cord. (Reproduced with permission from Partsch H: Compression therapy of the legs: a review, J Dermatol Surg Oncol 17:799, 1991.)

capillary pressure varies with posture and exercise. When a bandage is applied, it should be wrapped tighter at the foot and ankle, and looser proximally. Unfortunately, the bandage tends to work loose with movement and only maintains the initial pressure in the posture in which it was applied.

Because the degree of compression with manual bandages is unpredictable, arterial ischemia can occur. This is of concern particularly in the presence of venous leg ulcers during treatment. Two studies estimated the frequency of unsuspected arterial insufficiency among patients with chronic leg ulcers at 21%[34] and 31%.[35] Callam et al.[36] surveyed consultants in general surgery in Scotland regarding their experience with compression therapy in the previous 5 years and found 147 cases of cutaneous ulceration caused by the compression bandage. Of these consultants, 32% reported at least one case of ulceration or cutaneous necrosis aggravated by compression bandages; 21% reported more than one experience. Compression bandages accounted for 73 of 147 cases reported, with elastic and antiembolism stockings accounting for 36 and 38 cases respectively. Also, eight patients were reported who required amputations of the digits or feet as a direct result of arterial ischemia caused by an excessively tight compression bandage or stocking.[34] Finally, it has been estimated that up to 50% of patients over 80 years of age with leg ulcerations also have significant arterial disease.[34] Therefore, one should always check arterial pulses before and after applying a compression bandage or fitting a compression stocking, especially in the elderly. Low-stretch bandages offer some safety in patients with arterial disease because these bandages produce a high working pressure during ambulation and a low resting pressure during nonambulation.

Excessive or nongraduated compression can also result in iatrogenic compartment syndrome in patients with normal arterial function. Four cases of iatrogenic compartment syndrome were reported in patients who underwent surgery (stripping of the GSV) for varicose veins.[37] The type of compression bandage was not specified in the article. The damages varied from extensive irreversible neuromuscular defects to lesser functional handicaps. Of note is that all of the patients complained of pain postoperatively with total or partial removal of the stocking performed after 24 hours. Clinical and electromyographic studies indicated ischemic neuromuscular damage of the peroneal, posterior tibial, and/or sural nerves. Palpable pulses of the posterior tibial and dorsal foot arteries did not

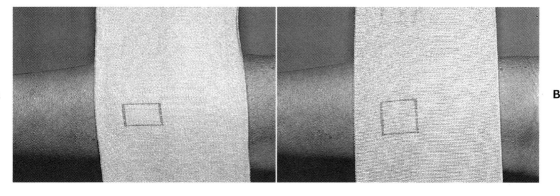

Fig. 6-8 Appearance of a 30 mm Hg medium-stretch compression bandage without tension (Setopress, Seton Healthcare Group plc, Oldham, England). **A,** Note rectangular boxes. **B,** Same bandage stretched to provide approximately 30 mm Hg compression. Note that the rectangular boxes have now assumed a square shape.

exclude increased intracompartmental pressure because the flow of the dorsal artery is normal up to 80 mm Hg of intracompartmental pressure.[38] Thus sensory disturbances should be warning for reevaluating the degree of compression in the posttreatment period (see Chapter 8).

In addition, bandages tend to lose a significant degree of compression pressure with time and body position. A study of elastic, minimal stretch and nonelastic (Circaid, Shaw Therapeautics, Inc.) demonstrated that 4 hours after application, elastic bandages had 94% of initial pressure, compared with 70% for minimal stretch and 63% for nonelastic bandages.[39] In the supine position, the decrease at 4 hours was 72% for elastic, 59% for minimal stretch, and 44% for nonelastic compression. Elastic bandages provided the highest sustained compression, but caused the risk of excess pressure on lying down. However, at least one study of a multilayered bandage demonstrated no loss in compression pressure at 1-week follow-up.[40] This bandage consists of an inner layer of orthopedic wool (Velband, Johnson & Johnson), compressed with a crepe bandage (Elset, Seton Healthcare Group plc, Oldham, England), topped with a lightweight elasticated cohesive bandage (Coban, 3M, UK). The bandage was applied at midstretch so that compression was achieved more by elasticity and overlap than by the tension applied by the bandager. Thus the technique and type of bandage(s) are important in ensuring consistent, prolonged compression.

As stated earlier, application of compression bandages requires skillful technique. The reader is referred to multiple authors for further information.[41,42] A number of different bandage companies have developed a built-in guide to help maintain uniform pressure. One type is the Setopress high-compression bandage (Seton Healthcare Group plc, Oldham, England). This medium-stretch bandage is marked with rectangles that become squares when the bandage is stretched to its proper length (Fig. 6-8). Depending on the circumference of the limb, this bandage will apply pressure of 20 to 50 mm Hg, with the average pressure being approximately 30 mm Hg.

Important points to consider when applying a bandage:
1. Graduation in pressure is ensured by applying even pressure on the bandage, which is stretched to a uniform degree while wrapping from the distal to the proximal direction. This occurs according to Laplace's law, that smaller diameters have increased pressures as long as tension remains

constant and the leg increases in diameter from a distal to proximal direction (Fig. 6-9).

2. Cotton wool padding or a thin polyurethane foam bandage underwrap (Mueller Sports Medicine, Prairie de Sac, WI 53578) should be placed on the anterior tibial and retromalleolar area both to protect thin-skinned areas and to distribute pressure evenly.

3. Oblique (not circular) turns of the bandage avoid constriction of the skin.[42,43]

4. Bandage materials must be nonallergic to avoid the development of dermatitis.

5. The bandage must be applied with no gaps so that each turn overlaps 50% to 70% of the previous turn.

6. The ankle joint should be maximally extended dorsally when the bandage is applied.

7. Although short-stretch lengthwise (one-way) elastic bandages are preferred, at the ankle and knee a two-way stretch elastic bandage better conforms to the shape of the joints and is thus more comfortable.

8. Local compression should be applied 5 to 10 cm beyond the treated areas to avoid bruising, hematoma, edema, and inflammatory reactions.

9. Listen to the patient, who will let you know immediately if the bandage is too tight. Pain indicates arterial ischemia.

A 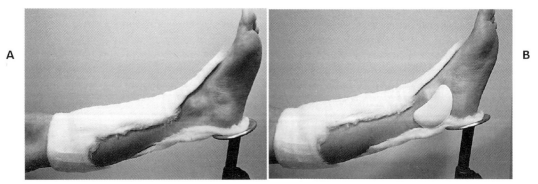 B

Fig. 6-9 Preferred method for applying compression bandages. **A,** All areas with a pronounced curvature, such as ankles, Achilles tendon, instep, and sharp edges of the tibia, are leveled and protected with cotton wool. **B,** The retromalleolar space is raised with a foam pad to prevent excess pressure on the medial and lateral malleoli. **C,** Cotton wool and pads are fixed to the leg with a light, absorbent dressing. **D,** Bandaging is begun at the medial dorsal foot with the foot in pronounced dorsiflexion. **E,** With each spiral turn, two-thirds of the bandage is covered, except for the turn at the knee (**F**) where there is no circular bandaging, but the bandage turns across the leg and the contour of the leg is followed naturally. Uniform stretch on the bandage is applied at all times. **G,** Appearance of the completed first bandage. **H,** If a second bandage is to be applied, it is started from the opposite direction from the lateral dorsal superior calf. (Reproduced with permission from Neumann HAM and Tazelaar DJ: Compression therapy. In Bergan JJ and Goldman MP, editors: Varicose veins and telangiectasia: diagnosis and treatment, St. Louis, 1993, Quality Medical.)

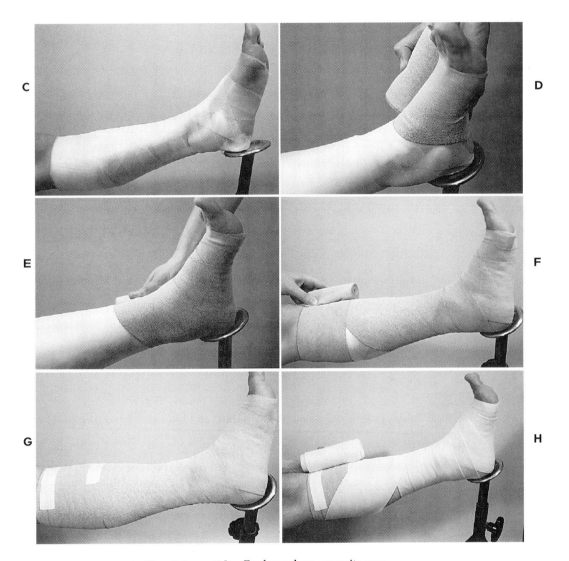

Fig. 6-9, cont'd For legend see opposite page.

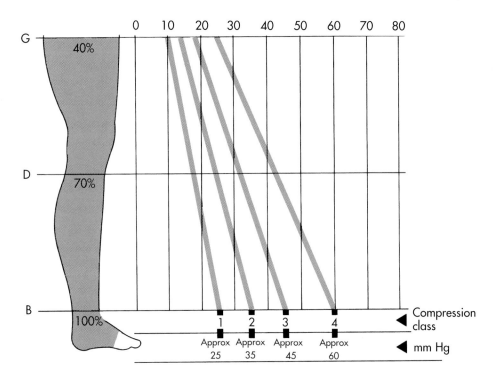

Fig. 6-10 Diagram comparing the degree of compression exerted at various locations on the leg with different compression class stockings. *B* is the pressure generated at the ankle; *D* is the pressure generated at the knee; *G* is the pressure generated at the superior thigh. Note that there is a graduation of pressure with all classes of stockings with the highest pressure exerted at the ankle. Also note that the most significant difference in pressure generated by the different classes of stockings is at the ankle. (Courtesy Julius Zorn, Inc.)

Compression stockings. Graduated compression stockings are required for long-term therapy. Here they provide an external support to constrict dilated veins to restore valvular competency, thus impeding reflux of blood from the deep to the superficial veins. By virtue of their "graduation," compression stockings help to propel blood toward the heart (Fig. 6-10). Unlike nonelastic bandages, they do not lose compression with time, and they work well as part of the calf muscle pump. Compression stockings should be used only when the leg diameter has stabilized and edema is no longer a factor. When used in this manner, the stocking will correspond to the leg dimensions over a long period to prevent a renewed increase in leg circumference. In addition, compression stockings function best when fitted early in the day when edema is reduced. Some types of elastic stockings may rarely cause an allergic reaction. This has been reported to occur with Scholl Soft Grip elastic stockings (composed of 76% nylon and 24% elastane) in less than 1% (2 of 126) of patients.[44]

CHARACTERISTICS OF MEDICAL GRADUATED COMPRESSION STOCKINGS

Compression stockings are almost exclusively two-way stretch stockings—elastic in both the longitudinal and transverse directions. This provides the stretch needed to apply a stocking that has the smallest diameter at the ankle to be drawn over the heel. Two-way stretch stockings also have the characteristics of longitudinal bandages. The longitudinal elasticity of the stocking compensates for differences in limb length, thereby facilitating joint movements.

Terminology

To understand the basic properties of the various compression stockings, the physician should be familiar with the following terms.

Resting pressure. Pressure from the bandage itself with the muscles at rest.

Working pressure. Pressure coming from inside the bandages from contracting muscles.

Stretch resistance. Stretch resistance is a measure of the tensile force required to elongate an elastic material. This represents the amount of resistance the wearer must overcome to don the support stocking. Of note is that an easy way to decrease the stretch resistance while increasing the degree of elastic support is to don two low-pressure stockings, one over the other. The end pressure will be equal to the pressure of both stockings added together, but each will be easier to don because of its individually lower stretch resistance.

Stress relaxation. Stress relaxation is the decrease in tensile force that occurs when an elastic yarn is held in an expanded state. This is a natural realignment of the molecular bonds within the framework of the elastomer. The amount of relaxation decay is different for each material and for the composition of the final elastic yarn.

Holding power. Holding power is the force exerted by an elastic material in an attempt to revert to its original length. This is the true reading of the support power available for applying pressure to a limb. The holding power is determined by the unloading portion of the stress/strain curve and is less than the stretch resistance.

Hysteresis. Hysteresis is a measure of the energy loss that occurs between loading (stretching) and unloading (relaxing) (Fig. 6-11). Yarns with minimal hysteresis are best because they have maximum holding power with minimal stretch resistance.

Available stretch. The available stretch is a measure of the amount of additional stretch available for donning and for joint mobility. It is a measure of the garment's ability to adapt to body movements.

Modulus. The ratio of change in the stress (force) to the change in the unit strain (percent stretch) is called the modulus. It is a measure of the rate of increased holding power with increased stretch.

Stretch recovery. Stretch recovery is the ability of an elastic material to return to its original shape after deformation and subsequent removal of an applied stress.

Ready-Made or Customized, Made-To-Measure Stockings

Ready-made stockings

Ready-made or off-the-shelf stockings are manufactured in fixed sizes. Most manufacturers have 12 sizes varying in both length and width at various points on the ankle, calf, and thigh (Table 6-1). Although the sizes are standardized to some degree by associations of stocking manufacturers, such as the Gutezeichengemeinschaft Medizinischer Gummistrumpfe e. V. (Quality Seal Association for

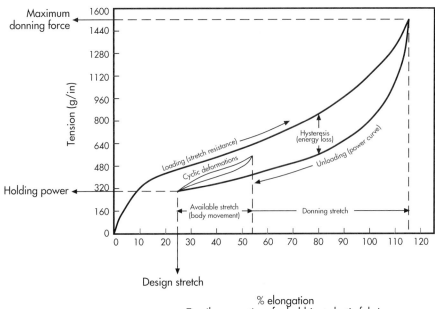

Fig. 6-11 Hysteresis curve generated by a Bobbinet elastic fabric. (Courtesy of the Jobst Institute, Inc.)

Medical Compression Stockings) in Europe, there may be considerable variation between the sizing of different manufacturers (Fig. 6-12). Therefore, it may be prudent for distributors to carry multiple brands of stockings in the event that some patients experience a poor fit. One study has estimated that 90% of patients seeking treatment for venous disease could be fitted with ready-made stockings.[45]

Made-to-measure stockings

Prescription guidelines. Made-to-measure stockings are custom-made according to the length and circumference measurements of the patient's leg. Adjustments are made either by hand on flat-knitting machines, where shaping is achieved by altering the width of the knit, or by machine in a circular-knit manner, in which changes in the pressure and width are achieved by varying the tension of the weft and stitch size. Made-to-measure stockings should be prescribed under the following circumstances:

1. For very large or small patients
2. When there is a significant difference in the length between the right and left leg
3. For patients with partial amputations or deformities of the leg or foot
4. When a special pressure gradient is required (for example, increased pressure over the thigh)
5. When the measurements of ready-made stockings do not correspond to the leg length and girth measurements of a patient (for example, when there is a difference of more than 3 cm between the lower leg length and the standard 39-cm length used for ready-made stockings); this may not be applicable for all brands of stockings
6. For patients who have very large instep to heel circumferences

Table 6-1 Characteristics and care of graduated class II compression stockings

Stocking brand name	Composition	Number of sizes Total/ankle/calf/foot/length	Toe Open/closed
Camp Classic 1600	Nylon/spandex (synthetic rubber)	24/6/2/1/2	Open
Camp 1800	Nylon/spandex	12/6/1/1/2	Open/closed
Jobst Camp 1900	Nylon/spandex/cotton	12/6/2/1/2	Open
Vairox	Rubber/nylon (knee-length)	12/3/2/1/2	Open
	(other lengths)	12/3/2/1/1	Open
Vairox (Zipper)	Spandex/nylon	6/3/1/1/2	Open
Fast fit	Spandex/nylon	3/3/1/1/1	Open/closed
Ultimate	Lycra/nylon (knee-length)	4/4/1/1/1	Closed
	(uncovered) (thigh-high)	3/3/1/1/1	Closed
Sheer	Spandex/nylon (panty hose)	6/6/1/1/1	Closed
Relief	Spandex/nylon	4/4/1/1/1	Closed
JuZo			
Hostess	Syn elastomers (coated)	12/6/1/1/3	Closed
Varin Soft	Syn elastomers (coated)	12/6/2/1/2	Open/closed
Varin Soft Cotton	23.5% Lycra 45.5% Nylon 31% Cotton	12/6/1/1/2	Open/closed
Varin Super	Syn elastomers (coated)	12/6/1/1/2	Open/closed
Varin Soft-in silk	27% Lycra 64% Nylon 9% Silk	12/6/1/1/2	Open/closed
Varilastic	Syn elastomers (coated)	12/6/1/1/2	Open
Medi 75	Spandex/nylon (uncoated)	12/6/1/2/2	Closed
Medi Plus	Spandex/nylon (uncoated)	14/7/2/1/2	Open
Medi Lastex	Spandex/nylon (uncoated)	14/7/1/1/2	Open
Sigvaris 202	Syn rubber (cotton-covered)	12/3/2/1/2	Open
Sigvaris 503/504/505	Natural rubber (nylon-covered)	12/3/2/1/2	Open
Sigvaris 601	Syn rubber (nylon-covered)	12/3/2/1/2	Open
Sigvaris 801/802	Syn rubber (nylon-covered)	12/3/2/1/2	Closed
Sigvaris 902	Syn rubber (nylon-covered)	12/3/2/1/2	Open/closed
Venosan 1000	Lycra 28% Nylon 72%	12/3/2/1/2	Open/closed
Venosan 2000	Lycra 25% Cotton 15% Nylon 60%	12/3/2/1/2	Open
Venosan 3000	Lycra 25% Cotton 75%	12/3/2/1/2	Open
Venosan Boutique	Lycra 16% Nylon 84%	4/4/1/1/1	Closed
Ibici/Italy	Polyamide 74% Elasteine 26%	10/5/2/1/1	Closed/open
Sirlex Radiante-France	Polytamide 75% Elasteine 25%	10/5/1/1/2	Closed/open

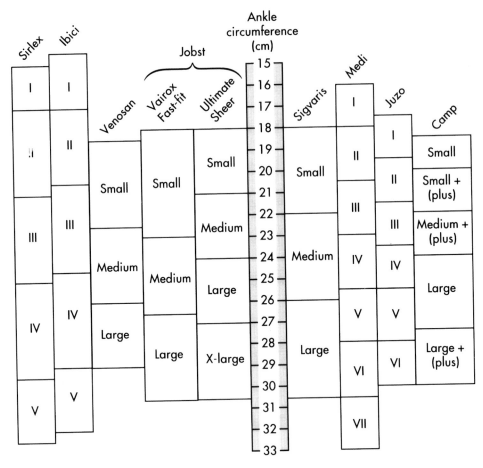

Fig. 6-12 Conversion chart based on the primary measurement around the smallest circumference above the ankle.

Measurement

The most important measurement location is at the ankle (Fig. 6-13, point *b*) where a graduated stocking exerts the greatest degree of pressure. Therefore, all ready-made stockings include this point as one of the measuring points. Measurements taken at various levels of the calf and thigh must conform to the manufacturer's guidelines. If a calf or thigh diameter does not conform to the manufacturer's guide for that particular stocking size, then a made-to-order stocking should be used.

A common error made by the physician to avoid prescribing a made-to-measure stocking is that of prescribing the next larger size of a ready-made stocking. This results in a lower pressure being exerted at the ankle; in addition, the counterpressures are altered because the wider stocking is designed at all levels for different leg measurements.

Proper measurement and fit of a compression stocking becomes increasingly important when higher compression classes are required. Therefore, made-to-measure stockings have particular application for compression classes above 40 mm Hg.

One should note that differences of more than 15 mm Hg can occur among different stocking manufacturers not only by virtue of different types and

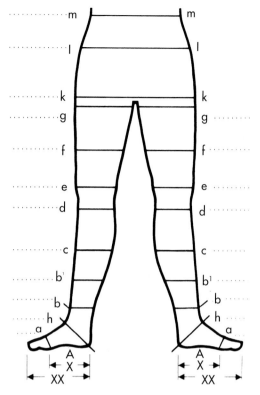

Fig. 6-13 Diagram of the points of measurement for fitting graduated support stockings. Measurement b is the most important measurement. Each stocking manufacturer has its own set of required measuring points to ensure proper fit of the ready-made stocking. Points c and f are usually required as well as the length points, a to f or a to g. Points k, l, and m are only required for fitting compression leotards. (Courtesy Julius Zorn, Inc.)

strengths of elastic materials, but also by different methods of measuring the stocking to fit the leg.[46] Some manufacturers provide only three ankle sizes of stockings, whereas others provide up to 6 or more ankle sizes. Thus there may be a large variation of applied pressure for different-sized legs among different stocking brands as dictated by Laplace's law (see p. 203).

Stocking lengths

Up to six styles of medical compression stockings are available, depending on the manufacturer: knee-length, midthigh, thigh, panty hose or leotard, one-legged panty hose, thigh with waist attachment, and maternity panty hose (Fig. 6-14). Regardless of the style, most stockings are available in three lengths: knee-length, midthigh, and thigh length. According to the standardized figure, a knee-length stocking is designated as A-D, a midthigh stocking as A-F, and a thigh-length stocking as A-G.

There are specific indications and contraindications for the various stocking lengths. Knee-length stockings should be prescribed only if the "c" circumference is approximately 2 cm greater than the "d" circumference; otherwise it will have no hold on the leg and tend to slide down (see Fig. 6-13). In addition, if the a to d length is too great, the excessive length interferes with movement at the knee. The patient will then usually fold the excess stocking down below the knee; this doubles the counterpressure at d and thus may reverse the "graduated pressure."

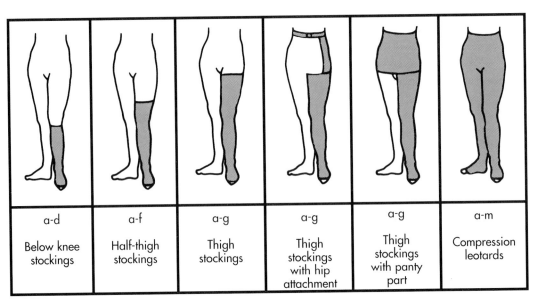

a-d	a-f	a-g	a-g	a-g	a-m
Below knee stockings	Half-thigh stockings	Thigh stockings	Thigh stockings with hip attachment	Thigh stockings with panty part	Compression leotards

Fig. 6-14   Six types of graduated compression stockings widely available. (Courtesy Julius Zorn, Inc.)

Likewise, if the a to d length is too short, the patient will try to stretch the stocking beyond its natural point, thereby decreasing the effective circumferential pressure and thus defeating the purpose of wearing the stocking.

In patients with marked adiposity of the knee region, the upper edge of the stocking may produce skin bulging, which may be particularly bothersome on the inner aspect of the knee. In these cases it may be necessary to fit the patient with a midthigh stocking.

Proper fit and position

Because the efficacy of compression stocking is directly related to a proper fit, its adherence to the leg to prevent vertical movement is important. Panty hose stockings are the most expensive method to ensure the stocking remains in place by virtue of its attachment at the panty line. The only disadvantages are the increased constriction and the heat generated by an additional undergarment.

With single-leg, thigh, or calf stockings, various inexpensive methods, such as adhesive tape, glues, clips, or garter belts, serve to ensure proper positioning. Diadvantages of tapes or glues include the pain on removal of tape from hairy legs and irritation of allergy caused by the adhesive portion of the tape. Various types of clips that secure the stocking to underwear are available. Disadvantages include tearing or stretching out the undergarment and cutaneous pressure and/or irritation by the clip itself.

Garter belts comprise a more elegant and practical yet perhaps unfashionable method for ensuring correct stocking placement. These belts may be built into the stocking as a waist attachment or purchased separately in various styles. Disadvantages include the digging in of the belt into an obese thigh if the belt is too narrow and the possibility of the garter itself producing a tourniquet effect.

Finally, a new type of silicone top-band on thigh or midthigh length stockings is now available from many manufacturers of graduated compression stockings. It keeps the stocking in place without the disadvantages of glues, clips, or garter belts.

THE RATIONALE FOR THE USE OF COMPRESSION IN VARICOSE VEIN SCLEROTHERAPY

Postsclerotherapy compression primarily eliminates a thrombophlebitic reaction and substitutes a "sclerophlebitis" with the production of a firm fibrous cord.[47] Compression serves at least six purposes:

1. Compression, if adequate, may result in direct apposition of the treated vein walls to produce a more effective fibrosis (Figs. 6-15 and 6-16).[17,48] Therefore, weaker sclerosing solutions may be used successfully.

2. Compressing the treated vessel will decrease the extent of thrombus formation, which inevitably occurs with the use of all sclerosing agents;[49-52] it is hoped this will decrease the subsequent risk of recanalization of the treated vessel.[18,53,54]

3. A decrease in the extent of thrombus formation may also decrease the incidence of postsclerosis pigmentation (see Chapter 8).[48,55-57]

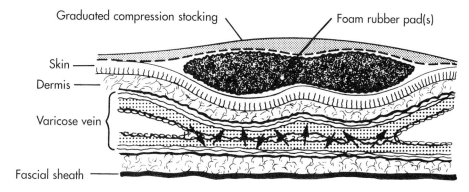

Fig. 6-15   Schematic diagram demonstrating idealized compression of a treated varicose vein segment using foam rubber pads under a compression stocking. (Redrawn from Wenner L: Vasa 15:180, 1986.)

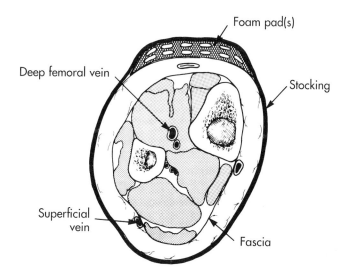

Fig. 6-16   Schematic cross section of a superficial varicose vein compressed with a foam rubber pad under a compression stocking. Note that superficial varicosities lateral to the foam rubber pad are only slightly compressed, and veins deep to the fascia are not compressed. (Redrawn from Reid RG and Rothnie NG: Br J Surg 55:889, 1968.)

4. The limitation of thrombosis and phlebitic reactions may prevent the appearance of telangiectatic matting (see Chapter 8).[54]

5. The physiologic effect of a graduated compression stocking is to improve the function of the calf muscle pump, which is accompanied by subjective improvement.[58]

6. Compression stockings increase blood flow through the deep venous system.[59,60] This acts to rapidly clear any sclerosing solution that has inadvertently made its way into the deep venous system and thus prevents damage to valves in the deep venous system.

Externally supporting untreated varicose veins will narrow their diameter, restoring competent valvular function and thereby decreasing retrograde blood flow.[61] External pressure will also retard the reflux of blood from incompetent perforating veins into the superficial veins.[62] Theoretically, because dermal collecting veins have been found histologically to contain one-way valves,[63] external pressure may also provide a normalization of cutaneous blood flow. In support of this theory, improvement in cutaneous oxygenation has been demonstrated with the use of compression in patients with venous stasis after only 10 to 15 minutes.[64]

Patients with varicose veins note relief of aching symptoms with all classes of compression stockings.[65,66] Patients with postphlebitic limbs find that the 30- to 40- and 40- to 50-mm Hg stockings control their edema and symptoms better than 20- to 30-mm Hg stockings. It is interesting to note that although symptoms are improved with all classes of compression stockings, patients with varicose veins achieve physiologic improvement only when 30- to 40- and 40- to 50-mm Hg compression stockings are worn. Therefore, 30- to 40-mm Hg graduated compression stockings are best used for conservative treatment of varicose veins, and 40- to 50-mm Hg compression stockings are best used for conservative treatment of chronic venous insufficiency.

How Much Pressure is Necessary for Varicose Veins?

The optimum cutaneous pressure required to compress the varicose vein after sclerotherapy has yet to be defined. Venous ambulatory pressures of 48 mm Hg have been recorded from the superficial dorsal foot veins in patients with venous insufficiency.[62] A pressure of at least 30 mm Hg is required to reduce the capacity by 96% of a model distended to similar venous pressures.[62] Initial compression measurements taken during manual wrapping of the leg with Crevic crepe bandages by multiple surgeons using the technique of Fegan[18] average between 20 and 100 mm Hg with a mean of 54 mm Hg at calf level.[67] In addition, experimental varicose vein models have shown this level of compression to result in a reduction of the vessel lumina by 94% even in veins distended to 90 mm Hg.[67] Thus the classic technique for compression sclerotherapy is theoretically sound.

The posture of the patient should also be taken into consideration when prescribing compression stockings. If higher compression pressures are used (through the use of double stockings), care must be taken to inform patients to remove the outer stocking when not ambulatory. Ankle pressures greater than 20 mm Hg have been reported to produce an impairment of calf muscle and cutaneous blood flow in some nonambulatory patients.[68-70] Recent studies concerning peripheral blood circulation and skin temperature demonstrate a significant impairment of blood when external pressures above 30 mm Hg are applied to the leg of supine patients.[32] This may be perceived by patients as achiness in the ankle area that occurs during sleep and resolves with walking after 30- to 40-mm Hg compression stockings are worn to bed following sclerotherapy.

By having compression of 30 to 40 mm Hg at the ankle, the compressive strength at other locations on the leg may be between 10 and 20 mm Hg depending on the site and amount of underlying bone, adipose tissue, and muscle.[71] Experimental models have demonstrated that external pressures of 8.5 mm Hg reduce the capacity of the underlying varicose vein by only 22%.[67] Therefore, with the use of this degree of compression, one does not attempt to completely empty intravascular blood from the treated veins. However, according to Laplace's law, the pressure exerted upon an individual superficial vein will be greater than that exerted on the limb as a whole because the vein radius is much smaller than the radius of the limb. Thus varicose veins will be decreased in diameter with smaller degrees of pressure than that calculated. In addition, any degree of compression will decrease the effective vein diameter to some extent, thus theoretically minimizing subsequent thrombus formation. This supports the rationale for the use of compression in the treatment of both varicose veins and leg telangiectasias.

How Long Should Compression Be Maintained?

In addition to the degree of compression needed to effect optimal sclerotherapy, the time duration needed to maintain compression is also open for debate. The classic technique for sclerosis of varicose veins described by Fegan[18,53] and used by Hobbs[72] and Doran and White[73] is to continue compression for 6 weeks. This period was not arrived at randomly, but through multiple histologic examinations of sclerotherapy-treated varicose veins at intervals of 30 seconds; 1 and 5 minutes; 12, 24, and 36 hours; 6, 8, 12, and 14 days; 3, 4, 7 , 10, 16, and 20 weeks; and $1/2$, 1, and 5 years.[26] Fegan concluded that organization of the fibrous occlusion required at least 6 weeks. However, a randomized study found no difference in clinical results at 2 years when compression was maintained for 3 weeks as compared with 6 weeks.[74] Thus many phlebologists recommend a maximum of 3 weeks of compression.[75-79]

Unfortunately, no randomized, properly performed, long-term studies have been performed to clearly define the optimal length of time for postsclerotherapy compression. Studies have shown that compression bandages maintain significant compression for only 6 to 8 hours while patients are ambulatory[80] and lose up to 50% of their initial compression pressure in recumbent patients at 24 hours,[81] thus questioning the rationale for prolonged use. Indeed, it has been shown that there is no significant clinical difference at 60 days between patients treated with 8 hours and those treated with 6 weeks of compression after sclerotherapy of below-the-knee varices without saphenofemoral incompetence.[82] Unfortunately, long-term follow-up examination of these patients to determine the ultimate success of therapy has not been reported. A study on the treatment of varicose veins less than 1.5 cm in diameter without saphenofemoral incompetence using compression with elastic bandages for 48 hours demonstrated good to excellent results at 1- and 5-year follow-up intervals.[83] A prospective randomized study comparing postambulatory phlebectomy bandaging for 1, 3, and 6 weeks found no difference in efficacy at 2 months postoperatively.[84] However, in this study, compression with an elastic bandage was given to all groups for only 1 week, with the variable being a Tubigrip tubegauze (Seton Products, Montgomeryville, PA) applied only during the day, which provided minimal compression. Finally, a randomized study of the use of compressive bandages in the treatment of varicose veins with a 3-month follow-up was reported.[85] The study demonstrated through both subjective and objective findings that 3 days of compression equaled the results at 6 weeks. Unfortunately, this study used a Coban bandage dressing that may not maintain effective pressure beyond 8 hours.

A corollary to the amount of time necessary to effect adequate compression is whether it is necessary to continue compression while the patient is lying down or asleep. The author recommends that some degree of compression be maintained at all times to ensure optimal contraction of the treated vein. In fact, studies have demonstrated that veins become more distensible during sleep.[86] This has been postulated to occur as a result of respiratory factors or emotional factors during dream states. In addition, thrombogenesis after the sclerotherapy-induced injury to vascular endothelium is maximal 8 hours after treatment, which may be when the patient wishes to lie down (see Chapter 8). Compression here speeds deep venous blood flow to prevent thrombosis in the deep system after treatment. Finally, it may be impractical for patients to remove and reapply the stocking at night if they must get out of bed for any reason. Therefore, if a high degree of compression is required after treatment, the use of double stockings appears practical since one of the stockings can be removed while the patient is lying down.

Practical Considerations

To optimize patient acceptability and compliance, a medium-strength compression stocking of 30 to 40 mm Hg is recommended. One study of two unnamed brands of 10- to 20-mm Hg graduated compression stockings demonstrated no significant difference in preference among 50 patients.[87] Another study demonstrated that approximately 80% of patients with varicose veins who use Sigvaris 30- to 40-mm Hg graduated compression stockings find them comfortable to wear, and symptoms are improved.[88] However, patients with varicose veins demonstrate a compliance of 67% when fitted with 30- to 40-mm Hg Medi Plus and a compliance of 41% when fitted with a 30- to 40-mm Hg Sigvaris graduated compression stocking.[89] Therefore, if patients refuse to wear the initially prescribed stockings, another brand of stockings should be recommended.

Some anatomic sites require inventive measures to effect compression of the underlying varicose veins. Perhaps the most difficult area to compress on the leg is the vulvar region. The author has found the "vulvar pad" described by Nabatoff to be effective in this region.[90]

THE RATIONALE FOR THE USE OF COMPRESSION IN THE TREATMENT OF TELANGIECTASIAS

In short, compression sclerotherapy is now standard practice in the treatment of varicose veins. However, its use in the treatment of smaller abnormal leg veins and telangiectatic "spider" veins has never been uniformly adopted. Theoretically, the same justification for the use of compression in larger veins should hold true for its use in smaller veins.

Duffy[91] has recently classified unwanted leg veins into six types based on clinical (and possibly functional) appearance (see p. 73). Types 1, 1A, and 1B are probably dilated venules, possibly with intimate and direct communication to underlying larger veins from which they are direct tributaries.[92] Both Bodian[93] and Faria and Moraes[94] have found on biopsy examination that such "telangiectasias" are actually ectatic veins. However, Duffy[91] and Biegeleisen[95] believe that the Duffy types 1, 1A, 1B, and 2 vessels may become dilated by virtue of their proximity to small arteriovenous communications. Indeed, multiple investigators[96-99] have demonstrated arteriovenous communications in association with larger varicose veins. However, serial histologic examination from 26 biopsies in 16 patients with telangiectatic leg veins (all but two with associated varicose veins) demonstrated an arteriovenous anastomosis in only one vein.[94] Thus the vast majority of telangiectasias arise from the venous system (see Chapters 1 and 4).

Therefore, because a significant percentage of smaller spider veins occur in direct communication with larger varicose or reticular superficial veins, compression of the "feeder" vein should decrease, if not eliminate, the blood flow to the smaller connected vessels. Thus, in addition to the effects of compression on the treated vessels themselves, compression of the entire leg should lead to a relatively stagnant blood flow in the feeder veins, which should allow for more effective endosclerosis of the treated vessel and a subsequent decreased risk of recanalization.

How Much Pressure is Necessary to Compress Telangiectasia?

The only reported study measuring the pressure necessary to empty superficial "capillaries" (telangiectasias) on the leg demonstrated that a sudden emptying of superficial cutaneous capillaries occurs between 40 and 60 mm Hg at a point 5 cm above the medial malleolus while the patient is recumbent.[100] However, 80 mm Hg was required to produce a complete emptying of blood with the patient in a standing position. Unfortunately, this degree of pressure is difficult to obtain with graduated compression stockings on areas of the leg above the ankle.

Interestingly, even graduated stockings with an ankle pressure of 7 to 8 mm Hg have been demonstrated in 6% of patients to control small superficial varices.[101] In this limited trial of women whose jobs entail standing for prolonged periods, this degree of ankle pressure was enough to produce a significant degree of symptomatic improvement in 74% of those studied. Whether these findings are real or are merely a placebo effect await further study. However, they do emphasize that at the very least, graduated compression stockings, properly fitted and applied, can be perceived as beneficial for a large number of people.

As previously explained, compression of the leg should be applied in a *graduated* manner to ensure and aid in the optimal unidirectional flow of blood toward the heart and to avoid a proximal tourniquet effect.

Multiple studies have demonstrated a pressure drop of 26% to 59% from the ankle to the thigh with graduated medical stockings.[62,71,102] Indeed, studies using photoplethysmography to evaluate the efficiency of venous return from the lower leg demonstrate a significant worsening when nongraduated, commercially available "support" pany hose are worn.[103] Therefore, obtaining a pressure high enough to empty telangiectasias on the thigh would require a cutaneous pressure at least 30% higher at the ankle for the stocking to be graduated.[104,105] The degree of pressure required to empty a thigh telangiectasia completely would likely result in cutaneous ischemia, especially with recumbency, thereby increasing the likelihood of cutaneous ulcerations.[106]

Therefore, in order to increase pressure in a localized area, the use of narrow foam rubber pads under compression stockings will result in an increase in cutaneous pressure under the pad by 15%[67] to 50%[80] over compression with the stocking alone. Foam Sorbo pads (STD Pharmaceuticas, Hereford, England) are widely used in Great Britain (see Fig. 13-15).[47] In addition to producing an increase in cutaneous pressure, their use, especially in the popliteal region, has decreased the incidence of abrasions from pressure stockings and tape, thereby improving patient comfort. Thus a localized relative increase in pressure on areas of the leg above the ankle may be possible.

Foam rubber pads have been noted to produce minor skin irritation (erythema) in up to 28% of patients in one physician's practice.[107] In these patients,

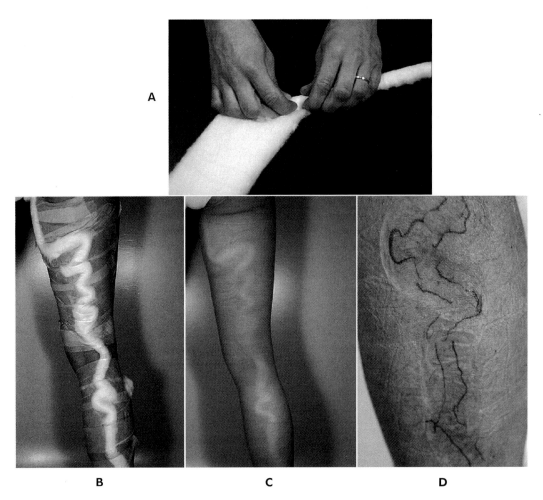

Fig. 6-17 **A,** a flat piece of cotton wool is twisted into a firm cotton wool roll with a diameter of approximately 2 m. **B,** The cotton wool roll follows the course of the varicose vein and is secured to the skin with 5 cm wide Leukopor® bandage. **C,** Appearance after application of a 30- to 40-mm Hg compression stocking. **D,** Appearance after stocking and cotton wool are removed in 2 weeks. Note compression of both the varicose vein and overlying tissues. (Reproduced with permission from Tazelaar DJ and Neumann HAM: Compression and sclerotherapy.)

substitution of another type of compression pad or cotton wool is necessary. Another device for increasing local pressure is Molefoam (Scholl®). This product comes in sheets of 7 mm thickness that may be easily cut to size. The adhesive side is covered with paper that is peeled away. Molefoam has a decreased incidence of local irritation (14% versus 28% for Sorbo pads). One study that compared the efficacy of sclerotherapy with Sorbo versus Molefoam showed no difference between the two groups.[107]

Another clever method for increasing local pressure is the use of rolls of cotton wool. The roll is secured with a nonelastic material (Fig. 6-17). This method is advantageous for compressing long lengths of veins.

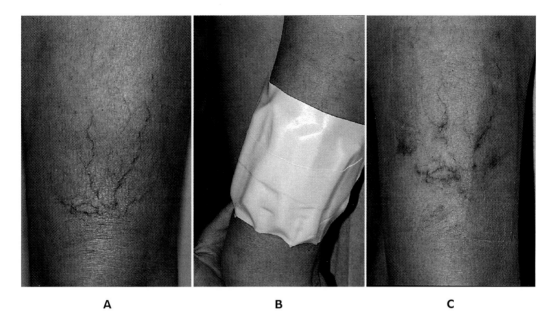

A   **B**   **C**

Fig. 6-18   **A,** Clinical appearance of venules and telangiectasia on anterior thigh of a 42-year-old woman measuring 0.2 to 0.6 mm in diameter without evidence of obvious feeding reticular or perforating vein. **B,** Immediately after sclerotherapy with POL 0.5%, STD foam pads were applied over the injected veins and secured with Microfoam tape under a 30 to 40 mm Hg graduated compression stocking. **C,** Three days after treatment, immediately after the removal of both the stocking and the pads. There is significant thrombosis of the treated veins even with a high degree of compression as noted by the indentation of the foam pad on the skin overlying the vessel.

Unfortunately, efforts to increase local compression through the use of foam rubber pads to effect *complete* emptying of telangiectatic leg veins are rarely successful. Follow-up of patients with Duffy types 1 and 2 veins treated with sclerotherapy and a combination of foam pads under a 30- to 40-mm Hg compression stocking demonstrates limited thrombus formation in the treated vessels (Fig. 6-18).

How Long Should Compression Be Maintained?

Formal studies on the use of compression in the treatment of leg telangiectasias have not been reported to my knowledge. However, a 3-day period for compression of leg telangiectasias is chosen based on the empirical report of Ouvry and Davy,[54] who advised a minimum of 3 days to limit the development of peripheral inflammation and intravascular thrombosis. Without supporting information, Harridge[51] recommends a 1-week period of compression for spider veins, using a local pressure band of elastic adhesive only.

Inadequacies of Compression

One limitation to the use of compression stockings in treating leg telangiectasias is the lack of complete emptying of the treated telangiectasias when only one stocking is used. Theoretically, the incorporation of foam pads directly over the injected vessels and a double layer of compression stockings for daytime use, with one stocking removed on recumbency, should produce a more complete vascular occlusion (see Figs. 6-15 and 6-16). However, even this technique will not completely close the treated vessel, as demonstrated by persistent thrombosis (see Fig. 6-18).

A multicenter, bilateral comparative study through the North American Society of Phlebology examined the necessity for the use of a single stocking when treating leg telangiectasias.[108] In short, 37 women with bilaterally symmetrical telangiectatic leg veins less than 1 mm in diameter were evaluated. One set of vessels was compressed for 3 days with a 30- to 40-mm Hg compression stocking* over cotton ball dressing. The alternate set of vessels had a cotton ball dressing applied for 2 hours with no overlying compression stocking. A greater clinical resolution of vessels occurred after treatment with one sclerotherapy injection on vessels located on the distal leg, or when vessels were greater than 0.5 mm in diameter. Vessels located elsewhere or less than 0.5 mm in diameter showed no significant difference when this form of compression was used (Table 6-2).

The main benefit of compression treatment was noted in the evaluation of adverse sequelae. The most significant finding in this study was that compression produced a relative decrease in postsclerotherapy hyperpigmentation, which fell from an incidence of 40.5% to 28.5% with the use of compression. In addition, ankle and calf edema were lessened if a graduated compression stocking was worn immediately after sclerotherapy. An additional nonrandomized study of 386 patients with leg telangiectasias was conducted without bilateral paired comparison.[57] In this study, 436 legs received graduated elastic stockings (compression class not stated) for 48 to 96 hours, and 182 legs were not compressed. Disappearance of more than 70% of telangiectasias occurred in one treatment in 85.7% of patients who wore compression stockings versus 72.5% of patients without compression ($P < 0.01$). In addition, compression reduced the incidence of pigmentation from 12.2% to 6.7%.

The major limitation of the above mentioned studies was the lack of complete emptying of the treated telangiectasia with the compression stocking used. Future studies may wish to incorporate different compression techniques to empty the treated vessels more completely. Also, these studies should address the optimal length of time needed for postsclerosis compression of telangiectasias.

*Medi USA, Arlington Heights, IL 60005.

Table 6-2   Adverse sequelae of sclerotherapy

	Pigmentation	Ankle edema	Calf edema
Compression	28.5%	33%	0%
Noncompression	40.5%	66%	40%

Modified from Goldman MP et al: Compression in the treatment of leg telangiectasia, J Dermatol Surg Oncol 16:332, 1990.

DONNING MEDICAL COMPRESSION STOCKINGS

Before donning the stocking, the patient should be advised of the following considerations. Hand jewelry should be removed to avoid damaging the stockings. Fingernails should be smooth and relatively short. Rubber gloves are helpful and recommended both to prevent damage to the stockings from long fingernails and to grip the stocking. Talcum powder may be applied to the leg or a light perlon panty hose or stocking may be worn under the compression stocking to create a smoother leg over which to slide the stocking. Finally, satin foot "socks" provided by the stocking manufacturer are helpful in getting an open-toe stocking over the ankle (Fig. 6-19).

After preparing the foot and leg, turn the stocking inside out with the foot from the heel to the toe tucked into the stocking (Fig. 6-20, *A*). Stretch the foot opening with the fingers or thumbs of both hands and pull the stocking foot over the foot up to the instep. Draw the stocking upward over the heel until pulling becomes difficult (Fig. 6-20, *B*). Push the fold that forms across the instep and heel of the stocking over the heel. Finally, pull the stocking up in sections, always remembering not to pull it over long distances all at once but to proceed in small steps (Fig. 6-20, *C*). When the stocking is applied without folds over the calf, the thigh section is then pulled over the knee (Fig. 6-20, *D*). Finally, remove the foot "sock" (Fig. 6-20, *E*).

It is very important for the physician or nurse to instruct and observe the patient applying the stocking. Effectiveness of compression will occur only when a stocking that has been fitted correctly is applied correctly. If the patient encounters difficulties in applying the stocking because of age, obesity, arthritis, etc., arrangements should be made to have an experienced helper on hand when needed. It is important to note that if patients have difficulty in applying higher-compression class stockings, wearing two layers of lighter stockings, one over the other, should be helpful. As discussed previously, the compressive effects of stockings are additive. Zippers in stockings also make donning them easier.

Recently, an application aid for compression stockings has been produced by various compression stocking companies. These devices are cleverly designed,

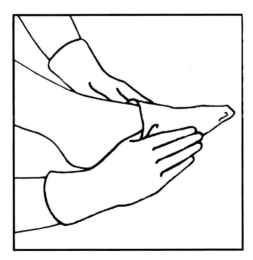

Fig. 6-19 Foot sock helpful for getting open-toe stocking over ankle. (Courtesy Julius Zorn, Inc.)

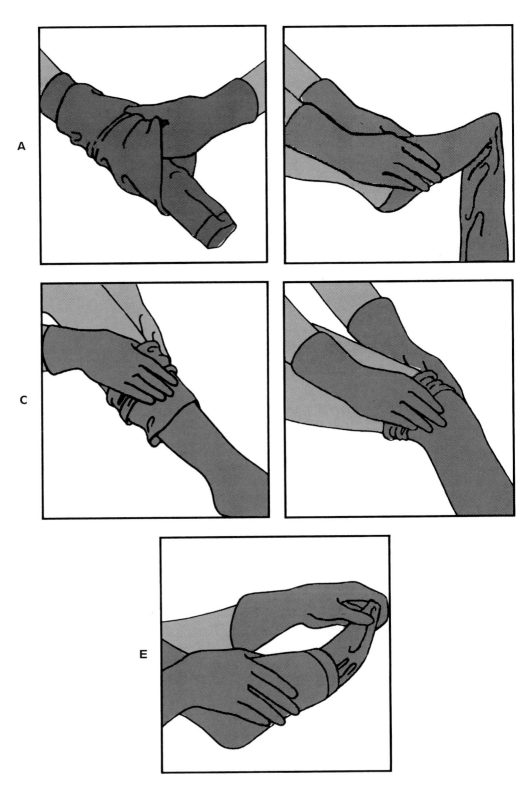

Fig. 6-20 Schematic diagram illustrating the proper method for donning the compression stocking. **A,** Turn the stocking inside out. Tuck in the foot from the heel to the toe. **B,** Using both hands, pull the stocking over the foot up to the instep, drawing it upward over the heel. **C,** Continue pulling the stocking up in small sections. **D,** Pull the thigh section over the knee. **E,** Remove the foot sock. (Courtesy Julius Zorn, Inc.)

simple metal supports that make donning compression stockings easier, even when the stockings must be placed over compression padding (Fig. 6-21). The compression stocking is pulled over the half-circle bracket located on the front (open) side of the device so that the heel portion of the stocking is 2 to 3 inches below the top on the half-circle bracket. The heel portion is positioned facing the user and the toe of the stocking is facing toward the open side of the device. The patient's foot is then placed into the foot of the stocking until the foot is completely on the floor or until the heel is in place. The metal grips on either side are

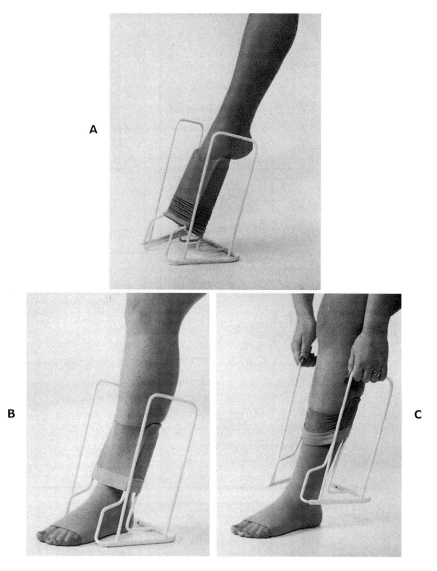

Fig. 6-21   The Medi Butler. **A,** After putting the compression stocking on the bracket, insert the foot. **B,** Continue until the foot is completely on the floor and the heel is in place. **C,** Pull up on the metal side grips until the Butler is above the calf, then remove it and continue until the stocking is in place. (Courtesy Medi USA)

then used to pull the rest of the stocking onto the leg. Once the stocking is above the calf, the device may be pulled away and the remainder of the stocking can then be easily pulled up.

CARE OF THE MEDICAL COMPRESSION STOCKING

Because these stockings are worn on a daily basis in extremely close contact with the skin, they are subjected to considerable wear. The chemical stresses from sweat, soaps, creams, and body oils, in addition to the physical stresses of the nearly continuous stretch and relaxation with movements of the leg, result in a gradual decline in the compressive effect of the stockings. Compression stockings, therefore, have a limited effective life. To ensure that they last as long as possible, special care is required.

The first lesson in proper stocking care is to avoid excessive trauma. Therefore, rubber gloves should be worn when the stocking is put on to avoid tearing the threads with fingernails. Likewise, toenails should be trimmed and hard calluses, verruca, or other rough spots on the feet should be softened or removed. Also, the stocking should be eased onto the leg, not pulled.

The stocking should not come into contact with ointments, creams, stain removers, or other solvents, especially if it is composed of rubber threads. These substances can damage the fine elastic yarns by causing them to swell and thus reducing the strength and elasticity of the fabric.

Regular and careful washing is necessary to maintain the elastic properties of the fabric. This is because of the harmful effects of sweat, skin oils, and environmental dirt that accumulate in the fabric while the stocking is worn. These substances will penetrate deeper into the elastic yarns if allowed to remain on the fabric for long intervals between washings. Environmental dust is damaging to the yarn by virtue of its abrasive action when the elastomers are stretched and relaxed.

Ideally, compression stockings should be washed every day. In fact, a study of six stocking types machine-washed 15 times at 40°C demonstrated no decrease in resting pressure or elasticity.[40] Therefore, if long-term use if required, it is best to provide the patient with two pairs of stockings that can be alternated between washings. Most compression stockings incorporating spandex can be machine-washed on a fine/gentle cycle with warm (40°C) water. This gives a better cleansing action than hand-washing. (Consult the manufacturer's guidelines for specific instructions.) Gentle detergents without bleach or alkali are best. Gentle spinning after the washing cycle is harmless to compression stockings and quickens the drying process. Rather than being hang-dried from a line, compression stockings should be laid flat on a drying rack or towel. Heat may be used in the drying process with most brands of compression stockings (see Table 6-1). With normal wear and proper care, compression stockings should have an effective life of 4 to 6 months.

REFERENCES

1. Orbach EJ: Compression therapy of vein and lymph vessel diseases of the lower extremities, Angiology 30:95, 1979.
2. Kohler H: Venous diseases of the leg and medical compression stockings and panty stockings, St Gallen, 1981, Ganzoni & Cie AG.
3. Johnson G Jr: The role of elastic support in venous problems. In Bergan J and Yao JST, editors: Surgery of the veins, 1985, Grune & Stratton.
4. Hohlbaum GG: The history of medical compression hoisery. In Hohlbaum GG et al, editors: The medical compression stocking, New York, 1989, Stuttgart.

5. Watson J: Observations on the nature and treatment of telangiectasis or that morbid state of the blood-vessels which gives rise to naevus and anuerism from anastamosis. Presented at the New York Medical and Surgical Society, March 2, 1839.

6. Christopoulos DG et al: Air-plethysmography and the effect of elastic compression on venous hemodynamics of the leg, J Vasc Surg 5:148, 1987.

7. Christopoulos D, Nicolaides AN, and Belcaro G: The long-term effect of elastic compression on the venous haemodynamics of the leg, Phlebology 6:85, 1991.

8. Gjores JE and Thulesius O: Compression treatment in venous insufficiency evaluated with foot volumetry, Vasa 6:364, 1977.

9. Pierson S et al: Efficacy of graded elastic compression in the lower leg, JAMA 249:242, 1983.

10. Gronbaek K et al: The effect of the Lastosheer stocking on venous insufficiency, Phlebology 6:198, 1991.

11. Matberry JC et al: The influence of elastic compression stockings on deep venous hemodynamics, J Vasc Surg 13:91, 1991.

12. Curri SB et al: Changes of cutaneous microcirculation from elasto-compression in chronic venous insufficiency. In Davy A and Stemmer R, editors: Phlebology '89, Montrouge, France, 1989, John Libbey Eurotext.

13. Fagrell B: Vital microscopy in the pathophysiology of deep venous insufficiency. In Eklof B et al, editors: Controversies in the management of venous disorders, London, 1989, Butterworths.

14. Ryan TJ, Mortimer PS, and Jones RL: Lymphatics and the skin: neglected but important, Int J Dermatol 25:411, 1986.

15. Brunstein IA: Prevention of discomfort and disability in the treatment of varicose veins, Am J Surg 54:362, 1941.

16. Sigg K: The treatment of varicosities and accompanying complications, Angiology 3:355, 1952.

17. Orbach EJ: A new approach to the sclerotherapy of varicose veins, Angiology 1:302, 1950.

18. Fegan WG: Continuous compression technique of injecting varicose veins, Lancet 2:109, 1963.

19. Partsch H and Mostbeck A: Constriction of varicose veins and improvement of venous pumping by dihydroergotamine, Vasa 14:74, 1985.

20. Mellander S and Nordenfelt I: Comparative effects of dihydroergotamine and noradrenaline on resistance, exchange, and capacitance functions in the peripheral circulation, Clin Sci 39:183, 1970.

21. Partsch H: Personal communication, 1990.

22. Fentem PH, Goddard M, and Gooden BA: The pressure exerted on superficial veins by support hoisery, J Physiol (Lond) 263(1):151P, 1976.

23. Horner J, Fernandes E, and Nicolaides AN: Valve of graduated compression stockings in deep venous insufficiency, Br Med J 280:820, 1980.

24. Siegel B et al: Type of compression for reducing venous stasis: a study of lower extremities during inactive recumbency, Arch Surg 110:171, 1975.

25. Horner J, Lowth LC, and Nicolaides AN: A pressure profile for elastic stockings, Br Med J 280:818, 1980.

26. Fegan WG: Varicose veins: compression sclerotherapy, London, 1967, Heinemann.

27. Norgren L, Austrell C, and Nilsson L: The effect of graduated compression hosiery on femoral blood flow during late pregnancy. Presented at the sixth Annual Meeting of the American Venous Forum, Maui, February 23-25, 1994.

28. Austrell C, Nilsson L, and Norgren L: Maternal and fetal haemodynamics during late pregnancy: effect of compression hosiery treatment, Phlebology 8:155, 1993.

29. O'Donnell TF Jr et al: Effect of elastic compression on venous hemodynamics in postphlebitic limbs, JAMA 242:2766, 1979.

30. Scurr JH, Coleridge-Smith P, and Cutting P: Varicose veins: optimum compression following sclerotherapy, Ann R Coll Surg (Engl) 67:109, 1985.

31. Partsch H: Improvement of venous pumping in chronic venous insufficiency by compression dependent on pressure material, Vasa 13:58, 1984.

32. Yamaguchi K et al: External compression with elastic bandages: its effect on the peripheral blood circulation during skin traction, Arch Phys Med Rehabil 67:326, 1986.

33. Tretbar LL and Pattisson PH: Injection-compression treatment of varicose veins, Am J Surg 120:539, 1970.

34. Callam MJ et al: Arterial disease in chronic leg ulceration: an underestimated hazard, Br Med J 294:929, 1987.

35. Cornwall JV, Dore CJ, and Lewis JD: Leg ulcers: epidemiology and aetiology, Br J Surg 73:693, 1986.

36. Callam MJ et al: Hazards of compression treatment of the leg: an estimate from Scottish surgeons, Br Med J 295:1382, 1987.

37. Danner R et al: Iatrogenic compartment syndrome, Clin Neurol Neurosurg 91:37, 1989.

38. Matsen RA et al: A model of compartment syndrome in man with particular reference to the quantification of nerve function, J Bone Joint Surg 59:648, 1977.

39. Callam MJ et al: Effect of posture on pressure profiles obtained by three different types of compression, Phlebology 6:79, 1991.

40. Blair SD et al: Sustained compression and healing of chronic venous ulcers, Br Med J 297:1159, 1988.

41. Neumann HAM and Tazelaar DJ: Compression therapy. In Bergan JJ and Goldman MP, editors: varicose veins and telangiectasia: diagnosis and treatment, St. Louis, 1993, Quality Medical.

42. Tazelaar DJ: Het compressieverband, keuze en techniek van aanleggen. The practitioner, Ned Uitg 973, 1987.

43. Schneider W and Fischer H: Die chronisch-venose Insuffizienz, Enke, 1969, Stuttgart, Germany.

44. Dinn E and Henry M: Treatment of venous ulceration by injection sclerotherapy and compression hosiery: a 5-year study, Phlebology 7:23, 1992.

45. von Beratung U: Die therapie venoser Beinleiden Kompressions therapie, medikamentos kombiniert? Der Bayerische Internist 1:46, 1987.

46. Hohlbaum GG: The use of medical compression stockings. In Hohlbaum GG et al, editors: The medical compression stocking, New York, 1989, Stuttgart, Germany.

47. Reid RG and Rothnie NG: Treatment of varicose veins by compression sclerotherapy, Br J Surg 55:889, 1968.

48. Wenner L: Sind endovarikose hamatische Ansammlungen eine Normalerscheinung bei Sklerotherapie? Vasa 10:174, 1981.

49. Orbach EJ: The importance of removal of postinjection coagula during the course of sclerotherapy of varicose veins, Vasa 3:475, 1974.

50. Lufkin H and McPheeters HQ: Pathological studies on injected varicose veins, Surg Gynecol Obstet 54:511, 1932.

51. Harridge H: The treatment of primary varicose veins, Surg Clin North Am 40:191, 1960.

52. Goldman MP et al: Sclerosing agents in the treatment of telangiectasia: comparison of the clinical and histologic effects of intravascular polidocanol, sodium tetradecyl sulfate, and hypertonic saline in the dorsal rabbit ear vein model, Arch Dermatol 123:1196, 1987.

53. Fegan WG: Continuing uninterrupted compression technique of injecting varicose veins, Proc R Soc Med 53:837, 1960.

54. Ouvry PA and Davy A: The sclerotherapy of telangiectasia, Phlebologie 35:349, 1982.

55. Goldman MP and Bennett RG: Treatment of telangiectasia: a review, J Am Acad Dermatol 17:167, 1987.

56. Goldman MP, Kaplan RP, and Duffy DM: Postsclerotherapy hyperpigmentation: a histologic evaluation, J Dermatol Surg Oncol 13:547, 1987.

57. Czaczka D et al: Contemporary approach to the telangiectasia of the lower extremity treatment in Poland. Proceedings of the European Congress of the IUP, Budapest, September 6-10, 1993, Essex, 1993, Multiscience.

58. Struckmann J et al: Venous muscle pump improvement by low compression elastic stockings, Phlebology 1:97, 1986.

59. Louis CE et al: Elastic compression in the prevention of venous stasis: a critical appraisal, Am J Surg 132:739, 1976.

60. Husi EA, Ximenes JOC, and Goyette EM: Elastic support of the lower limbs in hospital patients: a critical study, JAMA 214:1456, 1970.

61. Weber G: Manufacture, characteristics, testing, and care of medical compression hoisery. In Hohlbaum GG: The medical compression stocking, New York, 1989, Stuttgart, Germany.

62. Somerville JJ et al: The effect of elastic stockings on superficial venous pressures in patients with venous insufficiency, Br J Surg 61:979, 1974.

63. Braverman IM and Keh-Yen A: Ultrastructure of the human dermal microcirculation. IV. Valve Containing collecting veins at the dermal-subcutaneous junction, J Invest Dermatol 81:438, 1983.

64. Rooke TW et al: The effect of elastic compression on $TcPO_2$ in limbs with venous stasis, Phlebology 2:23, 1987.

65. Jones NAG et al: A physiological study of elastic compression stockings in venous disorders of the leg, Br J Surg 67:569, 1980.

66. Stoberl CH, Gabler S, and Partsch H: Indikationsgerechte bestrumpfung—messung der venosen pumpfunktion, Vasa 18:35, 1989.

67. Fentem PH et al: Control of distension of varicose veins achieved by leg bandages, as used after injection sclerotherapy, Br Med J 2:725, 1976.

68. Campion EC, Hoffmann DC, and Jepson RP: The effects of external pneumatic splint pressure on muscle blood flow, Aust N Z J Surg 38:154, 1968.

69. Chant ADB: The effects of posture, exercise, and bandage pressure on the clearance of Na from the subcutaneous tissues of the foot, Br J Surg 59:552, 1972.

70. Lawrence D and Kakkar VV: Graduated, static, external compression of the lower limb: a physiological assessment, Br J Surg 67:119, 1980.

71. Partsch H: Do we need firm compression stockings exerting high pressure? Vasa 13:52, 1984.

72. Hobbs JT: Surgery and sclerotherapy in the treatment of varicose veins, Arch Surg 109:793, 1974.

73. Doran FSA and White M: A clinical trial designed to discover if the primary treatment of varicose veins should be by Fegan's method or by an operation, Br J Surg 62:72, 1975.

74. Batch AJG et al: Randomized trial of bandaging after sclerotherapy for varicose veins, Br Med J 281:423, 1980.

75. Conrad P: Continuous compression technique of injecting varicose veins, Med J Aust 1:1011, 1967.

76. Orbach J: A new look at sclerotherapy, Folia Angiologica 25:181, 1977.

77. Weissberg D: Treatment of varicose veins by compression sclerotherapy, Surg Gynecol Obstet 151:353, 1980.

78. Tolins SH: Treatment of varicose veins: an update, Am J Surg 145:248, 1983.

79. Sladen JG: Compression sclerotherapy: preparation, technique, complications, and results, Am J Surg 146:228, 1983.

80. Raj TB, Goddard M, and Makin GS: How long do compression bandages maintain their pressure during ambulatory treatment of varicose veins? Br J Surg 67:122, 1980.

81. Coleridge-Smith PD, Scurr JH, and Robinson KP: Optimum methods of limb compression following varicose vein surgery, Phlebology 2:165, 1987.

82. Raj TB and Makin GS: A random controlled trial of two forms of compression bandaging in outpatient sclerotherapy of varicose veins, J Surg Res 31:440, 1981.

83. Chou FF et al: The treatment of leg varicose veins with hypertonic saline-Heparin injections, J Formosan Med Assoc 83:206, 1984.

84. Rodrigus I and Bleyn J: For how long do we have to advise elastic support after varicose vein surgery? A prospective randomized study, Phlebology 6:95, 1991.

85. Fraser IA et al: Prolonged bandaging is not required following sclerotherapy of varicose veins, Br J Surg 72:488, 1985.

86. Shepard JT: Reflex control of the venous system. In Bergan JJ and Yao JST, editors: Venous problems, Chicago, 1978, Year Book.

87. Williamson M et al: Graduated compression stockings in the prevention of post-operative deep vein thrombosis: a comparative study of pressure profiles and patient compliance, Phlebology 5:135, 1990.

88. Chant ADB, Magnussen P, and Kershaw C: Support hose and varicose veins, Br Med J 290:204, 1985.

89. Chant ADB et al: Support stockings in practical management of varicose veins, Phlebology 4:167, 1989.

90. Nabatoff RA: Vulval varicose veins during pregnancy: new support for effective compression, JAMA 173:1932, 1960.

91. Duffy DM: Small vessel sclerotherapy: an overview. In Callen JP et al, editors: Advances in dermatology, vol 3, Chicago, 1988, Year Book.

92. Bean WB: Vascular spiders and related lesions of the skin, Springfield, 1958, Thomas.

93. Bodian EL: Techniques of sclerotherapy for sunburst venous blemishes, J Dermatol Surg Oncol 11:696, 1985.

94. de Faria JL and Moraes IN: Histopathology of telangiectasias associated with varicose veins, Dermatologica 127:321, 1963.

95. Biegeleisen K: Primary lower extremity telangiectasias—relationship of size to color, Angiology 38:760, 1987.

96. Schalin L: Reevaluation of incompetent perforating veins: a review of all the facts and observations interpreted on account of a controversial opinion and our own results. In Tese M and Dormandy JA: Superficial and deep venous diseases of the lower limbs, Torino, Italy, 1984, Edizioni Panminerva Medica.

97. Schroth R: Venose sanerstoffsattigung bei Varicen, Arch Klin Chir 300:419, 1962.

98. Haeger KHM and Bergman I: Skin temperature of normal and varicose legs and some reflections on the etiology of varicose veins, Angiology 14:473, 1963.

99. Gins JA: Arteriovenous anastomoses and varicose veins, Arch Surg 81:299, 1960.

100. Allan JC: The micro-circulation of the skin of the normal leg, in varicose veins and in the post-thrombotic syndrome, S Afr J Surg 10:29, 1972.

101. Dinn E and Henry M: Value of lightweight elastic tights in standing occupations, Phlebology 4:45, 1989.
102. Berg EVD et al: A new method for measuring the effective compression of medical stockings, Vasa 11:117, 1982.
103. Godin MS, Rice JC, and Kerstein MD: Effect of commercially available pantyhose on venous return in the lower extremity, J Vasc Surg 5:844, 1987.
104. Bassi GL and Stemmer R: Traitments mecaniques fonctionnels en phlebologie, Ed Piccin, 1983, Padova.
105. Hohlbaum G: Mass-order Konfektionsstrumpf? Phlebol u Proktol 11:42, 1982.
106. Ashton H: Effect of inflatable plastic splints on blood flow, Br Med J 2:1427, 1966.
107. Stanley PRW, Brickerton DR, and Campbell WB: Injection sclerotherapy for varicose veins—a comparison of materials for applying local compression, Phlebology 6:37, 1990.
108. Goldman MP et al: Compression in the treatment of leg telangiectasia, J Dermatol Surg Oncol 16:322, 1990.

Production Methods and Materials for Medical Compression Stockings

In general, graduated compression stockings must satisfy two requirements. First, they must be manufactured in such a way that the pressure generated at the ankle is highest with a progressive decrease toward the thigh. Second, the stocking must have a high degree of elasticity so that it can slide over the heel and instep of the foot (an area one and a half times as wide as the ankle) as easily as possible, yet retain its compressive strength at the ankle.

The first mechanism for meeting the above requirement is that, without exception, all compression hosiery is knitted. Knitting is defined as a method of constructing fabric from one or more yarns by an interlocking series of loops (Figs. 6-A, 6-B, and 6-C). Knitted stockings are far more supple than woven textiles by virtue of the loop construction of their stitches. They can stretch both lengthwise and crosswise and return to their original shape. In other words, knitted fabric imparts elasticity.

Knitted elastic fabrics are made up of two or three yarn systems (see Figs. 6-A, and 6-B). A textile stitch-forming yarn with limited or no elasticity holds the knit together and determines its physical durability. This is usually a nylon, cotton, or synthetic cotton yarn. A stitch-forming elastic yarn renders the material elastic in the lengthwise direction. This is usually natural rubber or synthetic rubber (Spandex or Lycra®). A thicker, lateral laid-in or tied-in (nonstitch forming) elastic weft yarn is responsible for compression. This latter thread is referred to as the "woof." It is usually composed of natural rubber, Spandex, or Lycra® covered (coated) or uncovered (uncoated) yarns. The diameter of this elastic "woof" thread is important for exerting the required degree of compression by the stocking. The other threads can be considerably finer than the woof thread (Fig. 6-D).

The second mechanism for ensuring proper taut elasticity is to use a textile yarn. These yarns are woven into the hosiery in a crosswire (circumferential) direction. The yarns are either composed of natural rubber, synthetic elastic fibers such as spandex, or a combination of fibers (elastomer covered with cotton or silk).

Yarn Construction

Natural rubber yarns are derived from the milky juice (latex) of the rubber tree, *Hevea brasiliensis*. Latex is a high molecular hydrocarbon compound consisting of filiform macromolecules. Plasticizers, antiaging agents, antioxidants, fillers, and pigments are added. It is then shaped into threads. The threads are then vulcanized (heating the mixture with sulfur) to stabilize the material. Rubber yarns exhibit very good power with little loss of energy (low hysteresis). They possess a high degree of stretch and can be manufactured in large diameter sizes with resulting high compressive power. Rubber threads have been thought to have more elasticity than do synthetic elastomers. Therefore, rubber may be used in some ready-made stockings to allow them to fit a larger variation in leg size yet give the same compression. This is why Sigvaris® 500 series compression stockings (made with natural rubber) only come in three ankle sizes. Rubber may also be used in high compression class stockings (50 to 60 mm Hg). However, new generations of synthetic elastic fibers have been developed that Dupont now claims are superior to rubber in elasticity. In addition, as a natural product, rubber is subject to variations in composition and tends to deteriorate under certain environmental conditions, such as the effects of oils, sweat, chemicals, ointments, heat, light, and mechanical stress.[1] To protect the rubber core from external factors, crimped nylon is wrapped around it. Covered rubber is also said to retain its elasticity better for heavy compression requirements.[2]

Spandex (Perlon; Lycra® is manufactured by Dupont) is the generic name for a family of synthetic polyurethane elastomers developed as an alternative to natural rubber.

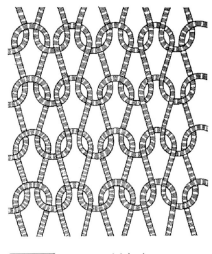

☗☗☗☗☗☗☗ Elastic yarn, stitch-forming

Fig. 6-A Drawing of a single-yarn knit. (Reproduced with permission from Gutezeichengemeinschaft Medizinsche Gummistrumpfe E V: The medical compression stocking. Schattauer, New York, 1989, Stuggart.)

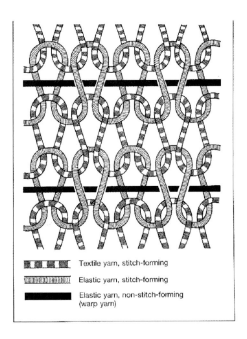

☗☗☗☗☗ Textile yarn, stitch-forming

⫟⫟⫟⫟⫟⫟ Elastic yarn, stitch-forming

▬▬▬▬ Elastic yarn, non-stitch-forming (warp yarn)

Fig. 6-B Diagram of a three-yarn knit with knitted-in elastic weft. (Reproduced with permission from Gutezeichengemeinschaft Medizinsche Gummistrumpfe E V.: The medical compression stocking, Schattauer, New York, 1989, Stuggart.)

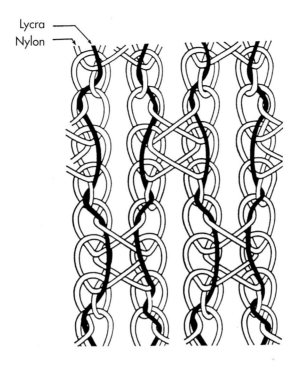

Lycra
Nylon

Fig. 6-C Diagram of a "typical" power-net fabric construction. (Courtesy Jobst Institute, Inc.)

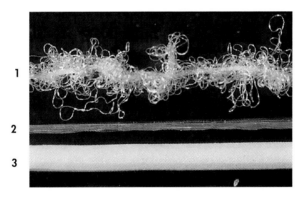

1

2

3

Fig. 6-D Photograph of three types of yarns found in compression stockings (×50 magnification). *1* = Covered spandex (Lycra® core with a nylon covering), used commonly as a knitting thread. *2* = Natural uncovered rubber. *3* = Uncoated Lycra®. (Courtesy Medi USA)

These elastomers are composed of various combinations of methane, acetylene, ethylene, and polyethylene to form polyamides of which at least 85% are segmented polyurethane. They are most commonly used in the rows of stitches for the elastic yarns. Elastomers are long-chain synthetic polymers comprised of at least 85% segmented polyurethane. They have the properties of natural rubber but are less prone to degradation from heat, oils, or other environmental factors. They are lighter in weight, more durable, and more supple than conventional elastic threads and have between 2 and 3 times the resting power. They can be repeatedly stretched to more than 5 times their length without breaking and still recover instantly to their original length. However, polyurethane elastomers are somewhat sensitive to hypochlorites and long-term exposure to moisture.[3] It has been stated that the

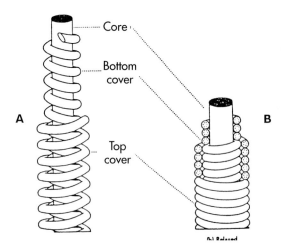

Fig. 6-E   Schematic drawing of double-covered yarn. a = stretched state, b = relaxed state. (Courtesy Jobst Institute, Inc.)

stretchability, or elasticity, of synthetic rubber is 20% less than that of natural rubber. Therefore, a compression stocking incorporating natural rubber has a maximum stretchability of 225% to 300%; one made with synthetic rubber is at most 175% to 250%.[4] However, newer synthetic rubber threads are said to have the same stretchability as natural rubber threads (Medi USA, personal communication, 1990). In addition, stockings incorporating uncoated synthetic threads have a higher stretchability than stockings incorporating coated threads, whether they are of a natural or synthetic rubber core.

Helanca, a synthetic cotton thread, is a crimped (wavy) and consequently slightly elastic nylon. Mutifiber Lycra® (Dupont) can be used with machine sewing because its threads are more resistant to fraying when manipulated. It is usually used in a covered state to improve its elastic memory. Lycra® is used for compression pressures up to 30 to 40 mm Hg. Nylon is virtually nonelastic and is therefore used mainly in coated elastic threads. Rubber weaving threads or stronger synthetic threads are used for higher-pressure stockings.

To utilize the positive characteristics of these materials and to provide prescribed pressures consistently, the bare synthetic or rubber core is covered with inelastic yarns such as cotton, silk, nylon, or Helenca (Fig. 6-E). The threads are covered while stretched to prescribed degrees and then treated to remove any electrostatic charges that occurred in the wrapping process. Then they are respooled with no tension or are allowed to lie in piles prior to their use in stocking construction. This method of stretch covering enables the designer to utilize the most desirable portion of the power curve (see Chapter 6, Fig. 6-11, p. 214), in addition to providing physical protection and/or a degree of comfort to the inner core fiber. Yarns may be double-covered in opposing turns to balance the torque applied to the core and to ensure positive entrapment. In high-stretch yarns, the elastic core provides the majority of stretch resistance and return power. In low-stretch yarns, the coverings provide the majority of stretch resistance.

Bare (uncoated) spandex threads may also be utilized in the construction of compression stockings. This is a key feature of the Medi brand of compression stocking. Possible benefits to the use of bare spandex threads include a greater two-way stretch; a softer, more comfortable feel; sheer quality; and greater washability. Greater two-way stretch is available from uncoated threads by the nature of the construction of coated threads. When elastomers are coated they are stretched to apply the coating or wrapping material. With this procedure, depending on the modulus of the thread, its stretch or extension may be decreased by up to 50%. The extent of elasticity lost may be difficult to estimate in coated

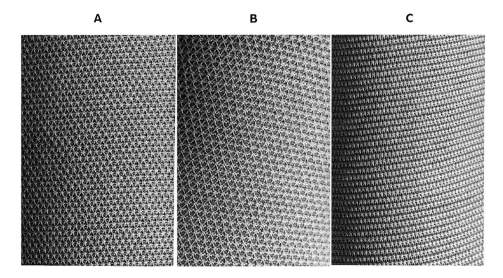

Fig. 6-F Photograph of the weave of a Juzo-Varen soft 30- to 40-mm Hg stocking taken from the midcalf aspect of the stocking. **A,** Outer view of the stocking. **B,** Texture of the fabric from the inner aspect with a silk thread woven in. **C,** Texture of the external aspect of the fabric with a silk thread woven in. (Courtesy Julius Zorn, Inc.)

threads. The Jobst Institute (personal communication, 1990) states that limitations of the covering materials and equipment place the maximum stretch of the final yarn near 300%. Because the bare elastomers are capable of repeat elongations in excess of 650%, the covering operation significantly reduces the ultimate stretch. Covering, though, is used to trap fine denier elastic threads at the higher end of their power curves, enabling higher compression levels with lighter cores. This results in a noticeable difference between stockings made with coated threads and those made with uncoated threads. Stockings with covered yarns tend to be wider in diameter at a given location and are more difficult to stretch. This is secondary to the loss of elasticity of the spandex or rubber threads produced by the coating/covering process.

Increased two-way stretch or elasticity allows the compression stocking to be more easily donned. In addition, the uncoated thread is stated by Medi to have a softer consistency and to "grip" the skin well, making the stocking less likely to slip down the leg.

Cleaning a fabric made with uncoated threads may allow for easier, quicker removal of dirt and debris. Coated threads may trap dirt in the nylon wrapping. When uncoated, the stocking is machine washable, can withstand machine drying, and dries more quickly.

Finally, coated threads are bulkier than uncoated threads. Stockings manufactured with uncoated threads are therefore more sheer. The weave is more open, which allows the skin to "breathe."

Cotton yarns are also used for lighter-weight compression stockings. Cotton yarns are less durable than polyamide yarns. Cotton has the ability to swell and absorb fluid, which may be useful for the absorption of sweat. Unfortunately, this same absorptive quality may also permit dirt and other particles to lodge in the porous cotton threads. However, newer polyamide fibers can also be manufactured to have a comparable moisture-transporting capacity. Although cotton fibers have a softer feel than synthetic fibers, polyamide fibers are usually textured to give them a higher stretch and a pleasant feel.

Silk, wool, and cotton threads may be incorporated into the stocking as an extra thread on the skin surface (Fig. 6-F, *A-C*). Here the threads serve to impart a pleasant feel to the stocking. They may also impart thermal characteristics to the stocking, making it more suitable for cold weather. Finally, they may act to absorb perspiration and skin oils.

The core type and coverings of the yarns determine the individual characteristic of the stocking. Low modulus, high-stretch yarns allow for easier donning of the stocking over the large heel to the instep circumference. Because the prescribed power must be obtained, it is the remaining holding power following the large deformation and subsequent stress relaxation that is of primary importance. In addition, low modulus stockings have been shown to deliver a more uniform pressure over a greater range of leg circumferences than do high modulus stockings.[5] However, fine, low modulus yarns may not possess sufficient holding power to effectively manage high-compression stockings.

Although the preceding description is simplified, the final construction of the stocking can be quite complex. Usually, stockings are composed of many different types of threads. For example, a Hostess Varien (Juzo) is composed of 10 different threads: three diameters of Lycra®, three diameters of spandex, and different covering threads according to the style. In addition, approximately 1.5 million stitches are required to manufacture a medium-sized thigh stocking. The following section describes the manufacturing process.

Stocking Construction

Medical compression stockings are manufactured by two different methods: flat-knitting and circular-knitting.

The flat-knitting technique was the first to be developed for the mass production of stockings. The fabric is woven by means of a carriage that is moved back and forth by hand or machine. The carriage holds the cams on which up to 20 latch needles per square inch are moved up and down. A yarn guide serves to lay the elastic weft yarns without tension between the front and rear needle beds in the parallel rows of stitches along the length of material. The width of the fabric is altered by changing the number of needles. A 25-cm width requires two sets of 83 needles at the ankle. The number of needles is then increased to two sets of 137 to produce the required 45-cm width at midcalf. Producing the heel section requires a similar change in needle placement. Therefore, although an infinite number of sizes can be manufactured, this type of construction is very labor intensive. One calf stocking requires almost 30 minutes to produce, with approximately 80% of that time used to make the heel.

Another type of flat-bed construction is called bobbinet. With this type, the resulting power is produced in one direction, with little contribution from tie in yarns (Fig. 6-G).

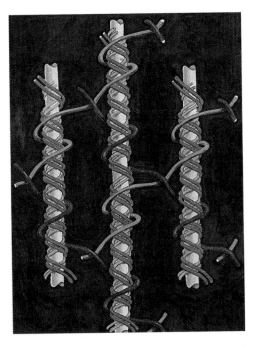

Fig. 6-G Diagram of Jobst's Bobbinet fabric with resulting one-direction power. (Courtesy Jobst Institute, Inc.)

When on the body, the high-power elastic yarns are oriented horizontally, enabling precise engineering to a specific body shape or custom design. Profiles of the required shape are cut from the flat fabric to the appropriately reduced measurements (based on graduated compression) and sewn into the shape of the leg. Bidirectional independent compression can be obtained by weaving latex and nylon threads in a patented manner.

An advantage of flat-knitting is that the width of the knitted fabric can be varied by adding or removing needles on either side. This is the way the prescribed dimensions of width are made. This method allows for a stocking to be made easily for legs that vary significantly in heel, calf, and thigh circumference. Modern overlock looping machines allow the fabric to be closed without seams and without damaging the yarns, producing a durable compression stocking.

The disadvantage of this knitting technique is that the stitches are relatively coarse, and the process is labor intensive and thus relatively expensive.

Circular-knitting of fashion stockings first occurred in the 1930s and was improved for use in medical compression stockings during the 1950s. On circular-knitting machines, the needles are arranged in a circle and interloop the yarns in a spiral succession as the cylinder spins. More than 500 needles (depending on machine size) are used in each machine. A sheer 30- to 40-mm Hg medium-sized Hostess compression stocking (Juzo) or a Medi 75 or Plus or Venosan requires up to 500 needles. An elastic yarn is fed into the looping sequence and lies between successive levels or courses of loops in a continuous spiral (Fig. 6-H). The body or construction yarns may contain a fine elastic yarn, imparting a high stretch in the longitudinal direction of the stocking. This biaxial stretch enables a good "fit" to be obtained over a variety of contours and allows for ease of motion.

Because the cylinder diameter and number of needles cannot be changed with this technique, it is not possible to widen or narrow the fabric. Therefore, with circular knitting, the hosiery is shaped to the leg in two ways—by varying the stitch size so that it is shorter and tighter at the heel and longer and looser at the thigh, and by varying the tension in the weft yarns during the knitting process (Fig. 6-I, *A-D*). With this method, the tension of the fabric is precisely controlled by a computer. The higher the pretension of the weft yarn, the more the stocking contracts upon removal from the knitting cylinder. To prevent a limitation in horizontal stretch from occurring with this knit, alternating nylon, rubber, or spandex threads are woven together.

Unlike the flat-knitting technique, these machines can produce a finely woven fabric with up to 450 needles in a cylinder diameter of $3\frac{1}{2}$ to 6 inches. With circular-knitting,

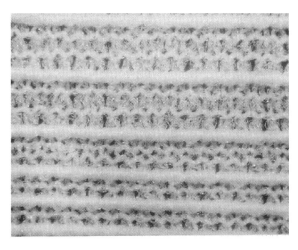

Fig. 6-H   Photograph of circular-knit construction showing the area of density distribution change of major elastic yarn of a Kendall T.E.D. ($\times 8$ magnification). (Courtesy Jobst Institute, Inc.)

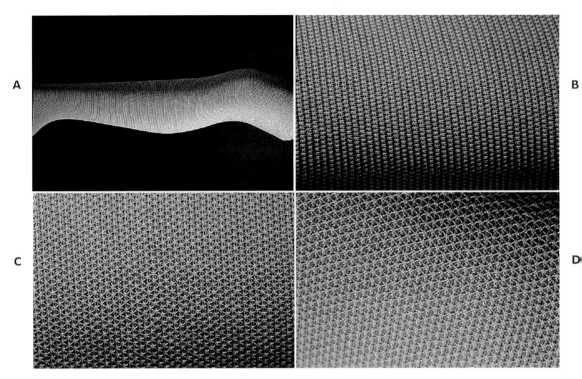

Fig. 6-1 **A,** Photograph of a Medi 30-to-40 mm Hg thigh stocking made on a circular-knitting machine. **B,** Close-up view of the knit pattern at the midthigh level. **C,** Close-up view of the knit pattern at the midcalf level. **D,** Close-up view of the knit pattern at the ankle level. Note how the knit changes to decrease the compression of the stocking as it goes up the leg. (All close-up photographs were taken under similar stretch pressure of the stocking.) (Courtesy of Medi U.S.A.)

the finest mesh used in compression stockings is approximately 32 needles/inch as compared with 20 needles/inch with flat-knitting machines.

The advantage of the circular-knitting technique is that a more attractive, finely knit stocking can be inexpensively produced. In fact, when worn by an individual who has been fitted correctly, even ready-made 20- to 30-mm Hg graduated stockings have been demonstrated to produce an improvement in symptomatology and a reduction in calf diameter and leg volume.[6] The disadvantage is that, as a general rule, this technique can be used only to manufacture compression stockings for patients whose thigh diameter is up to 2.5 to 3.5 times their ankle diameter.

In summary, all graduated compression stockings are manufactured using slightly different techniques and materials with their unique advantages and disadvantages. The patient can choose the best stocking by direct comparison of the various brands and styles. Stockings are often worn not only for a few days after treatment, but also when patients are traveling by car or plane (resulting in relative immobilization and stagnation of venous flow) or during everyday work (if patients are required to stand for long periods).

REFERENCES

1. Weber G: Manufacture, characteristics, testing and care of medical compression hoisery. In Hohl-baum GG et al, editors: The medical compression stocking, New York, 1989, Stuttgart.
2. Johnson G Jr: The role of elastic support in venous problems. In Bergan JA and Yao JST, editors: Surgery of the veins, New York, 1985, Grune & Stratton.
3. Bergan JJ: Conrad Jobst and the development of pressure gradient therapy for venous disease. In Bergan JA and Yao JST, editors: Surgery of the veins, New York, 1985, Grune & Stratton.
4. Kohler H: Venous diseases of the leg and medical compression stockings and panty stockings, St. Gallen, 1981, Ganzoni & Cie. AG.
5. Johnson Jr G et al: Graded compression stockings, Arch Surg 117:69, 1982.
6. Pierson S et al: Efficacy of graded elastic compression in the lower leg, JAMA 249:242, 1983.

MECHANISM OF ACTION OF SCLEROTHERAPY

GENERAL MECHANISM FOR PRODUCING ENDOTHELIAL DAMAGE

Sclerotherapy refers to the introduction of a foreign substance into the lumen of a vessel causing thrombosis and subsequent fibrosis (Fig. 7-1). This procedure, when performed on telangiectasias, is referred to as microsclerotherapy.[1]

The mechanism of action for sclerosing solutions is that of producing endothelial damage (endosclerosis) that eventuates in endofibrosis. The extent of damage to the blood vessel wall determines the effectiveness of the solution. Endothelial cells are highly complex and represent the largest "organ" of the human body. In addition to their function as a conduit for blood, these cells react to mechanical forces and multiple substances produced locally or circulating in the blood. They have a broad range of metabolic activities including, but not limited to, uptake and degradation of circulating norepinephrine, epinephrine, brady-kinin, and serotonin; the conversion of angiotensin I to the vasoconstrictor angiotensin II; production of plasminogen activator inhibitor; production of heparin and/or heparin-like substances; production of prostacyclin, which acts both on vascular smooth muscle and on platelet aggregation; production of endothelium-derived relaxing factor; storage and secretion of histamine; synthesis of basic fibroblast growth factor (FGF); and modulation of inflammation through interactions with tumor necrosis factor (TNF) and interferon-γ.[2-5] Thus it is miraculous that sclerotherapy treatment is not without significant adverse sequelae (see Chapter 8).

Total endothelial destruction results in the exposure of subendothelial collagen fibers causing platelet aggregation, adherence, and release of platelet-related factors. This series of events initiates the intrinsic pathway of blood coagulation by activating factor XII. Ideally, sclerosing solutions should not otherwise cause activation or release of thromboplastic activity because this would initiate the extrinsic pathway of blood coagulation.

Excessive thrombosis is detrimental to the production of endofibrosis because it may lead to recanalization of the vessel and excessive intravascular and perivascular inflammation and its resulting sequelae (see Chapter 8). This can be prevented or at least minimized with postsclerotherapy compression (see Chapter 6). However, thrombosis usually occurs to some degree as a result of sclerotherapy. If a thrombus is formed, it should be well anchored to the venous wall to ensure against embolization. Wolf[6] in 1920 established that effective sclerosis results in thrombosis that penetrates the full thickness of the adventitia of the vessel wall. Schneider[7] has shown in histologic examinations of sclerosed varices that the strongest fixation of a thrombus occurs in areas where the entire endothelium is destroyed. Therefore, endothelial damage must be complete and should result in minimal thrombus formation with subsequent organization and fibrosis (Fig. 7-2). In addition, after sclerotherapy, maximal full-thickness fibrosis of the treated segment occurs after 6 weeks of compression.[8] Therefore, in addition to limiting the extent of thrombosis, compression may facilitate endofibrosis (see Chapter 6).

Endothelial damage can be provoked by a number of mechanisms, such as changing the surface tension of the plasma membrane or modifying the

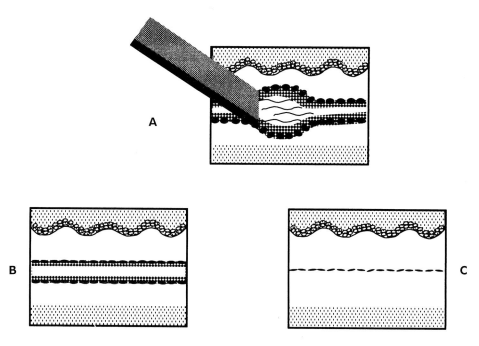

Fig. 7-1 Diagrammatic representation of the mechanism of action for sclerotherapy. A, Proper placement of needle into the vein and release of sclerosing solution. B, Early stage of endothelial destruction and minimal organizing thrombosis. C, Late stage demonstrating fibrous cord formation.

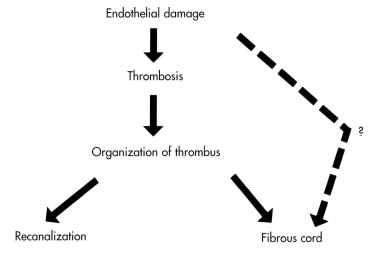

Fig. 7-2 Chain of events occurring after sclerotherapy. Ideally, the treated vessel will progress directly from damaged endothelium to a fibrous cord. However, some degree of intravascular thrombosis usually occurs.

physical/chemical milieu of the endothelial cell through a change of intravascular pH or osmolality. The endothelium can be directly destroyed by caustic chemicals or by other physical factors such as heat and cold. For sclerotherapy to be effective without recanalization of the thrombotic vessel, the endothelial damage and resulting vascular necrosis must be extensive enough to destroy the entire blood vessel wall.[9]

Destruction of the entire vessel wall and not just the endothelium is necessary, as demonstrated in animal studies that are described later in this chapter. The reason may relate to the multifunctional nature of vascular smooth muscle cells. These cells, which are found in significant concentration within superficial veins (see Chapter 2), have a large number of functions including the synthesis of collagen, elastin, and proteoglycans.[10] It is hypothesized that if they remain viable, they can regenerate a foundation that promotes migration of undamaged adjacent endothelial cells that allow recanalization of the treated vessel.[11]

In addition, for effective destruction of a varicosity or telangiectasia, the entire vessel must be sclerosed to prevent recanalization. Recanalization occurs easily in vessels where only a section of endothelium is damaged. This is due to rapid endothelial regeneration, which has been measured at a turnover rate of 0.1% to 10%/day or higher.[12] Endothelial migration has been estimated to proceed at a rate of 0.07 mm/day in the circumferential direction and 6 times faster in an axial direction in rat aorta.[13] In fact, endothelial cell regeneration may be sufficiently rapid to replace dying endothelium after small areas are denuded.[14] In the future, one may be able to estimate total endothelial destruction as a marker for effective sclerosis by counting circulating endothelial cells.[15]

CATEGORIES OF SCLEROSING SOLUTIONS

All sclerosing solutions can be placed into three broad categories based on their mechanisms for producing endothelial injury: detergent, osmotic, or chemical. There are an infinite number of potential solutions that when injected intravascularly can cause endothelial and vascular wall necrosis. In addition, an infinite variety of various combinations or mixtures of solutions can be used to produce endosclerosis. The ideal sclerosing solution should be painless to inject, free of all adverse effects, and specific for damaged (varicose) veins. Although such a solution has not been discovered for all types of veins, this chapter examines solutions commonly in use for this purpose.

Detergent Solutions

Detergent sclerosing solutions commonly used to treat varicose and telangiectatic veins include sodium morrhuate (SM), ethanolamine oleate (EO), sodium tetradecyl sulfate (STS), and polidocanol (POL). They produce endothelial damage through interference with cell surface lipids (Fig. 7-3). Strong detergents, such as STS and SM, produce maceration of the endothelium within 1 second of exposure.[16] The intercellular "cement" is disrupted, resulting in desquamation of endothelial cells in plaques. Because the hydrophilic and hydrophobic poles of the detergent molecule orient themselves so that the polar hydrophilic part is within the water and the hydrophobic part is away from the water, they appear as aggregates in solution or fixed onto the endothelial surface (Fig. 7-4). Because one cannot ensure that the solution is entirely in contact with the endothelial surface (if the injected vein contains blood), the decrease in surface tension on the endothelial cells may not be in direct proportion to the concentration of the solution. Strong detergent sclerosants therefore have a low safety margin.[16]

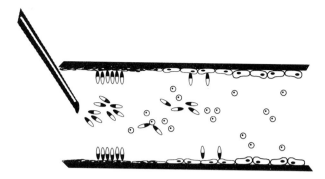

Fig. 7-3 Diagrammatic representation of the action of a detergent sclerosing solution on the vessel wall, showing formed elements of the blood.

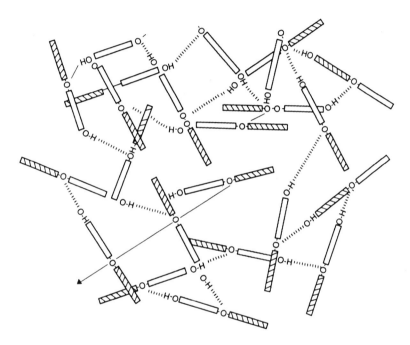

Fig. 7-4 Diagrammatic representation of the probable molecular orientation of detergent sclerosing solutions into aggregates.

Detergent sclerosing agents have also been studied regarding their direct toxic effects on the formed elements of blood. One study found that the addition of SM, EO, STS, or POL to citrated plasma did not cause clotting or shorten the prothrombin time (PT) or the partial thromboplastin time (PTT).[17] However, all of the sclerosing agents examined were directly toxic to both granulocytes and red blood cells at dilutions of up to 1:1000. When tested against cultured endothelial cells, all solutions were toxic to approximately 60% to 80% of endothelial cells at 1:100 dilutions, but only SM and EO were toxic at a further dilution of 1:1000. None of these tested solutions were toxic at 1:10,000 dilutions. Therefore, this study confirms that effective endosclerosis occurs through damage to endothelium and not through thrombosis induced by destruction or damage to red and/or

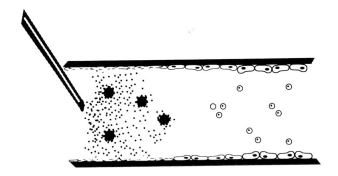

Fig. 7-5   Diagrammatic representation of the action of a hypertonic sclerosing solution on the vessel wall, showing formed elements of the blood.

white blood cells. Another in vitro study, however, found that activated partial thromboplastin time (PTT) was prolonged in proportion to the fall of factor XII and prekallikrein activity when POL was added to citrated serum.[18] This indicates that in addition to its action on endothelial cells, POL is capable of acting on blood coagulation through activation of the early phase of the intrinsic pathway. The clinical relevance of this finding is unclear because additional studies have failed to demonstrate its significance, as explained later in this chapter.[19,20]

Osmotic Solutions

Hypertonic solutions such as hypertonic saline (HS) probably cause dehydration of endothelial cells through osmosis, resulting in endothelial destruction[18] (Fig. 7-5). It is speculated that fibrin deposition with thrombus formation on the damaged vessel wall occurs through modification of the electrostatic charge of the endothelial cells.[16] For the vessel wall to be completely destroyed, the osmotic solution must be of sufficient concentration to diffuse throughout the entire vein wall.[21] In contrast to the immediate action of detergent sclerosing solutions, experimental studies have shown that endothelial destruction with HS 22% or glucose 66% occurs only after 3 minutes.[16] The destroyed endothelial cells do not appear to be desquamated as with detergent sclerosing solutions.[16]

Hypertonic solutions have a predictable destructive power that is proportional to their osmotic concentration. This was demonstrated in a comparative study of multiple hypertonic solutions used on the superficial and internal saphenous veins of 27 dogs.[22] The degree of endothelial damage was assessed histologically at multiple times from 30 minutes to 8 weeks after sclerotherapy. The authors ranked the solutions from strongest to weakest as:

Sodium salicylate 40%
Sodium chloride 10% + sodium salicylate 30%
Invert sugar 75%
Saccharose 5%
Phenol 1%
Dextrose 66%
Sodium chloride 20%
Sodium salicylate 30%

The authors concluded that maximal endothelial destruction occurred as early as 30 minutes to 4 days after injection, after which time the injected vessel went through either a reparative or fibrotic process.

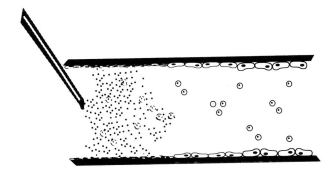

Fig. 7-6 Diagrammatic representation of the action of a caustic chemical sclerosing solution on the vessel wall, showing formed elements of the blood.

Because dilution occurs with intravascular serum and blood, osmotic solutions have their greatest effect at or near the site of injection. In contrast, detergent sclerosing solutions can exert effective sclerosis for 5 to 10 cm along the course of the injected vessel. Sadick recently examined the sclerosing effect of HS 23.4% and POL 0.5%.[23] He found equal sclerosing effect (length) for these two solutions injected in a similar type of veins using identical techniques. Unfortunately, HS 23.4% is more potent (about 2×) than POL 0.5%. Therefore, he inadvertently demonstrated that detergent solutions have about twice the therapeutic efficacy of osmotic solutions. A better comparison would have been with HS 11.7%.

Chemical Solutions

Chemical irritants also act directly on endothelial cells to produce endosclerosis. Lindemayr and Santler[24] studied the sclerosing effect of 4% polyiodinated ions (PII, Variglobin) with standard and immunofluorescent microscopy and demonstrated fibrin deposition on the sclerosed veins only. Platelets fixed only to elastin, collagen, the basement membrane, and the amorphous material of the subendothelial layer—not to intact endothelial cells. It is also thought that the chemical destruction is in part related to the dissolution of intercellular cement, which has been demonstrated to occur after 30 seconds of exposure.[16] Thus this chemical irritant sclerosing solution produces its end result of vascular fibrosis through the irreversible destruction of endothelial cells with resultant thrombus formation on the subendothelial layer (Fig. 7-6).

The aforementioned mechanism of action has also been visually demonstrated with scanning electron microscopy of sclerosed rabbit veins (agent not noted) by Merlen.[25] He demonstrated intimal cracks and fissures that left intimal connective tissue fibers and elastic lamina exposed. Ultrastructural damage involving stasis of blood and platelet aggregation on intact endothelial intima occurred in 5 minutes in the dorsal rabbit ear vein.

FACTORS PREDISPOSING TO THROMBOSIS

As discussed previously, optimal clinical results occur when sclerotherapy-induced thrombosis is minimized. Factors predisposing to thrombus formation include decreased velocity of blood flow, hypercoagulability, and endothelial cell damage.[26] The velocity of blood flow is unaffected by the sclerosing agent itself, but flow in general is usually slower in varicose veins and telangiectasia. This relative decrease in blood flow may predispose to thrombus formation in varicose veins and may be a significant contributing factor to the increased incidence of thrombophlebitis and deep vein thrombosis (DVT) in patients with varicose veins (see Chapter 2). However, decreased blood flow probably does not play a significant role in thrombus formation after sclerosing treatment.

Hypercoagulability also predisposes one to thrombus formation. Wuppermann[27] studied fibrinolysis in subjects injected with POL and found a slight, statistically insignificant hyperfibrinolysis in blood drawn from the antecubital vein. He hypothesized that because coagulation factors II, VII, VIII, and IX and platelet function are damaged directly by the sclerosing solution, coagulation at the injection site is delayed. Endosclerosis as measured by fibrinogen gradually occurred over 5 days only at the injection site and did not result in systemic hypercoagulability. Therefore, sclerotherapy should not result in a sudden thrombosis. In fact a hemolytic effect was detected with STS even at a 0.1% concentration, with POL at a 0.05% dilution and with PII at 2% concentration.[19] PTT, PT, and thrombin times (TT) were unchanged with injection of these agents into whole blood. Earlier work also demonstrated the lack of effect of POL on coagulation parameters in rabbits.[28] MacGowen et al.[29] combined STS with whole normal blood, resulting in a homogeneous red cell lysate without the formation of thrombin. In vivo studies have also demonstrated a lack of hypercoagulability from sclerosing solutions. Cepelak found that platelet aggregation occurs only at the site of the sclerosing solution injection, with aggregation-inhibiting effects occurring in the efferent deep veins distally to the femoral vein.[20] Thus endothelial damage probably causes a release of various factors that produce anticoagulant effects, lowering the risk of thrombotic complications of sclerosing therapy. This effect was confirmed by Raymond-Martimbeau and Leclerc, who measured fibrinopeptide A and fibrin degradation of D-dimer fragments after injection of sodium iodine.[30] They found no evidence for activation of blood coagulation. Therefore, experimental findings do not support the theory of intrinsic hypercoagulability of sclerosing solutions as the mechanism of action for thrombus formation during sclerotherapy (see Chapter 1).

This lack of hypercoagulability also correlates with clinical experience using POL. When POL is used in patients who are taking systemic anticoagulants, a decrease in its sclerosing action does not occur.[31] The addition of heparin to STS also has had no effect on the sclerotherapy results in a paired comparison of 100 patients.[32] Thus it appears that the mechanism of action of POL and STS is to produce endothelial damage,[33] but not thrombus formation associated with platelet aggregation. This mode of action is also seen with other (nondetergent) sclerosing agents.

FACTORS PREDISPOSING TO ENDOFIBROSIS

Whether altered vessels are more susceptible to the action of sclerosing agents than normal vessels is unknown. At times, human varicose and telangiectatic vessels are noted to sclerose focally after the injection of various solutions. The focal nature of endothelial necrosis and thrombus formation may be related to toxic effects of the sclerosing solutions on the surrounding media. This effect is commonly observed when injecting varicose veins under duplex control. With this technique (described in Chapter 9) the sclerosing solution is injected and/or held in place until the varicosity is seen to spasm. This indicates effective sclerosis. Venograms of varicose veins injected with STS demonstrate segmental, intense, and diffuse spasm, both proximally and distally, at the time of injection and 6 minutes after injection.[34] Effective endosclerosis occurs at points of vessel spasm where the entire endothelium is adherent. This agrees with the clinical impression that total compression of the sclerosed vessel is necessary for ideal, long-lasting, and complication-free sclerosis.[35,36]

At one time it was thought that "any solution which will not produce a slough when injected perivenously will generally not be strong enough to obliterate a vein."[37] However, some very effective sclerosing solutions are thought to act selectively on "damaged" varicose endothelium. In fact, experimental studies have documented that effective sclerosing solutions do not have to produce tissue necrosis on intradermal injection (see Chapter 8). The manufactures of POL state that this agent acts selectively on damaged vessels.*† In addition, a number of histologic studies of the effect of sclerotherapy on varicose veins have also concluded that damaged varices are preferentially sclerosed.‡[7,16,25] However, experimental injection of sclerosing agents on normal dorsal rabbit ear veins yields effective vessel sclerosis in a concentration-dependent manner.[38,39] Therefore, in addition to the type and concentration of sclerosing solution, other factors, including vessel diameter, rate of blood flow, and anatomic site of the vessel, may also be important.

Sclerosing solutions affect arteries in a different manner than they do veins. Although thrombosis occurs, intimal damage may not. MacGowen et al.[29] studied the local effects of intraarterial injection of STS. They injected STS 3.0% into the central auricular artery at the base of the rabbit ear and visualized the resulting chain of events through a perplex ear chamber with high-power and oil immersion lenses. Spasm was not noted in any vessels, but within minutes the erythrocytes appeared distorted and broken, with the formation of a central homogeneous thrombus that moved down the arteriole and lodged in a capillary. Intimal damage did not occur. Thus the major effect of STS was on the blood cell mass that it destroyed and converted into an intravascular embolus. Subsequent biopsies of the ears at 1 hour and 5 days demonstrated thrombus only, without evidence of intimal damage. These results are distinctly contrary to the effects of sclerosis on veins.

The reason for this different mechanism of action is unknown but may relate to the difference in velocity of blood flow in arteries and veins. Specifically, STS injected intraarterially may not have enough time to react with endothelium, being both absorbed and inactivated by formed elements in the blood and serum factors and thereby being diluted to a "safe" concentration by the more rapid arterial flow. *Safe* is a relative term since inadvertent intraarterial injections of STS have produced gangrene through thrombosis of vessels downstream of injection (see Chapter 8).

EXPERIMENTAL EVALUATION OF SCLEROSING SOLUTIONS

Since physicians in the United States are especially limited in the type of sclerosing solutions available, an analysis of the following studies was performed to compare the efficacy of various sclerosing agents.

An important question regarding these studies is whether the experimental animal model is an appropriate system in which to compare the efficacy of various sclerosing solutions. The dorsal marginal rabbit ear vein is similar in size

---

*Dexo SA Pharmaceuticals, France: Product description on hydroxypolyethoxydodecane, May 1985.
†Product insert for aethoxysklerol (1985) from Chemische Fabrik Kreussler & Co GmbH Wiesbaden-Biebrich, West Germany.
‡Henschel O: Sclerosing of varicose veins sclerotherapy with aethoxysklerol-Kreussler (product booklet), produced by Chemische Fabrik Kreussler & Co GmbH, Wiesbaden-Biebrich D-6202, Postfach 9105, West Germany.

(0.35 to 0.45 mm diameter) to telangiectasias in humans. Reiner[40] found that it was difficult to measure the rate of dilution of sclerosing solutions in the rabbit ear vein because of the greater number of collaterals and rapid blood flow caused by the thermoregulatory nature of the ear. Therefore, after injection of the solution, firm pressure for 20 seconds of occlusion on the proximal and distal aspects of the injected vein wall help simulate the more sluggish blood flow of human telangiectasias.[38,39] In vitro studies of the effect of sclerosing solution on saphenous veins harvested for coronary bypass surgery have confirmed the histologic effect of sclerosing solution type and concentration with the rabbit ear vein model.[41] However, study of an animal model may not produce accurate data because one is comparing the action of a sclerosing solution on a normal vessel. In addition, the injected vessels are not compressed in rabbit ear vein studies, thereby resulting in the formation of a larger thrombus, which may allow for a more rapid or increased incidence of recanalization. Finally, thrombogenesis and thrombolytic effects are different in the rabbit ear than in the human artery and vein.[42] However, with all these shortcomings, as a model the rabbit ear vein does allow one to compare the mechanism of action of various sclerosing solutions both clinically and histologically. On the basis of these studies, the physician can achieve a similar therapeutic effect in humans by varying the concentration and type of solution (Table 7-1).

In the 1920s the first studies to elucidate the mechanism of action of sclerosing agents were performed using the dorsal vein of the rabbit ear. Sclerosing agents tested included 1% bichloride of mercury,[43] 30% sodium chloride and

Table 7-1 Relative potency of sclerosing solutions

Vein diameter	Sclerosing solution
<0.4 mm	Glycerin 70%
	Chromated glycerin 50%
	Polidocanol 0.25%
	Sodium tetradecyl sulfate 0.1%
	Hypertonic saline 11.7%
	Sclerodex
	Ethanolamine oleate 2%
	Polyiodinated iodine 0.1%
	Polidocanol 0.5%
	Sodium morrhuate 0.25-0.5%
0.6-2 mm	Chromated glycerin 100%
	Sodium tetradecyl sulfate 0.25%
	Polidocanol 0.75%
	Polyiodinated iodine 0.5-1%
	Ethanolamine oleate 5%
	Hypertonic saline 23.4%
	Sodium morrhuate 1-2.5%
3-5 mm	Polidocanol 1-2%
	Sodium tetradecyl sulfate 0.5-1%
	Sodium morrhuate 5%
	Polyiodinated iodine 2%
>5 mm	Polidocanol 3-4%
Perforators	Sodium tetradecyl sulfate 2-3%
Saphenofemoral/popliteal Junctions	Polyiodinated iodine 3-12%

50% grape sugar,[44,45] 30% sodium salicylate,[46] 50% to 60% calorose,[47,48] and SM.[49,50] All of the above solutions achieved venous obliteration through endothelial cell alteration, with inflammation resulting in thrombus formation and eventual production of a fibrous cord.

Sodium Tetradecyl Sulfate

The mechanism of sclerosis for intravascular sodium tetradecyl sulfate (STS) was elucidated by Schneider[7] and Schneider and Fischer[50] in human varicose veins, by Dietrich and Sinapius[51] in rabbit external jugular veins, and by Imhoff and Stemmer[6] in the dorsal rabbit ear vein. With STS, endothelial damage is concentration dependent and occurs immediately after injection with resulting rapid thrombus formation leading to vascular sclerosis.

In two recent studies, sclerosis with STS produced similar results in a concentration-dependent manner.[38,39] Endothelial damage occurred within 1 hour (Fig. 7-7), followed by the rapid onset of vascular thrombosis with subsequent organization (Fig. 7-8). Histologic recanalization occurred after 30 days with solution concentrations of 0.1% to 0.5%. The histologic findings explained the clinical appearance that demonstrated initial thrombosis followed by partial reappearance of the vessel injected with STS 0.1%. Therefore, there may be a

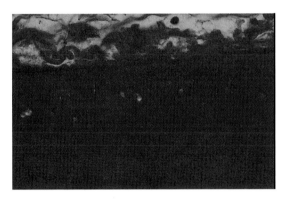

Fig. 7-7 Endothelial cells and the vascular wall are entirely destroyed 1 hour after injection with STS 0.5%. Hemolysis of red blood cells and early thrombosis are also present. (Hematoxylin-eosin, ×200.)

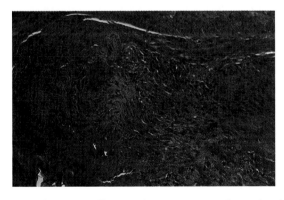

Fig. 7-8 Microangiopathic recanalization is apparent 14 days after injection with STS 0.5%. (Hematoxylin-eosin, ×100.) (From Goldman MP et al: Arch Dermatol 123:1196, 1987.)

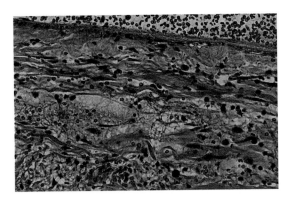

Fig. 7-9   Vessel 2 days after injection with SM 1%. Note large numbers of perivascular mast cells. (Hematoxylin-eosin, ×400.)

concentration gradient in which an ideal concentration depends on many factors, including vessel diameter, rate of blood flow, animal model, and anatomic region within each animal model.

Sodium Morrhuate

Sodium morrhuate* (SM), a mixture of sodium salts of the saturated and unsaturated fatty acids present in cod liver oil, has been studied in the rabbit ear vein model.[52] SM 0.5% produced no clinical evidence of endothelial damage. Temporary histologic evidence of thrombosis was noted at 1 hour only with a mild perivascular mixed cellular infiltrate (MCI). There was no evidence for extravasation of red blood cells (RBCs). Vessels injected with SM 1.0% were thrombosed between 2 and 10 days, after which the vessels normalized. Histologically, the SM 1.0% injected vessel demonstrated a partially destroyed endothelium with extravasation of RBCs. The vessels injected with SM 2.5% demonstrated clinical fibrosis with histologic evidence of microangiopathic recanalization through a fibrotic cord at 45 days after injection. A unique finding noted with injection of SM, both 1.0% and 2.5%, was the presence of large numbers of perivascular mast cells (Fig. 7-9). This finding may correlate with the increased inflammatory nature and allergenicity of SM as compared with other sclerosing solutions.

Ethanolamine Oleate

Ethanolamine oleate (EO), a synthetic mixture of ethanolamine and oleic acid, is another sclerosing solution that has been studied in the rabbit ear vein model (see Figs. 7-13 and 7-14).[52] No histologic or clinical changes were noted with injection of EO 0.5%. Although an organizing thrombus was produced, complete recanalization occurred in the vessel injected with EO 1%, resulting in the returned clinical appearance of the injected vessel. Vessels injected with EO 2.5% had a partially destroyed endothelium followed by luminal recanalization. Evidence of phagocytosis of lipidlike material was noted in a vessel injected with EO 2.5% at 48 hours (Fig. 7-10). This may indicate extravasation of sclerosing solution either during injection or with endothelial destruction. Large numbers of perivascular mast cells were also noted 2 days after injection with EO 1% and 2.5%. Ex-

---

*Omega; Montreal, Canada.

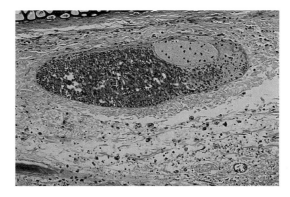

Fig. 7-10   Vessel 2 days after injection with EO 2.5%. Note extensive phagocytosis of lipidlike globules. (Hematoxylin-eosin, ×200.)

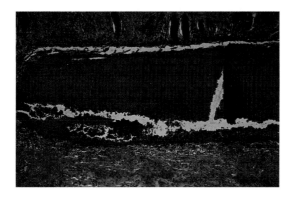

Fig. 7-11   Partially damaged endothelial cells with thrombosis is seen 8 hours after injection with POL 0.25% in the rabbit ear vein. (Hematoxylin-eosin, ×40.)

travasated RBCs occurred in vessels injected with EO 1% and 2.5% at 1 hour and 2 days, but not in vessels injected with EO 0.5%.

A previous study comparing EO with STS was performed using the rat tail vein model.[53] In this model EO 5% was compared to STS 3% and 1%. Solution measuring 0.1 ml was injected and the veins were biopsied at 4 weeks. In this study EO 5% was effective only in sclerosing 25% of the treated veins, as opposed to a 73% efficacy with STS 1% and a near 100% efficacy with STS 3%. Therefore, results in the rabbit ear vein compare well with those in the rat tail vein.

Polidocanol

A concentration gradient was also demonstrated in a study of polidocanol (POL) in concentrations of 0.25, 0.5, and 1.0%.[38] Only vessels injected with POL 0.5% and 1% were clinically sclerosed, and only the vessels injected with POL 1% maintained sclerosis without revascularization by 60 days.

An examination of the histologic effects of POL on the endothelium specifically between 1 hour and 4 days after injection illustrates the effect of varying the concentration of sclerosing solutions. Endothelial cells exposed to POL 0.25% were at first only partially damaged (Fig. 7-11). Mitotic figures indicating endothelial regeneration were noted 4 days after injection (Fig. 7-12). Likewise, with POL 0.5%, partial luminal recanalization occurred through an initial fibrotic cord in vessels (Fig. 7-13). Only vessels sclerosed with POL 1.0% developed complete endosclerosis (Fig. 7-14). Therefore, POL is probably a weaker detergent type of sclerosing solution than STS, and higher concentrations are necessary to produce complete vascular sclerosis.

Hypertonic Saline

The sclerosing effect of hypertonic saline (HS) was histologically examined in the external jugular vein of the dog by Kern and Angle,[54] and in human varicose veins by McPheeters and Anderson.[48] These investigators noted endothelial damage with thrombus formation within 1 hour of injection, with ultimate conversion into a fibrous cord within 2 to 4 weeks. This was confirmed in the rabbit ear vein model[38] both clinically and histologically. Examination of the marginal ear vein 1 hour after exposure to HS 23.4% demonstrated complete endothelial destruction (Fig. 7-15).

However, subsequent evaluation of HS 11.7% in the rabbit ear vein model[52] demonstrated an immediate thrombosis that lasted only 48 hours before complete normalization. Endothelial destruction was patchy at 1 hour with perivascular and intraluminal marginization of polymorphonuclear (PMN) cells and eosinophils (EOS). There was no evidence of extravasation of RBCs in the veins injected with HS 11.7% as opposed to extravasation that was noted in 30% of vessels injected with HS 23.4%. Therefore, the degree of endothelial damage and resulting extravasation of RBCs is proportional to the concentration of HS used.

Hypertonic Glucose/Saline

Sclerodex* (SX), a mixture of dextrose, sodium chloride, propylene glycol, and phenethyl alcohol, when studied in the rabbit ear vein model,[52] produced an immediate thrombosis that lasted for 2 days, after which the vessel recanalized. At 1 hour, perivascular and intraluminal marginization of PMNs and EOS were present with patchy endothelial destruction. Endothelial mitoses were present at 2 days within a regenerative endothelium. Extravasation of RBCs was not noted. Therefore, SX has a potency similar to HS 11.7%.

Chromated Glycerin

The effect of chemical irritant sclerosing solutions has also been studied in the rabbit ear model.[39] Chromated glycerin (CG, Scleremo, Laboratories Boutile, Lemogue, France), 50% and 100%, was injected into the dorsal marginal rabbit ear vein producing clinical and histologic thrombosis that lasted only 2 to 8 days, after which the vessel appeared clinically and histologically normal. As noted with POL 0.25% above, the endothelium 1 hour after biopsy was almost undamaged. Therefore, in this experimental model, CG is a weak solution with a sclerosing effect similar to POL 0.25%. This correlates well with its clinical profile.

Polyiodinated Iodine

Various iodine solutions with or without hypertonic solutions have been examined in the rabbit ear vein model. Sclerodine (Omega Laboratory, Montreal) is a mixture of iodine USP (60 mg/ml, sodium iodide, USP 90 mg/ml). This

---

*Omega; Montreal, Canada.

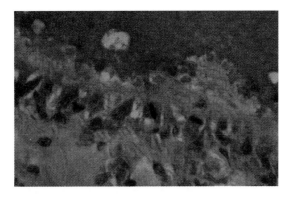

Fig. 7-12   Endothelial regeneration is apparent 4 days after injection with POL 0.25% in the rabbit ear vein. (Hematoxylin-eosin, ×100.)

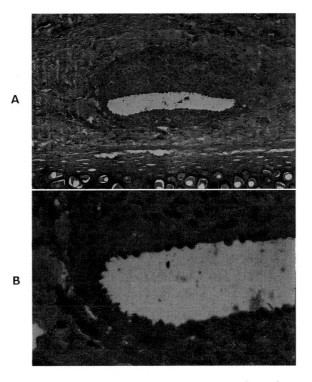

Fig. 7-13   Advanced luminal recanalization is present 60 days after injection with POL 0.5%, as seen in cross section. **A**, ×100; **B**, ×200; note endothelial lining on recanalized lumen. (Hematoxylin-eosin.) (**A** from Goldman MP et al: Arch Dermatol 123:1196, 1987.)

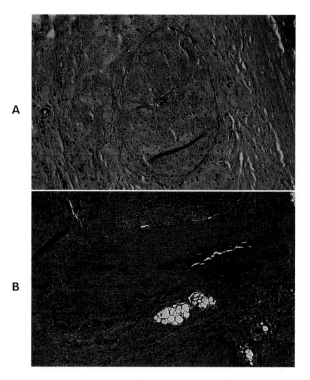

Fig. 7-14 Fibrous cord formation is present 30 days after injection with POL 1.0%. The darker areas within the fibrous cord represent hemosiderin-laden macrophages. **A,** Longitudinal section, ×40. **B,** Cross section, ×100. (Hematoxylin-eosin). (**B** from Goldman MP et al: Arch Dermatol 123:1196, 1987.)

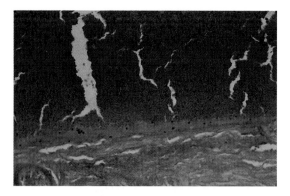

Fig. 7-15 The endothelial cells and vascular wall structure are completely homogenized 1 hour after injection of the rabbit ear vein with HS 23.4%. Longitudinal section, ×40. (Hematoxylin-eosin.)

solution was compared to an American iodine formula consisting of iodine sodium iodide of identical composition, compounded by Women's Hospital of Texas in Houston, mixed with either normal saline, Sclerodex (Omega Laboratories, Montreal) or dextrose 250 mg/ml + sodium chloride 100 mg/ml (compounded by Women's Hospital of Texas in Houston). There was virtually no difference between the Omega solutions and those compounded at Women's Hospital. Solutions of 0.1% and 0.5% iodine were used. Thrombosis occurred in all solutions at 1 hour with an attenuated endothelium and focal endothelial necrosis in all solutions. A mild perivascular mixed cellular infiltrate consisting of eosinophils and polymorphonucleocytes was present with margination along the endothelial border. In the 0.1% solutions the endothelium was hyperplastic with regenerative changes noted by 8 days (Fig. 7-16) and complete normalization by 28 days. In the 0.5% solutions, the endothelium was necrotic with multiple brown spherules approximately 1 μm in diameter seen within the endothelial wall (Fig. 7-17). These may represent iodine crystals. By 28 days a fibrous cord was present without inflammation. Interestingly, veins treated with iodine/normal saline mix showed a greater incidence and extent of extravasated erythrocytes as compared with iodine/Sclerodex (hypertonic saline/dextrose) solutions.

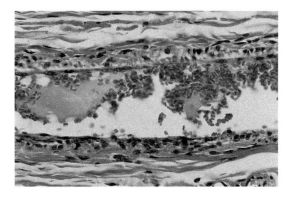

Fig. 7-16   Regenerating hyperplastic endothelium is present 8 days after injection of the rabbit ear vein with 0.1% PII diluted with SX. (Hematoxylin-eosin, ×20.)

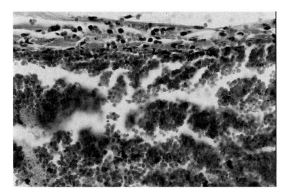

Fig. 7-17   Multiple brown spherules approximately 1 μm in diameter are noted within necrotic endothelium at 8 days in rabbit ear vein injected with 0.5% PII. (Hematoxylin-eosin, ×40).

The PII 0.1% solution had an experimental efficacy equivalent to HS 11.7%, SM 2.5%, STS 0.25%, and POL 0.5%. The PII 0.5% had an experimental efficacy similar to HS 23.4%, STS 0.5%, and POL 1.0%.

Comparative Efficacy in the Animal Model

The mechanism of action for all sclerosing solutions injected into veins in these studies was basically similar; that is, endothelial damage and simultaneous thrombus formation occurred almost immediately after injection. Endothelial damage was less in the vessels injected with CG, POL 0.25%, SX, and EO 0.5%, which showed early recanalization and a continued normal clinical appearance. POL 0.5%, SM 0.5% and 1%, EO 1%, and HS 11.7% produced endothelial attenuation, not necrosis. Although an organizing thrombus was produced, recanalization occurred resulting in the returned clinical appearance of the injected vessel. Vessels injected with PII 0.1%, STS 0.5%, SM 2.5%, and EO 2.5% also demonstrated recanalization, although endothelial necrosis was demonstrated. In contrast to the luminal recanalization that occurred with POL 0.5% and EO 2.5%, recanalization with STS 0.5% and SM 2.5% occurred with multiple minute vascular channels. Vessels sclerosed with STS 0.25% and 0.5% and SM 2.5% never totally reappeared clinically in the 60-day span of this study. The only vessels to histologically demonstrate fibrous cord formation that did not recanalize were sclerosed with PII 0.5%, HS 23.4%, and POL 1.0%. Therefore, there is a minimal sclerosant concentration (MSC) that is essential to produce endosclerosis. This term, coined by Neil Sadick, is useful in determining which solution and concentration is best at sclerosing a specific vessel.[52]

Comparative Efficacy in the Human Model

In an effort to assess the effect of sclerosing agents in human leg telangiectasias, I injected 0.1 ml of either POL 0.5% or STS 0.5% into two nearly identical telangiectasias 0.4 mm in diameter over the anterior tibia in a 65-year-old man. This vessel did not have any associated "feeding" reticular veins, and there was no evidence of associated varicose veins or signs of venous insufficiency. The injected vessel was not compressed, and a biopsy of it was taken 48 hours after treatment.

The vessel injected with POL 0.5% demonstrated a blue thrombus (Fig. 7-18) that was histologically confirmed and an endothelium that was relatively intact with extensive cellular vacuolization (Fig. 7-19).

The vessel injected with STS 0.5% demonstrated a deep blue thrombus (Fig. 7-20). Histologically, the endothelium was totally destroyed, showing extensive intravascular thrombosis and early organization (Fig. 7-21). Therefore, this limited human study correlates with the above-mentioned studies on the marginal rabbit ear vein demonstrating that STS is a stronger sclerosing agent than POL.

CLINICAL USE OF SCLEROSING AGENTS

The only sclerosing agents approved for use in the United States by the Food and Drug Administration (FDA) are sodium morrhuate (SM), ethanolamine oleate (EO), and sodium tetradecyl sulfate (STS). All of these agents were approved for use before 1950 and thus have never been subjected to the rigorous toxicity and efficacy studies that would be required by the FDA today. Hypertonic saline (HS) in a 23.4% concentration is available and approved for use as an abortifacient. However, it is commonly used in various concentrations with and without the addition of heparin, procaine, or lidocaine for sclerosis of telangiectasias and superficial varicosities. POL, widely used in the United States today, is in the final stages of investigative trials and should be approved in the very near future.

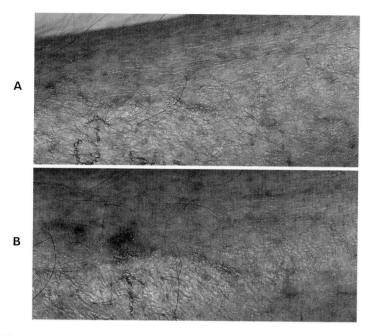

Fig. 7-18   Anterior tibial telangiectasia. **A**, Before treatment. **B**, 48 hours after injection with POL 0.5%.

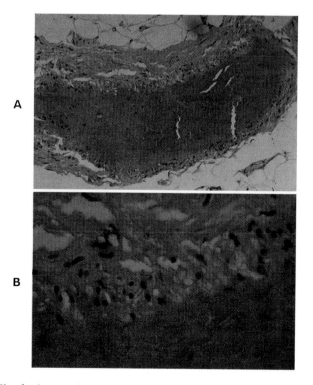

Fig. 7-19   Histologic examination of vein in Fig. 7-9. **A**, ×40. **B**, ×100; shows endothelial cell vacuolization with thrombosis. (Hematoxylin-eosin.)

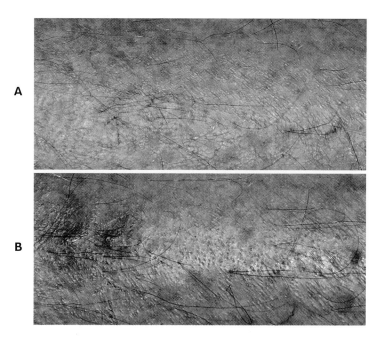

Fig. 7-20   Anterior tibial telangiectasia. **A,** Before treatment. **B,** 48 hours after injection with STS 0.5%.

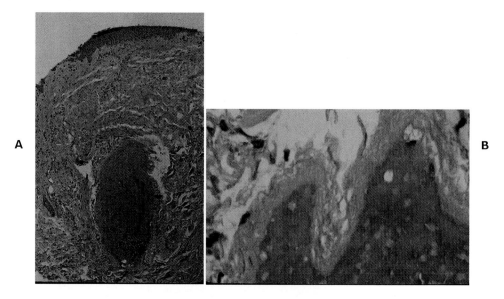

Fig. 7-21   Histologic examination of vein in Fig. 7-20. **A,** ×40. **B,** ×100; shows endothelial cell homogenization/necrosis with thrombosis. (Hematoxylin-eosin.)

Sclerodex (SX), a solution of dextrose 5% and sodium chloride 10%, is commonly used in Canada for sclerosis of superficial varicosities and telangiectasias. Chromated glycerin (CG) is perhaps the most widely used sclerosing agent worldwide for the treatment of leg telangiectasias. It has been popularized in the English literature by Ouvry.[55] Polyiodinated iodine (PII) is the most powerful sclerosing agent and is commonly used outside of the United States for sclerotherapy of the saphenofemoral junction. It is not yet approved for use by the FDA in the United States but will be discussed because of its importance in sclerotherapy. Another solution rarely used outside of the United States, sodium salicylate, is not widely used or available here and is briefly discussed.

Osmotic Agents

Hypertonic saline

Hypertonic saline (HS) was first used to sclerose varicose veins by Linser[16] in 1926 and Kern and Angle[54] in 1929. With the advent of more effective synthetic detergent sclerosing solutions in the 1940s, its use declined. Renewed interest in its use occurred in the 1970s, spurred on by numerous publications in the dermatology literature and multiple lectures on its use presented at major medical meetings.

A double-blind, paired-comparison study of various concentrations of HS with and without heparin was performed in different sized varicose and telangiectatic leg veins.[56] Sadick found that an 11.7% HS solution was as effective in treating vessels less than 8 mm in diameter as a 23.4% solution, and more effective than a 5.8% solution, with less burning, pigmentation, and cramping. The addition of heparin only decreased thrombosis formation, requiring puncture evacuation in vessels greater than 4 mm in diameter. This demonstration of MSC produced superior cosmetic results with an improved therapeutic-to-complication index.

Advantage

Part of the currently experienced popularity stems from the lack of allergenicity of unadulterated HS solution compared with the exaggerated claims of allergenicity associated with all other sclerosing agents. However, HS is not without significant adverse sequelae (see Chapter 8).

Disadvantages

Unlike detergent sclerosing solutions, all hypertonic solutions act nonspecifically to destroy all cells (including RBCs) within their osmotic gradients. Osmotic agents damage cellular tissues and readily produce ulceration if injected extravascularly or if diffused through the vessel extravascularly (see Chapter 8). Therefore, injection technique is critically important when using this sclerosing agent.

Because HS diffuses to some extent through the blood vessel wall, nerves in the adventitia of the vein may be stimulated, causing pain (see Chapter 3). This diffusion may also lead to transient muscle cramping. Hemolysis of RBCs occurs via hyperosmosis, resulting in the release of hemosiderin, which may readily diffuse across the damaged endothelium. This may lead to posttreatment hyperpigmentation, especially in a punctate pattern. Finally, because osmotic agents are rapidly diluted in the bloodstream, they lose their potency within a short distance of injection. Thus these agents are only rarely effective in treating veins larger than 3 to 4 mm in diameter.

Modification of the solution and the technique

Various modifications of the HS solutions have been made in an effort to increase the efficacy and decrease the pain of injection and other adverse sequelae.

In 1975 Foley[57] described the microinjection of "venous blemishes" with a 30-gauge needle using 20% hypertonic saline, 100 U/ml of heparin, and 1% procaine, which he patented as Heparsal. He reported no allergic or anaphylactic reactions and only rare pigmentary problems in more than 1000 treatments to more than 100 patients. Foley theorized that the addition of heparin helped to prevent thrombi in larger vessels, and the addition of procaine helped alleviate the pain on injection. Sadick,[56,58] in randomized, blinded 800-patient and 600-patient double-blind, paired comparison studies, found that the addition of heparin to HS provided no benefit in the treatment of varicose and telangiectatic veins less than 4 mm in diameter. Bodian,[59,60] because of his personal clinical comparison experience, also does not believe that the addition of heparin is necessary for effective sclerosis. Finally, it has been demonstrated that the addition of heparin to the culture medium enhances proliferation and increases the life span of endothelial cells.[61] Therefore, its use may be counterproductive.

A number of modifications in injection technique have also been made to limit the pain of HS. Bodian has found that muscle cramps occurring at the site of injection last 3 to 5 minutes and are relieved with gentle massage or ambulation. To limit the risk of extravasation, he recommends injecting a small air bolus before injecting 0.5 to 1 ml of HS to ensure undiluted contact of the HS with the intima to produce maximal irritation of the vessel. He believes that hemolysis caused by the sclerosing solution may lead to or exacerbate hemosiderin staining and thus should be lessened by the prior injection of air, which washes out the RBCs from the vessel.[62] Finally, regarding the possible exacerbation of hypertension with injection of a large sodium bolus, he states that 1.0 gm of sodium chloride injected during a "long treatment session" (5 ml of a 20% HS solution) is well tolerated.

Alderman[63] was the first to advocate dilution of the HS solution to better adjust the osmotic damage to the caliber of the vessel. From his experience with 150 patients with telangiectasias treated over 8 years with 18% to 30% HS, he recommends the following HS concentrations for sclerosis of varicose and telangiectatic veins: 18% to 25% HS for "venous telangiectasias" (blue telangiectasias), 22% to 25% HS for "arterial lesions" (red telangiectasias), and 30% HS for rare large "arterial" lesions. He dilutes the saline with lidocaine to achieve a 0.4% concentration of lidocaine. The only adverse side effects reported were mild, temporary burning at injection and residual brownish pigmentation that occurred in up to one third of patients. The pigmentation usually resolved, for the most part, over 1 year.

Lidocaine, when used as a diluent, can be used with or without epinephrine. Animal studies have demonstrated that solution concentrations with less than a 1% concentration of lidocaine are vasoconstrictive.[64,65] In addition, I routinely use it with epinephrine as a diluent to enhance vasospasm and partially stabilize perivascular mast cells.

Hypertonic glucose/saline

Sclerodex* is a mixture of dextrose 250 mg/ml, sodium chloride 100 mg/ml, propylene glycol 100 mg/ml, and phenethyl alcohol 8 mg/ml (as a local anesthetic/preservative) at a pH of 5.9, mainly used in Canada for sclerosis of telangiectasias and small-diameter superficial varicosities.[66] It is essentially a hypertonic solution with a mechanism of action similar to HS. The manufacturer states that the sodium chloride reinforces the sclerosing potency of dextrose.

---

*Omega; Montreal, Canada.

It is interesting to note that a similar product was manufactured by Abbott Laboratories (Abbott Park, IL) in the 1950s and 1960s under the trade name Varisol. This compound consisted of 30% invert sugar and 10% sodium chloride, with a mixture of preservatives and stabilizers (benzylcarbonate phenethyl, propylene glycol) in water. It was withdrawn from the market in 1963 in conjunction with the FDA's new requirements for efficacy and toxicity testing. Correspondence with Abbott Laboratories has not spurred their interest in development or production of this solution (Diane Rennpferd, Coordinator, External Technology Evaluation, Aug. 15, 1991).

The manufacturer of Sclerodex recommends that the maximum quantity to be injected during one visit is 10 ml in divided doses, with a 5-cm interval between each site of injection.* (The maximum recommended amount to be injected at any one site is 1 ml.) The average dose per treated vein varies between 1 ml in the upper thigh and 0.1 ml in the lower leg. The reason for these recommended doses by the manufacturer is unclear.

Advantage

Omega Laboratories, which produces SX, claims that the addition of dextrose allows for a reduction of the concentration of sodium chloride, thereby minimizing the pain and local discomfort that would occur with injection of sodium chloride alone.* However, it is probably the decrease in osmolarity relative to 23.4% HS that allows Sclerodex to produce less pain and muscle cramping.

Disadvantages

Despite its lower osmolarity, like HS, it is slightly painful for the patient on injection.[67] Superficial necrosis may occur rarely, with an incidence of less than HS.†[66,68] I have noted postsclerosis pigmentation to occur with a frequency similar to that of other sclerosing agents, although Mantse[68] notes a decreased incidence of complications with Sclerodex as compared with POL and STS (see Chapter 8).

Another disadvantage of its use is that the solution becomes sticky in the syringe when blood is withdrawn to ensure an intravenous position. Unfortunately, unlike unadulterated HS, allergic reactions may occur to the phenethyl alcohol component of the solution.† Mantse[44] notes one allergic reaction in 500 patients treated with Sclerodex, for an incidence of 0.2%.

Sodium Salicylate

Sodium salicylate (SS [Saliect, Omega, Montreal, Canada]) is provided in a 10 ml multiuse vial. Each ml contains 570 mg of sodium salicylate with benzyl alcohol 1% and sodium metabisulfate 0.1% added as preservatives. Since it is very painful upon injection, especially if it diffuses or is injected extravascularly, it is recommended that it be diluted with lidocaine 1% without epinephrine. The manufacturer recommends a maximum daily total quantity of 8 to 10 ml be used. It may also be added to other sclerosing solutions such as glycerin (see p. 275) to achieve a final concentration of between 6% and 30%. In this concentration it can be used for telangiectasia <1 mm in diameter.

---

*Correspondence (1986) received from Laboratories Ondee Ltee; 280 Milice Longueuil; Montreal, Canada.

†Scleremo product information (1987) from Laboratories E. Bouteille; 7 rue des Belges; Limoges 8100, France.

This solution causes muscle cramping after use, especially if volumes greater than 0.1 ml are injected in a single location. Like other osmotic agents, SS also will produce necrosis on extravasation in a concentration-dependent manner. Because of the intense pain produced with arterial or extravascular injection, it is often mixed with STS to ensure that injection of STS is intravascular (STS is nearly painless when injected extravascularly).

Chemical Irritants
Chromated glycerin

Chromated glycerin (CG) 72% (Sclermo [Laboratories E. Bouteille, Limoges, France], Chromex [Omega Laboratories, Montreal, Canada]) is a sclerosing solution that is popular in Europe, whereas clinical experience in the United States remains limited. The French manufacturer has recently gone out of business, leaving Omega Laboratories as the sole producer. The maximum recommended amount per injection session is 0.1 ml of pure solution. Concentrations of 25% to 100% have been used.*[69] Its clinical efficacy has been shown to be dose dependent. CG, although not approved by the FDA, is the most widely used sclerosing agent for leg telangiectasias in the world; 500,000 vials were sold in 1986.*

The glycerin component of CG is rapidly absorbed by the intestine and transformed into carbon dioxide or glycogen, or is directly used for the synthesis of fatty acids.[70] Therefore, this solution must be used with caution in diabetic patients. One case of reactive hypoglycemia to an infusion of glycogen occurred in a child, resulting in a comatose state within 4 minutes of infusion.[71]

The sclerosing quality of glycerin was first studied in 1925 by Jausion, Carrot, and Ervais,[72] who found that it induced a mild, rapid, and complete endosclerosis. Isosmotic glycerol (2.6% m/v) produces 100% hemolysis in 45 minutes.[70,73] This usually occurs with rapid infusions of 60 gm in 15 minutes, 70 gm in 30 minutes, and 80 gm in 60 minutes.[74] However, a review of 500 patients who received glycerol intravenously (at 50 gm/500 ml) 6 hours a day for 7 to 10 days demonstrated hemoglobinuria in less than 1% of patients.[75,76]

The chromium alum component of CG is a potent coagulating factor that increases the sclerosing power of glycerin. It also prevents somewhat the mild hematuria induced through the use of glycerin alone.[70,77,78]

Mihael Georgiev (personal communication, 1994) has produced a 70% glycerin solution sterile for injection and has seen a sclerosing effect with this agent that is identical to CG. Multiple animal and human studies with 70% glyercin are being conducted currently to confirm this experience.

Advantages

The relatively weak sclerosing power of CG corresponds to its promotion as a mild sclerosing solution with more versatile usage and a low incidence of side effects. Pigmentation and cutaneous necrosis are exceedingly rare at recommended dosages, and minimal extravascular injection causes only a small temporary ecchymosis without any cutaneous damage.[79,80] Reportedly, the incidence of adverse sequelae is very low.*[36,69]

Disadvantages

The disadvantages of CG include its high viscosity and local pain at injection.[81,82] Both of these drawbacks can be partially overcome by dilution with lidocaine. Hy-

---

*Sclermo product information (1987) from Laboratories E. Bouteille; 7 rue des Belges; Limoges 8100, France.

persensitivity is a very rare complication.[83,84] Hematuria associated by ureteral colic can occur transiently after injection of large doses. Ocular manifestations, including blurred vision and a partial visual field loss, have been reported by a single author, with resolution in less than 2 hours.[85] These latter two complications may be a result of excessive, nonspecific destruction of RBCs.

Polyiodinated iodine

Polyiodinated iodine* (PII, Variglobin [Globopharm, Switzerland], Sclerodine [Omega Laboratories, Canada]) is a stabilized water solution of diatomic iodine (I^2), sodium iodine, and benzyl alcohol. The solution was invented by Imhoff and was first used by Sigg in Switzerland in 1958. Others had reported on the use of iodine solutions in sclerotherapy; however, stabilization of the mixture by Imhoff produced a standardized solution that could be easily obtained. The active sclerosing ingredient is elemental iodine. Sodium and potassium help to make it water soluble. Benzyl alcohol is added as a preservative/stabilizer. Variglobin is available in concentrations of 2%, 4%, 8%, and 12% as a dark-brown solution contained in brown glass vials.

When diluted in blood, molecular iodine produces iodinated proteins. The redox potential of blood rapidly converts any remaining iodine to its reduced iodide, which is devoid of any sclerosing action.[86] Thus its sclerosing effect is very localized.

After 1 minute, iodine cannot be measured radiographically at the injected site but is rapidly distributed through all vascular spaces. In 15 to 60 minutes, an accumulation occurs in the liver with renal excretion occurring over the next 3 to 4 days in zero-order kinetics.[86] This is important because daily injections can increase total body iodine stores to saturation.

Wenner[87] states that PII should be used only in the manufactured concentrations because dilution may allow the chemical effect to propagate away from the injection site. However, others mix it with normal saline or Sclerodex.† Raymond-Martimbeau[88] claims that the addition of Sclerodex to the solution potentiates the action and causes a more localized destruction with less risk of diffusion of the sclerosing solution. Mixing with ethanol has been advocated by Wenner[87] to increase the sclerosing potency.[87] Wenner believes that the addition of ethanol delays inactivation of the solution by blood proteins in addition to increasing the potentiating action of ethanol, which directly damages the lipoprotein component of the endothelial surface. He recommends the addition of 50% ethanol to an equal amount of Variglobin 12%. The amount of ethanol injected is likened to a "large glass of wine."

Omega Laboratories recommends that concentrations of 0.15% are optimal to sclerose telangiectasia and recommends 6% to sclerose truncal varicose veins. They recommend an injection of 2 ml of a 3% solution into the proximal "internal saphena" and 0.5 ml of a 0.5% solution into the ankle "internal and external saphena." The maximum quantity that can be injected in a single session is 3 ml of a 6% solution.† Kreussler Pharma‡ recommends the following concentrations: 4%, 8%, or 12% for injection to the saphenofemoral junction; 4% for the saphenopopliteal junction; 4% to 8% for perforating veins and varicosities greater than 8 mm in diameter; 2% to 4% for varicose veins 4 to 8 mm in diameter; and

---

*Varigloban (Chemische Fabrik Kreussler & Co, Wiesbaden-Biebrich, West Germany); Variglobin (Globopharm, Switzerland); Sclerodine (Omega, Montreal, Canada).
†Product information on Sclerodine 6 (1989) from Omega; Montreal, Canada.
‡Product information (June 1987) from Kreussler Pharma; Wiesbaden 12, D-6200, West Germany.

2% for varicose veins 2 to 4 mm in diameter. They do not recommend its use in smaller veins.

Advantage

The sclerosing effect of PII is based on direct destruction of the endothelium. It destroys the entire vessel wall through diffusion at the point of injection. It is very short acting because it is neutralized within a few seconds by binding to different blood components, especially proteins.[87] PII is primarily used for large varicosities, including the saphenofemoral junction. Sigg[89] performed more than 400,000 injections with Variglobin. Sigg and Zelikovski reported performing over 560,000 injections in 58,000 patients without any serious complications or allergic reactions.[90]

Disadvantage

Paravenous injections will readily produce tissue necrosis; therefore, its injection should be performed with utmost care. Sigg, Horodegen, and Bernbach[89] and Sigg and Zelikovski[91] never used more than 0.5 ml per injection site. Fortunately, PII is painful when injected outside a vein so that improper injection technique is immediately apparent. To prevent nonspecific damage, the concentration, not the volume of solution, is increased to enhance the sclerosing power.

Detergent Sclerosing Solutions

Sodium morrhuate

Sodium morrhuate (SM, [Palisades Pharmaceuticals, Inc., Tenafly, NJ; American Regent Laboratories, Inc., Shirley, NY]) is a mixture of sodium salts of the saturated and unsaturated fatty acids present in cod-liver oil (see box below). It is prepared by the saponification of selected cod-liver oils. Each milliliter contains morrhuate sodium, 50 mg; benzyl alcohol 2% (as a local anesthetic); water for injection (as much as will suffice); and pH adjusted to approximately 9.5 with hydrochloric acid and/or sodium hydroxide. It is available as a 5% concentration that can be diluted with normal saline to the appropriate concentration for the vessel to be treated.

SM was first prepared for injection by Ghosh[92] or Cutting.[93] This sclerosing agent was met with enthusiasm in the United States by Biegeleisen[49] and others. However, extensive cutaneous necrosis occurs when it is inadvertently injected perivascularly. Many cases of anaphylactic reactions within a few minutes after injection have been reported. More commonly, these reactions occur when therapy is reinstituted after a few weeks. Anaphylaxis has resulted in fatalities, albeit rarely (see Chapter 8). SM is approved by the FDA for sclerosis of varicose veins. However, because of its extremely caustic nature, it is not recommended for use

---

FATTY ACID COMPOSITION OF SODIUM MORRHUATE

Linoleic acid	28.2%	Palmitic acid	8.1%
Unknown	20.8%	Myristic acid	4.2%
Eicosadienoic acid	15.5%	Oleic acid	1.8%
Palmitoleic acid	12.1%	Stearic acid	1.1%
Arachidonic acid	8.2%		

From Monroe P et al: Acute respiratory failure after sodium morrhuate esophageal sclerotherapy, Gastroenterology 85:693, 1983.

as a sclerosing agent for telangiectasias, although Gallagher advocates its use diluted to a 0.25% to 0.5% concentration.[94]

Most patients have minimal discomfort after injection, with an occasional tenderness at the injected site for a few days.[94] Gallagher's 25-year experience with 20,000 patients treated with SM is notably free of significant adverse sequelae, with only one episode of "full anaphylactoid reaction." He describes more than 20 patients who had immediate postinjection "early anaphylactoid reactions" manifesting as chest pain, shortness of breath, tachycardia, and hypotension, who responded to intravenous dexamethasone and intramuscular Benadryl. Gallagher states that STS has a higher incidence of adverse reactions than SM, so he prefers the latter for telangiectasia.

Ethanolamine oleate

Ethanolamine oleate (EO) (Ethamolin) is a synthetic mixture of ethanol-amine and oleic acid with an empirical formula of C_{20}-H_{41}-NO_3. It is available as a 5% aqueous solution containing approximately 50 mg ethanolamine oleate per milliliter. Benzyl alcohol, 2% by volume, is used as a preservative. The pH ranges from 8.0 to 9.0. The minimum lethal intravenous dose in rabbits is 130 mg/kg.[95] The oleic acid component is responsible for the inflammatory action. Oleic acid may also activate coagulation in vitro by release of tissue factors and Hageman factor XII.

Advantage. EO was first reported to be an ideal sclerosing agent by Biegeleisen[96] in the medical literature in 1937. No toxic effects were noted in 500 injections. EO is thought to have a decreased risk of allergic reactions compared with SM or STS.[97] However, pulmonary toxicity has been associated with this sclerosing agent (see Chapter 8).

The sclerosing action is thought to occur as a dose-dependent extravascular inflammatory reaction caused by diffusion of EO through the venous wall.* Autopsy findings regarding its use in esophageal varix injection demonstrated that variceal obliteration occurred as a result of mural necrosis, followed by fibrosis, and that thrombosis was a transient phenomenon.[98,99]

Disadvantage. EO is a viscous solution that can be injected only through a 30 gauge needle with dilution. Some degree of nonspecific RBC hemolysis may occur with its use. A hemolytic reaction occurred in 5 of 900 patients with injection of over 12 ml of 0.5% EO per patient per treatment session.[100] Acute renal failure with spontaneous recovery followed injection of 15 to 20 ml of Ethamolin in two women.† The patients were described as "feeling generally unwell and shivery, with aching in the loins and passage of red-brown urine. All rapidly recovered with bed-rest and were perfectly normal the next day." Injections of less than 12 ml per treatment session did not result in this reaction.

Sodium tetradecyl sulfate

Sodium tetradecyl sulfate (STS [Wyeth-Ayerst Laboratories, Philadelphia]) is a synthetic, surface-active substance first described by Reiner[40] in 1946 (Fig. 7-22). It is composed of sodium 1-isobutyl-4-ethyloctyl sulfate plus benzoyl alcohol 2% (as an anesthetic agent) and phosphate buffered to a pH of 7.6. It is

---

*Product information (1989) from Glaxo Pharmaceuticals; Research Triangle Park, NC. (Ethanolamine now available from Block Drug Company, Piscataway, NJ.)

†Ethanolamin injection, 5%; product information (Dec 1988) from Glaxo Pharmaceuticals Inc.

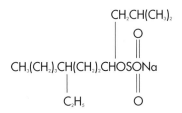

Fig. 7-22   Structural formula of sodium tetradecyl sulfate.

recommended that solutions be protected from light. It is a long-chain fatty acid salt of an alkali metal with the properties of a soap. The solution is clear, nonviscous, has a low surface tension, and is readily miscible with blood, leading to a uniform distribution after injection.[101] It primarily acts on the endothelium of the vein because, if diluted with blood, the molecules attach to the surface of RBCs, causing hemolysis. The recommended maximal dosage suggested by the British manufacturer in a treatment session is 4 ml of a 3% solution.* The recommended maximum dosage by the United States and Canadian manufacturers is 10 ml of a 3% solution with intervals between treatments of 5 to 7 days.†

This solution should not be mixed with other anesthetic solutions because it will become turbid and form a new compound.[102] Approximately 60% to 70% of the sclerosing "activity" of this compound is undiluted STS. In addition, heparin should not be included in the same syringe as STS because the two are incompatible (product insert revised October, 1988). Yet a paired comparison study of STS with and without heparin disclosed no difference in the therapeutic effect between the two solutions.[32]

It is available as a 1% or 3% solution that can be diluted with sterile water or normal saline to achieve an appropriate therapeutic concentration. The Canadian manufacturer recommends dilution with phosphate-buffered saline to preserve the original pH level.† (This also prevents pain from injection.) It is limpid and does not stick to the syringe cylinder when blood is withdrawn to ensure accurate needle placement. Concentrations of 0.1% to 0.3% are commonly used for the treatment of telangiectatic veins 0.2 to 1.0 mm in diameter; 0.5% to 1% for treatment of uncomplicated varicose veins 2 to 4 mm in diameter; and 1.5% to 3% for the treatment of larger varicose veins, incompetent perforating veins, or an incompetent saphenofemoral junction.

Advantages. STS became widely used in the 1950s after its introduction in 1946 by Reiner.[40] Tretbar[103] in 1978 first reported the injection of a 1% solution into spider angiomata. He noted excellent results in virtually all 144 patients treated. He also noted an unspecified number of episodes of epidermal necrosis without significant sequelae and a 30% incidence of postsclerosis pigmentation that resolved within a few months.

Shields and Jansen[104] in 1982 were the first to describe microsclerosis of telangiectasias with STS in the dermatologic literature. They injected STS 1% in 105 patients and reported only 1 episode of necrosis in more than 600 treatments

*S.T.D. Injection product data sheet (1977) from S.T.D. Pharmaceuticals Products Ltd., Hereford, England.

†Tromboject product information (rev 10/87) from Omega; Montreal, Canada.

in vessels less than 5 mm in diameter. There were no systemic reactions, and the majority of postsclerosis pigmentary changes resolved in 3 to 4 months. However, as more experience with its use in the treatment of leg telangiectasias occurred, even further dilutions (0.1% to 0.3%) were recommended, both to achieve clinical efficacy and to limit adverse sequelae (see Chapter 11).

Disadvantages. STS, approved for use by the FDA for vein sclerosis, has a number of disadvantages. Epidermal necrosis frequently occurs with extravasation of concentrations higher than 1%. Allergic reactions occur rarely. Postsclerotherapy hyperpigmentation is frequent (see Chapter 8). Therefore, its dilution is critical. The above-mentioned percentages per diameter of treated vein provide only a preliminary guide for effective treatment. In addition, the Canadian and United States manufacturers recommend that as a precaution against anaphylactic shock, 0.3 ml of a 1% solution should be injected into the varicosity, and then the patient should be observed for several hours before proceeding with further injections.* The reason for this recommendation is unclear, impractical, and potentially hazardous; it is discussed further in Chapter 8.

The intravenous LD50 in mice is 90 ± 5 mg/kg and between 72 and 108 mg/kg in the rat. When tested in the L5178YTK $\pm$ mouse lymphoma assay, STS did not induce a dose-related increase in the frequency of thymidine kinase-deficient mutants. However, long-term animal carcinogenicity studies have not been reported (product insert revised October, 1988).

Polidocanol

Polidocanol (POL), manufactured by Chemische Fabrik Kreussler & Co. GmbH (Wiesbaden-Biebrich, Germany), is composed of a mixture of hydroxy-polyethoxydodecane dissolved in distilled water, to which 96% ethyl alcohol is added to a concentration of 5% to ensure emulsification of POL micelles (which provides a clear solution) and to decrease foaming during the production process. Thus 1 ml of POL contains 40.5 mg of ethyl alcohol, and patients taking disulfiram (Antabuse†) should be warned about a possible alcohol-disulfiram reaction. Sclerovein (manufactured by Globopharm AG, Switzerland) contains chlorobutanolum as a preservative, 0.5 g/100 ml. Its pH varies from 4.8 to 6.1. The manufacturer has no stability data on POL when diluted with bacteriostatic water or normal saline, but Sadick and Farber have determined that it remains sterile for at least 3 months following dilution.[105] The sterility is confirmed even when used daily through a multiple-use vial.

POL was synthesized by BASF and introduced in 1936 as a local and topical anesthetic under the trade name Sch 600. Unlike the two main groups of local anesthetics, esters (procaine, benzocaine, and tetracaine) and the amides (lidocaine, prilocaine, mepivacaine, procainamide, and dibucaine), POL has a noncyclic chemical structure. The anesthetic effect is not a direct function of its concentration but is optimum at a concentration between 3% and 4%.‡ Animal trials on its use as a local anesthetic demonstrated the occurrence of obliteration of vessels as a side effect. Henschel, the former medical director of Kreussler

---

*Trombojet product information (rev 10/87) from Omega; Montreal, Canada.
†Wyeth-Ayerst Laboratories, New York, NY.
‡Henschel O: Sclerosing of varicose veins sclerotherapy with aethoxysklerol-Kreussler (product booklet), Chemische Fabrik Kreussler & Co GmbH, Wiesbaden-Biebrich D-6202, Postfach 9105, West Germany.

Table 7-2 Maximum daily doses of polidocanol

Concentration of POL	Dose (ml) according to body weight of patient				
	50 kg	60 kg	70 kg	80 kg	90 kg
0.5%	20 ml	24 ml	28 ml	32 ml	36 ml
1.0%	10 ml	12 ml	14 ml	16 ml	18 ml
2.0%	5 ml	6 ml	7 ml	8 ml	9 ml
3.0%	3.3 ml	4 ml	4.6 ml	5.3 ml	6 ml

From Kreussler & Co GmbH: Product insert for Aethoxysklerol, Wiesbaden-Biebrich, West Germany, 1985, Chemische Fabrik.

Pharma, first started clinical trials of several concentrations of POL to treat varicose veins (correspondence from B. Olesch, 1992).

The maximum daily dose recommended by Kreussler Pharma is found in Table 7-2. Blenkinsopp[106] recommends a higher maximum daily dosage of 10 ml of a POL 6% solution for an average person based on toxicity experiments extrapolated from rats. However, rats are much less sensitive to POL. Since the lethal dose in 50% of the population (LD_{50}) of rabbits is approximately 11.7 mg/kg, Blenkinsopp's minimal dose may be toxic.[107]

POL is unique among local anesthetics in its lack of an aromatic ring. As an aliphatic molecule it is composed of a hydrophilic chain of polyethylene glycolic ether and a liposoluble radical of dodecylic alcohol. It is used as a topical anesthetic agent in ointments and lotions for mucous membranes, including hemorrhoidal treatment.[108] It is also used as a local anesthetic for skin irritation, burns, and insect bites and as an epidural anesthetic.[109-111] The subcutaneous anesthetic effect of a 0.4% solution is equal to a 2% solution of novocaine.[109] The LD_{50} in rabbits at 2 hours is 0.2 gm/kg, which is three to six times greater than the LD_{50} for novocaine.[110] The LD_{50} in mice has been found to vary between 1.2 gm/kg[112] and 110 mg/kg (correspondence from Kreussler Pharma, 1992). The systemic toxicity was similar to procaine and lidocaine.[113] Thus POL was considered an ideal local anesthetic. However, it soon became apparent that intravascular and intradermal instillation produced sclerosis of small diameter blood vessels and "moderate, clinically unimportant reversible damage to healthy tissue."* Therefore, compound Sch 600 was considered for use as a sclerosing agent. The polidocanol preparation Aethoxysklerol was registered at the German health authority, the Bundesgesundheitsaumt (BGA), in 1967.[111]

Experimental evaluation of absorption, distribution, metabolism, and excretion of POL has been studied in dogs, rats, and humans.[111] POL is rapidly distributed throughout the body within minutes of injection.[111] The compound is rapidly metabolized and eliminated, having a terminal elimination half-life of 1.4 to 1.7 hours in dogs. After 72 hours, 97% of the administered compound is excreted (61% in urine, 37% in feces).

In humans the elimination half-life is 4 hours, with 89% of the dose eliminated from the blood within 12 hours. Amounts excreted in the urine and feces are equal, and almost 80% of the injected compound is excreted via respiration through a breakdown into low molecular weight products. POL is completely

---

*Henschel O: Sclerosing of varicose veins sclerotherapy with aethoxysklerol-Kreussler (product booklet), Chemische Fabrik Kreussler & Co GmbH, Wiesbaden-Biebrich D-6202, Postfach 9105, West Germany.

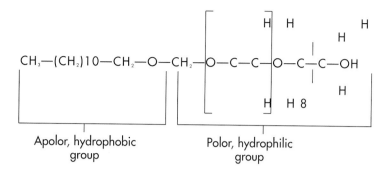

Fig. 7-23   Structural formula of polidocanol.

eliminated from body organs whether the patient receives one dose or repeated doses. Therefore, no accumulation takes place. Polidocanol also does not cross the blood-brain barrier.[111]

The capacity of POL to cross the placental barrier was investigated in rats. Of radioactivity from labeled POL, 15% to 87% was recovered from fetal tissue after 13 days.[111] The striking variations in an earlier differentiation phase may come from weight differences between fetuses. The fetus of day 19 accumulated less activity per gm of tissue than those of day 13 and showed only 18% to 19% of the maternal blood values. From the data obtained, it is evident that the placenta is a partial barrier for POL, and its penetration capacity declines upon increasing differentiation of the fetus.

POL belongs to the class of detergent sclerosing solutions that are nonionic compounds. It consists of an apolar hydrophobic part, dodecyl alcohol, and a polar hydrophilic part, polyethylene-oxide chain, which is esterified (Fig. 7-23). In solution POL is associated as macromolecules through electrostatic hydrogen bonding between the H– atom of the OH– group in one molecule, and the free electron-pair of an O– atom of a second molecule. This bonding results in the formation of a network (see Fig. 7-4). The sclerotherapeutic activity results from this double hydrophobic and hydrophilic action, and thus POL is a "detergent." The optimal efficacy of the compound coincides with the highest concentration that still permits the existence of nonaggregated molecules, 3%.* However, Kreussler Pharma states that POL 4% is also optimal and soluble (personal correspondence, 1992).

Telangiectasias are treated with concentrations of 0.25% to 0.75%. Recently a randomized study determined that a 0.5% concentration may be ideal for sclerosis of leg telangiectasia.[114] Varicose veins are treated with concentrations of 1% to 4%. Small vessels and telangiectasias respond well. Efficacy is decreased in the treatment of large or medium-sized varicose veins. Kreussler Pharma† recommends the use of POL forte (4%) for treatment of the saphenofemoral and saphenopopliteal junctions, perforating veins, and varicosities greater than 8 mm in diameter. POL 3% is recommended for varicose veins 4 to 8 mm in diameter. POL 2% is recommended for varicose veins 2 to 4 mm in diameter and 1% solution for veins 1 to 2 mm in diameter. The concentration of solution for

---

*Dexo SA Pharmaceuticals, France: Product description on hydroxypolyethoxydodecane. Received with correspondence, May 1985.

†Product information (June 1987) from Kreussler Pharma; Wiesbaden 12, D-6200, West Germany.

telangiectasia ranges from 0.5% to 1%. One should take care not to exceed the maximum dose of POL, which is 2 mg/kg/day.

Advantages. The safety and efficacy of this agent is such that a derivative of POL, polyoxyethylene dodecanol, was developed by the Vick Chemical Company in the 1950s as a mucolytic wetting agent for use in vaporizers.[115] Toxicity studies on rats demonstrated a lack of sensitization to cutaneous application and no toxicity with oral ingestion or with exposure to steaming electric vaporizers. A clinical study carried out on 168 infants and children treated with this compound in vaporizers showed no harmful effects.[112]

Henschel* states that the selective activity on damaged endothelium results from the steric structure of POL. "The macromolecules retard the individual molecules and thus shield the tissue from their uninhibited action." This damage is therefore said to be reversible in normal tissue. Henschel goes on to claim that since the surface-active—induced absorption on the varix wall is greatest at the point of injection and falls off rapidly with increasing distance, large quantities can be injected without danger of damage to the deep venous system. He recommends the injection of a maximum of 2 ml of POL 3% at each site with a maximum of 6 ml POL 3% injected in one sclerotherapy session. However, Goldman et al.[38] have demonstrated that POL will sclerose normal vessels (rabbit ear vein) and that the concentration injected is critical to the final outcome of vein sclerosis. POL is a weaker detergent-type sclerosing solution than STS. These experimental studies indicate that its sclerosing power is approximately 50% of the strength of STS.

POL is unique among sclerosing agents in that it is both painless to inject and will not produce cutaneous ulcerations, even with intradermal injection of concentration less than 1.0% (see Chapter 8). Allergic reactions rarely have been reported. The degree of pigmentation produced may be less than that of other detergent sclerosing agents (see Chapter 8).

An open clinical trial comparing STS with POL is being conducted by 120 physicians in Australia. The results at 2 years were reported recently.[116] Fifty-five of 65 physicians found that POL had a better efficacy than STS, with two claiming decreased efficacy, and 8 seeing no difference. When compared to HS, 49 of 58 claimed better efficacy, with 1 physician reporting decreased efficacy, and 8 physicians finding no difference. Pain of injection with POL was less than STS in the experiences of 54 of 65 physicians, with pain being less than HS as reported by 56 of 58 physicians. Finally, the physicians' perceptions of complications were that POL had fewer overall complications (pigmentation, ulceration, phlebitis, telangiectatic matting) according to 58 of 65 physicians as compared with STS, and according to 43 of 58 physicians as compared with HS.

Other Sclerosing Solutions/Combinations

As mentioned in the introduction and previously in this chapter, almost any caustic substance can be or has been used to sclerose blood vessels. Although this chapter has detailed those commonly used, commercially available solutions, it is by no means complete.

Another method for sclerosing varicose veins is to combine solutions either together or in a sequential manner. Certainly, diluting PII with HS or SX increases

---

*Henschel O: Sclerosing of varicose veins sclerotherapy with aethoxysklerol-Kreussler (product booklet), Chemische Fabrik Kreussler & Co GmbH, Wiesbaden-Biebrich D-6202, Postfach 9105, West Germany.

the potency and localizes the sclerosing effect to the point of injection. This technique may be useful when sclerosing junctions between the superficial and deep systems (saphenofemoral/saphenopopliteal junctions and/or perforating veins).[117]

Stemmer (personal communication, 1993) found that a mixture of sodium salicylate 0.30 mg—glycerin 1.80 mg in 5 ml distilled water giving a final concentration of 6% sodium salicylate and 26% glycerin—is an excellent sclerosing solution for telangiectasia less than 1 mm in diameter. My limited experience with this solution in humans confirms Stemmer's observation. According to the rabbit ear model, this solution has an equivalent clinical and histologic effect to undiluted 72% CG (unpublished observations, Goldman MP, 1994).

Sequential injections may be useful to enhance the efficacy of milder sclerosing solutions either by increasing its potency or by the act of sequentially damaging endothelium. After mechanical trauma, endothelial cells are unable to generate various substances or to respond to circulating or locally produced substances.[118] In this damaged state, further injury may produce irreparable damage. In addition, combining solutions may produce an additive effect on its potency.

Since STS 3% is presently the strongest solution approved by the FDA, pretreating a large varicose vein or an area of high reflux with HS produces a stronger, synergistic effect. This technique has been reported recently using ultrasound guidance to sclerose the saphenofemoral junction.[119] One-year follow-up of 66 patients treated with STS 3% alone under ultrasound guidance at the SFJ demonstrated a recanalization rate of 25%. When a second group of 70 patients with similar pathology was treated with STS, 3% immediately followed by HS 23.4%, only 12% demonstrated recanalization at one-year follow-up. Thus the sclerosing effect was enhanced. Further experience varying the order of injection is needed, as are longer follow-up times.

REFERENCES

1. Green D: Compression sclerotherapy techniques, Dermatol Clin 7:137, 1989.
2. Hoeffner U and Vanhoutte PM: Endothelial factors and regulation of vascular tone. In Vanhoutte PM, editor: Return circulation and norepinephrine: an update, Paris, 1991, John Libbey Eurotext.
3. Ralevic V, Lincoln J, and Burnstock G: Release of vasoactive substances from endothelial cells. In Ryan U and Rubanyi GM, editors: Endothelial regulation of vascular tone, New York, 1992, Marcel Dekker.
4. van Hinsbergh VWM et al: Tumor necrosis factor increases the production of plasminogen activator inhibitor in human endothelial cells in vitro and in rats in vivo, Blood 72:1467, 1988.
5. Munro JM, Pober JS, and Cotran RS: Tumor necrosis factor and interferon-gamma induce distinct patterns of endothelial activation and associated leukocyte accumulation in skin of papio anubis, Am J Pathol 135:121, 1989.
6. Wolf E: Die histologischen Veranderungen der venen nach intravenosen sub limatein Spritzungen, Med Klin 16:806, 1920.
7. Schneider W: Contribution to the history of the sclerosing treatment of varices and to its anatomo-pathologic study, Soc Fran Phlebol 18:117, 1965.
8. Fegan WG: Varicose veins: compression sclerotherapy, London, 1967, Heinemann.
9. Hanschell HM: Treatment of varicose veins, Br Med J 2:630, 1947.
10. Campbell GR et al: Arterial smooth muscle: a multifactorial mesenchymal cell, Arch Pathol Lab Med 112:977, 1988.
11. Thulesius O: Physiological and pathophysiological variations of smooth muscle. European Congress of the International Union of Phlebology, Budapest, September 6, 1993, Mutiscience Publishing.
12. Schwartz SM et al: Maintenance of integrity in aortic endothelium, Fed Proc 39:2618, 1980.
13. Haudenschild CC and Schwartz SM: Endothelial regeneration II. Restitution of endothelial continuity, Lab Invest 41:407, 1979.
14. Schwartz SM, Gajdusek CM, and Selden SC: Vascular wall growth control: the role of endothelium, Arteriosclerosis 1:107, 1981.

15. Bouvier CA et al: Circulating endothelium as an indication of vascular injury. In Koller F et al, editors: Vascular factors and thrombosis, Stuttgart, 1970, Schattauer Verlag.

16. Imhoff E and Stemmer R: Classification and mechanism of action of sclerosing agents, Soc Fran Phlebol 22:143, 1969.

17. Stroncek DF et al: Sodium morrhuate stimulates granulocytes and damages erythrocytes and endothelial cells: probable mechanism of an adverse reaction during sclerotherapy, J Lab Clin Med 106:498, 1985.

18. Cacciola E et al: Activation of contact phase of blood coagulation can be induced by the sclerosing agent polidocanol: possible additional mechanism of adverse reaction during sclerotherapy, J Lab Clin Med 109:225, 1987.

19. Brenn H, Imhoff E, and Duckert F: Wirkung verschiedener Sklerosierungsmittel auf einige Gerinnungsparameter in vitro und bei Patienten wahrend Varizenverodung, Vasa 5:199, 1976.

20. Cepelak V: Effect of sclerosing agents on platelet aggregation, Folia Angiologica 30:363, 1982.

21. Cooper WM: Clinical evaluation of sotradecol, a sodium alkyl sulfate solution, in the injection therapy of varicose veins, Surg Gynecol Obstet 83:647, 1946.

22. Oscher A and Garside E: Intravenous injection of sclerosing substances: experimental comparative studies of changes in vessels, Ann Surg 96:691, 1932.

23. Sadick N: Hyperosmolar vs detergent sclerosing agents in sclerotherapy: effect on distal vessel obliteration, J Dermatol Surg Oncol 1994 (in press).

24. Lindemayr H and Santler R: The fibrinolytic activity of the vein wall, Phlebologie 30:151, 1977.

25. Merlen JF et al: Histological changes in sclerosed vein, Phlebologie 31:17, 1978.

26. Virchow R: Gesammelte Abhandlungen zur wissenschaftlichen Medicin, Frankfurt, 1856, Meidingersohn.

27. Wuppermann TH: Study of sclerosis of varicose veins: comparison between the natural fibrinolysis in the blood of the antecubital vein and the test with labelled fibrinogen in the sclerosed leg, Phlebologie 30:145, 1977.

28. Soehring K and Nasemann TH: Beitrage zur Pharmakologie der Alkylpolyathylenoxyderivate. III. Gerinnungszeit bei wiederholtzer Applikation, hamolytische Wirkungen, Arch Int Pharmacodyn 91:96, 1952.

29. MacGowen WAL et al: The local effects of intra-arterial injections of sodium tetra-decyl sulfate (STD) 3%: an experimental study, Br J Surg 59:101, 1972.

30. Raymond-Martimbeau P and Leclerc JR: Effects of sclerotherapy on blood coagulation: a prospective study, 445 In Phlebologie '92, Rayomond-Martinbeau P, Prescott R, Zummo M (eds), p. 445. John Libbey Eurotext, Paris, 1992.

31. Dastain JY: Sclerotherapy of varices when the patient is on anticoagulants, with reference to 2 patients on anticoagulants, Phlebologie 34:73, 1981.

32. Kanter AH: Complications of sotradecol sclerotherapy with and without heparin. In Raymond-Martimbeau P, Prescott R, and Zummo M, editors: Phlebologie '92, Paris, 1992, John Libbey Eurotext.

33. Klein-Fein J: What happens during the injection of sclerosant, Phlebologie 30:165, 1977.

34. Williams RA and Wilson E: Sclerosant treatment of varicose veins and deep vein thrombosis, Arch Surg 119:1283, 1984.

35. Wenner L: Sind endovarikose hamatische Ansammlungen eine normalerscheinung bei Sklerotherapie? Vasa 10:174, 1981.

36. Fegan WG: Continuous compression technique of injecting varicose veins, Lancet 2:109, 1963.

37. Schmier AA: Clinical comparison of sclerosing solutions in injection treatment of varicose veins, Am J Surg 36:389, 1937.

38. Goldman MP et al: Sclerosing agents in the treatment of telangiectasia: comparison of the clinical and histologic effects of intravascular polidocanol, sodium tetradecyl sulfate, and hypertonic saline in the dorsal rabbit ear vein model, Arch Dermatol 123:1196, 1987.

39. Martin DE and Goldman MP: A comparison of sclerosing agents: clinical and histologic effects of intravascular sodium tetradecyl sulfate and chromated glycerine in the dorsal rabbit ear vein, J Dermatol Surg Oncol 16:18, 1990.

40. Reiner L: The activity of anionic surface active compounds in producing vascular obliteration, Proc Soc Exp Biol Med 62:49, 1946.

41. Rotter SM and Weiss RA: Human saphenous vein in vitro model for studying the action of sclerosing solutions, J Dermatol Surg Oncol 19:59, 1993.

42. Feied C and Kessler CM: Personal communication, 1993.

43. Regard GL: The treatment of varicosities by sclerosing injections, Rev Med de la Suisse Rom, Geneve 65:102, 1925.

44. Doerffel J: Klinisches und Experimentelles uber Venenverodung mit Kochsalzlosung und Traubenzucker, Deutsche Med Wohnschr 53:901, 1927.

45. Binet L and Verne J: Evolution histo-physiologie de la veine ala suite de son obliteration experimentale, Presse Med 1:761, 1925.

46. Schwartz E and Ratschow M: Experimentelle und klinische Erfahrungen bei der kunstlichen Verodung von Varicen, Arch Klin Chir 156:720, 1929.

47. Biegeleisen HI: Fatty acid solutions for the injection treatment of varicose veins: an evaluation of 4 new solutions, Ann Surg 105:610, 1937.

48. McPheeters HO and Anderson JK: Injection treatment of varicose veins and hemorrhoids, Philadelphia, 1938, FA Davis.

49. Biegeleisen HI: The evaluation of sodium morrhuate therapy in varicose veins: a critical study, Surg Gynecol Obstet 57:696, 1933.

50. Schneider W and Fischer H: Fixierung und bindegewebige organization artefizieller Thromben bei der Varizenuerodung, Dtsch Med Wschr 89:2410, 1964.

51. Dietrich VHP and Sinapius D: Experimental endothelial damage by varicosclerosation drugs, Arznittel-Forsh 18:116, 1968.

52. Goldman MP: A comparison of sclerosing agents: clinical and histologic effects of intravascular sodium morrhuate, ethanolamine oleate, hypertonic saline (11.7%), and Sclerodex in the dorsal rabbit ear vein, J Dermatol Surg Oncol, 1991 (in press).

53. Blenkinsopp WK: Comparison of tetradecyl sulfate of sodium with other sclerosants in rats, Br J Exp Pathol 49:197, 1968.

54. Kern HM and Angle LW: The chemical obliteration of varicose veins: a clinical and experimental study, JAMA 93:595, 1929.

55. Ouvry PA: Telangiectasia and sclerotherapy, J Dermatol Surg Oncol 15:177, 1989.

56. Sadick NS: Sclerotherapy of varicose and telangiectic leg veins: minimal sclerosant concentration of hypertonic saline and its relationship to vessel diameter, J Dermatol Surg Oncol 17:65, 1991.

57. Foley WT: The eradication of venous blemishes, Cutis 15:665, 1975.

58. Sadick N: Treatment of varicose and telangiectatic leg veins with hypertonic saline: a comparative study of heparin and saline, J Dermatol Surg Oncol 16:24, 1990.

59. Bodian EL: Techniques of sclerotherapy for sunburst venous blemishes, J Dermatol Surg Oncol 11:696, 1985.

60. Bodian EL: Sclerotherapy, Sem Dermatol 6:238, 1987.

61. Thornton SC, Mueller SN, and Levine EM: Human endothelial cells: use of heparin in cloning and long-term serial cultivation, Science 222:623, 1983.

62. Bodian E: Sclerotherapy, Dialogues Dermatol 13(3), 1983 (tape recording).

63. Alderman DB: Therapy for essential cutaneous telangiectasias, Postgrad Med 61:91, 1977.

64. Haines PC et al: Effects of lidocaine concentration on distal capillary blood flow in a rabbit ear model, Microsurgery 8:54, 1987.

65. Johns RA, DiFazio CA, and Longnecker DE: Lidocaine constricts or dilates rat arterioles in a dose-dependent manner, Anesthesiology 62:141, 1985.

66. Mantse L: A mild sclerosing agent for telangiectasias, J Dermatol Surg Oncol 11:9, 1985.

67. Nguyen VB: Sklerotherapie des varices des membres inferieurs etude de 522 cas, Le Saguenay Medical 23:134, 1976.

68. Mantse L: More on spider veins, J Dermatol Surg Oncol 12:1022, 1986.

69. Ouvry PA: Telangiectasia and sclerotherapy, J Dermatol Surg Oncol 15:177, 1989.

70. Martindale: The extra pharmacopoeia, ed 28, London, 1982, Pharmaceutical.

71. Maclaren NK et al: Glycerol intolerance in a child with intermittent hypoglycemia, J Pediatr 86:43, 1975.

72. Jausion H, Carrot E, and Ervais A: Une methode simple de phlebosclerose: la cure des varices par les injections de glycerine diluee, Bull Soc Fran Dermatol Syph 38:171, 1931.

73. Hammarlund ER and Pedersen-Bjergaard L: Hemolysis of erythrocytes in various iso-osmotic solutions, J Pharm Sci 50:24, 1961.

74. Hagnevik K et al: Glycerol-induced haemolysis with haemoglobinuria and acute renal failure, Lancet 1:75, 1974.

75. Welch KMA et al: Glycerol-induced hemolysis (letter), Lancet 1:416, 1974.

76. Welch KMA et al: Glycerol-induced hemolysis, Lancet 1:416, 1974.

77. Jausion H: Glycerine chromee et sclerose des ectasies veineuses, La Presse Medicale 53:1061, 1933.

78. Jausion H et al: La sclerose des varices et des hemorroides par le glycerine chromee, Bull Memoires Soc Med Hospitaux Paris, p 587, 1932.

79. Hutinel B: Esthetique dans les scleroses de varices et traitement des varicosites, La Vie Medicale 20:1739, 1978.

80. Nebot F: Quelques points techniques sur le traitement des varicosites et des telangiectasies, Phlebologie 21:133, 1968.

81. Ducros R and Gruffaz J: Indications, techniques et resultats du traitement sclerosant, La Revue du Praticien 20:2027, 1970.

82. Stemmer R, Kopp C, and Voglet P: Etude physique del injection sclerosante, Phlegologie 22:149, 1969.

83. Ouvry P and Arlaud R: Le traitement sclerosant des telangiectasies des membres inferieurs, Phlebologie 32:365, 1979.

84. Ouvry P and Davy A: Le traitement sclersant des telangiectasies des membres inferieurs, Phlebologie 35:349, 1982.

85. Wallois P: Incidents et accidents de la sclerose. In Tournay R, editor: La sclerose des varices, ed 4, Paris, 1985, Expansion Scientifique Francaise.

86. Bernier E, Savoie C, and Escher E: Pharmacokinetics of sclerosing iodine injections. In Raymond-Martimbeau P, Prescott R, and Zummor M, editors: Phlebologie '92, Paris, 1992, John Libbey Eurotext.

87. Wenner L: Anwendung einer mit Athylalkohol modifizierten Polijodidjonenlosung bei skleroseresistenten Varizen, Vasa 12:190, 1983.

88. Raymond-Martimbeu P: Personal communication, 1990.

89. Sigg K, Horodegen K, and Bernbach H: Varizen-Sklerosierung: Welchos ist das wirUsamste Mittel? Deutsohes Arzteblatt 34/35:2294, 1986.

90. Sigg K and Zelikovski A: "Quick treatment"—a modified method of sclerotherapy of varicose veins, Vasa 4:73, 1975.

91. Sigg K and Zelikovski A: Kann die Sklerosierungotherapie der Varizen obne Oparation in jedem Fallwirksam vein? Phlebol Proktol 4:42, 1975.

92. Ghosh S: Chemical investigation in connection with leprosy inquiry, Indian J Med Res 8:211, 1920.

93. Cutting RA: The preparation of sodium morrhuate, J Lab Clin Med 11:842, 1926.

94. Gallagher PG: Varicose veins—primary treatment with sclerotherapy, J Dermatol Surg Oncol 18:39, 1992.

95. Meyer NE: Monoethanolamine oleate: a new chemical for obliteration of varicose veins, Am J Surg 40:628, 1938.

96. Biegeleissen HI: Fatty acid solutions for the injection treatment of varicose veins: evaluation of four new solutions, Ann Surg 105:610, 1937.

97. Hedberg SE, Fowler DL, and Ryan LR: Injection sclerotherapy of esophageal varices using ethanolamine oleate: a pilot study, Am J Surg 143:426, 1982.

98. Ayres SJ et al: Endoscopic sclerotherapy for bleeding esophageal varices: effects and complications, Ann Intern Med 98:900, 1983.

99. Evans DMD et al: Osophageal varices treated by sclerotherapy: a histopathological study, Gut 23:615, 1982.

100. Reid RG and Rothine NG: Treatment of varicose veins by compression sclerotherapy, Br J Surg 55:889, 1968.

101. Nabatoff RA: Recent trends in the diagnosis and treatment of varicose veins, Surg Gynecol Obstet 90:521, 1950.

102. Orbach EJ: Histopathological findings of telangiectasies treated with sodium tetradecyl sulfate-procaine precipitate, Angiopatias (Brasil) 8:103, 1968.

103. Tretbar LL: Spider angiomata: treatment with sclerosant injections, J Kansas Med Soc 79:198, 1978.

104. Shields JL and Jansen GT: Therapy for superficial telangiectasias of the lower extremities, J Dermatol Surg Oncol 8:857, 1982.

105. Sadick NS and Farber B: A microbiologic study of diluted sclerotherapy solutions, J Dermatol Surg Oncol 19:450, 1993.

106. Blenkinsopp WK: Choice of sclerosant: an experimental study, Angiologica 7:182, 1970.

107. Pfahler B, Kreussler and Co, GMBH: Personal communication, March 29, 1990.

108. Schulz KH: Uber die Verwendung von Alkyl-polathylenoxyd-derivaten als Oberflachenanaesthetica, Dermatol Wochen 126:657, 1952.

109. Soehring K et al: Beitrage zur Pharmakologie der Alkylpolyathylerioxyd derivate. I. Untersuchungen uber die acute und subchronische Toxizitat bein verschiedenen Tierarten, Arch Int Pharmacodyn 87:301, 1951.

110. Siems KJ and Soehring K: Die Ausschaltug sensibler nerven duren peridurale und paravertebrale injektion von alkylpolyathylenoxydathern bei meerschweinchen, Arzneimittelforsche 2:109, 1952.

111. Olesch B: Neuere Erkenntnisse zur Pharmakokinetik von Polidocanol (Aethoxysklerol), Vasomed Aktuell 4:22, 1990.

112. Larkin V De P: Polyethylene dodecanol vaporization in the treatment of respiratory infections of infants and children, NY State J Med 57:2667, 1957.

113. Soehring K and Frahm M: Studies on the pharmacology of alkylpolyethyleneoxide derivatives, Arzneimittelforsche 5:655, 1955.
114. Carlin MC and Ratz JL: Treatment of telangiectasia: comparison of sclerosing agents, J Dermatol Surg Oncol 13:1181, 1987.
115. Grubb TC, Dick LC, and Oser M: Studies on the toxicity of polyoxyethylene dodecanol, Toxicol Appl Pharmacol 2:133, 1960.
116. Conrad P and Malouf GM: The Australian polidocanol (aethoxysklerol) open clinical trial results at two years. Presented at the 8th annual meeting of the North American Society of Phlebology, Maui, February 24, 1994.
117. Raymond-Martimbeau P: Intravascular ultrasound and evaluation of treatment results. Presented at the 50th Annual Meeting of the American Academy of Dermatology, Dallas, December 11, 1991.
118. Vanhoutte PM: The endothelium—modulator of vascular smooth-muscle tone, N Engl J Med 319:512, 1988.
119. Mauriello J and Zygmunt J Jr: Synergistic effect of sclerosing agents. Presented at the 8th annual meeting of the North American Society of Phlebology, Maui, February 22, 1994.

COMPLICATIONS AND ADVERSE SEQUELAE OF SCLEROTHERAPY

Primum non nocere—above all else do no harm. This has always been a watchword in medicine and should always be considered before embarking on any form of treatment. Rarely in medicine does the physician have the luxury of administering a totally benign therapy, one that has absolutely no chance of harm. Rather, after establishing that the treatment is truly in the best interest of the patient, one should become familiar with the potential hazards of the proposed therapy and be prepared to treat those hazards should they occur. Further, in this era of pervasive medical-legal conflicts, it is advisable to inform the patient of the various potential complications and adverse sequelae of therapy. A cognizant patient can better recognize a problem early and can more willingly participate in the necessary treatment.

Unfortunately, as with any therapeutic technique, sclerotherapy carries with it a number of potential adverse sequelae and complications. Fairly common, and often self-limiting, side effects include perivascular cutaneous pigmentation, edema of the injected extremity, a flare of new telangiectasias, pain with injection of certain sclerosing solutions, localized urticaria over injected sites, blisters or folliculitis caused by postsclerosis compression, recurrence of previously treated vessels, stress-related problems, and localized hirsutism. Relatively rare complications include localized cutaneous necrosis; systemic allergic reactions; thrombophlebitis of the injected vessel; arterial injection with resultant distal necrosis; deep vein thrombosis (DVT), which may result in chronic venous insufficiency or pulmonary emboli; nerve damage; compartmental syndrome; and air emboli. This chapter addresses the pathophysiology of these reactions, methods for reducing their incidence, and treatment of their occurrence.

ADVERSE SEQUELAE
Postsclerotherapy Hyperpigmentation

Cutaneous pigmentation to some degree is a relatively common occurrence after sclerotherapy of veins varying in size from varicose to capillary. This complication has been reported in 30%[1] to 80%[2] of patients treated with sodium tetradecyl sulfate (STS), although a recent report found an 11% incidence when using a 0.1% STS concentration.[3] Percentages of incidence range from 10% to 30% in patients treated with hypertonic saline (HS),[3-7] 10.7%[8] to 30%[5,9] in patients treated with polidocanol (POL), and 35% in 7200 patients treated with POL, ethanolamine oleate (EO), or iodine-iodide solution.[10] Therefore the incidence appears to depend on technique and concentration (as discussed below) and not solely on solution type. However, certain sclerosing solutions may have an inherent lower incidence of pigmentation (discussed below).

A recent evaluation of patients in one practice found a 1% incidence of pigmentation persisting after 1 year.[11] Pigmentation is usually linear along the course of the treated blood vessel. I use the term *ghost of the blood vessel* to explain to patients that it represents a resolving and not intact vessel. However, in addition to linear lines of pigmentation, osmotic sclerosing solutions may produce punctate pigmentation at points of injection, which may be related to their mechanism of action through an osmotic gradient that produces maximal osmolality and resultant endothelial destruction at the injection site. In contrast, detergent-type sclerosing solutions destroy the treated vessel for a few centimeters along its length, giving a more linear golden-brown color (Fig. 8-1).

Etiologic factors

The etiology of this pigmentation is subject to much conjecture. It was once believed that this pigmentation results from a *combination* of postinflammatory hyperpigmentation (incontinence of melanin pigment) and hemosiderin deposition.[12-14] However, histologic examination has demonstrated that this pigmentation is caused only by hemosiderin staining of the dermis.[15-17] Defects in iron storage or transport mechanisms or both have also been found in a significant number of patients who developed postsclerotherapy pigmentation.[18]

Histologic studies have examined the etiology of postsclerotherapy hyperpigmentation. One study examined biopsies from 14 patients 6 to 54 months after sclerotherapy treatment of varicose veins and demonstrated hemosiderin without melanin incontinence.[16] A second histologic study performed after injection of varicose veins in patients with spontaneous pigmentation associated with chronic venous insufficiency was reported by Cuttell and Fox.[19] They treated seven patients with STS, using 6 weeks of compression followed by an additional 2 months of wearing elastic stockings. Patients underwent biopsies both before sclerotherapy and from 10 to 23 months after sclerotherapy. Full-thickness skin biopsies were stained with hematoxylin and eosin, hexamine silver, and Perls' reagent and then blindly reviewed by two histopathologists. All patients demon-

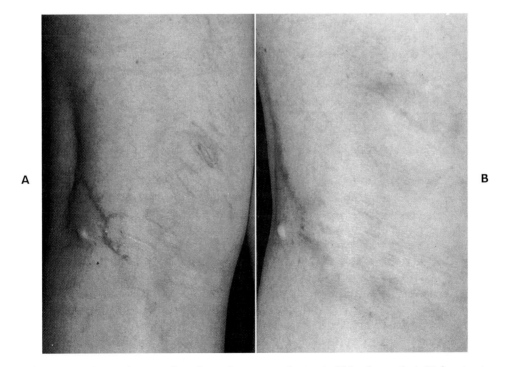

Fig. 8-1   Linear pigmentation along the course of a treated blood vessel. **A,** Before treatment. **B,** 8 weeks after treatment with POL 0.5%.   *Continued.*

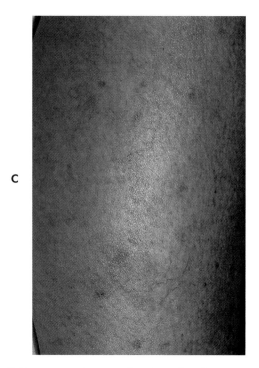

Fig. 8-1, cont'd C, Punctuate pigmentation 8 weeks after treatment with Sclerodex. (C from Goldman MP: Adverse sequelae of sclerotherapy treatment of varicose and telangiectatic leg veins. In Bergan JJ and Goldman MP, editors: Varicose veins: diagnosis and treatment, St. Louis, 1993, Quality Medical Publishing, Inc.)

strated a decrease in melanin. Dermal hemosiderin was increased in two patients, unchanged in one patient, and curiously decreased in four patients. These authors concluded that "residual pigmentation following sclerotherapy of varicose veins occurs where there has been extravasation of blood at the injection site."

Goldman, Kaplan, and Duffy[17] microscopically examined this pigmentation in six patients 6 weeks to 6 months after treatment of leg telangiectasias with POL, HS, and STS. Treatment and biopsy characteristics of this study and an additional three patients are listed in Table 8-1. Analysis of these patients shows that postsclerotherapy pigmentation occurred 6 to 12 weeks after treatment. There were no apparent histologic differences in the degree of pigmentation between the three sclerosing agents. In each biopsy specimen scattered foci of golden-brown refractile pigment were noted on hematoxylin-eosin–stained specimens (Fig. 8-2). Perls' reagent revealed iron deposition in the dermis. Fontana's stain demonstrated a normal pattern of melanocytes along the dermal-epidermal junction. Diapedesis of red blood cells (RBCs) was noted only on biopsy specimens taken from the ankle (at 6 and 8 months after injection). Interestingly, periadnexal hemosiderin was prominent in this location and in the popliteal fossae. The depth of hemosiderin ranged from 0.2 to 2.8 mm from the granular layer.[18]

Each specimen differed somewhat in the degree of dermal hemosiderin; the more darkly pigmented cutaneous lesions exhibited a greater extent of dermal hemosiderin. In this limited study apparently a greater amount of hemosiderin staining occurred in biopsy specimens taken from the ankle as opposed to the calf or thigh. In addition, darkly pigmented patients did not demonstrate melanin incontinence.

Table 8-1 Postsclerotherapy hyperpigmentation treatment characteristics

Agent	Patient's race	Time of biopsy	Result
POL 0.25%	White	6 wk after injection	Heme
POL 0.75%	White	6 wk after injection	Heme
POL 0.75%	Hispanic	6 mo after injection	Heme
POL 0.75%	White	12 mo after injection	Heme
SM ?	White	7 yr after injection	Heme
HS 18%	White	8 mo after injection	Heme
HS 20%	White	2 mo after injection	Heme
STS 0.5%	White	5 mo after injection	Heme
STS 0.25%	Hispanic	3 mo after injection	Heme

POL, polidocanol; *SM,* sodium morrhuate; *HS,* hypertonic saline; *STS,* sodium tetradecyl sulfate; *Heme,* hemosiderin.

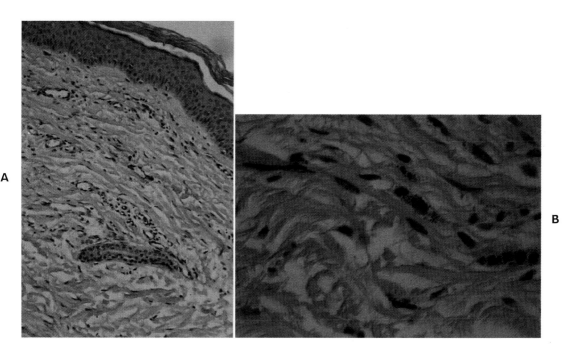

Fig. 8-2 Section stained with hematoxylin-eosin taken 6 months after injection with POL 0.75%. Note scattered foci of golden-brown pigment. **A,** Original magnification ×50. **B,** Original magnification × 200. (From Goldman MP, Kaplan RP, and Duffy DM: J Dermatol Surg Oncol 13:547, 1987.) *Continued.*

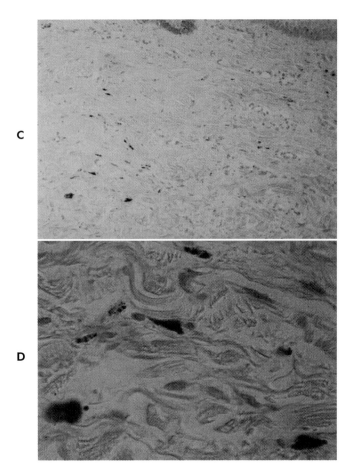

Fig. 8-2, cont'd. Perls-stained section from the same patient as in Fig. 8-1. Note scattered foci of green-blue granules within siderophages. **C,** Original magnification ×50. **D,** Original magnification ×200. (From Goldman MP, Kaplan RP, and Duffy DM: J Dermatol Surg Oncol 13:547, 1987.)

Hemosiderin deposition predominantly occurs in the superficial dermis, although it may be present in periadnexal and middermal locations, particularly in the ankle area. This phenomenon probably occurs when RBCs extravasate into the dermis after the rupture of treated vessels.[20] Erythrocyte diapedesis is a regular finding in patients with chronic venous insufficiency in whom it is not caused by inflammatory wall alterations but solely by a pressure rise within the cutaneous vessels.[21] Erythrocyte diapedesis may also occur after inflammation of the vessel and is commonly seen after thrombophlebitis. Perivascular inflammation is presumed to promote degranulation of perivascular mast cells. Released histamine leads to endothelial cell contraction, which results in widening of endothelial gaps through which extravasation of RBCs can occur.[22-26] Thus injecting a sclerosing solution both dilates the vessel directly through pressure generated by the syringe and indirectly through histamine-induced endothelial cell contraction.

Perivascular phagocytosis of RBCs occurs either by intact cells or piecemeal after fragmentation by macrophages.[27,28] The intracellular fragments in the macrophage cytoplasm are further compartmentalized into hemoglobin-containing globules. They are referred to as *secondary lyposomes.* Since hemosiderin is an indigestible residue of hemoglobin degradation, it may appear as aggregates up to 100 μm in diameter.[29] Hemosiderin has a variable concentration. Iron concentrations vary from 24% to 36%.[30] Iron hydroxide contained in hemosiderin occurs in different forms, with differing amounts of ferritin.[31] On unstained tissue it appears golden and is 30% iron by weight. Its elimination from the area may take years if it ever occurs.

In addition to being insoluble, hemosiderin may directly affect cellular function. Histologic examination with x-ray fluorescence analysis of patients with varicose ulceration disclosed an elevation of mean iron levels in periulcerated skin.[32] The authors speculate that free radical formation resulting from local iron accumulation may cause melanocytic stimulation, thereby augmenting brown pigmentation. Indeed multiple authors have demonstrated melanin incontinence in the presence of venous stasis, complicated by extravascular RBCs.[33-35] Whether melanocytic stimulation plays a role in the early appearance of postsclerotherapy pigmentation is unlikely, but it may contribute to the persistence of pigmentation in certain patients.

Pigmentation resolves from a gradual resorption of ferritin particles from macrophage digestion. It is hypothesized that the patient's iron storage and transport mechanisms may influence the rate of clearance of dermal hemosiderin.[36] A preliminary study of 16 patients with age-matched controls disclosed that patients who developed pigmentation had higher serum ferritin levels. Serum ferritin levels correlate with total body iron stores.[37] To clarify the relationship between serum ferritin and postsclerotherapy pigmentation, a prospective study of 233 consecutive patients was performed.[38] Serum ferritin levels were determined before sclerotherapy, and patients were assessed 3, 6, and 12 months after treatment for evidence of pigmentation. A linear relationship between the occurrence of pigmentation and pretreatment serum ferritin levels was found at each posttreatment assessment date. This supports the hypothesis that high total body iron stores increase the susceptibility toward hyperpigmentation. Therefore serum ferritin levels may be used to identify patients at risk for this complication. These patients may require special attention with meticulous microthrombectomy, and an increase in time and extent of posttreatment compression is advocated.

Regardless of its etiology, the incidence of pigmentation apparently is related to multiple factors, including (1) sclerosing solution type and concentration, (2) sclerotherapy technique, (3) gravitational and other intravascular pressures, (4) innate tendency toward cutaneous pigmentation (total body iron stores and/or altered iron transport and storage mechanisms, innate enhanced histamine release or hypersensitivity, and vessel fragility), (5) postsclerotherapy treatment, (6) vessel diameter, and (7) concomitant medication.

Solution type and concentration

The type and concentration of the sclerosing solution affect the degree of endothelial destruction. The extent of endothelial destruction with resulting inflammation and extravasation of RBCs is thought to influence the development of postsclerotherapy hyperpigmentation. Cloutier and Sansoucy[39] and Tournay[1] state that STS has the highest incidence of pigmentation among sclerosing solutions. Although Duffy[5] and Goldman, Kaplan, and Duffy[17] have noted a similar incidence of pigmentation between use of HS and STS solutions, Weiss and Weiss[40] note a 10.8% incidence of pigmentation with HS solution compared to a 30.7% incidence with 1% POL solution.

Foley[41] claims that the addition of 100 U/ml of heparin decreases the incidence of pigmentation, but in a large series of patients Duffy[5] and Sadick[42] have not found this to occur. Sclerosing solutions reported to have the lowest incidence of postsclerotherapy pigmentation are chromated glycerin (CG)[11,39,43-47] and sodium salicylate.[11,14] A retrospective study of 135 patients investigated whether replacing POL with CG would lower the incidence of pigmentation.[48] CG was used as the sclerosing agent in the first session. CG was continued according to the degree of inflammation, or if no reaction occurred POL was begun. CG caused a strong inflammatory reaction and was continued in 27% of patients, with the remaining patients continuing treatment with POL. Postsclerotherapy hyperpigmentation developed in only 8% of CG-treated patients and in none of the POL-treated patients. The author concluded that patients who developed a strong inflammatory reaction to CG were predisposed to pigmentation by virtue of an enhanced vascular sensitivity to sclerotherapy. Thus using POL in "non-sensitive" patients eliminated the development of pigmentation. The highly sensitive patients developed pigmentation but in a low number (8% of their group), even with the use of a mild sclerosing agent. This trial argues for the use of preliminary sclerotherapy tests before proceeding with definitive treatment.

In addition to the sclerosing solution itself, its concentration may also affect development of pigmentation. Norris, Carlin, and Ratz[49] have observed an increased incidence of pigmentation (60%) in patients treated with 1% POL compared with those treated with 0.5% POL (20%). Weiss and Weiss[40] noted a similar decrease in pigmentation between 1% POL (30.7%) and 0.5% POL (10%). Therefore excessive endothelial destruction, caused by either high concentrations of sclerosing solutions or the use of extremely caustic agents, increases perivascular inflammation. This may produce melanocytic changes in the skin or potentiate extravasation of RBCs through endothelial disruption as previously described.

Technique

To limit the degree of intravascular pressure, larger feeding varices, incompetent varices, and points of high pressure reflux should be treated first. Doing so minimizes the extent of proximal intravascular pressure, which should decrease the risk for extravasation of RBCs. C. Guarde[50] has found a greater incidence of pigmentation if vessels distal to the saphenofemoral junction (SFJ) are treated before successful closure of the junction. Marley[51] has also reported a decreased incidence of pigmentation in his practice since he began treating legs by injecting veins in order from proximal to distal.

Because telangiectasia and small venules are composed essentially of endothelial cells with a thin (if any) muscular coat and basement membrane, excessive intravascular pressure from injection may cause vessel rupture. In addition, endothelial pores and spaces between cells in the vascular wall will dilate in response to pressure, leading to extravasation of RBCs. It is therefore important to inject intravascularly with minimal pressure. Since injection pressure is inversely proportional to the square of the piston radius, using a syringe with a larger radius will result in less pressure. The average piston radius is 8 mm for a 2-ml syringe and 5 mm for a 1-ml syringe. The calculated pressure with an implied force of 250 g is 180 mm Hg for a 2-ml syringe and more than 300 mm Hg for a 1-ml syringe.[52] This is one reason I recommend using a 2- to 3-ml syringe for sclerotherapy.

Gravitational and other intravascular pressures

Postsclerotherapy pigmentation appears most commonly in vessels treated below the knee[14] but can occur anywhere on the leg, probably as a result of a combination of increased capillary fragility and increased intravascular pressure by gravitational effects in this location. Chatard[14] also has observed an increased incidence of pigmentation when blue venulectases are treated as opposed to the treatment of red telangiectasias. The explanation for this latter observation is unknown but may be related to vessel diameter. An evaluation of 113 patients treated with sclerotherapy demonstrated rare pigmentation in vessels less than 1 mm in diameter.[53]

Predisposition to pigmentation

The reason certain individuals are predisposed to the development of pigmentation is unknown. Pigmentation has been reported as more common and pronounced in patients with dark hair and "dark-toned" skin.[12] This is believed to be caused by an increased incidence of postinflammatory hyperpigmentation in patients with these colorings. However, Chatard[14] reported that pigmentation is unrelated to skin or hair color. I agree with this assessment. As described previously, iron storage and transfer mechanisms and histamine hypersensitivity may also predispose toward pigmentation.[36]

If histamine-induced endothelial contraction promotes extravasation of RBCs or hemosiderin or both, histamine antagonists should prevent or limit its occurrence. The catecholamines norepinephrine and isoproterenol antagonize histamine-induced edema in canine brachial artery preparations.[54] Similarly, corticosteroids decrease the size of histamine-induced endothelial gap junctions.[55] Terbutaline also inhibits macromolecular leakage from postcapillary venules in hamster femoral veins.[56] Cimetidine blocks histamine-induced widening of endothelial gaps in rat femoral veins.[57] Therefore patients who develop postsclerotherapy pigmentation may be pretreated with one or a combination of these medications to block or limit histamine effects.

Vessel fragility may also result in an innate predisposition toward pigmentation. Capillary strength has been related to both menstrual cycles and circulating estrogen.[58] Capillary fragility was measured as a suction blister technique during 42 menstrual cycles in 32 nurses and was found to correlate with both ovulation and menses.[58] Decreased capillary strength occurred 3 to 5 days before and 2 days after menses and during ovulation. Fragility improved with intravenous (IV) and oral administration of conjugated equine estrogen (Premarin) in 26 postmenopausal women examined. Interestingly, one patient normalized her premenstrual drop in capillary strength when surreptitiously taking vitamin C. This interesting archival study hopefully will be verified by additional prospective studies. However, until its verification physicians may wish to consider timing sclerotherapy treatment accordingly.

Patients taking minocycline develop postsclerotherapy pigmentation.[59,60] Unlike the golden to deep brown color characteristic of typical sclerotherapy-induced pigmentation, pigmentation from minocycline is typically blue-grey. In one of these patients pigmentation developed after superficial ulceration. Therefore the ulcer itself with its coincidental inflammation and vascular disruption may explain the pigmentation.

Minocycline produces pigmentation in a variety of organs and structures.[61,62] One form of minocycline pigmentation develops in depressed acne scars or at other sites of inflammation.[7,63-67] A second form of pigmentation has been described on UV-exposed legs.[68] The pigment involved in minocycline hyperpigmentation is hemosiderin or some other iron-chelating compound.[66,68-71] It is hypothesized that minocycline or a metabolite interferes with degradation of hemosiderin through lysosomal disruption, leading to macrophage death and deposition of pigment.[67] Therefore it may be prudent to withhold minocycline therapy in sclerotherapy patients. Futher studies are needed to establish this direct relationship.

Postsclerotherapy coagula

Removal of postsclerotherapy coagula may decrease the incidence of pigmentation. Thrombi to some degree are thought to occur after sclerotherapy of all veins, regardless of size, because of the inability to occlude the vascular lumen completely with external pressure. The persistence of a small vascular lumen even with maximal external pressure has been predicted with experimental models of vein wall.[21] This has also been directly observed with fiberoptic varicography.[72]

Persistent thrombi are thought to produce a subacute "perivenulitis" that can persist for months.[73-75] The perivenulitis favors extravasation of RBCs through a damaged endothelium or by increasing the permeability of treated endothelium. In addition, intratissue fixation of hemosiderin may occur.[14] This provides a rationale for drainage of all foci of trapped blood 2 to 4 weeks after sclerotherapy. Sometimes blood can be released even 2 months after sclerotherapy.

Thrombi are best removed by gentle expression of the liquefied clot through a small incision made with a 21-gauge needle, no. 11 blade, or lancet (Fig. 8-3). A rocking action applied around the clot may aid in its expulsion. This should be

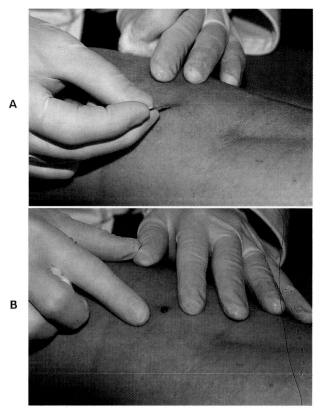

Fig. 8-3 Method for evacuation of a thrombosis in a 1-mm diameter reticular varicose vein 2 weeks after sclerotherapy. **A,** Small incision. **B,** Expelling clot (see text for details).

continued until all dark blood is removed. The art of this procedure is to find the right place to puncture, which is best perceived as a soft, fluctuating spot. If the thrombosis is in the deep dermis, the area should be marked, and 1% lidocaine can be infiltrated around the area to facilitate a less painful removal. Compression pads and/or stockings are then worn an additional 3 days to prevent further thrombosis formation and to aid in adherence of the opposing endothelial walls to establish effective endosclerosis.

An alternate technique for extraction of larger segments of thrombotic vein is to remove the thrombus with aspiration through a 16- or 18-gauge needle. This technique usually requires local infiltration with use of an anesthetic along the course of the thrombotic vessel.

Perchuk[76] raises the possibility of infection occurring from stab incisions. This danger was presumed to be caused by the presence of bacteria in varicose veins—a belief commonly held by physicians 40 to 50 years ago.[77,78] However, there have been no reports of infections occurring in patients treated with stab incisions into postsclerotherapy clots in the modern medical literature. This problem has not occurred in my practice, in which this procedure is used routinely.

Duration

Despite therapeutic attempts, pigmentation often lasts from 6 to 12 months.[17] Rarely pigmentation may last more than 1 year. Georgiev[11] estimates that 1% of his patients and Duffy[5] estimates that up to 10% of his patients have pigmentation lasting more than 1 year. In certain patients this pigmentation may be present over superficial varicosities and telangiectasias before sclerotherapy is performed.[11,14] Hyperpigmentation as a result of "physiologic" diapedesis of RBCs through fragile vessels is common in patients with venous stasis or over varicose veins. Therefore preoperative documentation, including photographs, may be beneficial during follow-up patient visits.

Prevention

Although never formally studied, apparently there is a decreased incidence of postsclerosis pigmentation after injection treatment of deep varicose veins. This may occur because sclerosis of vessels in the deeper dermis results in a more efficient reabsorption of extravasated heme, eventuating in a decreased incidence of overlying pigmentation.

Thibault and Wlodarczyk[38] recommend that patients avoid taking all iron supplements during the course of treatment and for 1 month after treatment. This presumably will decrease serum ferritin levels. Alternatively, patients' serum ferritin levels may be assessed before sclerotherapy to determine if iron chelation therapy is warranted. Obviously this latter recommendation awaits further study.

To prevent the development of pigmentation, sclerotherapy should produce limited endothelial necrosis and not total destruction with its resulting diapedesis of RBCs. This may be achieved by using meticulous technique, avoiding excessive injection pressures, selecting the appropriate solution concentration, and treating areas of reflux venous return in a proximal-to-distal manner.

Treatment

Treatment of pigmentation, once it occurs, is often unsuccessful. Because this pigmentation primarily is caused by hemosiderin deposition and not melanin incontinence, bleaching agents that affect melanocytic function are usually ineffective. Exfoliants (trichloroacetic acid) may hasten the apparent resolution of this pigmentation by decreasing the overlying cutaneous pigmentation, but they carry a risk of scarring, permanent hypopigmentation, and postinflammatory hyperpigmentation. However, some physicians have reported apparent success with this therapeutic modality.[79]

Effective treatments for this pigmentation have only rarely been reported. Chatard[14] has found that using light cryotherapy to exfoliate the epidermis and "evict the pigment" is helpful. I have not found cryotherapy useful in my practice.

Terezakis[80] has found the use of topical retinoic acid enhances resolution of the pigmentation. She speculates that retinoids enhance fibroblastic removal of hemosiderin. I have treated patients with topical tretinoin (Retin-A 0.1% Cream) who have pigmentation beyond 3 months. Although formal placebo control studies have not been completed, it appears this therapy may be effective. It does not appear to have any adverse sequelae and has the advantage of bringing the patient into active therapy.

A seemingly logical form of treatment would be chelation of the subcutaneous iron deposition. Myers[81] reported the use of a 150 mg/ml ointment of disodium ethylenediamine tetraacetic acid (EDTA) in the treatment of 10 patients with pigmentation after sclerotherapy or vein stripping or with pigmentation in chronic postphlebitic legs. He reported a consistent reduction in the shade of the pigmentation in every patient treated. Unfortunately, this was an uncontrolled study, and there have been no further reports of this form of treatment since its presentation in 1965. In my experience intradermal injections of deferoxamine in an attempt to cause chelation of the hemosiderin have not proved uniformly beneficial.

Graduated elastic compression with coadministration of the anabolic steroid stanozolol decreased pigmentation from lipodermatosclerosis in 34 legs of 23 patients who also had varicose veins.[82] There was no change in skin pigmentation when patients used graduated compression stockings alone. The authors suggest that stanozolol exerts its effect through reduction in perivascular fibrin from fibrinolytic enhancement. Unfortunately, additional studies have not been published to support these claims. In addition, compression alone improves lipodermatosclerotic skin changes, including hyperpigmentation (Partsch H, personal communication, 1992). Although it seems reasonable to promote wearing graduated support stockings after treatment, further studies are needed before recommending systemic stanozolol therapy.

Finally, laser treatment has been demonstrated as efficacious in 45%[18] to 69%[36] of patients with pigmentation of 12 or 6 months duration, respectively. Hemosiderin has an absorption spectrum that peaks at 410 to 415 nm, followed by a gradually sloping curve throughout the visible spectrum[83,84] (Fig. 8-4). The copper vapor (CV) laser at 511 nm in a continuous air-brush technique and the flashlamp-excited pulsed dye (FLPD) laser at 510 nm should interact relatively specifically with the hemosiderin absorption spectrum. Competition from oxygenated hemoglobin (peak absorption at 577 nm) should be low. But interaction with epidermal melanin, which has a higher absorption rate at these wavelengths, may be significant. These lasers are thought to result in physical fragmentation of pigment granules, which are later removed by phagocytosis. However, penetration of laser energy at 510 and 511 nm is limited to 1 mm below the granular layer (Anderson R, personal communication, 1991). Since hemosiderin may occur up to 2.8 mm below the granular layer, nonthermal effects may result in clinical resolution. An inflammatory reaction from thermal and/or photoacoustic effects may stimulate hemosiderin absorption. Although CV laser–treated pigmentation responded better than that treated with FLPD laser therapy, thermal relaxation times used by the latter laser system

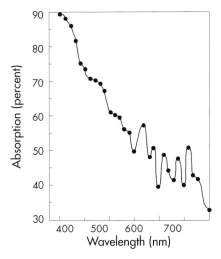

Fig. 8-4   Absorption spectra for hemosiderin (freshly frozen, average of two determinations). (From Wells CI and Wolken JJ: Nature 193:977, 1962.)

should be more selective. Further expanded studies should resolve this discrepancy.

The recommended treatment is "flashbulb therapy" or "chronotherapy." Since the majority of patients will have a resolution of pigmentation within 1 year, time and photographic documentation usually are very satisfactory for the understanding patient.

Temporary Swelling
Etiologic factors

Multiple factors are responsible for swelling of a treated area. These factors include changes in the pressure differential between the intravascular and perivascular space and changes in endothelial permeability. Edema is most common when varicose veins or telangiectasias below the ankle are treated. This relates both to the increase in gravitational intravascular pressure in this area and the relative sparsity of perivascular fascia at the ankle. Riddock[85] speculates that edema is caused by an unduly prolonged reflex spasm spreading to some of the subfascial (deep) veins. Reflex vasospasm is thought to increase proximal intravascular pressures.

The extent of edema is also related to the strength of the sclerosing solutions used. This result apparently correlates with the degree of perivascular inflammation produced by the sclerosing solution. The by-products of inflammation, including release of histamine and various mediators, increase endothelial permeability. In addition to the degree of inflammation induced by sclerotherapy itself, the innate sensitivity of a patient's perivascular mast cells (possibly related to their atopic or asthma history), concomitant medications that may promote or inhibit mast cell degranulation (e.g., corticosteroids, antihistamines, nonsteroidal antiinflammatory agents), and previous exposure sensitivity to the sclerosing agent may all contribute to edema. Duffy[5] and Goldman[9] estimate the occurrence of pedal edema as 2% to 5%. They do not note a difference in the incidence of pedal edema between HS and POL use.

Edema may also occur if compression is not applied in a graduated manner. Edema may be produced when application of localized pressure on the thigh over an injected vein is attempted with the addition of a tape dressing over or under a graduated compression stocking. If patients are informed of the possibility of the production of a tourniquet effect by the extra compression, they can be advised to remove the dressing at the first sign of edema distal to the dressing.

Prevention and treatment

Two techniques may limit temporary swelling. First, limit perivascular inflammation. Ankle edema occurs much less frequently if the quantity of sclerosing solution is limited to 1 ml per ankle. Application of pharmacologic agents either topically or systemically may be beneficial in patients with excessive postsclerotherapy edema. Methylprednisolone acts both to stabilize mast cell membranes, preventing histamine release, and to exert part of its antiinflammatory action directly on the endothelial cell, rendering it less responsive to various mediators.[86] Ruscus extract inhibits macromolecular permeability, increasing the effect of histamine in the hamster cheek pouch model.[87] This effect is due to stabilization of endothelial pore size. Beta-receptor agonists such as terbutaline and theophylline counteract histamine-induced venular permeability. This effect also occurs with verapamil and glucocorticoids.[88]

A second method for limiting the degree of pedal or ankle edema is to apply a graduated pressure stocking routinely after injections in this area. A recent study on the use of 30 to 40 mm Hg compression hosiery in the treatment of leg telangiectasia found a significant decrease in the incidence of ankle edema when a 30 to 40 mm Hg graduated compression stocking was worn for 3 days after sclerotherapy.[89]

Telangiectatic Matting

The new appearance of previously unnoticed fine red telangiectasias occurs in a number of patients after either sclerotherapy or surgical ligation of varicose veins and leg telangiectasias (Fig. 8-5). This occurrence has been termed *flares* by Arenander and Lindhagen,[90] *distal angioplasia* by Terezakis,[91] and *telangiectatic matting* (TM) by Duffy.[5] The reported incidence varies from 5%[9] to 75%.[49,90] Two retrospective analyses of 2120 and 7200 patients with leg telangiectasias each reported a 16% incidence.[10,92] This incidence has been confirmed in a random sample of 113 female sclerotherapy patients.[40] The incidence of TM increased with increasing patient age in one report,[90] but this correlation was not seen in another report.[92] Although most authors do not comment on a sexual predisposition,[5] I have seen the development of TM in only one male patient with leg telangiectasias. Because of the small number of men seeking treatment, an accurate appraisal of the sexual incidence of TM cannot be stated.

TM may appear anywhere on the leg. One detailed study found that most TM occurred on the medial ankle and the medial and lateral calves.[90] However, TM has also been reported to occur more frequently on the thighs.[93]

Etiologic factors

Postsclerosis TM was first described in the 1960s by Ouvry and Davy.[94] They observed that the incidence of matting was proportional to the degree of inflammation and thrombus formation. The etiology of TM is unknown but is believed to be related either to angiogenesis[5,95] or to a dilation of existing subclinical blood vessels by the promotion of collateral flow through arteriovenous anastomoses.[95,96] One or both of these mechanisms may occur. Terezakis[91] believes that TM refers to the "survival of the fittest," with new blood vessels developing after occlusion of neighboring vessels. Experimentally, a number of etiologic factors can initiate or contribute to angiogenesis (see box on p. 293).

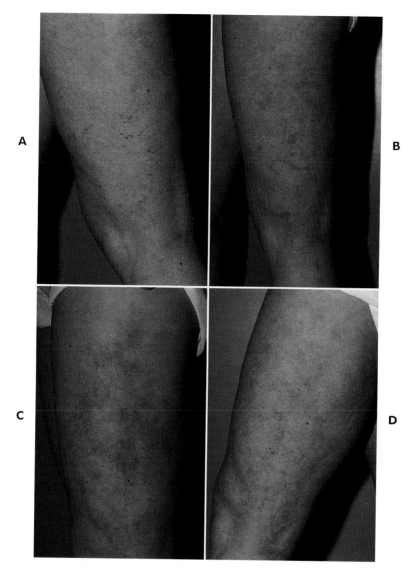

Fig. 8-5 Typical telangiectatic matting (TM) in a 36-year-old woman. **A,** Before sclerotherapy treatment, left lateral thigh. **B,** 3 months after treatment of reticular veins with POL 0.75%. **C,** 6 weeks after treating telangiectatic veins with POL 0.5%; note development of extensive TM. **D,** 6 weeks later; note complete resolution of TM without treatment. (From Goldman MP: Adverse sequelae of sclerotherapy treatment of varicose and telangiectatic leg veins. In Bergan JJ and Goldman MP, editors: Varicose veins: diagnosis and treatment, St. Louis, 1993, Quality Medical Publishing, Inc.)

ANGIOGENIC FACTORS

Obstruction of blood flow—thrombosis, anoxia

Disruption of endothelial continuity

Heparin secretion by mast cells

Endothelial leakage of fibrinogen

Inflammation

Estrogen receptors

Probable risk factors for the development of TM in patients with leg telangiectasia include obesity, use of estrogen-containing hormones, pregnancy, and a family history of telangiectatic veins. Excessive standing does not appear to influence the incidence of TM.[92] Excessive postsclerotherapy inflammation may also predispose toward development of TM.

The development of new vessels can occur in 2 to 3 days. Observations of mammalian systems have demonstrated the development of a vein from a capillary, an artery from a vein, a vein from an artery, or from either back to a capillary.[97,98] In coronary vessels increased numbers of arterioles and capillaries occur within 1 week after injury.[99]

Angiogenesis. Angiogenesis is a complex process in which capillary blood vessels grow in an ordered sequence of events. Angiogenic factors either act directly on the endothelium to stimulate locomotion and mitosis or indirectly by mobilization of host helper cells (mast cells and macrophages) with release of endothelial growth factors (see below). When a new capillary sprout grows from the side of a venule, endothelial cells degrade basement membrane, migrate toward an angiogenic source, proliferate, form a lumen, join the tips of two sprouts to generate a capillary loop, and manufacture new basement membrane.[100] Obstruction of outflow from a vessel (which is the end result of successful sclerotherapy) is one of the most important factors contributing to angiogenesis.[101] Initiation of angiogenesis also follows disruption of endothelial continuity or intercellular contact. This contact results in endothelial cell sprouting and migration.[102]

In addition, endothelial damage leads to the release of heparin and other mast cell factors that both promote the dilation of existing blood vessels and stimulate angiogenesis.[103-106] Finally, neovascularization may be promoted by numerous other angiogenic factors, including but not limited to heparin-binding fibroblast growth factor (FGF),[11,107,108] tumor necrosis factor (TNF),[104,109,110] platelet-derived endothelial mitogen,[111] endothelial cell growth factor (ECGF),[112] and other macrophage-derived growth factors.[113-115] These factors and many others are released from perivascular mast cells.[116] FGF is released at cell death and is essential for the stimulation of angiogenesis and wound repair.[117,118] Thus sclerotherapy through endothelial damage promotes both the release of endothelial angiogenic factors and perivascular mast cell angiogenic factors that provide multiple mechanisms for new blood vessel formation to occur. Indeed, it is remarkable that a greater incidence of postsclerosis TM does not occur.

Heparin both binds to endothelial cells and promotes endothelial proliferation in vitro and produces angiogenesis in vivo through an affinity for growth factors.[103] Heparin potentiates angiogenesis in vivo by stimulating endothelial cell plasminogen activator, endothelial cell chemotaxis, or both.[119] Therefore it is interesting to speculate that the high incidence of TM reported by Duffy[5] may be related to his use of heparin in the HS sclerotherapy solution. Bodian[93] notes a 10% incidence of TM in his patients with the use of HS saline solution without the addition of heparin. Weiss and Weiss[3] note an 11% incidence of TM in their patient population treated with HS solution without heparin.

Sclerotherapy produces some degree of perivascular inflammation.[20] Inflammation may be considered a hypermetabolic state, with new vessel growth occurring as a result of increased metabolic demand.[120] In addition, mast cells are found in increased numbers in inflammatory states such as allergic contact dermatitis or delayed hypersensitivity reactions.[121] Since mast cell heparin is one factor responsible for capillary endothelial cell migration,[103] in an attempt to decrease angiogenic stimuli one should try to limit the degree of inflammation as much as possible. This is achieved by choosing an appropriate solution concentration for each type of vessel treated and limiting the quantity of solution to the amount that will not produce excessive endothelial damage. This was confirmed by Weiss and Weiss[40] who found that in a random sample of 113 sclerotherapy patients, 10 developed TM with injection of POL 1% into vessels less than 1 mm in diameter. When POL 0.5% was used for subsequent treatments in these patients, none developed further areas of TM.

As noted previously, assuming a role for the perivascular mast cell in the etiology of TM is intriguing. With aging, a 50% decrease in cutaneous mast cells occurs, associated with a 35% decrease in subepidermal venules.[53] Thus if TM develops predominantly from mast cell factors, its incidence should be decreased in the elderly. This has not been noticed in two studies.[90,92] Cutaneous mast cells usually occur perivascularly, with a distribution ranging from 7000/mm[5] to 20,000/mm.[5,122-125] This represents 0.2% to 0.7% of normal skin. In telangiectatic macules associated with mastocytosis, mast cells account for 3.5% ($\pm$1.8 SEM) of cells, whereas telangiectasias not associated with mastocytosis have a mast cell volume of 0.4% ($\pm$0.1 SEM).[126] An analysis of mast cell content in TM lesions is needed.

Ouvry and Davy[94] and Mantse[127] note a decreased incidence of TM when the pressure of injection is minimized and the extent of dispersion of sclerosing solution is limited to a 1-cm diameter with each injection. These techniques may minimize the degree of perivascular inflammation with sclerotherapy. However, these procedural cautions are discounted by Duffy[5] who advocates the injection of up to 1.5 ml of solution through each injection site and by Lary[128] who advocates injection of up to 3 ml per injection site. Duffy[5] has reported that TM occurs in 20% to 35% of his patients. Lary[128] does not remark on the development of TM in his patients.

Estrogen may play a role in the development of TM. It appears that there may be an increased incidence of persistent TM among patients taking systemic estrogen preparations.[5,40,92] Weiss and Weiss[40] found a relative risk of 3.17 (P <.003) for development of TM while patients were receiving exogenous estrogen. The mechanism for promotion of TM by estrogen is speculative. However, estrogens have been implicated in modulating mast cell responses.[129]

Estrogen receptors have been found in a number of tumors, including angioma of the nose, soft-tissue sarcoma, breast carcinoma, endometrial carcinoma, and unilateral nevoid telangiectasia syndrome. Estrogens also play a role in the development of vascular tissues. In vitro estrogen and estradiol have promoted endothelial cell migration and proliferation.[130] Spider angiomas develop during pregnancy and resolve after delivery.[31,132] Spider nevi also occur in patients with hepatic cirrhosis associated with elevated serum estradiol levels.[133] In addition, Davis and Duffy[92] have reported on the virtual disappearance of leg telangiectasia and TM in a 51-year-old woman with estrogen-receptor–positive breast carcinoma after initiation of antiestrogen therapy with tamoxifen citrate (Nolvadex). However, Sadick and Niedt[134] could not demonstrate estrogen receptors in a number of biopsy specimens from leg telangiectasias. An evaluation of estrogen receptors in TM lesions is needed. Since estrogen receptors have been implicated in the promotion of angiogenesis,[135] it may be prudent, albeit premature, to withhold estrogen therapy during sclerotherapy treatment.

Prevention and treatment

Regardless of the etiology of TM, since patients come for treatment to have leg telangiectasia eliminated, it is disconcerting for the sclerotherapist to produce new areas of telangiectasia. Therefore any technique that may limit this side effect, such as limiting the injection blanch to 1 to 2 cm, should be used. Further recommendations await further studies. Unfortunately, despite one's best efforts, TM will occur in a significant percentage of patients. Fortunately, TM usually resolves spontaneously over 3 to 12 months.[5,40] It has been estimated that 10% to 20% of patients will have permanent TM.[92,136]

Treatment modalities for TM are limited. Reinjection with hypertonic solutions may be helpful. Because of the extremely small diameter of these vessels, use of a 33-gauge needle ($^1/_2$-cc disposable insulin syringe) is helpful. Injection of any feeding reticular veins or venulectases is also helpful. In addition, the pulsed dye laser is useful in treating these vessels.[137] Unfortunately, even with all of these therapeutic modalities, TM may be resistant to treatment.

In the future, modifications of present treatment techniques may minimize this complication. Experimentally, protamine blocks the ability of mast cells and heparin to stimulate migration of capillary endothelial cells.[138] Protamine also prevents the neovascularization induced by an inflammatory agent when it is applied locally or given systemically.[139] It has no effect on established capillaries that are not proliferating.[140] In addition, beta-cyclodextrin tetradeasulfate administered with cortexolone is a potent inhibitor of angiogenesis.[141] Thus preventive topical preparations or the use of additives with the sclerosing solution may limit the development of TM.

Systemic treatment before or during sclerotherapy may also be helpful in limiting TM. Through its ability to suppress the synthesis of TNF, pentoxifylline (Trental) may minimize angiogenesis.[142,143] Inhibition of mast cell mediators with the cell wall stabilizing medication Ketotifen may also be useful for preventing TM, edema, and localized urticaria. Ketotifen, a benzocycloheptathiophene derivative, has H_1 antihistaminic properties in addition to decreasing mast cell mediator release.[144,145] Ketotifen may also exert its effect by depleting mediators in cutaneous mast cells and so require multiple doses over a few days to have maximal effect.[146] Its clinical beneficial effect in patients with chronic idiopathic urticaria, cutaneous mastocytosis, and urticaria pigmentosa has been established.[146-150] Unfortunately, the pharmaceutical company in the United States, Sandoz, has no plans to release this agent in the near future (personal communication, 1994).

Pain

Since a great number of patients who come for treatment of cosmetic leg telangiectasia require multiple treatment sessions, each consisting of numerous injections, an attempt should be made to minimize the unpleasantness of the procedure.

Prevention

Certain areas are slightly more painful, especially the ankles, upper medial thighs, and medial knees. Two variables that can be adjusted to minimize pain are the type and size of the needle used for injection and the type of sclerosing solution used.

Type and size of needle. Using the smallest possible diameter needle for injection is the most obvious way to minimize injection pain. Another factor to consider is the shape of the needle bevel. Needles, even those of the same gauge, are shaped differently and may or may not be coated with a layer of silicone. Acutely tapered needles, especially when tribeveled, and those that are silicone coated usually are perceived by the patient as less painful in my experience. Finally, with some agents that are inherently painful to inject (e.g., hypertonic solutions), pain can be minimized with slow infusion.[3,5] Slow injection produces a slower distention of tissue and may minimize endothelial cell separation, which may decrease perivascular nerve stimulation. Therefore choice of needle type and size is important in minimizing the pain of injection.

Type of sclerosing solution. The second method for reducing pain is to choose the least painful sclerosing solution. Hypertonic solutions are notorious for causing pain on injection. The cramping pain that may develop after correct IV injection usually occurs a few minutes after injection. Weiss and Weiss[3] report that 72% of their patients injected with HS 23.4% experience pain that lasts less than 5 minutes; 4.5% of patients have pain that lasts more than 5 minutes. This pain probably occurs at the time the hypertonic solution reaches the nerve fibers of the adventitia, either through the wall of the vein or through the capillaries. Subsequently, because of stimulation of sympathetic perivenous nerve fibers, an active contraction of the muscle occurs that may also produce a cramping pain.[151] In addition, vascular spasm caused by direct effects of the hypertonic solution itself may occur.

Hypertonic solutions also produce muscle cramping after injection. With the injection of 5 to 10 ml of Heparsal (20% HS plus heparin, 10 U/ml) per injection site into varicose veins, Chou et al.[152] noted that 16% of 310 patients could not tolerate the pain associated with the procedure. Duffy[5] estimates that 82% of his patients treated with HS note moderate cramping or aching. This can be limited somewhat by keeping the volumes injected to 0.1 ml or less per injection site and by massaging the area immediately after injection. Also adding lidocaine to the sclerosing solution may lessen muscle cramping and allow placement of additional injections into the same area with less pain.[5,6] However, the addition of lidocaine to a hypertonic solution is associated with two problems. First, lidocaine if acidified (in a multidose bottle) is painful during the injection. Therefore nonacidified lidocaine (found in single dose "cardiac" ampules) should be used as an additive. Second, the addition of lidocaine gives the sclerosing solution the potential to produce an allergic reaction (discussed below).

Chromated glycerin solutions are also painful during injection and may produce mild muscle cramping if more than 1 ml of solution is injected into a single vein.[45]

Two relatively painless solutions are POL and STS. STS has the advantage of being painful only when it is injected into perivascular tissues, thereby providing a noticeable check on inadvertent perivascular injection. POL is painless with both intradermal and IV injection. Therefore one does not have the additional sign of pain to ensure accurate placement of the sclerosing solution. In a double-blind comparison of STS, HS, and POL, patients preferred injection with POL.[153] Finally, despite optimal technique and the use of mild sclerosing agents, posttreatment soreness for 1 or 2 weeks after injection occurs in 20% of patients.[5] With the use of nonosmotic sclerosing solutions and the use of graduated compression stockings after treatment, I have *not* seen soreness in most patients after treatment. If patients do complain of soreness, the cause usually is thrombosed and/or inflamed vessels. Although relatively painless to inject, STS does produce a dull ache a few minutes after injection. This ache resolves in a few minutes. POL does not produce posttreatment aching.

Localized Urticaria

Localized urticaria occurs after injection of all sclerosing solutions (Fig. 8-6). It is usually transient (lasting approximately 30 minutes) and is probably the result of

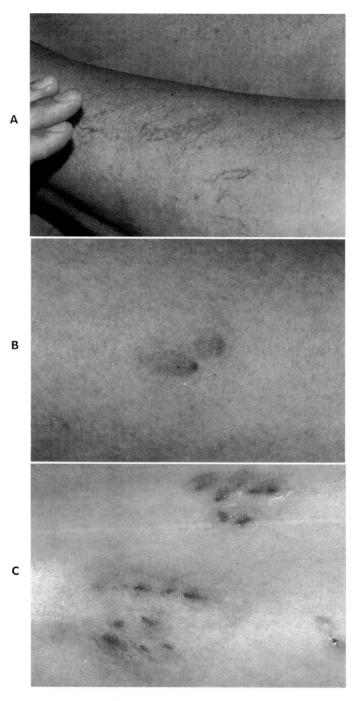

Fig. 8-6 **A,** Urtication immediately after sclerotherapy with HS 23.4%. **B,** Urtication immediately after sclerotherapy with STS 0.1%. **C,** Urtication immediately after sclerotherapy with POL 0.5%.

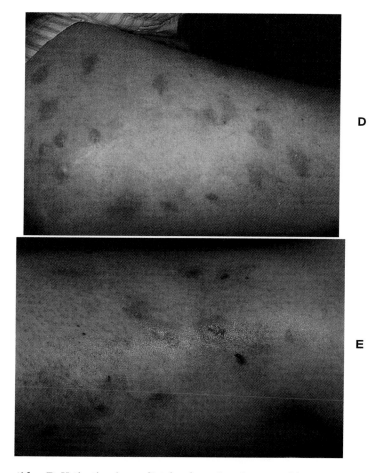

Fig. 8-6, cont'd   D, Urtication immediately after sclerotherapy with CG. **E,** Urtication immediately after sclerotherapy with Sclerodex.

endothelial irritation. Localized urticaria is not likely an allergic response since it occurs even after injection of 23.4% unadulterated HS. It is probably related to the release of endothelial factors after these cells have been destroyed by the sclerosing solution. Alternatively, it may occur as the earliest manifestation of perivascular inflammation, again through release of endothelial- or platelet-derived factors or perivascular mast cell degranulation[154] (see previous discussion in sections on pigmentation and edema).

Approximately 40% of patients studied by Norris, Carlin, and Ratz[49] described temporary itching after injections with POL regardless of drug dosage. Duffy[5] reports an almost 100% occurrence of urticaria with injection of either POL or HS-heparin-lidocaine solutions. The urtication is usually more intense when more concentrated solutions are used.[5,9] Urtication may also be more intense with repeat injection sessions, especially when POL or STS is used.

Treatment

In my experience localized urticaria and itching can be diminished by applying topical steroids immediately after injection and by limiting the injection quantity per injection site. This is particularly helpful in patients who will wear a graduated support stocking after treatment.

Tape Compression Blister

The relatively uncommon cutaneous lesion, tape compression blister (Fig. 8-7), occurs when a tape dressing is applied in an area of tissue movement and/or on thin elderly skin. The blister usually appears as a flaccid fluid-filled sack overlying normal-appearing skin. It is usually not associated with induration or erythema of the adjacent skin. Common sites of occurrence are the posterior calf, medial thigh, and popliteal fossae.

Blisters may occur with the use of any tape but appear more commonly when one uses 3M Microfoam tape (3M Medical Surgical Division, St. Paul, Minn.) as opposed to hypoallergenic paper tape (Dermilite II, Johnson & Johnson, New Brunswick, NJ) over foam pads or cotton balls, probably because of the greater adhesiveness of the Microfoam tape. In addition, Microfoam tape is usually placed over the foam dressing with a slight amount of tension, thus increasing the tension on either end of the tape. Blistering is also more common in the summer months when the weather is hotter and in elderly patients with thinner, more fragile skin.

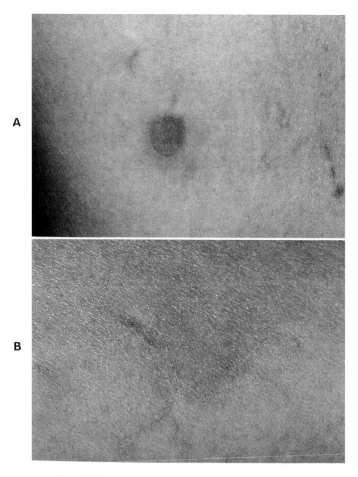

Fig. 8-7 **A,** Superficial blister that developed 1 week after sclerotherapy treatment; compression of the treated area was produced with an STD pad overlaid with Microfoam tape and a 30 to 40 mm Hg graduated thigh-length compression stocking (seen pulled down below the knee). **B,** Complete resolution 3 weeks later.

The only problem with blistering is that it must be distinguished from early cutaneous necrosis, cutaneous infection, or an allergic reaction. Early cutaneous necrosis may appear as a superficial blister. In this situation the underlying and adjacent tissue is usually indurated and erythematous. Bullous impetigo can also have a similar physical appearance. With it the blister is usually overlying warm, erythematous skin. If not warned beforehand, patients may think that the blister is the result of an allergy to the sclerosing solution. A detailed explanation of the cause of the blister is usually required before treatment can continue.

Prevention

If compression pads will be used under graduated stockings in a patient susceptible to blistering, a Tubigrip tubular support bandage (Seton Products, Inc., Montgomeryville, Penn.) can be used over the pad to hold it in place while the stocking is being applied. Although somewhat costly, this dressing (similar to a net dressing used in burn patients) helps prevent blister formation. (It can also be used in patients with allergies to tape.)

Treatment

Resolution of the blister occurs within 1 or 2 weeks without any adverse sequelae. To aid healing and prevent infection of the denuded skin, the use of an occlusive hydroactive dressing such as Duoderm (Convatec, Princeton, NJ) is helpful. Occlusive dressings may also help alleviate any pain associated with the blister.

Tape Compression Folliculitis

Occlusion of any hairy area can promote the development of folliculitis (Fig. 8-8). If they do not have secondary alopecia associated with chronic venous insufficiency, men seeking treatment for varicose veins usually have hairy legs. If a tape dressing is placed over foam or cotton ball pads under a graduated compression stocking, a follicular inflammation or infection may occur. Folliculitis is more likely to occur in the summer months or when patients are active and perspire under the dressing.

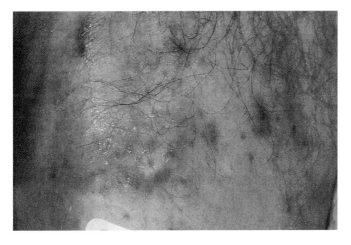

Fig. 8-8 Folliculitis apparent 7 days after sclerotherapy; compression of the treated area was produced with STD foam pads overlaid with Microfoam tape.

Treatment

Treatment consists of removal of the occlusive dressing and application of topical treatment with an antibacterial soap such as chlorhexidine gluconate (Hibiclens Antimicrobial Skin Cleanser) or a topical antibiotic gel such as erythromycin 2% (Erygel Topical Gel) or clindamycin phosphate topical solution 1% (Cleocin T). The folliculitis usually resolves within a few days. Only rarely will use of systemic antibiotics be necessary.

Recurrence

Recurrence of sclerotherapy-treated vessels has been estimated to occur in 20% to nearly 100% of leg telangiectasias at 5-year follow-up.[155] Recanalization of initially thrombosed leg veins is procedure dependent. The larger the extent of intravascular thrombosis, the greater is the likelihood of recanalization of the thrombosis during organization.[156,157] The recanalization of injected varices without subsequent compression or with inadequate compression is caused by clot contraction and the formation of sinuses that may become lined with endothelium; central clot liquefaction and the formation of vascular tunnels through the thrombosis; formation of vascular organization of the thrombosis and collateral vessel formation of the newly formed capillaries; and formation of peripheral sinuses filled with sludged blood (Figs. 8-9 through 8-11).[157,158] Therefore the most important factor in preventing recurrence is the limiting of intravascular thrombosis.

Treatment

Tournay[159] was the first physician to stress the importance of postinjection removal of blood clots in 1938. The importance of draining these postsclerotherapy thrombi has since been emphasized by Sigg,[160] Pratt,[161] and Hobbs.[162] Orbach[156] advocates the compulsive removal of all postinjection clots, both fluctuating and hard cords. After administration of local anesthesia, he uses a no. 11 blade to make an incision over the vein and a von Graefe cataract knife to dissect the clot

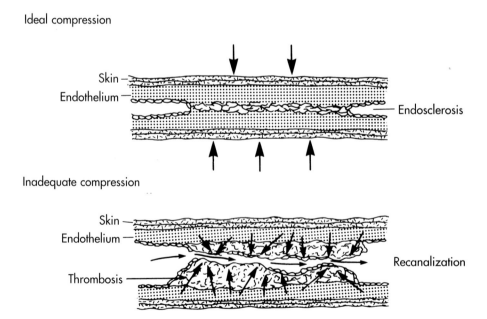

Fig. 8-9 Diagrammatic representation of recanalization of a varicose vein through a sclerotherapy-induced thrombosis. (Redrawn from Wenner L: Vasa 15:180, 1986.)

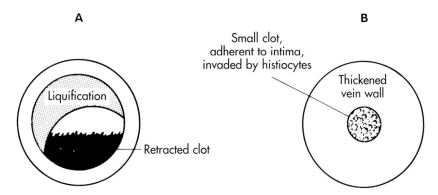

Fig. 8-10   Diagrammatic representation of a histologic study from Fegan WG[158] demonstrating the appearance of a varicose vein after sclerotherapy treatment. **A**, Without compression. **B**, With continuous compression for 6 weeks. (From Orbach EJ: Vasa 3:475, 1974.)

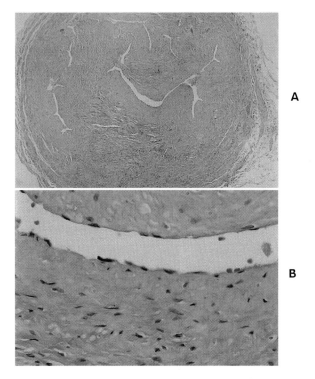

Fig. 8-11   This 50-year-old male had a varicose greater saphenous vein (GSV) fed by an incompetent Hunterian perforator vein without evidence of saphenofemoral junction (SFJ) reflux. The vein recurred 1 year after successful closure with 2 ml of STS 3% and was subsequently removed with ambulatory phlebectomy. **A**, Appearance of recanalized sclerosed vein (Hematoxylin-eosin, ×10). **B**, At ×400 magnification, endothelial slits are lining a newly recanalized channel.

completely from the vein wall. This is followed by continuous compression until resolution of the vein occurs.

With proper technique, recurrence of varicose veins only rarely occurs. A biopsy study of six patients with "recurrence" of previously treated veins demonstrated that the veins thought to have recurred were in reality new varicose veins.[163] When high recurrence rates are reported, the patients have usually been treated with minimal compression.[156] For example, in one recent study of 310 patients, 83% required reinjection of a treated varicosity. These patients received only 48 hours of compression with elastic bandages.[152]

Unlike recanalization through a varicose vein cord, recanalization is not common through a sclerosed telangiectasia. Posttreatment histologic studies have demonstrated only fibrosis in an area treated with sclerotherapy.[4]

Stress-Related Symptoms
Vasovagal reflex

The vasovagal reflex is a common adverse sequela of any surgical or invasive procedure. It has been estimated to occur in 1% of patients during sclerotherapy[164] and is more frequent when using the technique of Fegan or Sigg.[165] With these latter two techniques, 21- to 25-gauge needles are inserted while the patient is sitting or standing, and blood is allowed to flow freely from the punctured vein. Duffy,[5] who performs sclerotherapy with 30-gauge needles in reclining patients, estimates the incidence of vasovagal reactions as 0.001%. Interestingly, the percentage of men who experience this response far exceeds the percentage of women.

Vasovagal reactions have typical clinical findings. The usual symptoms include light-headedness, nausea, and sweating. The patient may also experience shortness of breath and palpitations. Syncope rarely occurs but usually provokes the most concern in the physician and staff. Vasovagal reactions are most often preceded by painful injection but may occur from the patient's seeing the needle or smelling the sclerosing solution.

Prevention. The main concern in a vasovagal reaction is that the patient will fall and be injured. Therefore both the nurse and physician should watch the patient closely for signs of restlessness and excessive perspiration. All patients should be warned to sit down if they become dizzy. It is also helpful when needle placement is performed on a standing patient for the patient to hold onto an arm rail or other support. All such reactions are easily reversible when the patient assumes the supine or Trendelenburg position. Preventive measures consist of recommending that the patient eat a light meal before the appointment, maintaining good ventilation in the treatment room, and maintaining constant communication with the patient during the procedure.

The physician must recognize the vasovagal response in a patient and not assume that an allergic reaction is occurring. If subcutaneous epinephrine is given in the mistaken belief that an anaphylactic reaction is occurring, the symptoms will become both exaggerated and obscured. This only further confuses the clinical situation and adds to patient apprehension about further treatment sessions.

Underlying medical disease

More serious stress-induced problems include exacerbation of certain underlying medical diseases. Patients with a history of asthma may experience wheezing, which can be treated with bronchodilator therapy such as metaproterenol sulfate (Alupent, Proventil) or over-the-counter epinephrine bitartrate or metered dose inhalers (Primatene).

Patients with cardiovascular disease may develop angina, which is treatable with sublingual nitroglycerin tablets. Urticaria is easily treated with an oral antihistamine but may be a sign of systemic allergy. Therefore the use of the sclerosing agent in future treatment sessions should be carefully evaluated. It is intriguing that urticaria and periorbital edema have occurred even with injection of unadulterated HS solution.[166] This may be related to histamine release from irritated perivascular mast cells. Finally, triggering of frequent migraine headaches has also occurred after sclerotherapy.[5]

Localized Hirsutism

Localized hypertrichosis developing after sclerotherapy with the use of multiple sclerosing agents has been described. The etiology is believed to be the result of an improved cutaneous oxygen content stimulating increased hair growth or of a long-standing low-grade inflammatory reaction that increases vascularity. In support of this phenomenon, patients with chronic venous insufficiency have been reported to have developed localized hair growth after surgical treatment.[167]

Hair growth at the site of injection has been described in three patients treated with STS.[168] All patients were given injections of 1 to 6 ml of STS over 5 to 10 sessions. Localized hair growth developed 4 to 7 months after the last injection. The site of hair growth was related to the area of skin most damaged by venous incompetence. Weissberg[169] has also reported on the development of localized hirsutism in one of 62 patients. The hair growth occurred at the site of injection 1 month after treatment. It lasted 4 months and then subsided. Sclerotherapy with polyiodinated iodine has also been associated with hypertrichosis at the injection site in three cases.[163]

COMPLICATIONS
Cutaneous Necrosis
Etiology

Cutaneous necrosis may occur with the injection of any sclerosing agent even under ideal circumstances and does not necessarily represent physician error (Fig. 8-12). Fortunately, its occurrence is both rare and usually of limited sequelae. Its cause may be the result of (1) extravasation of a sclerosing solution into the perivascular tissues, (2) injection into a dermal arteriole or an arteriole feeding into a telangiectatic or varicose vein, (3) a reactive vasospasm of the vessel, or (4) excessive cutaneous pressure created by compression techniques.

Extravasation

Extravasation of caustic sclerosing solutions may directly destroy tissue. The final clinical appearance of the skin may not be apparent for several days; thus therapeutic intervention must be undertaken as soon as possible in all cases. With certain extravasation injuries, the formation of small epidermal blisters does not predict a partial-thickness injury but may precede eventual full-thickness necrosis.[170]

During injection of an abnormal vein or telangiectasia, even the most adept physician may inadvertently inject a small quantity of sclerosing solution into the perivascular tissue (Fig. 8-13). A tiny amount of sclerosing solution may be left in the tissue when the needle is withdrawn, and sclerosing solution may leak out of the injected vessel, which has been traumatized by multiple or through-and-through needle punctures. Rarely, the injection of a strong sclerosing solution into a fragile vessel may lead to endothelial necrosis and rupture, producing a

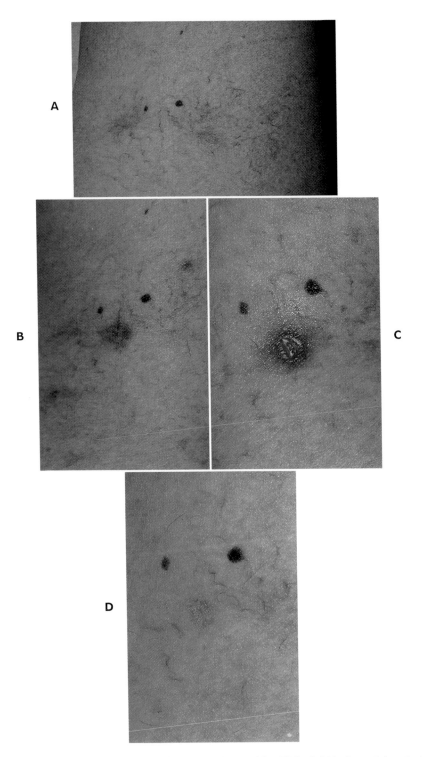

Fig. 8-12 Cutaneous necrosis after injection with POL 0.5% into telangiectasia. **A**, Preinjection. **B**, Early atrophie blanche 10 days after injection. **C**, 5 weeks after injection superficial ulceration is present. **D**, Complete resolution occurred in 12 weeks; clinical appearance 24 weeks after injection.

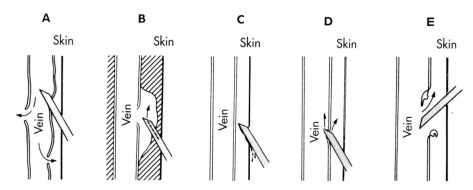

Fig. 8-13   Mechanism for extravasation of sclerosing solution. **A,** Extravasation through multiple needle puncture holes. **B,** Extravasation from injection of sclerosing solution after slight withdrawal of the needle. **C,** Extravasation of sclerosing solution along needle shaft. **D,** Extravasation from injection with needle bevel both in and out of the vein. **E,** Extravasation through excessive destruction of the vein wall. (Redrawn from Biegeleisen HI: Varicose veins, related diseases, and sclerotherapy: a guide for practitioners, Montreal, 1984, Eden Press.)

"blow-out" of the vessel and perivascular extravasation of sclerosing solution (Fig. 8-14). Therefore injection technique is an important but not foolproof factor in avoiding this complication even under optimal circumstances.

Sclerosing solutions vary in the degree of cellular necrosis they produce. If minimal tissue necrosis is caused by a sclerosing agent, it may even be suitable for perivascular injection in the treatment of telangiectatic mats whose vessels cannot be cannulated even with a 33-gauge needle.

Hyperosmotic agents with an osmolality greater than that of serum (281 to 289 mOsm/L) can cause tissue damage as a result of osmotic factors. Epidermal necrosis has even occurred from extravasation of solutions containing 10% dextrose.[171] HS 23.4% is a caustic sclerosing agent as demonstrated in intradermal injection experiments. Clinically, small punctate spots of superficial epidermal damage occur at points of injection, especially when a small bleb of the solution escapes from the vein. However, subcutaneous injection of up to 1 ml of HS 23.4% (by mistake) in lieu of lidocaine into the neck or cheek has been reported to result in no adverse sequelae.[172] In this situation cutaneous necrosis was most likely avoided by rapid physiologic dilution of HS. Alternatively, dermal tissue may be more resistant to the caustic effects of hypertonic solutions. However, the increasing frequency of cutaneous necrosis occurring after extravasation of inadvertent subcutaneous injection of HS has moved the Department of Health and Human Services and the product manufacturer (American Regent Laboratories, Inc.) to recommend that storage of HS be only in pharmacies where all dilutions would be performed before dispensing. This would eliminate the possibility of an iatrogenic medication error outside the pharmacy (Mary Helenek, American Regent Laboratories, Inc., written communication, May 1990). It is recommended that storage of HS be in a location separate from other injectable solutions to avoid this potential complication.

Experimentally, POL apparently is minimally toxic to subcutaneous tissue. Although some physicians advocate the use of intradermal POL 0.5% to treat tiny telangiectatic leg veins,[173,174] POL in sufficient concentration will cause cutaneous necrosis. Solutions of POL greater than 1.0% may produce superficial necrosis with intradermal injection.[173] This unfortunately occurred with the mistaken

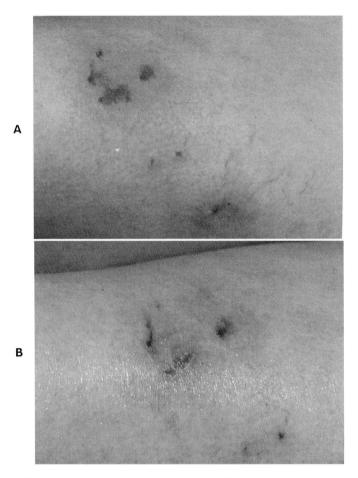

Fig. 8-14 Cutaneous necrosis after injection of STS 0.5%. **A,** Immediately after injection. Note "hyperemic burn reaction." **B,** Necrotic epidermis 2 weeks after injection.

injection of 0.1 ml POL 5% solution into a leg telangiectasia 0.2 mm in diameter in my practice. This injection resulted in extensive overlying cutaneous necrosis that took 8 weeks to heal. Therefore POL is not without the risk of cutaneous necrosis if a strong enough concentration is injected.

Glycerin or chromated glycerin (CG) solutions have not been reported to produce cutaneous necrosis with extravasation. Duffy (personal communication, 1992) has shown that injection of "full strength" CG will not produce cutaneous necrosis when it is injected into the mid-dermis. Histologic examination of his patient showed no evidence of dermal or epidermal damage.

Even when sclerotherapy is performed with expert technique, using the safest sclerosing solutions and concentrations, cutaneous ulceration may occur (see Figs. 8-12 and 8-15). Therefore it appears that extravasation of caustic sclerosing solutions alone is not totally responsible for this complication.

Arteriolar injection

De Faria and Moraes[175] have observed that one in 26 leg telangiectasias is associated with a dermal arteriole. It is my opinion that inadvertent injection into or near this communication is the most common cause of cutaneous ulcerations.

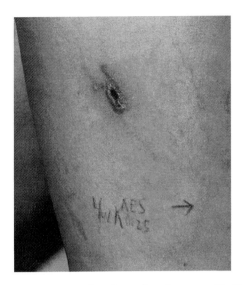

Fig. 8-15   Cutaneous necrosis 6 weeks after sclerotherapy with POL 0.25%. Note that 2 ml of solution was injected into a feeder vein approximately 10 cm distal to the necrotic area.

POL has been injected intradermally to effect sclerosis of TM in my practice without the development of cutaneous ulceration, even with the injection of 0.5 ml of a 0.75% solution. However, I have noted the development of 3- to 6-mm diameter ulcerations in approximately 0.0001% of injections with POL 0.5%. Five consecutive ulcerations that appeared over the course of 12 months were excised. In these patients each cutaneous ulceration developed as the result of the occlusion of the feeding dermal arteriole. This produced a classic wedge-shaped arterial ulceration (Fig. 8-16). The Australian Polidocanol Open Clinical Trial at 2 years reported 43 ulcers on 32 legs after sclerotherapy treatment of varicose and telangiectatic leg veins on 12,544 legs for an incidence of 0.23%.[176] Therefore it appears that this complication may be unavoidable to some extent.

Vasospasm

Rarely after injection of the sclerosing solution an immediate porcelain-white appearance to the skin is noted at the site of injection (Fig. 8-17). A hemorrhagic bulla usually forms over this area within 2 to 48 hours (Fig. 8-18) and progresses to an ulcer.[73] This cutaneous reaction might represent an arterial spasm. In an attempt to reverse the spasm, vigorous massage when the white macule appears has sometimes averted ulceration. However, prevention of the ulceration with massage alone is not always successful. Massaging in a nitroglycerin ointment 2% has prevented the development of ulcerations in this setting.

The major systemic action of nitrates is a direct reduction in venous smooth muscle tone.[177] Nitrates also relieve spasm of angiographically normal and diseased arteries.[178] Topical nitroglycerin ointment has been reported as beneficial in treating both dopamine extravasation and vasoconstriction necrosis.[179,180] Although more experience from other investigators needs to be reported, it seems prudent to use this technique.

Arterial spasm may also explain the development of cutaneous ulceration upstream from the injection site (see Fig. 8-15). In this latter case 2 ml of POL 0.25%

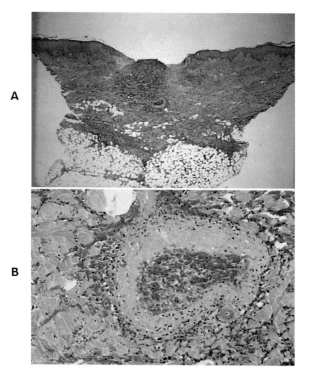

Fig. 8-16 **A,** Low-power view showing skin ulceration and focal inflammation extending into the subcutaneous fat. A thrombosed vessel, most likely an artery, is present directly under the area of necrosis. (Hematoxylin-eosin, ×25.) **B,** Higher magnification of same area as in **A** showing a thrombosed artery that caused the infarct. The arterial lumen is completely occluded by fresh thrombus. (Hematoxylin-eosin, ×200.)

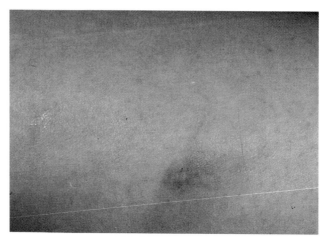

Fig. 8-17 Porcelain-white cutaneous reaction immediately after injection with POL 0.25%. This area progressed into a punctate cutaneous ulceration.

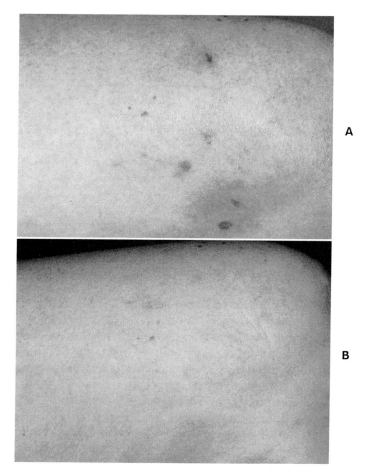

Fig. 8-18   A, Hemorrhagic macular reaction 1 week after injection with POL 0.5%. B, Appearance after 2 months. This area healed without any complication.

was injected into a feeding reticular vein as shown by the arrow. That was the only injection given to the patient in that sclerotherapy session.

Lymphatic injection

Injection into a lymphatic vessel may also lead to cutaneous necrosis. Histologic studies have disclosed evidence of lymphovenous anastomoses in humans.[181] It is possible that injection into such an anastomosis could result in necrosis of the associated lymphatic vessel and infiltration of the sclerosing solution extravascularly. If the sclerosing solution is caustic to extravascular tissues, this may result in tissue necrosis.

Excessive compression

Excessive compression of the skin overlying the treated vein may produce tissue anoxia with the development of localized cutaneous ulceration. Subcutaneous tissue flow in the leg is decreased when cutaneous pressure exceeds 20 mm Hg.[182] In addition, external pressure greater than 30 mm Hg reduces muscle blood flow in some patients.[183] Therefore excessive compression may produce tissue ischemia. However, both of these studies used indirect measurements of subcutaneous tissue flow and calf muscle blood flow and thus must be viewed with caution. A more physiologic method for measuring the effect of compression on blood flow was recently performed through determination of femoral blood flow.[184] These authors demonstrated that in the recumbent patient, static, graduated external compression of approximately 20 mm Hg at the ankle, reduced to approximately 10 mm Hg in the upper thigh, produces an increase in femoral flow of up to 75%. However, if calf pressures exceed 30 mm Hg when the patient is recumbent, a progressive fall in subcutaneous tissue flow and deep venous velocity occurs. Therefore it is recommended that patients not wear a graduated compression stocking of greater than 30 to 40 mm Hg when lying down for prolonged periods of time.

One method for applying compression to treated veins that could be varied with patient position is that of using a double layer of graduated compression stockings. This would ensure that maximal pressure over the vein is maintained while the patient is ambulatory. When the patient is recumbent, the outer stocking is removed, thereby decreasing the cutaneous pressure to 20 to 30 mm Hg at the ankle, which should prevent a reduction in cutaneous and subcutaneous blood flow.

Prevention

If extravasation of sclerosing solution occurs, the solution must be diluted as soon as possible. Hypertonic solutions should be diluted with copious amounts of normal saline solution. At least 10 times the volume of extravasated solution should be injected to limit osmotic damage. However, one study in Sprague-Dawley rats demonstrated increased incidence and size of ulcers after intradermal HS injection.[185] This may be secondary to spread of the sclerosant without adequate dilution. Unfortunately, this animal model may not accurately mimic human cutaneous tissue. Higher extravascular pressure in this animal model may compromise tissue perfusion.

Detergent sclerosing solutions of adequate strength may also be toxic to tissues. Dilution is again of paramount importance. In the above-mentioned study[185] dilution with hyaluronidase in normal saline solution limited the extent and prevented development of cutaneous necrosis from 3% STS.

It seems prudent to dilute the concentration of a caustic solution with hyaluronidase (Wydase, lyophilized, 150 USP U/ml) in the diluent. Hyaluronidase enzymatically breaks down connective tissue hyaluronic acid. This is hypothesized to disrupt the normal interstitial fluid barrier to allow rapid diffusion of solution through tissues, thereby increasing the effective absorption.[186,187] This beneficial effect has been demonstrated in limiting IV extravasation injuries from 10% dextrose, calcium and potassium salts, contrast media, sodium bicarbonate, aminophylline, hyperalimentation solution, and doxorubicin.[186,188-191] In addition to its enhanced dilutional ability, hyaluronidase may have an independent cellular preservation function. Hyaluronidase injection improves skin flap survival[192] and reduces myocardial infarction.[193] This has been postulated to occur through enhanced nutritive flow. Enhanced healing with resolution of painful induration was observed when 250 U of hyaluronidase was injected in an area where neoasphenamine and mapharsen were extravasated subcutaneously.[194] Finally, hyaluronidase promotes wound repair in fetal skin, contributing to scarless repair of wounds by as yet unclear mechanisms.[195] In summary, accelerated dilution, cellular stabilization, and wound repair properties of hyaluronidase appear useful in preventing cutaneous necrosis from inadvertent sclerosing solution extravasation.

Side effects from hyaluronidase use are rare and generally of the urticarial type.[196,197] Because of its limited stability, it should be reconstituted with 0.9%

sodium chloride solution immediately before use. The ideal concentration and quantity to inject after extravasation have not been determined. I recommend injecting 300 USP U of hyaluronidase diluted in 5 ml of 0.9% sodium chloride solution into multiple sites around the extravasated area. Studies have demonstrated that hyaluronidase solution must be injected within 60 minutes of extravasation to be effective.[198]

Treatment

Whatever the cause of the ulceration, it must be dealt with when it occurs. Fortunately, ulcerations, when they do occur, are usually fairly small, averaging 4 mm in diameter in my practice. At this size primary healing usually leaves an acceptable scar (Fig. 8-19). In addition to various topical therapies directly applied to the ulcer, elevation of the affected extremity and systemic pentoxifylline may be helpful in minimizing the ulcer size. In a series of 26 extravasation sloughs, less tissue damage occurred when limbs were elevated.[199]

Bodian,[93] who uses 23.4% HS, notes that ulceration usually takes 3½ months to heal, even when judicious wound care is given. He advocates treatment with a daily application of 20% benzoyl peroxide powder (Vanoxide Acne Lotion) under moist dressings cut to fit snugly over the ulcer. However, benzoyl peroxide is cytotoxic for newly growing epidermis. Therefore its use cannot be recommended. I have found that the use of occlusive or hydrocolloid dressings results in an apparent decrease in wound healing time. Occlusive dressings do not speed healing of full-thickness ulcers until granulation tissue has formed. Hydrocolloid gel dressings enhance debridement of wounds, possibly through their pectin-gelatin base. Nongelatin, nonpectin hydrocolloid dressings only act to stimulate fibrin

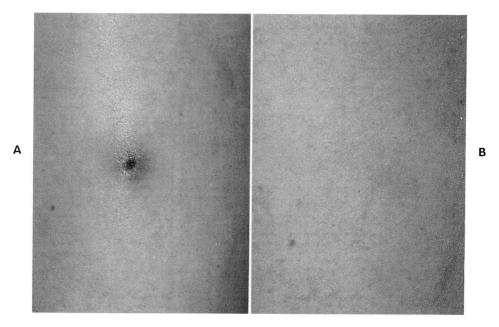

A   **B**

Fig. 8-19 Cutaneous ulceration on the posterolateral thigh. **A,** Three weeks after treatment with POL 0.5%. **B,** After 6 months. Treatment consisted of a duoderm dressing that was changed every 4 days until complete healing occurred in 5 weeks. Note the cosmetically acceptable stellate scar.

lysis. Thus its enhanced efficacy may be related to wound debridement, which should always be used either medically or surgically to promote granulation tissue formation.

More importantly, the use of occlusive dressings decreases the pain associated with an open ulcer. However, because an ulcer may take 4 to 6 weeks to heal completely even under ideal conditions, if possible, excision and closure of these lesions are recommended at the earliest possible time. This affords the patient the fastest healing and an acceptable scar.

Systemic Allergic Reaction or Toxicity

Systemic reactions caused by sclerotherapy treatment occur very rarely.

Minor reactions

Minor reactions such as urticaria are easily treated with an oral antihistamine such as diphenhydramine (Benadryl), 25 to 50 mm by mouth, or hydroxyzine (Atarax), 10 to 25 mg by mouth. Rarely the addition of corticosteroids is needed if the reaction does not subside readily. A short course of prednisone, 40 to 60 mg per day for 1 week, in conjunction with systemic antihistamine every 6 to 8 hours is helpful. Suppression of the adrenal axis is not a problem with this short course, so a tapering schedule is not necessary.

Because of the possibility of angioedema or bronchospasm, each patient with evidence of an allergic reaction should be examined for stridor and wheezing by auscultating over the neck and chest while the patient breathes normally. Supine and sitting blood pressure and pulse should be checked to rule out orthostatic changes, hypotension, or tachycardia that might result from the vasodilation that precedes anaphylactic shock.

Minor degrees of angioedema can be treated with oral antihistamines; however, if stridor is present, an intramuscular (IM) injection of diphenhydramine and IV corticosteroids should be administered, and a laryngoscope and endotracheal tube should be available.

Bronchospasm is estimated to occur after sclerotherapy in 0.001% of patients.[5] It usually responds to the addition of an inhaled bronchodilator or IV aminophylline, 6 mg/kg over 20 minutes, or to the antihistamine-corticosteroid regimen already noted.

Wheezing has been reported to occur in up to 5% of patients treated with hypertonic saline solution (personal communication, Michael Coverman, 1991). Coverman notes wheezing that resolves spontaneously occurring 15 minutes after the completion of sclerotherapy. He has found that if treatment sessions are performed with the patient sitting at a 45-degree angle, wheezing can be aborted. This is probably not an allergic reaction but an irritant phenomenon on the airways. Alternatively, it may be related to rapid infusion of histamine from perivascular mast cell degranulation with damage from the hyperosmotic solution.

Major reactions

Four types of potentially serious systemic reactions specific to the type of sclerosing agent have been noted: anaphylaxis, pulmonary toxicity, cardiac toxicity, and renal toxicity. These reactions are discussed both in general and separately for each sclerosing solution.

Anaphylaxis is a systemic hypersensitivity response caused by exposure or, more commonly, reexposure to a sensitizing substance. Anaphylaxis is usually an IgE-mediated, mast cell–activated reaction that occurs most often within minutes of antigen exposure. Other classes of immunoglobulin such as IgG may also produce anaphylaxis.[200] Since the risk of anaphylaxis increases with repeated exposures to the antigen, one should always be prepared for this reaction in every patient.[201]

The principal manifestations of anaphylaxis occur in areas where mast cell concentrations are highest: skin, lungs, and gastrointestinal (GI) tract. Histamine release is responsible for the clinical manifestations of this reaction. Although urticaria and abdominal pain are common, the three principal manifestations of anaphylaxis are airway edema, bronchospasm, and vascular collapse. Urticaria alone does not constitute anaphylaxis and should not be treated as such because of the potential side effects of treatment with epinephrine, especially in the older patient.

The signs and symptoms of anaphylaxis initially may be subtle and often include anxiety, itching, sneezing, coughing, urticaria, and angioedema. Wheezing may be accompanied by hoarseness of the voice and vomiting. Shortly after these presenting signs, breathing becomes more difficult, and the patient usually collapses from cardiovascular failure resulting from systemic vasodilation. One helpful clue toward distinguishing between anaphylaxis and vasovagal reactions is heart rate. Sinus tachycardia is almost always present in a patient with anaphylaxis, whereas bradycardia or cardiac rhythm disturbances are commonplace in vasovagal reactions.

The recommended treatment is to give epinephrine, 0.2 to 0.5 ml 1:1000 subcutaneously. This can be repeated three to four times at 5- to 15-minute intervals to maintain a systolic blood pressure above 90 to 100 mm Hg. This should be followed with establishment of an IV line of 0.9% sodium chloride solution. Diphenhydramine hydrochloride, 50 mg, is given next along with cimetidine, 300 mg; both the IV solution and oxygen are given at 4 to 6 L/minute. An endotracheal tube or tracheotomy is necessary for laryngeal obstruction. For asthma or wheezing, IV theophylline, 4 to 6 mg/kg, is infused over 15 minutes. At this point it is appropriate to transfer the patient to the hospital. Methylprednisolone sodium succinate, 60 mg, is given IV and repeated every 6 hours for four doses. Corticosteroids are not an emergency medication since their effect only appears after 1 to 3 hours. They are given to prevent the recurrence of symptoms 3 to 8 hours after the initial event. The patient should be hospitalized overnight for observation.

Allergic Reactions to Sclerosing Agents
Sodium morrhuate

Although touted by the manufacturer as "the natural sclerosing agent," SM causes a variety of allergic reactions, ranging from mild erythema with pruritus[202-204] to generalized urticaria[204-206] to GI disturbances with abdominal pain and diarrhea[202,203] to anaphylaxis. It has been estimated that "unfavorable reactions" when treating varicose leg veins occur in 3% of patients.[207] The incidence of allergic reactions when treating esophageal varices ranges from 11% to 48%.[208] The reason for the high number of allergic reactions with this product may be related to the inability to remove all the fish proteins that are present in SM. In fact, 20.8% of the fatty acid composition of the solution is unknown.[209]

Many cases of anaphylaxis have occurred within a few minutes after the drug is injected or more commonly when therapy is reinstituted after a few weeks.[204,210-212] Most of these cases occurred before 1950. Rarely anaphylaxis has resulted in fatalities,[206,207,213] many of which have not been reported in the medical literature.[202]

Pleural effusions with pulmonary edema and acute respiratory failure appearing as *adult respiratory distress syndrome* (ARDS) are common with esophageal injection.[209] It has been estimated that pleural effusions occur in 46% of patients with an esophageal injection.[214] With injection into esophageal varices, the sclerosing solution rapidly enters the pulmonary circulation, causing increased permeability of the pulmonary microvasculature.[209] There have been no reports of pleural effusions with injection into varicose veins of the legs.

Prolonged dysrhythmia requiring placement of a permanent pacemaker has been reported in two cases.[215] This complication has been attributed to a direct cardiotoxic effect of SM.

Ethanolamine oleate

EO (Ethamolin) is a synthetic mixture of ethanolamine and oleic acid with an empirical formula of $C_{20}H_{41}NO_3$. The minimal lethal IV dose in rabbits is 130 mg/kg.[205] The oleic acid component is responsible for the inflammatory action. Oleic acid may also activate coagulation in vitro by release of tissue factor and Hageman factor. This agent was first reported in the medical literature as an ideal sclerosing agent in 1937 by Biegeleisen.[216] He observed no toxic effects in 500 injections. EO is thought to have a decreased risk of allergic reactions compared with SM or STS.[217] However, pulmonary toxicity and allergic reactions have been associated with this sclerosing agent.

Pleural effusion, edema, and infiltration and pneumonitis have been demonstrated in human trials with the injection of esophageal varices. Pleural effusion or infiltration has been estimated by the product manufacturer to occur in 2.1% of patients and pneumonia in 1.2% of patients. One study of 75 patients treated for esophageal varices disclosed abnormal chest x-ray films showing infiltration or effusion in 45 patients for an incidence of 60%.[218] These conditions usually resolve spontaneously within 48 hours.[218]

Anaphylactic shock has been reported by the product manufacturer after injection in three cases (product information [1989] from Glaxo Pharmaceuticals, Research Triangle Park, NC). Another case of a nearly fatal anaphylactic reaction during the fourth treatment of varicose leg veins with 1 ml of solution has also been reported.[219] In one additional case a fatal reaction occurred in a man with a known allergic disposition (product information, [1989] from Glaxo Pharmaceuticals, Research Triangle Park, NC). Another episode of a fatal anaphylactic reaction occurred in a woman having her third series of injections.[202] This represented one reaction in 200 patients from that author's practice. Generalized urticaria occurred in approximately 1 in 400 patients; this symptom responded rapidly to an antihistamine.[220]

Acute renal failure with spontaneous recovery occurred after injection of 15 to 20 ml of EO in two women.[221] A hemolytic reaction occurred in five patients in a series of over 900 patients, with injection of over 12 ml of 0.5% EO per patient per treatment session.[220] The patients were described as "feeling generally unwell and shivery, with aching in the loins and passage of red-brown urine. All rapidly recovered with bed rest and were perfectly normal the next day." Injections of less than 12 ml per treatment session have not resulted in this reaction.

Transient chest pain has also been reported in 13 of 23 patients treated for esophageal varices.[222] However, pyrexia and substernal chest pain are considered common sequelae of esophageal varices injection with any sclerosing agent.[217]

EO has also been tested for carcinogenic activity in the albino rat by intradermal injection without induction of tumors.[223]

Sodium tetradecyl sulfate

A synthetic detergent developed in the 1940s, STS has been used throughout the world as a sclerosing solution. A comprehensive review of the medical literature (in multiple specialties and languages) until 1987 disclosed a total of 47 cases of nonfatal allergic reactions in a review of 14,404 treated patients. This included six case reports.[224] A separate review of treatment in 187 patients with 2249 injections disclosed no evidence of allergic or systemic reactions.[225] An additional report of 5341 injections given to an unknown number of patients found "no unfavorable reaction."[226] Fegan[227] has reviewed his experience with STS in 16,000 patients. He reported 15 cases of "serum sickness, with hot stinging pain in the skin, and an erythematous rash developing 30 to 90 minutes after injection." These patients subsequently underwent additional uneventful treatment with STS after premedication with antihistamines. Ten additional patients developed "mild anaphylaxis" that required treatment with an injection of epinephrine. If one were to combine only those reviews of over 1000 patients, the incidence of nonfatal allergic reactions would be approximately 0.3%.[6,220,228-230]

The product manufacturer notes two fatalities associated with the use of STS, both from the sclerotherapy procedure itself and not specifically related to STS. One fatality occurred in a patient who was receiving an antiovulatory agent. Another death (fatal pulmonary embolism) was reported in a 36-year-old woman who was not taking oral contraceptives. Four deaths attributed to anaphylactoid reactions were reported to the Committee on Safety of Medicines for the United Kingdom between 1963 and 1988, with 22 nonfatal allergic reactions such as urticaria noted over the same time period.[231]

A fatality has been reported after a test dose of 0.5 ml of STS 0.5% was given to a 64-year-old woman.[232] An autopsy performed by the Hennipin County, Minnesota coroner's office revealed no obvious cause of death. Subsequently, mast cell tryptase studies were performed on blood collected approximately 1 hour after the reaction while the patient was receiving life support. A normal tryptase level is less than 5 ng/ml; in experimental anaphylactic reactions induced in the laboratory, levels up to 80 ng/ml have been seen. In this patient the levels were extremely high at 6000 ng/ml, suggesting that an anaphylactoid reaction had caused her death. Unfortunately, tryptase levels are experimental at this time, and it is unclear how such a high level could be obtained. Therefore it is also unclear whether fatal anaphylaxis is a significant possibility with STS.

Since all reported cases of allergic reactions are of the IgE-mediated immediate hypersensitivity type, it is recommended that patients remain in or near the office for 30 minutes after sclerotherapy when STS is used. However, patients may also develop allergic reactions hours or days after the procedure.[230,233] For example, urticaria occurred 8 hours after treatment in one patient[233] and 2 weeks after treatment in two other patients.[230] Therefore patients should be warned about the possibility of allergic reactions and how to obtain care should a reaction occur.

In a review of 2300 patients treated over 16 years, four cases of allergic reactions were reported (0.17% incidence).[234] Reactions in this study were described as periorbital swelling in one patient and *urticaria* in three. All reactions were easily treated with oral antihistamines. It is of interest that French phlebologists advocate a 3-days-before and 3-days-after treatment course with an antihistamine. P. Flurie noted no episodes of allergic reactions in 500 patients treated in this manner.[235]

As of January 1990, a total of 37 reports of adverse reactions have been reported to the Drug Experience Monitoring Program of the Food and Drug Administration (FDA). However, this information cannot be used to estimate the incidence of adverse drug reactions since there was no central reporting agency before August 1985. A review of these adverse reactions was remarkable in that five cases of suspected anaphylaxis and two cases of asthma induced by injection were reported. One of the cases of anaphylaxis resulted in the death previously discussed. After a detailed review it is unclear to me whether anaphylaxis indeed occurred in every reported case.

The reports of the Clinical Drug Safety Surveillance Group of Wyeth-Ayerst Laboratories are compiled from voluntary reporting to the manufacturer and/or the FDA. The following are summaries of 3 years of reports. January to July 1991 disclosed one episode of erythema multiforme; one episode of ARDS; one episode of fever, lymphadenopathy, and rash; and three episodes of abdominal pain, nausea, vomiting, and diarrhea. From September 1991 to November 1992 there were five reports of urticaria and one episode of ARDS. From December 1992 to September 1993 there was only one case of a maculopapular rash (written correspondence, Paul Minicozzi, Wyeth-Ayerst Laboratories, October 1991 to 1993). The case report of erythema multiforme was reported in a woman after her thirteenth sclerotherapy treatment.[236] The patient developed pruritus the morning after the last injection, with the development of a generalized eruption beginning on the legs 4 days later. This was followed by fever the following day. A rapid tapering course of oral prednisone was given, with complete resolution of the rash in 2 weeks.

In short, anaphylaxis has been reported with rare fatal reactions.[237] The most common systemic reaction consists of transient low-grade fever and chills lasting up to 24 hours after treatment.[238] This has also been noted in one of my patients. Of note is that three patients with allergic systemic reactions to monoethanolamine oleate had no evidence of allergy to STS.[238]

An interesting dilemma develops with patients who have a history of allergy to sulfa medication. STS contains a sulfate; therefore one can assume that these patients would be at increased risk for an allergic reaction. However, a review of all reported cases of allergic reactions to STS has not disclosed an independent allergic history to sulfa-containing medications (correspondence from Tom Udicious, R.Ph., Wyeth-Ayerst Laboratories, November 1993). I have treated many patients with a history of sulfa allergy with STS without adverse sequelae.

A hemolytic reaction occurred in five patients in a series of more than 900 patients with injection of more than 8 ml of STS 3%.[220] Like a similar reaction that occurred with EO, patients were described as "feeling generally unwell and shivery, with aching in the loins and passage of red-brown urine. All rapidly recovered with bed rest and were perfectly normal the next day." Injections of less than 8 ml per treatment session did not result in this reaction. Intravascular hemolysis was also reported to the FDA after injection of STS into a hepatic artery feeding a hepatic tumor.

The IV median lethal dose (LD_{50}) in mice is 90 mg/kg.[239] The lethal volume after IV injection in the rat is approximately four to six times as high for STS as for POL in equivalent concentrations.[175]

Polidocanol

Allergic reactions to POL have been reported in four patients in a review of the world's literature up to 1987, with an estimated incidence of 0.01%.[224] Amblard[240] reported no allergic reactions in over 250 patients, including no allergic reactions in two patients who were intolerant to STS. Hoffer[174] reported no allergic reactions in over 19,000 cases. In addition, patients who are allergic to STS or iodine have no allergic manifestations to injections of POL.[240-242] However, rare allergic reactions have been reported, including a case of nonfatal anaphylactic shock to 1 ml of POL 2% injected into a varicose vein during the fourth treatment session.[234,243-245] Also, Ouvry, Chandet, and Guillerot[246] reported a patient who developed generalized urticaria with cough and dyspnea after receiving 2 ml of POL 2%; the condition resolved in 30 minutes with IV corticosteroid therapy.

Since the previous review, additional cases of allergic reaction have been reported or discovered. Guex[52] reported seven cases of minor general urticaria in nearly 11,000 patients treated over 12 years. These patients cleared completely in 1 to 2 days with antihistamine and topical corticosteroid therapy, with one patient requiring systemic corticosteroids. Kreussler and Company, the product manufacturer in Germany, has documented 35 cases of suspected sensitivity from 1987 to 1993 (personal correspondence, January 1994). Of these reports, most were either vasovagal events or unproven allergic reactions. Nine patients were given repeat challenges with polidocanol, with only three demonstrating an allergic reaction (urticaria or erythematous dermatitis). One patient died of anaphylactic shock 5 minutes after injection with 1 ml despite maximal intervention. Three serious cases of anaphylaxis were reported from the Netherlands.[247] These patients developed anaphylaxis within 15 minutes after injection of POL. Two of them received the drug for the first time. One patient was successfully resuscitated after cardiac arrest. She was a 70-year-old woman with a complicated medical history of two heart operations, two cerebrovascular accidents, and hyperthyroidism. She was receiving multiple medications, including digoxin, carbimazol, captopril, furosemide, mebeverine, and acenocoumerol. She was treated without complications four previous times with POL. The second patient showed signs of ARDS after being treated with epinephrine and systemic methylprednisolone for "shock." The third patient developed urticaria, dyspnea, parathesia, headache, and chest pain with electrocardiographic (EKG) findings of cardiac ischemia. No further studies were performed on these patients.

The Australian Polidocanol Open Clinical Trial at 2 years, with over 8000 treated patients, reported nine local urticarial reactions and three generalized reactions, with two patients developing a rash, for a frequency of approximately 0.2%. There were no cases of anaphylaxis.[176] A 5-year experience in 500 patients treated with POL 3% reported five cases of allergic reaction (1% incidence). One patient had nonfatal anaphylactic shock, with the other patients experiencing urticaria.[248]

Two additional patients were recently reported who developed an immediate-type hypersensitivity reaction with systemic pruritus and urticaria.[249] This represented two cases in 689 sequential patients for an incidence of 0.3% in their patient population and 0.91% for the "true" population. These two reactions occurred without prior exposure to POL as a sclerosing agent. Since POL is used as an emulsifying agent in preprocessed foods, prior exposure may have occurred from its ingestion. Both patients responded easily to either a single dose of oral diphenhydramine, 50 mg, or 0.3 ml of subcutaneous epinephrine plus 50 mg diphenhydramine IM.

Jaquier and Loretan[173] believe that the decrease in antigenicity is the result of the absence of a benzene nucleus and a paramine group and the presence of a lone free alcohol group. Dexo SA Pharmaceuticals, the product manufacturer in France, recommends that this substance not be used in patients with an allergic diathesis (e.g., asthma) (product description of hydroxypolyethoxydodecane [May 1985] received with correspondence from Dexo SA Pharmaceuticals, France). Thus allergic reactions to POL are much rarer than those reported with STS but do occur.

An interesting adverse effect may be noticed in patients in whom a near maximal dosage of POL is used. These patients report paresthesia or tingling of the tongue or a strange sensation in taste that resolves within 5 minutes. This has been reported to Kreussler five times from 1986 to 1993 (correspondence, January 1994) and has been noted in my practice as well. This sensation may be explained by particular effects of the anesthetic properties of POL.

Other unusual reactions reported to Kreussler (correspondence, January 1994) include rare episodes of short convulsive coughing, acute pressure sensation in the chest, acute difficulty with breathing, and one case of stabbing chest pain without demonstrable EKG changes or myoglobin band creatine phosphokinase fluctuations.

Like EO and SM, POL has demonstrated a dose-dependent cardiac toxicity when injected into esophageal varices. POL has a negative inotropic effect and reduces atrioventricular and intraventricular conduction. Animal studies demonstrate a reversible, dose-dependent decrease in myocardial contractility, blood pressure, and pulse rate and a prolongation of the PQ interval.[250] This effect may explain the cause of heart failure in three elderly patients with severe liver failure who were given massive quantities of POL during esophageal sclerotherapy (760 mg in a 74-year-old woman; 600 mg in a 70-year-old woman; 750 mg in a 76-year-old woman).[251,252]

The LD_{50} in rabbits at 2 hours is 0.2 g/kg, which is three to six times greater than the LD_{50} for procaine hydrochloride.[253] The LD_{50} in mice is 110 mg/kg.[254] The systemic toxicity level is similar to that of lidocaine and procaine.[255]

Chromated glycerin

CG 72% (Scleremo) is a sclerosing solution whose incidence of side effects is very low (Scleremo product information [1987]).[15,21,256] Hypersensitivity is a very rare complication.[257,258] Contact sensitivity to chromium occurs in approximately 5% of the population.[259] IV potassium dichromate leads to complete desensitization in chromium-sensitized guinea pigs. This effect occurs because chromium needs to bind to skin proteins to become an effective antigen.[260] This may be related to the necessity for epidermal Langerhans' cells to produce an allergic response, whereas T-lymphocyte-accessory cooperation is not optimal with IV injection and its resulting endothelial necrosis.

Hematuria accompanied by urethral colic can occur transiently after injection of large doses of CG. Ocular manifestations, including blurred vision and a partial visual field loss, have been reported by a single author, with resolution in less than 2 hours.[261]

An additional case recently was reported of transient hypertension and visual disturbance after the injection of 12 ml of 50% CG into spider and "feeder" leg veins in a fourth treatment session.[262] These symptoms occurred $2\frac{1}{2}$ hours after treatment and lasted over a 3-hour period without treatment. This may have represented a retinal spasm or an ophthalmic migraine.[262]

Polyiodide iodine

Polyiodide iodine (Varigloban; Variglobin; Sclerodine 6) is a stabilized water solution of iodide ions, sodium iodine, and benzyl alcohol. Sigg, Horodegan, and Bernbach[263] reported on their experience in over 400,000 injections with Variglobin. Paravenous injections readily produced tissue necrosis. In 1975 Sigg and Zelikovski[264] reported an incidence of side effects of 1.25 per 1000 injections, 0.13 allergic cutaneous reactions per 1000, 0.04 instances of localized necrosis per 1000, and 1 instance of varicophlebitis per 1000. No systemic allergic reactions were observed. Obvious contraindications to the use of Variglobin are hyperthyroidism and allergies to iodine and benzyl alcohol.

Iodine solutions may also produce bronchiomucosal lesions if used in high concentration. Therefore Wenner[265] recommends that a maximum of 5 ml of 12% solution be used in a single sclerosing session.

Hypertonic saline

Alone, hypertonic saline (HS) solution shows no evidence of allergenicity or toxicity. Complications that may arise from its specific use include hypertension that may be exacerbated in predisposed patients when an excessive sodium load is given, sudden hypernatremia, central nervous system disorders, extensive hemolysis, and cortical necrosis of the kidneys (Mary Helenek, written correspondence, American Regent Laboratories, Inc., May 1990). These complications among others have led one manufacturer (American Regent Laboratories) to add to its label the warning "FOR IV OR SC USE AFTER DILUTION" in bold red ink.

Dodd[266] has reported painless hematuria in five patients injected with HS. Sometimes blood appears in the urine after one to two acts of micturition and sometimes at additional times throughout the day. There are usually no other ill effects, and the hematuria resolves spontaneously. Hematuria probably occurs because of hemolysis of RBCs during sclerotherapy.

Recently Coverman[267] described two patients injected with up to 6 ml of HS 23.4% who developed "peculiar visual symptoms in just one eye." This was described as either blurred vision or an aura. There were no other symptoms, and each incidence passed quickly and spontaneously. Coverman speculates that this may have been caused by the addition of lidocaine to the HS solution.

Heparin in hypertonic saline

Whereas unadulterated hypertonic saline solutions in concentrations from 15% to 30% are used for the treatment of varicose and telangiectatic leg veins, adding heparin to the solution to prevent the theoretic risk of embolization associated with sclerotherapy has been advocated.[16] Although the necessity for heparin has been discounted in a well-controlled 800-patient randomized study,[19] Foley's solution, "Heparsal," consisting of HS 20% with heparin, 100 U/ml, and procaine 1%, is commonly used in the treatment of telangiectatic leg veins. Therefore the risk of adverse reactions to heparin should be mentioned.

Commercial preparations of heparin consist of straight-chain anionic polysaccharides of variable molecular weight (usually 7000 to 40,000). Heparin prepared from different tissues also appears to vary: more protamine is required to neutralize a unit of beef lung heparin than porcine mucosal heparin. Plasma lipolytic activity, antifactor Xa activity, and activated partial thromboplastin time ratios are significantly different.[268]

Fever, urticaria, and anaphylaxis occur occasionally after administration of heparin.[268-272] Necrosis has been reported in patients receiving subcutaneous heparin.[263,273-276] Necrosis usually occurred 3 to 10 days after multiple subcutaneous injections. Pruritus, local tenderness, and burning sensations associated with large, indurated, erythematous plaques were also reported to occur in six patients 10 to 20 days after beginning prophylactic doses of heparin.[277] Thus there is a measurable risk of toxicity to heparin.

Although heparin is not a totally benign substance, there have been no reports by those who use Heparsal of any adverse reactions that could be attributed to the heparin component.[5,16,19,152] The lack of side effects has been reported in one series of 310 patients when volumes of 10 to 20 ml have been injected into varicose veins.[152] In the doses used, heparin in Heparsal may be without significant side effects, but one must be aware of the potential dangers associated with its use.

Lidocaine in hypertonic saline

Alderman[6] and Duffy[5] advocate the addition of lidocaine (to achieve a 0.4% final concentration) to minimize patient discomfort during injection of HS. This addition means that this sclerosing mixture potentially can be allergenic. Although the most common causes of previous allergic reaction in a patient to lidocaine are psychogenic or vasovagal reactions,[278] allergic reactions may occur.

The amide class of anesthetics has a very low risk of allergic reaction.[279-284] Allergy is most likely caused by the methylparabens or sodium metabisulfite that is used as a preservative in the anesthetic solutions.[279,280,285-287] To keep the allergic risk as low as possible, single-dose vials of lidocaine without preservatives should be used.

Despite the low risk of allergenicity to lidocaine, multiple allergic reactions, including anaphylaxis, have been reported.[288-295] Thus HS, when adulterated with lidocaine, may place the patient at risk for allergic reactions.

Superficial Thrombophlebitis

Before the advent of modern day sclerotherapy, which uses graduated compression to limit thrombosis, thrombophlebitis, both superficial and deep, occurred in a significant number of sclerotherapy patients.[296] In fact, it was commonly thought that the incidence of phlebitis was so common a sequelae of sclerotherapy that there was doubt whether this form of therapy was legitimate.[297] With the use of compression and the realization that many adverse effects resulted from thrombus formation in treated veins, the incidence of thrombophlebitis has greatly decreased.

Certain patients may be predisposed to the development of thrombophlebitis (see the section on deep vein thrombosis and pulmonary emboli on p. 328). Fegan[298] states that this complication occurs more commonly if perforator veins in the region of treatment are undiagnosed and not treated.

Etiology

Superficial thrombophlebitis appears 1 to 3 weeks after injection as a tender erythematous induration over the injected vein (Fig. 8-20). Duffy[5] estimates that it occurs in 0.5% of his patients. Mantse[230] reported an incidence of 1% in the treatment of varicose (nontelangiectatic) veins despite the use of a tensor bandage for 6 weeks. Mantse notes that the patients who developed superficial thrombophlebitis found the bandage was too tight and reapplied it too loosely at home. In my experience this complication occurs in some degree in approximately 0.01% of patients. Severe cases requiring treatment with compression and anti-inflammatory agents occur very rarely (<0.001% of patients totaling more than 10,000 separate injections).

Prevention and treatment

The decreased incidence of superficial thrombophlebitis in my practice may be the result of the greater degree and length of compression used in treating all injected veins. Indeed, the cause of thrombophlebitis is related in part to treatment technique. An inadequate degree or length of compression results in excessive intravascular thrombosis. Sigg[299] notes that perivenous inflammation is observed only at those parts of the limb not covered by a compression dressing. Thus to avoid this complication, one should prevent or minimize the development of postsclerosis thrombosis by using compression pads and hosiery.

However, even when appropriate compression is used over treated varicose veins, thrombosis and perivascular inflammation may occur (Fig. 8-21). Ascend-

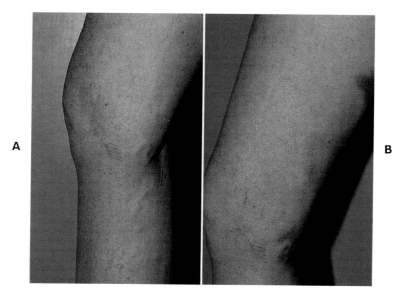

Fig. 8-20   A, This 45-year-old woman had incompetence of the SFJ and refused surgical ligation and stripping of the greater saphenous vein. Therefore all reticular, accessory, and tributary veins were treated with POL 0.75% for a total of 20 ml to the entire right leg. Localized compression, with STD foam pads and a short stretch bandage, was applied to the medial thigh only. She did not apply the graduated 30-40 mm Hg compression stocking until 30 to 45 minutes after leaving the office. **B,** Acute thrombophlebitis developed 3 days after sclerotherapy. Note ecchymosis from compression padding.

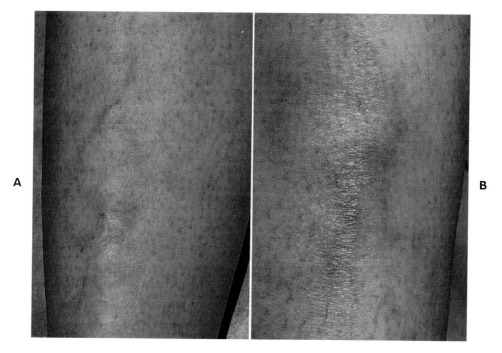

Fig. 8-21   A, Clinical appearance of the vein over the anterior tibia before injection. **B,** Acute thrombophlebitis developed 10 days after sclerotherapy with POL 0.5%.

ing phlebitis in the lesser saphenous vein (LSV) or its long tributaries starting at the upper edge of the compression stocking is relatively common. Here the sclerosing action continues up the abnormal vessel (even beyond what apparently is the extent of the abnormality). It is thought that the sclerosing solution destroys damaged endothelium to a greater extent than normal endothelium (product description on Hydroxypolyethoxydodecane received with correspondence, May 1985). Therefore the placement of a sorbo pad extending above the compression stocking or bandage to create a gradual transition of pressure from compressed to noncompressed vein may provide a safety margin. Also, it may prevent damage to the vein by the otherwise abrupt cutoff of the pressure stocking.

In addition to adequate compression, drainage of thrombi after liquefaction (approximately 2 weeks after sclerotherapy) will hasten resolution of the otherwise slow, painful resorption process.[299]

Thrombophlebitis is not a complication that should be taken lightly. If untreated, the inflammation and clot may spread to perforating veins and the deep venous system, which leads to valvular damage and possible pulmonary embolic events.[300-304] When thrombophlebitis occurs, the thrombus should be evacuated and adequate compression and frequent ambulation should be maintained until the pain and inflammation resolve. Aspirin or other nonsteroidal antiinflammatory agents may be helpful in limiting both the inflammation and pain.

Arterial Injection

The most feared complication in sclerotherapy is inadvertent injection into an artery. Fortunately, this complication is very rare.[305-307] Five examples of this complication had been reported to the Medical Defense Union in Great Britain by 1985.[308] Cockett[309] has reported 18 cases, including those reported to the two medical protection societies in the United Kingdom over a 10-year period. However, Cockett believes even this number is too low because many cases occur that never reach the courts or the medical literature. Biegeleisen, Neilsen, and O'Shaughnessy[310] have reported seven cases in their practice history of more than 10 years.[310] Forty cases over 17 years have been reported from France.[311]

Arterial injection of a sclerosing solution causes the development of an embolus. This has been experimentally confirmed in the canine femoral artery.[312] These experiments demonstrate little effect on the artery itself with injection. Spasm does not occur. The sclerosing solution acts to denature blood in smaller arteries, producing a sludge embolus that obstructs the microcirculation (Fig. 8-22).[313] Stagnant blood flow, secondary thrombosis, and necrosis soon follow.

Occlusion of small arteries may lead to the development of a compartmental syndrome. Intracompartmental pressures of 30 mm Hg or more in humans usually produce neural deficits characterized by pain during stretching of the muscles involved, paresthesia, and then paresis and anesthesia in the sensory distribution of the nerve that courses through the affected compartment. The end result is paralysis.[233] Muscle necrosis then leads to leg atrophy. Sensory deficit in the first web space (deep peroneal nerve) implicates anterior compartment syndrome. Sensory deficit on the dorsum of the foot (superficial peroneal nerve) implicates the lateral compartment. The superficial posterior compartment is indicated by sensory deficit of the sural nerve distribution (lateral foot). Deep compartment syndrome is likely if the sole of the foot is affected (posterior tibial nerve).

Unless large arteries are blocked, peripheral pulses will be intact, and capillary filling is easily identified since the compartmental pressure must be greater than 80 mm Hg to occlude large-artery flow.[314] This may lull the physician into a false sense of security, and the underlying compartmental syndrome may not be

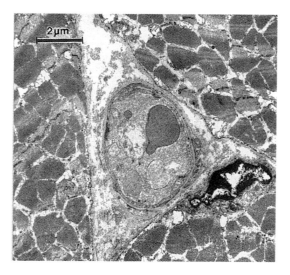

Fig. 8-22 Terminal arteriole from the adductor musculature of the rat hind limb 60 minutes after injection of 4% Varioglobin into the iliac artery through a Fogarty catheter. The lumen contains a large amount of cellular debris. Transmission electron micrograph, primary magnification ×3800; for final enlargement see scale. (From Staubesand J and Seydewitz V: Phlébologie 20:1, 1991.)

recognized. Intracompartmental pressures between 30 and 40 mm Hg for 6 to 12 hours can cause irreversible damage to the nervous tissue because of impairment of microcirculation.[233] Magnetic resonance imaging (MRI) examination of the affected limb has been able to distinguish muscle destruction (Fig. 8-23).

Etiology

The most common location for arterial injection to occur is in the posterior or medial malleolar region, particularly when an effort is made to inject the internal ankle perforator vein, specifically in the posterior tibial artery.[298,307,309,315] The patient will usually, but not always, note immediate pain. The pain slowly propagates down into the foot and outer toes over the following 2 to 6 hours. During this time arterial pedal pulses are palpable. Ten to 12 hours later the four outer toes are white, with the sole of the foot becoming painful. Cutaneous blanching of the injected area usually occurs in an arterial pattern associated with a loss of pulse and progressive cyanosis of the injected area.

Another area in which the artery and veins are in close proximity is the junction of the femoral and superficial saphenous veins. A review of one sclerotherapy practice over 20 years disclosed two cases of accidental arterial injection in this area, requiring thigh amputations.[316] This has also been the experience of Biegeleisen, Neilsen, and O'Shaughnessy[310] who reported seven cases of arterial injection during attempts to inject the greater or lesser saphenous veins at the groin or popliteal areas even under color-flow ultrasound control. In this location the external pudendal artery bifurcates and may surround the LSV shortly after the location of its connection with the femoral vein. In addition, the junction of the LSV with the popliteal vein has been demonstrated to have a tortuous and variably located satellite arteriole.[317] Because these collateral arteries vary anatomically in these locations, duplex scanning may be useful before sclerosing these vessels but does not guarantee absolute safety.

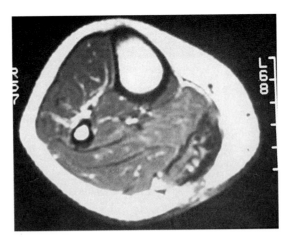

Fig. 8-23 Magnetic resonance image of the medial calf a few weeks after inadvertent intraarterial injection has produced muscular weakness and pain. Note atrophy of gastrocnemius muscles with significant edema within fascial compartments. (Courtesy Professor Jean Natali, Paris.)

With the onset of duplex-assisted sclerotherapy, small arteries in superficial and deep aspects of the thigh and calf have been inadvertently injected (Fig. 8-24). As described previously, the usual sequelae are both loss of tissue (cutaneous and subcutaneous) and nerve damage, which may result in muscle atrophy and or necrosis (see Fig. 8-23). Color-flow duplex scanning and the use of open needles when sclerosing these very tricky areas are recommended. A physician should be present at all times to give immediate treatment if needed.

Prevention and treatment

Arterial injection is a true sclerotherapy emergency. The extent of cutaneous necrosis usually is related to the amount of solution injected. Therapeutic efforts to treat this complication are usually unsatisfactory but should be attempted.[307] Because its occurrence is extremely rare, I recommend that an emergency flow sheet be readily accessible (see box on p. 327). Hobbs[166] recommends that on realization of arterial injection, blood and sclerosing solution should be aspirated back into the syringe to empty the needle of solution.[166] In addition, aspiration of the injected artery as rapidly and completely as possible, if performed immediately, may help remove the injected sclerosing solution. The needle should not be withdrawn, but the syringe should be replaced with one containing 10,000 U of heparin, which should be injected slowly into the artery. Unfortunately, this maneuver is difficult to accomplish since the patient is usually in considerable pain and may find it difficult to hold still (Hobbs, personal communication, 1991). In addition, some patients have no complaints of pain and only demonstrate a mild, sharply demarcated erythema that becomes dusky and cyanotic after a few hours.[310]

More practical treatments include periarterial infiltration with procaine 3%, 1 ml, which will form a complex with STS and render it inactive.[298,315] The foot should be cooled with ice packs to minimize tissue anoxia. Immediate heparinization (continued for 6 days) and administration of IV dextran 10%, 500 ml per dose, for 3 days is recommended. Use of IV streptokinase also may be considered if there are no contraindications for its use. Finally, use of oral prazosin, hydralazine, or nifedipine for 30 days should be considered. However, Cockett[309]

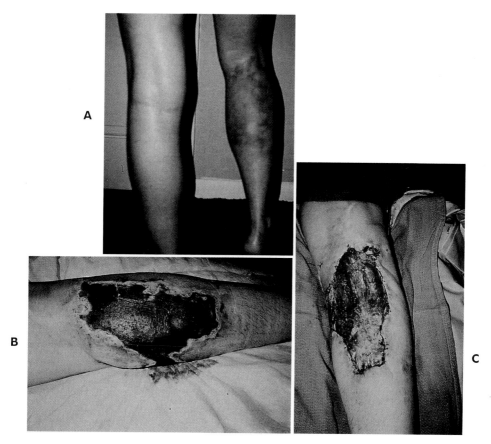

Fig. 8-24   **A,** Two days after duplex-assisted sclerotherapy with STS 1.0% into the gastrocnemial area to treat cutaneous telangiectasia. Note mottled skin. Treatment consisted of pain medication and local infiltration with lidocaine. **B,** 3 weeks after treatment a well-circumscribed necrotic area is apparent. **C,** Intraoperative debridement of all necrotic tissue to fascia.

ARTERIAL INJECTION TREATMENT

Arterial and periarterial infiltration with procaine 1% (inactivates STS)

Cooling of injected area with ice packs

Immediate heparinization (continue 6 days or longer)

Intravenous dextran 10%, 500 mg/day × 3 days

Consider direct thrombolytic therapy with streptokinase

Oral prazosin, hydralazine, or nifedipine × 30 days

has found that treatment that is delayed for more than an hour has no effect in limiting damage to the foot.

Use of IV heparin followed by subcutaneous heparin has been found to avert skin necrosis.[310] It was observed that warfarin (Coumadin) did not appear as effective as subcutaneous heparin in these patients. The protective effect of heparin may be unrelated to its anticoagulant activity. Postischemic endothelial cell dysfunction was prevented with heparin perfusion in the rat hind limb model.[318] Heparin infusion at 0.5 U/ml resulted in endothelial-dependent vasodilation. Serum levels less than 0.5 U/ml (the average serum heparin level in a patient undergoing therapeutic anticoagulation) were less effective. It is postulated that direct interactions of heparin with the endothelium, inducing maintenance of a strong luminal charge, may produce beneficial membrane-stabilizing effects. Heparin may also modulate TNF activity, contributing to this effect.[319] In addition, a favorable resolution of arterial injection occurred in one patient with injection of tissue-type plasminogen activator (t-PA).[320] In this patient promazine was injected into an artery. Use of heparin, axillary plexus blockade, and IV sodium nitroprusside was not successful. Brachial artery injection of t-PA (Actilyse, 50 mg over 8 hours) resulted in therapeutic efficacy. Thus local fibrinolytic therapy should be considered if conservative treatments prove ineffective.

Given the known relationship of injection site to the development of this problem, one must consider the necessity for injecting vessels in the vicinity of the medial malleolus. There is an interesting report in the *British Medical Journal* of a legal case brought against a physician for performing such an injection, which resulted in a transmetatarsal amputation.[305] The case was found in favor of the physician after several renowned sclerotherapists stated that if the patient would benefit from the injection, it should be attempted since the risks are infrequent and the benefits significant.

Prevention of this dreaded complication is best accomplished by visualization of the blood emanating from the needle. If it is pulsatile and continues to flow after the leg is horizontal, injection should not be attempted at this site. Mantse[230] advises that when the medial malleolar area is treated, placement of the sclerosing needle should be performed while the patient is standing so the varix is bulged and the distance between the artery and vein is increased.

Theoretically, visualization of arteries and veins with duplex-assisted sclerotherapy should negate this risk. Indeed, newer color-flow duplex imagery allows visualization of minute arteries and veins. However, a number of arterial ulcerations have occurred with this technique, even when injecting posterior calf, gastrocnemius, and saphenofemoral junctional varicose veins. Thus no technique is completely free from this complication.

Pulmonary Embolism and Deep Venous Thrombosis

Pulmonary emboli (PE) and deep vein thrombosis (DVT) occur very rarely after sclerotherapy. The literature contains many case reports but does not permit an exact estimate of the incidence of postsclerotherapy DVT or PE. A recent review by Feied[321] summarizes the major reports and risk factors for DVT.

The diagnosis of DVT is often clinically difficult, with up to 50% of cases going unnoticed. Embolization of a thrombus occurs in more than 50% of patients[322] and is not diagnosed in up to 70% of cases,[323] with a mortality rate approaching 35% without treatment.[324] Both the use of preventive measures and maintaining clinical suspicion are important in preventing this complication. The clinical diagnosis of DVT is only accurate 50% of the time as compared to the use of fibrinogen scanning.[325] Venous Doppler examination has a 30% to 96% accuracy, depending on the experience of the investigator.[326-328] Likewise, impedance phlebography has a 40% accuracy.[328] Thus the reported incidence of DVT post-sclerotherapy treatment is greatly underestimated.

In the 1930s and 1940s PE after sclerotherapy of varicose veins occurred in, at most, 0.14% of patients.[329,330] In a series of 45,000 injections given to 7500 patients, only one episode of PE was reported.[331] Sicard, in 1928, reported 325,000 injections without a pulmonary infarction.[332] Linser and Vohwinkel[333] reported four cases of PE after 75,000 injections, only one of which was fatal. More recently with the onset of compression techniques in combination with sclerotherapy, this complication has become even less common. Sigg[334] has reported PE occurring only once with 42,000 injections. A French vascular surgeon who treats approximately 75 sclerotherapy patients a week, amounting to 25,000 yearly injections, reported only one case of PE in 20 years.[306] Fegan[227] reported that he has never seen conclusive evidence of DVT after injection treatment of 16,000 patients in his clinic. The 2-year Australian Polidocanol Trial reported one case of major DVT and two cases of minor DVT that occurred after injection of 4 ml of 0.5% POL, 4 ml of 0.5% POL, and 0.5 ml of 1% POL, respectively, in 12,544 injected legs, for an incidence of approximately 0.02%.[176] In a review of 28 cases of PE after sclerotherapy, most cases occurred in patients at bed rest. PE occurred 1 to 21 days after the treatment session. The incidence in this series was estimated as one case of PE per 10,000 patients.[335]

To evaluate the true incidence more accurately, 13 patients undergoing compression sclerotherapy with Fegan's technique were studied with continuous-screening ascending venography. Not more than 1 ml of 3% STS was injected, with the total amount not exceeding 5 ml. Patients were seen in follow-up 1 week later for comparison venography. Patients did not develop radiographic evidence for DVT.[336]

An additional study using impedance plethysmography and Doppler ultrasonic examination was performed before and after sclerotherapy treatment by the classic Fegan technique in 67 legs.[337] This study confirmed that there were no alterations in deep venous blood flow at 1 and 2 weeks after injection treatment. This confirmed the clinical experience that sclerotherapy using the Fegan technique is highly unlikely to be complicated by the development of DVT. Venographic evaluation of the injection of 0.5 to 1.0 ml of sclerosing solution in 15 patients with incompetent perforator veins failed to demonstrate extension of radiocontrast media into the deep venous system.[336]

An additional reason why sclerotherapy treatment does not usually result in DVT may be related to platelet inhibition by sclerosing solutions.[338] One study found that platelet aggregation, the first step in thrombogenesis, is inhibited by the concentrations of sclerosing solution that usually occur in the deep venous system after sclerotherapy of superficial varicosities.[339,340]

Cause

The cause of DVT, with or without PE, after sclerotherapy is unclear. The three major factors responsible for DVT were first elucidated more than 100 years ago by Virchow[341]: (1) endothelial damage; (2) vascular stasis; and (3) changes in coagulability. Sclerotherapy treatment always produces the first two causes in the triad, with coagulability changes related to the unique properties of sclerosing solutions (see Chapter 7) in addition to the predisposing factors of the patient. Chemical endophlebitis produced by sclerotherapy should anchor the thrombus to the site of injection. Histologic examination of treated varicose veins has demonstrated that firm thrombosis occurs only on the damaged endothelium. Nonadherent thrombosis occurs on normal endothelium.[342] Therefore the most logical explanation for the development of emboli is damage to the deep venous system by migration of sclerosing solution or a partly attached thrombosis into deep veins from treated superficial veins. This may occur as a result of either injection of excessive volumes of sclerosing solution or physical inactivity after injection.[343]

An additional possibility concerns injection of tributary perforator veins, which may directly communicate with the deep venous system. In this situation inadequate compression or injection of even 0.5 ml of sclerosing solution may force nonadherent thrombi into the deep circulation with muscle contraction. Ascending venography and digital subtraction phlebography in women with leg telangiectasia found that 0.7 ml of contrast medium injected into telangiectatic branches spread into the saphenous system in 8 of 15 patients.[344] Two of the eight patients had telangiectasia as the only clinically perceptible abnormality. Therefore it is possible that up to 13% of patients with telangiectatic veins are at risk for the spread of sclerosing solution directly into the deep venous system. This further emphasizes the importance of limiting injection volumes.

Amount of injection per site

The circulation and direction of blood flow in varicose veins have been determined radiographically as stagnant or reversed (away from the heart) so that the chemically induced thrombus is forced distally toward the smaller branching veins.[345] However, cinematographic studies documented that a small amount of sclerosing solution entered the deep circulation after injection of 0.5 to 1.0 ml of solution into a superficial varicosity during 7 of 15 injections in nine subjects (see Figs. 9-2 and 9-3).[346] No adverse effects were noted in these patients treated with POL 2%. The lack of adverse effects was probably related to rapid compression and ambulation of treated individuals and the resulting rapid dilution of the sclerosing agent within the deep venous system.

Although studies demonstrating the rarity of DVT after sclerotherapy are reassuring, DVT and embolic episodes usually occur 4 to 28 days after the sclerotherapy treatment session.[329] Therefore longer follow-up is necessary. In addition, nearly 40% of patients with DVT have asymptomatic PE.[347]

DVT and PE have been reported to occur with injection of large quantities of sclerosing solution (12 ml) in a single site.[348] Two separate case reports of this complication, occurring with injection of less than 0.5 ml of POL 1% in two patients in each report, have been published.[176,349] In both reports the injected veins were leg telangiectasias. In addition, the injection of 0.5 to 1 ml of sclerosing solution above the midthigh resulted in a presumed thrombus at the saphenofemoral junction with resulting pulmonary emboli.[220] This prompted Reid and Rothine[220] to recommend that injections not be given above the midthigh.

Thus the quantity of sclerosing solution per injection site must be limited to ensure that the agent will remain within the superficial system, and blood flow in the deep venous system must be rapidly stimulated after sclerotherapy with compression and muscle movement.

Finally, sclerotherapy of pedal veins may be hazardous since the lack of valves or reversal of valves allow inward flow from superficial to deep veins.[350] This may produce DVT. Therefore when treatment is necessary, phlebectomy may be preferable to sclerotherapy.

Inappropriate compression

The inappropriate tourniquet effect of an excessively tight wrap on the thigh is a rare cause for the development of DVT.[35] Occlusion of deep venous flow results in popliteal vein thrombosis, which can be resolved with conservative treatment. The adverse effects of nongraduated compression emphasize the importance of using properly fitted graduated support stockings in sclerotherapy treatment.

Hypercoagulable states

A number of primary and secondary hypercoagulable states exist that can be ruled out through the use of an appropriate patient history and a review of systems in the presclerotherapy treatment evaluation (see box below). The prevalence of inherited thrombotic syndromes in the general population is 1 in 2500 to 5000 but increases to 4% in patients with a past history of thrombosis.[352] In addition, a past history of DVT raises the likelihood of new postoperative venous thrombosis from 26% to 68%, whereas a past history of both DVT and PE gives a near 100% incidence of thrombosis.[353] Thus sclerotherapy should be undertaken cautiously in patients with previous DVT. Further detail on all hypercoagulable states is beyond the scope of this chapter. The most common states are discussed below. The reader is referred to multiple review articles on this important subject.[321,352,354,355]

Oral Contraceptive Agents and Estrogen Replacement Therapy

The mechanism for thromboembolic disease in women who use oral contraceptives is multifactorial. Both estrogens and progestogens have been implicated in promoting thrombosis despite low-dose therapy.[356-358] All studies have indicated

---

HYPERCOAGULABLE STATES

PRIMARY HYPERCOAGULABLE STATES
Deficiency in inhibitors of coagulation
  Antithrombin III deficiency
  Protein C deficiency
  Protein S deficiency
Disorders of the fibrinolytic system
Plasminogen deficiency
Plasminogen activator excess
Dysfibrinogenemias
Vascular damage—homocystinuria
Platelet damage—paroxysmal nocturnal hemoglobinuria
  Lupus anticoagulant

SECONDARY HYPERCOAGULABLE STATES
Abnormalities of coagulation and fibrinolysis
  Pregnancy
  Malignancy
  Nephrotic syndrome
  Oral contraceptives
  Estrogen/progestin supplementation
  Inflammatory bowel disease
Infectious diseases
  Secondary syphilis
  Psittacosis

Platelet abnormalities
  Myeloproliferative disorders
  Diabetes mellitus
  Hyperlipidemia
  Paroxysmal nocturnal hemoglobinuria
  Lupus anticoagulant
  Heparin-associated thrombocytopenia
Stasis or aberrant blood flow
  Varicose veins
  Congestive heart failure
  Immobilization
  Obesity
  Advanced age
  Perioperative state
  Polycythemia vera, sickle cell disease
  Dehydration
  Paraproteinuria
Endothelial damage
  Intravenous catheters
  Intravenous solutions
  Intravenous drug abuse
  Vasculitis
    Behçet's disease
  Thromboangiitis obliterans

Modified from Thomas JH: Am J Surg 160:547, 1990; and from Samlaska CP and James WD: J Am Acad Dermatol 23:1, 1990.

that the increased risk occurs only while the preparations are actually in use and perhaps for 1 week or so after discontinuation.[359,360] The highest rates of thromboembolism occur with the use of higher levels of estrogen[356-359,361]; some studies show an elevenfold increase.[360,362] Nevertheless the risk of postoperative PE still appears increased in women who use oral contraceptive agents with minimal amounts of estrogen.[363] Interestingly, a detailed review of the statistical methodologies of these studies did not prove a *definite* risk.[364] However, it appears prudent to examine the available literature on this topic.

It has been estimated that oral contraceptives are responsible for one case of superficial or deep vein thrombosis per 500 women users per year.[365] This estimate of hypercoagulability may be low since an examination of plasma fibrinogen chromatography demonstrated a 27% incidence of silent thrombotic lesions in 154 new contraceptive users of either mestranol, 100 μg, or ethinyl estradiol, 50 μg.[366] Oral contraceptive users as a group have numerous alterations in their coagulation system that promote a hypercoagulable state. They include hyperaggregable platelets, decreased endothelial fibrinolysis,[367] decreased negative surface charge on vessel walls and blood cells,[368] elevated levels of procoagulants, reduced RBC filterability,[369] increased blood viscosity secondary to elevated RBC volume,[370] and decreased levels of antithrombin III.[371-373] Any of these factors, alone or in combination, may predominate in women taking oral contraceptives. The extent of this derangement in the hemostatic system determines whether thrombosis will occur. When endothelial damage with sclerotherapy is initiated in this population, an increased incidence of thrombosis may result.

The most important factors preventing clot propagation are antithrombin III and vascular stores of t-PA.[371,374-376] Antithrombin III levels have been demonstrated as 20% lower in some women taking oral contraceptive agents[374] and estrogen replacement therapy.[377] Of women using oral contraceptive agents who have thromboembolic events, 90% have a twenty-fivefold decrease in releasable t-PA[371,374-375]; 51.6% have an abnormally low plasminogen activator content in the vein walls.[376] Therefore a certain subgroup of women taking birth control pills is at particular risk for thromboembolic disease.

In addition, increased distensibility of peripheral veins may occur with use of systemic estrogens and progestins.[378] This may promote valvular dysfunction and a relative stasis in blood flow to add to the hypercoagulable state. Since it is practically impossible and also impractical at this time to determine which women are at risk, it would appear prudent to recommend that patients consider discontinuing this medication before sclerotherapy treatment.

An alternative for women who cannot discontinue oral estrogen replacement therapy is the use of transdermally administered 17 beta-estradiol. By delivering estrogen directly into the peripheral circulation, the "first-pass effect" of liver metabolism is eliminated. This decreases hepatic estrogen levels with subsequent minimization of estrogen-induced alteration of coagulation proteins. Thus it is recommended that transdermal estrogen be used in patients at risk for thromboembolism since alterations in blood clotting factors have not been demonstrated during such treatment.[379]

Tamoxifen

For multiple reasons, including prevention of breast cancer in high-risk populations, adjunctive treatment of breast cancer, and possibly treatment and/or prevention of osteoporosis, tamoxifen is not an uncommon medication for patients who also are seen for sclerotherapy or surgical treatment or both. An unusual and poorly understood complication of tamoxifen use is the development of thrombophlebitis and DVT. This occurs in up to 1% of treated patients.[380,381] Results from evaluation of various coagulation parameters and factors, including sex hormone binding globulin, antithrombin III fibrinogen level, platelet count, protein C, and fibrinopeptide A, have been normal.[381-385] Until more is known about this theoretical predisposing factor to thrombosis, note should be taken of patients receiving tamoxifen.

Pregnancy

It was common medical practice as early as 1579 not to tamper with varicose veins during pregnancy.[386] However, some physicians advocate removal of varicose veins to prevent postpartum venous thrombosis.[387] These authors report a distinct lack of complications to both mother and baby with this practice, even though treatment spanned between the first and eighth months of gestation. However, in addition to the possible effects on the fetus through passage of sclerosing solution through the placental barrier, there is a potential for stimulating thrombosis.

Endothelial cell damage (presumably through sclerotherapy) releases t-PA to promote coagulability on the already formed clot, which invariably occurs in the immediate postsclerotherapy period.[388] In addition, coexistent hypercoagulability may promote excessive (uncontrolled) thrombosis.

The hypercoagulable state in the immediate antepartum period is responsible in large part for the development of superficial thrombophlebitis and DVT in 0.15% and 0.04% of patients, respectively.[389] Even more important is the immediate postpartum period during which the incidence of superficial thrombophlebitis and DVT is 1.18% and 0.15%, respectively.[389] DVT developed by the second postpartum day in 50% of patients. This development may be due to the rapid decrease in coagulation factors at partum that normalizes in most patients on the third day.[390] However, additional factors must also play a role since an additional 21% developed DVT 2 to 3 weeks postpartum. Interestingly, two thirds of the patients who developed postpartum DVT had varicose veins. Age of the mother was also linked to venous thrombosis, with the rate changing from approximately 1:1000 in women younger than 25 years of age to 1:1200 in women over 35.[361]

During pregnancy an increase in most procoagulant factors and a reduction in fibrinolytic activity occur. Plasma fibrinogen levels gradually increase after the third month of pregnancy to double those of the nonpregnant state. In the second half of pregnancy factors VII, X, VII and IX are also elevated.[391] Decreased fibrinolytic activity probably is related to a decrease in circulating plasminogen activator.[392] In addition, a 68% reduction in protein S levels has been measured during pregnancy and in the postpartum period.[393] Protein S levels do not return to normal until 12 weeks postpartum. These changes are necessary to prevent hemorrhage during placental separation. Thus, in addition to the potential adverse effects on the fetus, sclerotherapy near term should be avoided until coagulability returns to normal 6 weeks postpartum.

Inherited Factor Deficiency

Another subgroup of patients is also at increased risk for DVT. Protein C and protein S are two vitamin K–dependent proteins that are important anticoagulant factors that prevent thrombosis. Protein S is a cofactor for activated protein C on factor Va. It has been estimated that the prevalence of heterozygous protein C deficiency is 1:300 to 1:60 healthy adults in the United States.[394] More than 95% of these subjects are asymptomatic and without a history of thrombotic disease. However, these deficiencies may predispose them to the development of DVT.

Seventy-five percent of patients homozygous for protein S deficiency will develop venous thrombosis before age 35.[395] It has been speculated that damaged endothelium in combination with this deficiency may be necessary for symptomatic thrombosis to occur.[396] In otherwise healthy patients under 45 years of age referred for evaluation of venous thrombosis, the prevalence of deficiencies of antithrombin III, protein C, and protein S is approximately 5% each.[397] A resistance to activated protein C has been found in approximately one third of patients referred for evaluation of DVT.[398] Precipitating factors for thrombosis, such as pregnancy and the use of oral contraceptives, were present in 60% of these patients. Therefore patients who exhibit excessive thrombosis with sclerotherapy and patients with a family history of thrombotic disease should be screened for deficiencies of protein C and protein S before treatment.

A rare cause of acquired protein S deficiency occurs from a transient circulating autoantibody. An 11-year-old boy with varicella was described with this transient abnormal immune response that resulted in severe thromboembolic disease.[399] With chickenpox, endothelitis that may disrupt normal production of protein S occurs.[400] In this patient thrombosis was resistant to heparin therapy, and it was postulated that infusions of protein S would have been therapeutic. Although this is an extremely rare cause of DVT, withholding sclerotherapy treatment in febrile patients, especially those with varicella, Rocky Mountain spotted fever, and vasculitis, is recommended.

Antithrombin III deficiency occurs in 1:2000 to 1:5000 people in the general population.[401,402] Acquired antithrombin III deficiency may occur during liver disease and from the use of oral contraceptives as previously discussed.

Defects in the fibrinolytic system, specifically plasminogen, occur in up to 10% of the normal population.[403] When they occur alone, there is little risk of thrombosis. Abnormal plasminogen levels may also predispose to thrombosis.

Lupuslike anticoagulants are present in 16% to 33% of patients with lupus erythematosus but are also associated with a variety of autoimmune disorders.[404-406] Thirty to 50% of patients with lupuslike anticoagulants develop thrombosis.[406-408]

Prevention

Because of the potentially lethal nature of excessive thrombosis, all attempts should be made to minimize its occurrence. The sclerosing solution quantity should be limited to 0.5 to 1 ml per injection site to prevent leakage of the solution into the deep venous system.[315] Other techniques that minimize damage to the deep venous system include rapid compression of the injected vein with a 30 to 40 mm Hg pressure stocking, followed by immediate ambulation or calf movement of the injected extremity and frequent ambulation thereafter to promote rapid dilution of the solution from the injected area. Full dorsiflexion of the ankle empties all deep leg veins, including muscular and soleal sinuses.[409] Using these recommendations, Fegan[410] reported no cases of DVT or pulmonary emboli in 13,352 patients when the sclerosing solution quantity was limited to 0.5 ml and rapid compression was used.

The critical time period for thrombus formation in sclerotherapy-treated vessels is approximately 9 hours after treatment (see Chapter 7). Therefore compression stockings or bandages are of most benefit during the night after sclerotherapy treatment and during other periods of relative vascular stasis when an intravascular thrombus is being formed.

Foley[41] advocates the addition of heparin, 100 U/ml, to HS to prevent the theoretical possibility of embolization associated with "microthrombus formation" in sclerotherapy. However, a well-controlled, randomized study of 800 patients treated with and without heparin in the sclerosing solution found no evidence for embolization and no difference in the incidence of thrombophlebitis or microthrombosis requiring puncture evacuation.[42]

Consideration must be given to treating elderly patients since they have a reportedly increased risk for DVT.[200,411-413] It is hypothesized that the major cause for this increased risk is the relative pooling of blood in the soleal venous sinuses, which occurs from decreased calf muscle pump infusion.[414] In the elderly population it may be best to perform small treatments, with calf pumping given manually immediately after injection.

Venous stasis is the most likely mechanism for DVT after sclerotherapy. This can occur from a tourniquet effect due to an improperly bandaged extremity or from immobilization of a treated limb. At least one case of fatal PE after sclerotherapy has been blamed on improper bandaging coupled with a prolonged car ride immediately after treatment.[415] If a patient becomes ill or injured after sclerotherapy, he or she must avoid immobilization. In this scenario it is strongly recommended that consideration be given heparin prophylaxis or anticoagulation until ambulation is restored.[321]

Treatment

Since DVT is a potentially life-threatening complication, its treatment must be rapid and decisive. After effective anticoagulation with IV heparin has been achieved, oral anticoagulation with warfarin and other inhibitors of vitamin K metabolism should begin. Alternatively, patients may continue receiving subcutaneous heparin. IV heparin should be continued for 3 to 5 days after initiation of warfarin to prevent an early reduction in anticoagulant protein C and protein S function before procoagulant activity is affected.

Peripheral infusions of lytic agents may be superior to anticoagulation in the rapidity of clot resolution, in the reduction of late symptoms, and in the reduction of the risk of recurrent thrombosis.[416] If peripheral systemic lytic therapy is ineffective, direct infusion of lytic agents into the thrombus may be useful.[417] To prevent recurrence, thrombolytic therapy should be followed by the use of antiplatelet agents such as aspirin or warfarin or both. A more complete discussion of the various lytic agents is beyond the scope of this chapter.

Nerve Damage

Because of their close proximity, the saphenous and sural nerves may be injected with solution during sclerotherapy. Injection into a nerve is reported as very painful and, if continued, may cause anesthesia and sometimes a permanent interruption of nerve function.[165] Five episodes of injection into a nerve were reported from France over 18 years.[310] Various degrees of nerve paralysis or paresis occurred.

Occasionally a patient complains of an area of paresthesia in the treated leg. This is probably caused by perivascular inflammation extending from the sclerosed vein to adjacent superficial nerves. Steps to limit inflammation, including therapy with nonsteroidal antiinflammatory medications and high-potency topical steroids, may hasten resolution of this minor annoyance. However, this complication may take 3 to 6 months to resolve.[227]

Air Embolism

When the air-block[418,419] or foam techniques are used to inject sclerosing solutions, the theoretical possibility of air embolism is raised. The danger would be that if enough air entered the heart at one time, it might lead to vascular collapse. In addition, if air enters a cerebral vascular artery, a cerebral vascular infarction may occur. More likely, transient ischemic symptoms might occur with this injection technique.

Introduction of air in small amounts into the venous system does not lead to clinical air embolism.[418,419] It appears that small amounts of air are absorbed into the bloodstream before the blood enters the pulmonic circulation. It has been estimated that it would be necessary to put 480 ml of air into the venous system within 20 to 30 seconds to cause death in a person weighing 60 kg.[420] This occurrence has never been reported in the medical literature and has not occurred in a series of 297 cases with the air-block technique.[418]

Scintillating Scotomata

Although not reported in the literature, many physicians have told me of patients who develop temporary blindness or unusual visual disturbances after sclerotherapy. These physical findings most likely suggest ischemia of the calcarine cortex, which may occur through either embolism of ophthalmic arteries via the internal carotid or a vasospastic event. Arterial embolism appears unlikely unless the patient has a patent foramen ovale since venous injection and possible embolic events terminate in the pulmonary system. Monocular retinal migraine may occur in patients with a migraine diathesis. In such a case the patient's history is helpful and the outcome usually benign. It is recommended that a complete ophthalmologic examination be obtained in these patients to rule out other more serious and treatable causative factors.

Membranous Fat Necrosis

A single patient with multiple tender, erythematous subcutaneous nodules that occurred after sclerotherapy with HS solution has recently been reported.[421] This rare dermatologic entity is secondary to subcutaneous inflammation with alteration and necrosis of adipose tissue. The etiology may also be secondary to trauma, thromboangiitis obliterans, arteriosclerosis, or scleroderma. It is essentially a diagnosis of exclusion made on biopsy. In the reported patient extravasation of HS solution or vessel rupture with subsequent exposure of HS to subcutaneous tissues was the probable causative event.

Table 8-2 Summary of complications of sclerosing agents

Solution	Pigmentation	Allergic reaction	Necrosis	Pain
Sodium morrhuate	++	++	+++*	+++
Sodium tetradecyl sulfate	++	+	++*	+
Ethanolamine oleate	+	++	++*	++
Polidocanol	+	+	+*	0
Hypertonic saline	+	0	+++*	+++
Sclerodex(10% saline + 5% dextrose)	+	0	+	++
Chromated glycerin	0	+	0	++
Polyiodinated iodine	++	+	+++*	+++

+, Minimal; ++, moderate; +++, significant.
*Concentration dependent.

Summary

In summary, sclerotherapy of varicose and telangiectatic leg veins may be associated with a number of complications and adverse sequelae, which may occur despite optimal treatment. Some adverse sequelae are preventable to a limited degree, but given a large enough number of procedures, these adverse sequelae will occur in any practice. Complications also are avoidable to some extent. As with any adverse procedure, however, sclerotherapy has inherent risks. Thus each patient should be evaluated and cautioned accordingly before initiating treatment. A summary of the common complications that can occur with the commonly used sclerosing agents is presented in Table 8-2.

REFERENCES

1. Tournay PR: Traitment sclerosant des tres fines varicosites intra ou saous-dermiques, Soc Fran Phlebol 19:235, 1966.
2. Tretbar LL: Spider angiomata: treatment with sclerosant injections, J Kans Med Soc 79:198, 1978.
3. Weiss R and Weiss M: Resolution of pain associated with varicose and telangiectatic leg veins after compression sclerotherapy, J Dermatol Surg Oncol 16:333, 1990.
4. Bodian EL: Techniques of sclerotherapy for sunburst venous blemishes, J Dermatol Surg Oncol 11:696, 1985.
5. Duffy DM: Small vessel sclerotherapy: an overview. In Callen JP et al, editors: Advances in dermatology, vol 3, Chicago, 1988, Year Book Medical Publishers, Inc.
6. Alderman DB: Surgery and sclerotherapy in the treatment of varicose veins, Conn Med 39:467, 1975.
7. White SW and Besanceney C: Systemic pigmentation from tetracycline and minocycline therapy, Arch Dermatol 119:1, 1983.
8. Cacciatore E: Experience of sclerotherapy with aethoxysklerol, Minn Cardioangiol 27:255, 1979.
9. Goldman P: Sclerotherapy of superficial venules and telangiectasias of the lower extremities, Dermatol Clin 5:369, 1987.
10. Avramovic A and Avramovic M: Complications of sclerotherapy: a statistical study. In Raymond-Martimbeau P, Prescott R, and Zummo M, editors: Phlebologie '92, Paris, 1992, John Libbey Eurotext.
11. Georgiev M: Postsclerotherapy hyperpigmentations: a one-year follow-up, J Dermatol Surg Oncol 16:608, 1990.
12. Biegeleisen HI and Biegeleisen RM: The current status of sclerotherapy for varicose veins, Clin Med 83:24, 1976.
13. Chrisman BB: Treatment of venous ectasias with hypertonic saline, Hawaii Med J 41:406, 1982.
14. Chatard H: Discussion de la question de J-C Allart: pigmentations post-sclotherapiques, Phlebologie 29:211, 1976.
15. Shields JL and Jansen GT: Therapy for superficial telangiectasias of the lower extremities, J Dermatol Surg Oncol 8:857, 1982.
16. Barner FR, Holzegel K, and Voigt K: Über Hyperpigmentation nach Krampfaderverödung, Phebol u Proktol 6:54, 1977.
17. Goldman MP, Kaplan RP, and Duffy DM: Postsclerotherapy hyperpigmentation: a histologic evaluation, J Dermatol Surg Oncol 13:547, 1987.
18. Goldman MP: Postsclerotherapy hyperpigmentation: treatment with a flashlamp excited pulsed dye laser, J Dermatol Surg Oncol 18:417, 1992.
19. Cuttell PJ and Fox JA: The etiology and treatment of varicose pigmentation, Phlebologie 35:387, 1982.
20. Goldman MP et al: Sclerosing agents in the treatment of telangiectasia: comparison of the clinical and histologic effects of intravascular polidocanol, sodium tetradecyl sulfate, and hypertonic saline in the dorsal rabbit ear vein model, Arch Dermatol 123:1196, 1987.
21. Moreno AH et al: Mechanics of distention of dog veins and other thin-walled tubular structures, Circ Res 27:1069, 1970.
22. Grega GJ, Svensjo E, and Haddy FJ: Macromolecular permeability of the microvascular membrane: physiological and pharmacological regulation, Microcirc 1:325, 1981-1982.
23. Majno G, Palade GE, and Schoefl GI: Studies on inflammation: the site of action of histamine and serotonin along the vascular tree: a topographic study, J Biophys Biochem Cytol 11:607, 1961.
24. Bjork J and Smedegard G: The microvasculature of the hamster cheek pouch as a model for studying acute immune-complex-induced inflammatory reactions, Int Arch Allergy Appl Immunol 74:178, 1984.

25. Fox J, Galey F, and Wayland H: Action of histamine on the mesenteric microvasculature, Microvasc Res 19:108, 1980.

26. Simionescu N, Simionescu M, and Palade G: Open junctions in the endothelium of the postcapillary venules of the diaphram, J Cell Biol 79:27, 1978.

27. Bessis M: Living blood cells and their ultrastructure, Berlin, 1973, Springer-Verlag, Inc.

28. Leu HJ et al: Veranderungen der transendothelialen Permeabilitat als Ursache des Odems bei der chronisch-venosen Insuffizienz, Med Welt 31:781, 1980.

29. Bessis M, Lessin LS, and Beutler E: Morphology of the erythron. In Williams WJ et al, editors: Hematology, ed 3, New York, 1983, McGraw-Hill Book Co.

30. Ludewig S: Hemosiderin. Isolation from horse spleen and characterization, Proc Soc Exp Biol Med 95:514, 1957.

31. Richter GW: The nature of storage iron in idiopathic hemochromatosis and in hemosiderosis, J Exp Med 112:551, 1960.

32. Ackerman Z et al: Overload of iron in the skin of patients with varicose ulcers, Arch Dermatol 124:1376, 1988.

33. Chatarel H and Dufour H: Note sur la nature mixtre, hématique et mélanique, des pigmentations en phlébologie, Phlébologie 36:303, 1983.

34. Merlen JF, Coget J, and Sarteel AM: Pigmentation et stase veinĕuse, Phlébologie 36:307, 1983.

35. Klüken N and Zabel M: La pigmentation est-elle un signe caractéristique de L'insuffisance veineuse chronique? Phlébologie 36:315, 1983.

36. Thibault P and Wlodarczyk J: Postsclerotherapy hyperpigmentation: the role of serum iron levels and the effectiveness of treatment with the copper vapor laser, J Dermatol Surg Oncol 18:47, 1992.

37. Pippard MJ and Hoffbrand AV: Iron. In Hoffbrand AV and Lewis SM, editors: Postgraduate haematology, 1989, Heinemann Medical Books.

38. Thibault P and Wlodarczyk J: Correlation of serum ferritin levels and postsclerotherapy pigmentation: prospective study. J Dermatol Surg Oncol 20:684, 1994.

39. Cloutier G and Sansoucy H: Le traitement des varices des membres inferieurs par les injections sclerosantes, L'Union Medicale du Canada 104:1854, 1975.

40. Weiss RA and Weiss MA: Incidence of side effects in the treatment of telangiectasias by compression sclerotherapy: hypertonic saline vs polidocanol, J Dermatol Surg Oncol 16:800, 1990.

41. Foley WT: The eradication of venous blemishes, Cutis 15:665, 1975.

42. Sadick N: Treatment of varicose and telangiectatic leg veins with hypertonic saline: a comparative study of heparin and saline, J Dermatol Surg Oncol 16:24, 1990.

43. Hutinel B: Esthetique dans les scleroses de varices et traitement des varicosites, La Vie Med 20:1739, 1978.

44. Nebot F: Quelques points tecniques sur le traitement des varicosites et des telangiectasies, Phlébologie 21:133, 1968.

45. Landart J: Traitment medical des varices des membres inferieurs, La Rev du Pract 26:2491, 1976.

46. Tournat R: La Sclerose des varices, Paris, 1980, Expansion Scientifique Francaise.

47. Lucchi M and Bilancini S: Sclerotherapy of telangiectasia (English abstract), Minerva Angiol 15:31, 1990.

48. Georgiev M: Postsclerotherapy hyperpigmentation: chromated glycerin as a screen for patients at risk (a retrospective study), J Dermatol Surg Oncol 19:649, 1993.

49. Norris MJ, Carlin MC, and Ratz JL: Treatment of essential telangiectasia: effects of increasing concentrations of polidocanol, J Am Acad Dermatol 20:643, 1989.

50. Guarde C: Personal communication, 1989.

51. Marley W: Low-dose sotradecol for small vessel sclerotherapy, Newsletter of North Am Soc Phlebol 3:3, 1989.

52. Guex J-J: Indications for the sclerosing agent polidocanol, J Dermatol Surg Oncol 19:959, 1993.

53. Gilchrest BA, Stoff JS, and Soter NA: Chronologic aging alters the response to ultraviolet-induced inflammation in human skin, J Invest Dermatol 79:11, 1982.

54. Marciniak DL et al: Antagonism of histamine edema formation by catecholamines, Am J Physiol 234:H180, 1978.

55. Svensjo E: Pharmacological modulation of venular permeability with some antiinflammatory drugs. Return circulation and norepinephrine: an update, Paris, 1991, Eurotext.

56. Svensjo E, Persson CGA, and Rutili G: Inhibition of bradykinin induced macromolecular leakage from post-capillary venules by a B₂-adrenoreceptor stimulant, terbutaline, Acta Physiol Scand 101:504, 1977.

57. Heltianu C, Simionescu M, and Simionescu N: Histamine receptors of the microvascular endothelium revealed in situ with a histamine-ferritin conjugate: characteristic high-affinity binding sites in venules, J Cell Biol 93:357, 1982.

58. Clemetson CAB, Blair L, and Brown AB: Capillary strength and the menstrual cycle, Ann N Y Acad Sci 93:277, 1962.
59. Jacoby WD: Comment 21, Schoch Lett 41:2, 1991.
60. Leffell DJ: Minocycline hydrochloride hyperpigmentation complicating treatment of venous ectasia of the extremities, J Am Acad Dermatol 24:501, 1991.
61. Poliak SC et al: Minocycline associated tooth discoloration in young adults, JAMA 254:2930, 1985.
62. Billano RA, Ward WQ, and Little WP: Minocycline and black thyroid (Letter), JAMA 249:1887, 1983.
63. Dwyer CM et al: Skin pigmentation due to minocycline treatment of facial dermatoses, Br J Dermatol 129:158, 1993.
64. Fenske NA, Millns JL, and Greer KE: Minocycline-induced pigmentation at sites of cutaneous inflammation, JAMA 244:1103, 1980.
65. Eedy DJ and Burrows D: Minocycline-induced pigmentation occurring in two sisters, Clin Exp Dermatol 16:55, 1991.
66. Basler RSW and Kohnen PW: Localized hemosiderosis as a sequela of acne, Arch Dermatol 114:1695, 1978.
67. Basler RSW: Minocycline therapy for acne (Letter), Arch Dermatol 115:1391, 1979.
68. Ridgway HA et al: Hyperpigmentation associated with oral minocycline, Br J Dermatol 107:95, 1982.
69. Sato S et al: Ultrastructual and x-ray microanalysis observations of minocycline-related hyperpigmentation of the skin, J Invest Dermatol 77:264, 1981.
70. Gordon G, Sparano BM, and Iatropoulos MJ: Hyperpigmentation of the skin associated with minocycline therapy, Arch Dermatol 121:618, 1985.
71. Okada N et al: Skin pigmentation associated with minocycline therapy, Br J Dermatol 124:247, 1989.
72. Muntlak H: Personal communication (Paris), 1989.
73. Wenner L: Sind endovarikose hamatische ansammlungen eine normalerscheinung bei sklerotherapie? Vasa 10:174, 1981.
74. Leu HJ, Wenner A, and Spycher MA: Erythrocyte diapedesis in venous stasis syndrome, Vasa 10:17, 1981.
75. Orbach EJ: Hazards of sclerotherapy of varicose veins—their prevention and treatment of complications, Vasa 8:170, 1979.
76. Perchuk E: Injection therapy of varicose veins: a method of obliterating huge varicosities with small doses of sclerosing agent, Angiology 25:393, 1974.
77. De Takats G: Problems in the treatment of varicose veins, Am J Surg 18:26, 1932.
78. Biegeleisen HI: Sclerotherapy: clinical significance, Clin Med Surg 47:140, 1940.
79. Bernier EC and Escher E: Treatment of postsclerotherapy hyperpigmentation with trichloracetic acid, a mild and effective procedure. Proceedings of the second annual International Congress of the North American Society of Phlebology, New Orleans, La, February 25, 1989.
80. Terezakis N: Personal communication, 1989.
81. Myers HL: Topical chelation therapy for varicose pigmentation, Angiology 17:66, 1966.
82. Burnand K et al: Venous lipodermatosclerosis: treatment by fibrinolytic enhancement and elastic compression, Br Med J 280:7, 1980.
83. Shoden A and Sturgeon P: Hemosiderin: I. A physio-chemical study, Acta Haematol (Basel) 23:376, 1960.
84. Wells CI and Wolken JJ: Biochemistry: microspectrophotometry of haemosiderin granules, Nature 193:977, 1962.
85. Riddock J: Treatment of varicose veins, Br J Med 2:671, 1947.
86. Bjork J et al: Methylprednisolone acts at the endothelial cell level reducing inflammatory responses, Acta Physiol Scand 123:221, 1985.
87. Bouskela E, Cyrino PZGA, and Marcelon G: Inhibitory effect of the ruscus extract and the flavanoid hesperidine methylchalcone (HMC) on increased microvascular permeability induced by various agents in the hamster cheek pouch, J Cardiovasc Physiol, 1994 (in press).
88. Svensjo E and Grega GJ: Evidence for endothelial cell-mediated regulation of macromolecular permeability by postcapillary venules, Fed Proc 45:89, 1986.
89. Goldman MP et al: Compression in the treatment of leg telangiectasia, J Dermatol Surg Oncol 16:322, 1990.
90. Arenander E and Lindhagen A: The evolution of varicose veins studied in a material of initially unilateral varices, Vasa 7:180, 1978.
91. Terezakis N: Sclerotherapy treatment of leg veins. Presented at the summer session of the American Academy of Dermatology, San Diego, Calif, June 17, 1989.

92. Davis LT and Duffy DM: Determination of incidence and risk factors for post-sclerotherapy telangiectatic matting of the lower extremity: a retrospective analysis, J Dermatol Surg Oncol 16:327, 1990.

93. Bodian EL: Sclerotherapy, Semin Dermatol 6:238, 1987.

94. Ouvry P and Davy A: Le traitement sclerosant des telangiectasias des membres inferieurs, Phlébologie 35:349, 1982.

95. Merlen JF: Telangiectasies rouges, telangiectasies bleues, Phlébologie 23:167, 1970.

96. Biegeleisen K: Primary lower extremity telangiectasias, relationship of size to color, Angiology 38:760, 1987.

97. Clark ER and Clark EL: Observations on living performed blood vessels as seen in a transparent chamber inserted into the rabbit's ear, Am J Anat 49:441, 1932.

98. Clark ER and Clark EL: Microscopic observations on the extracellular cells of living mammalian blood vessels, Am J Anat 66:1, 1940.

99. Yanagisawa-Miwa A et al: Salvage of infarcted myocardium by angiogenic action of basic fibroblast growth factor, Science 257:1401, 1992.

100. Shing Y et al: Angiogenesis is stimulated by tumor-derived endothelial cell growth factor, J Cell Biochem 29:275, 1985.

101. Ashton N: Corneal vascularization. In Duke-Elder S and Perkins ES, editors: The transparency of the cornea, Oxford, 1960, Blackwell Scientific Publications Inc.

102. Haudenschild CC: Growth control of endothelial cells in atherogenesis and tumor angiogenesis. In Altura BM, editor: Advances in microcirculation, vol 9, Basel, 1980, Karger.

103. Folkman J and Klagsbrun M: Angiogenic factors, Science 235:442, 1987.

104. Frater-Schroder M et al: Tumor necrosis factor type alpha, a potent inhibitor of endothelial cell growth in vitro, is angiogenic in vivo, Proc Natl Acad Sci USA 84:5277, 1987.

105. Fujita M et al: Improvement of treadmill capacity and collateral circulation as a result of exercise with heparin pretreatment in patients with effort angina, Circulation 77:1022, 1988.

106. Ryan TJ: Factors influencing the growth of vascular endothelium in the skin, Br J Dermatol 82(suppl 5):99, 1970.

107. Baffour R et al: Enhanced angiogenesis and growth of collaterals by in vivo administration of recombinant basic fibroblast growth factor in a rabbit model of acute lower limb ischemia: dose-response effect of basic fibroblast growth factor, J Vasc Surg 16:181, 1992.

108. Lindner V et al: Role of basic fibroblast growth factor in vascular lesion formation, Circ Res 68:106, 1991.

109. Leibovitch SJ et al: Macrophage-induced angiogenesis is mediated by tumor necrosis factor-alpha, Nature 329:630, 1987.

110. Piquet PF, Grau GE, and Vassalli P: Subcutaneous perfusion of tumor necrosis factor induces local proliferation of fibroblasts, capillaries, and epidermal cells, or massive tumor necrosis, Am J Pathol 136:103, 1990.

111. Miyazono K et al: Purification and properties of an endothelial cell growth factor from human platelets, J Biol Chem 262:4098, 1987.

112. Shing Y, Folkman J, and Haudenschild C: Angiogenesis is stimulated by tumor-derived endothelial cell growth factor, J Cell Biochem 29:275, 1985.

113. Leibovich SJ et al: Macrophage-induced angiogenesis is mediated by tumor necrosis factor-alpha, Nature 329:630, 1987.

114. Sporn MB et al: Transforming growth factor beta: biologic function and chemical structure, Science 233:532, 1987.

115. Martin BM, Gimbrone MA Jr, Unanue ER, et al: Stimulation of nonlymphoid mesenchymal cell proliferation by a macrophage-derived growth factor, J Immunol 126:1510, 1981.

116. Rothe MJ, Nowak M, and Kerdel FA: The mast cell in health and disease, J Am Acad Dermatol 23:615, 1990.

117. Flaumenhaft R et al: Role of extracellular matrix in the action of basic fibroblast growth factor: matrix as a source of growth factor for long-term stimulation of plasminogen activator production and DNA synthesis, J Cell Physiol 140:75, 1989.

118. Vlodavsky I et al: Endothelial cell-derived basic fibroblast growth factor: synthesis and deposition into subendothelial extracellular matrix, Proc Natl Acad Sci 84:2292, 1987.

119. Castellot JJ Jr et al: Heparin potentiation of $3T_3$-adipocyte stimulated angiogenesis: mechanisms of action on endothelial cells, J Cell Physiol 127:323, 1986.

120. Barnhill RL and Wolf JE Jr: Angiogenesis and the skin, J Am Acad Dermatol 16:1226, 1987.

121. Dvorak AM, Mihm MC Jr, and Dvorak HF: Morphology of delayed-type hypersensitivity reactions in man. II. Ultrastructural alterations affecting the microvasculature and the tissue mast cells, Lab Invest 34:179, 1976.

122. Enerback L: Mast cells in rat gastrointestinal mucosa. I. Effects of fixation, Acta Pathol Microbiol Scand 66:289, 1966.

123. Mikhail GR and Miller-Milinska A: Mast cell population in human skin, J Invest Dermatol 43:249, 1964.

124. Hellstrom B and Holmgren HJ: Numerical distribution of mast cells in human skin and heart, Acta Anat 10:81, 1950.
125. Eady RAJ et al: Mast cell population density, blood vessel density, and histamine content in normal human skin, Br J Dermatol 100:623, 1979.
126. Kasper CS, Freeman RG, and Tharp MD: Diagnosis of mastocytosis subsets using a morphometric point counting technique, Arch Dermatol 127:1017, 1987.
127. Mantse L: More on spider veins, J Dermatol Surg Oncol 12:1022, 1986.
128. Lary BG: Varicose veins and intracutaneous telangiectasia: combined treatment in 1500 cases, South Med J 80:1105, 1987.
129. Schiff M and Burn HF: The effect of intravenous estrogens on ground substance, Arch Otolaryngol 73:43, 1961.
130. Kleinman HK et al: Role of estrogens in inflammation and angiogenesis. Presented at The Joint Meeting of the Wound Healing Society and European Tissue Repair Society, Amsterdam, August 23, 1993.
131. Corbett DA: Discussion, Br J Dermatol 26:200, 1914.
132. Bean WB: The vascular spider in pregnancy. In Bean WB, editor: Vascular spiders and related lesions of the skin, Springfield, Ill, 1958, Charles C Thomas.
133. Pirovino M et al: Cutaneous spider nevi in liver cirrhosis: capillary microscopical and hormonal investigation, Klin Wochenschr 66:298, 1988.
134. Sadick NS and Niedt GW: A study of estrogen and progesterone receptors in spider telangiectasias of the lower extremities, J Dermatol Surg Oncol 16:620, 1990.
135. Saski GH, Pang CY, and Wittcliff JL: Pathogenesis and treatment of infant skin strawberry hemangiomas: clinical and in vitro studies of normal effects, Plast Reconstr Surg 73:359, 1984.
136. Puisseau-Lupo ML: Sclerotherapy—a review of results and complications in 200 patients, J Dermatol Surg Oncol 15:214, 1989.
137. Goldman MP and Fitzpatrick RE: Pulsed-dye laser treatment of leg telangiectasia: with and without simultaneous sclerotherapy, J Dermatol Surg Oncol 16:338, 1990.
138. Azizkhan RG et al: Mast cell heparin stimulates migration of capillary endothelial cells in vitro, J Exp Med 152:931, 1980.
139. Rakusan K and Turek Z: Protamine inhibits capillary formation in growing rat hearts, Circ Res 57:393, 1985.
140. Taylor S and Folkman J: Protamine is an inhibitor of angiogenesis, Nature 297:307, 1982.
141. Folkman J et al: Control of angiogenisis with synthetic heparin substitutes, Science 243:1490, 1989.
142. Zabel P, Schade FU, and Schlaak M: Pentoxyfylline—an inhibitor of the synthesis of tumor necrosis factor alpha, Ammun Infekt (Germany) 20:80, 1992.
143. Wang P et al: Mechanism of the beneficial effects of pentoxifylline on hepatocellular function after trauma hemorrhage and resuscitation, Surgery 112:451, 1992.
144. Martin U and Roemer D: Ketotifen: a histamine release inhibitor, Monogr Allergy 12:145, 1977.
145. Mansfield LE et al: Inhibition of dermographia, histamine, and dextromethorphan skin tests by ketotifen. A possible effect on cutaneous response to mediators, Ann Allergy 63:201, 1989.
146. Huston DP et al: Prevention of mast cell degranulation by ketotifen in patients with physical urticarias, Ann Intern Med 104:507, 1986.
147. Kuokkanen K: Comparison of a new antihistamine HC 20-511 (ketotifen) with cyproheptadine (Periactin) in chronic urticaria, Acta Allergica 32:316, 1977.
148. Saihan EM: Ketotifen and terbutaline in chronic urticaria, Br J Dermatol 104:205, 1981.
149. Shear NH and MacLeod SM: Diffuse cutaneous mastocytosis (DCM): Treatment with ketotifen and cimetidine, Clin Invest Med 6(suppl):36, 1983.
150. Czarnetzki BM: A double-blind cross-over study of the effect of ketotifen in urticaria pigmentosa, Dermatologica 166:44, 1983.
151. De Takats G and Quint H: The injection treatment of varicose veins, Surg Gynecol Obstet 50:545, 1930.
152. Chou F-F et al: The treatment of leg varicose veins with hypertonic saline–heparin injections, J Formosan Med Assoc 83:206, 1984.
153. Carlin MC and Ratz JL: Treatment of telangiectasia: comparison of sclerosing agents, J Dermatol Surg Oncol 13:1181, 1987.
154. Natbony SF et al: Histologic studies of chronic idiopathic urticaria, J Allergy Clin Immunol 71:177, 1983.
155. Alderman DB: Therapy for essential cutaneous telangiectasias, Postgrad Med 61:91, 1977.
156. Orbach EJ: The importance of removal of postinjection coagula during the course of sclerotherapy of varicose veins, Vasa 3:475, 1974.
157. Orbach EJ: A new approach to the sclerotherapy of varicose veins, Angiology 1:302, 1950.
158. Fegan WG: Sound film: varicose veins—compression sclerotherapy. Produced by Pharmaceutical Research Limited, 6-7 Broad St, Hereford HR4 9AE, England.

159. Tournay R: Collections hematiques intra ou extra-veineuses dans les phlebites superficielles ou apres injections sclerosantes de varicies a quel moment la thrombectomie? Soc Fran Phlebol 19:339, 1966.

160. Sigg K: Varizenverodung am hochgelgerten Bein. Deutsches Arzteblatt—Arztliche Mitteilungen. 69. Jahrang, Heft 14, S. 809-818. 6. April 1972, Postverlagsort Koln.

161. Pratt D: The technique of injection and compression. Stoke Mandeveille Hospital Symposium: The treatment of varicose veins by injection and compression, October 15, 1971.

162. Hobbs JT: The management of recurrent and residual veins. Stoke Mandeville Hospital Symposium: The treatment of varicose veins by injection and compression, October 15, 1971.

163. Holzegel VK: Uber Krampfaderverodugen, Dermatol Wocheuschr 153:137, 1967.

164. Winstone N. In The treatment of varicose veins by injection and compression. Proceedings of the Stoke Mandeville Symposium, Hereford, England, Pharmaceutical Research STD Ltd.

165. Browse NL, Burnard KG, and Thomas ML: Diseases of the veins: pathology, diagnosis, and treatment, London, 1988, Edward Arnold.

166. Duffy DM: Personal communication, 1989.

167. Schraibman IG: Localized hirsuties, Postgrad Med J 43:545, 1967.

168. Marks G: Localized hirsuties following compression sclerotherapy with sodium tetradecyl sulphate, Br J Surg 61:127, 1974.

169. Weissberg D: Treatment of varicose veins by compression sclerotherapy, Surg Gynecol Obstet 151:353, 1980.

170. Upton J, Mulliken JB, and Murray JE: Major extravasation injuries, Am J Surg 137:489, 1979.

171. Yosowitz P et al: Peripheral intravenous infiltration necrosis, Ann Surg 182:553, 1975.

172. Eaglstein W: Inadvertent intracutaneous injection with hypertonic saline (23.4%) in two patients without complications, J Dermatol Surg Oncol 16:878, 1990.

173. Jaquier JJ and Loretan RM: Clinical trials of a new sclerosing agent, aethoxysklerol, Soc Fr Phlebol 22:383, 1969.

174. Hoffer AE: Aethoxysklerol (Kreussler) in the treatment of varices, Minn Cardioang 20:601, 1972.

175. de Faria JL and Moraes IN: Histopathology of the telangiectasias associated with varicose veins, Dermatologia 127:321, 1963.

176. Conrad P and Malouf GM: The Australian polidocanol (aethoxysklerol) open clinical trial results at two years. Presented at the Annual Meeting of the North American Society of Phlebology, Maui, Hawaii, February 21, 1984.

177. Dinkler JA and Cohen BE: Reversal of dopamine extravasation injury with topical nitroglycerin ointment, J Plast Reconstr Surg 84:811, 1989.

178. AMA Drug Evaluation, ed 6, Chicago, Ill, 1986, American Medical Association.

179. Franks AG: Topical glyceryl trinitrate as adjunctive treatment in Raynaud's disease, Lancet 1:76, 1982.

180. Ross M: Dopamine-induced localized cutaneous vasoconstriction and piloerection, Arch Dermatol 127:586, 1991.

181. Chavez CM: The clinical significance of lymphatico-venous anastomoses, Vasc Dis 5:35, 1968.

182. Chant ADB: The effects of posture, exercise, and bandage pressure on the clearance of 24Na from the subcutaneous tissues of the foot, Br J Surg 59:552, 1972.

183. Campion EC, Hoffman DC, and Jepson RP: The effects of external pneumatic splint pressure on muscle blood flow, Aust N Z J Surg 38:154, 1968.

184. Lawrence D and Kakkar V: Graduated, static, external compression of the lower limb: a physiological assessment, Br J Surg 67:119, 1980.

185. Zimmet SE: The prevention of cutaneous necrosis following extravasation of hypertonic saline and sodium tetradecyl sulfate, J Dermatol Surg Oncol 19:641, 1993.

186. Senk KE: Management of intravenous extravasation, Infusion 5:77, 1981.

187. Dorr RT and Alberts DS: Vinca alkaloid skin toxicity: antidote and drug disposition studies in the mouse, JCNI 74:113, 1985.

188. Laurie SWS et al: Intravenous extravasation injuries: the effectiveness of hyaluronidase in their treatment, Ann Plast Surg 13:191, 1984.

189. Zenk KE, Dungy CL, and Greene GR: Nafcillin extravasation injury: use of hyaluronidase as an antidote, Am J Dis Child 135:1113, 1981.

190. Razka WV et al: The use of hyaluronidase in the treatment of intravenous extravasation injuries, J Perinatol 10:146, 1990.

191. Dorr RT and Alberts DS: Pharmacologic antidotes to experimental doxirubicin skin toxicity: a suggested role for beta-adrenergic compounds, Cancer Treat Rev 65:1001, 1981.

192. Grossman JA et al: The effects of hyaluronidase and DMSO on experimental flap survival, Ann Plast Surg 11:222, 1983.

193. Campbell CA, Przyklenk K, and Kloner RA: Infarct size reduction: a review of the clinical trials, J Clin Pharmacol 26:317, 1986.

194. Haire RD: Use of alidase in prevention of painful arm in accidental perivascular injection of neoasphenamine and mapharsen, Rocky Mt Med J 600, 1950.
195. Lorenz HP and Adzick NS: Scarless skin wound repair in the fetus, West J Med 159:350, 1993.
196. Britton RC and Habif DV: Clinical uses of hyaluronidase. A current review, Surgery 33:917, 1953.
197. Schwartzman J: Hyaluronidase: a review of its therapeutic use in pediatrics, J Pediatr 39:491, 1951.
198. Heckler FR and McCraw JB: Calcium related cutaneous necrosis, Plast Surg 27:553, 1976.
199. Brown AS, Hoelzer DJ, and Piercy SA: Skin necrosis from extravasation of intravenous fluids in children, Plast Reconstr Surg 64:145, 1979.
200. Beall GN, Casaburi R, and Singer A: Anaphylaxis—everyone's problem (Specialty Conference), West J Med 144:329, 1986.
201. Wasserman SI: Anaphylaxis. In Middleton E, Reed CE, and Ellis EF, editors: Allergy: principles and practice, ed 2, 1983, CV Mosby.
202. Shelley J: Allergic manifestations with injection treatment of varicose veins: death following injection of monoethanolamine oleate, JAMA 112:1792, 1939.
203. Schmier AA: Clinical comparison of sclerosing solutions in injection treatment of varicose veins, Am J Surg 36:389, 1937.
204. Zimmerman LM: Allergic-like reactions from sodium morrhuate in obliteration of varicose veins, JAMA 102:1216, 1934.
205. Meyer NE: Monoethanolamine oleate: a new chemical for obliteration of varicose veins, Am J Surg 40:628, 1938.
206. Lewis KM: Anaphylaxis due to sodium morrhuate, JAMA 107:1298, 1936.
207. Dick ET: The treatment of varicose veins, N Z Med J 65:310, 1966.
208. Sarin SK and Kumar A: Sclerosants for variceal sclerotherapy: a critical appraisal, Am J Gastroenterol 85:641, 1990.
209. Monroe P et al: Acute respiratory failure after sodium morrhuate esophageal sclerotherapy, Gastroenterology 85:693, 1983.
210. Dale ML: Reaction due to injection of sodium morrhuate, JAMA 108:718, 1937.
211. Ritchie A: The treatment of varicose veins during pregnancy, Edinburgh Med J 40:157, 1933.
212. Probstein JG: Major complications of intravenous therapy of varicose veins, J Missouri Med Assoc 33:349, 1936.
213. Dodd H and Oldham JB: Surgical treatment of varicose veins, Lancet 1:8, 1940.
214. Kilby A et al: Abnormal chest roentgenograms following endoscopic injection sclerosis of esophageal varices, Hepatology 2:709, 1982.
215. Perakos PG, Cirbus JJ, and Camara S: Persistent bradyarrhythmia after sclerotherapy for esophageal varices, South Med J 77:531, 1984.
216. Biegeleisen HI: Fatty acid solutions for the injection treatment of varicose veins: evaluation of four new solutions, Ann Surg 105:610, 1937.
217. Hedberg SE, Fowler DL, and Ryan LR: Injection sclerotherapy of esophageal varices using ethanolamine oleate: a pilot study, Am J Surg 143:426, 1982.
218. Hughes RW Jr et al: Endoscopic variceal sclerosis: a one-year experience, Gastrointest Endosc 28:62, 1982.
219. Foote RR: Severe reaction to monoethanolamine oleate, Lancet 390-95, 1942.
220. Reid RG and Rothine NG: Treatment of varicose veins by compression sclerotherapy, Br J Surg 55:889, 1968.
221. Clin-Alert correspondence, 1992.
222. Harris OD, Dickey JD, and Stephenson PM: Simple endoscopic injection sclerotherapy of esophageal varices, Aust N Z J Med 12:131, 1982.
223. Shubik P and Hartwell JL: Survey of compounds which have been tested for carcinogenic activity, US Department of Health, Education, and Welfare Public Health Service, 1969.
224. Goldman MP and Bennett RG: Treatment of telangiectasia: a review, J Am Acad Dermatol 17:167, 1987.
225. Steinberg MH: Evaluation of sotradecol in sclerotherapy of varicose veins, Angiology 6:519, 1955.
226. Nabatoff RA: Recent trends in the diagnosis and treatment of varicose veins, Surg Gynecol Obstet 90:521, 1950.
227. Fegan G: Varicose veins: compression sclerotherapy, London, 1967, Heinemann Medical.
228. Wallois P: Incidents et accidents au cours du traitement sclerosant des varices et leur prevention, Phlébologie 24:217, 1971.
229. Mantse L: A mild sclerosing agent for telangiectasias, J Dermatol Surg Oncol 11:855, 1985.
230. Mantse L: The treatment of varicose veins with compression sclerotherapy: technique, contraindications, complications, Am J Cosmetic Surg 3:47, 1986.

231. Tibbs DJ: Treatment of superficial vein incompetence. 2. Compression sclerotherapy. In Tibbs, DJ, editor: Varicose veins and related disorders, Oxford, 1992, Butterworth-Heineman Ltd.

232. Clinical Case 1. Presented at the third annual meeting of the North American Society of Phlebology, Phoenix, Ariz, February 21, 1990.

233. Mubarak SJ et al: Acute compartment syndromes: Diagnosis and treatment with the aid of the wick catheter, J Bone Joint Surg 60-A:1091, 178.

234. Fronek H, Fronek A, and Saltzbarg G: Allergic reactions to sotradecol, J Dermatol Surg Oncol 15:684, 1989.

235. Passas H: One case of tetradecyl-sodium sulfate allergy with general symptoms, Soc Fran Phlebol 25:19, 1972.

236. Shick LA and Laing K: Possible allergic reaction to agent used in sclerotherapy, Clin Cases Dermatol 4:2, 1992.

237. Schneider W: Contribution al'historique du traitment sclerosant des varices et a son etude anatomo-pathologique, Soc Fran Phlebol 18:117, 1965.

238. Dingwall JA, Lin W, and Lyon JA: The use of sodium tetradecyl sulfate in the sclerosing treatments of varicose veins, Surgery 23:599, 1948.

239. Reiner L: The activity of anionic surface active compounds in producing vascular obliteration, Proc Soc Exp Biol Med 62:49, 1946.

240. Amblard P: Our experience with Aethoxysklerol, Phlébologie 30:213, 1977.

241. Hartel S: Complications and side effects of sclerotherapy, Zarztl Furtbild (Jena) 78:331, 1984.

242. Heberova V: Treatment of telangiectasias of the lower extremities by sclerotization: results and evaluation, Cs Dermatol 51:232, 1976.

243. Eichenberger H: Results of phlebosclerosation with hydroxypolyethoxydodecane, Zentralbl Phlebol 8:181, 1969.

244. Jacobesen BH: Aethoxysklerol: a new sclerosing agent for varicose veins, Ugeskr Laeg 136:532, 1974.

245. Feuerstein W: Anaphylactic reaction to hydroxypolyaethoxydodecon, Vasa 2:292, 1973.

246. Ouvry P, Chandet A, and Guillerot E: First impressions of Aethoxysklerol, Phlébologie 31:75, 1978.

247. Stricker BHCh et al: Anafylaxie na gebruik van polidocanol, Ned Tijdschr Geneeskd 135:240, 1990.

248. Tombari G et al: Sclerotherapy of varices: complications and their treatment. In Raynard-Martimbeau P, Prescott R, and Zummo M, editors: Phebologie '92, Paris, 1992, John Libbey Eurotext.

249. Feied CF and Jackson JJ: Allergic reactions to polidocanol for vein sclerosis: two case reports, J Dermatol Surg Oncol, 1994 (in press).

250. Thies E, Lange V, and Iven H: Cardiac effects of polidocanol, a sclerotherapeutic drug—experimental evaluations, Chir Forum 192:313, 1982.

251. Imperiali G et al: Heart failure as a side effect of polidocanol given for esophageal variceal sclerosis, Endoscopy 18:207, 1986.

252. Paterlini A et al: Heart failure and endoscopic sclerotherapy of variceal bleeding, Lancet 2:1241, 1984.

253. Siems KJ and Soehring K: Die Ausschaltug sensibler nerven duren peridurale und paravertebrale injektion von alkylpolyathylenoxydathern bei meerschweinchen, Arzneimittelforschung 2:109, 1952.

254. Soehring K et al: Beitrage zur pharmakologie der alkylpolyathylenoxyd-derivate. I: Untersuchungen uber die acute und subchronische toxizitat bei verschiedenen tierarten, Arch Int Pharmacodyn Ther 87:301, 1951.

255. Soehring K and Frahm M: Studies on the pharmacology of alkylpolyethyleneoxide derivatives, Arzneimittelforschung 5:655, 1955.

256. Nguyen VB: Sclerotherapie des varices des membres inferieurs etude de 522 cas, Le Saguency Med 23:134, 1976.

257. Ouvry P and Arlaud R: Le traitement sclerosant des telangiectasies des membres inferieurs, Phlébologie 32:365, 1979.

258. Ouvry P and Davy A: Le traitement sclerosant des telangiectasias des membres inferieurs, Phlébologie 35:349, 1982.

259. Jager H and Pelloni E: Tests epicutanes aux bichromates, posotofs dan l'eczema au ciment, Dermatologica 100:207, 1950.

260. Polak L, Turk JL, and Frey JR: Studies on contact hypersensitivity to chromium compounds, Prog Allergy 17:145, 1973.

261. Wallois P: Incidents et accidents de la sclerose. In Tournay R, editor: La sclerose des varices, ed 4, Paris, 1985, Expansion Scientifique Francaise.

262. Zimmet SE: Letter to the editor, J Dermatol Surg Oncol 16:1063, 1990.

263. Sigg K, Horodegen K, and Bernbach H: Varizen-Sklerosierung: Welchos ist das wirUsamste Mittel? Deutsohes Arzteblatt 34/35:2294, 1986.

264. Sigg K and Zelikovski A: Kann die Sklerosierungotherapie der Varizen obne Oparation in jedem Fallwirksam sein? Phlebol Proktol 4:42, 1975.

265. Wenner L: Anwendurg einer mit Athylalkahol modifizierten Polijodidjonenlosung bei skleroseresistenten Varizen, Vasa 12:190, 1983.

266. Dodd H: The operation for varicose veins, Br Med J 2:510, 1945.

267. Coverman M: Personal communication, 1989.

268. Anticoagulants. In Bennett R, editor: AMA drug evaluations, ed 5, Chicago, 1983, American Medical Association.

269. Zinn WJ: Side reactions of heparin in clinical practice, Am Cardiol 14:36, 1964.

270. Gervin AS: Complications of heparin therapy, Surg Gynecol Obstet 140:789, 1975.

271. White PW, Sadd JR, and Nensel RE: Thrombotic complications of heparin therapy, including six cases of heparin-induced skin necrosis, Ann Surg 190:595, 1979.

272. Dukes MNG, editor: Meyler's side effects of drugs: an encyclopaedia of adverse reactions and interactions, ed 9, Amsterdam, 1980, Excerpta Medica Foundation.

273. O'Toole RD: Heparin: adverse reaction, Ann Intern Med 79:759, 1973.

274. Hume M, Smith-Petersen M, and Fremont-Smith P: Sensitivity to intrafat heparin, Lancet 1:261, 1974.

275. Hall JC, McConahay D, and Gibson D: Heparin necrosis: an anticoagulation syndrome, JAMA 244:1831, 1980.

276. Shelley WB and Ayen JJ: Heparin necrosis: an anticoagulant-induced cutaneous infarct, J Am Acad Dermatol 7:674, 1982.

277. Tuneu A, Moreno A, and de Moragas JM: Cutaneous reactions secondary to heparin injections, J Am Acad Dermatol 12:1072, 1985.

278. DeShago RD and Nelson HS: An approach to the patient with a history of local anesthesia hypersensitivity: experience with 90 patients, J Allergy Clin Immunol 63:387, 1979.

279. de Jong RH: Local anesthetics, ed 2, Springfield, Ill, 1977, Charles C Thomas.

280. Swanson JG: Assessment of allergy to local anesthetic, Ann Emerg Med 12:316, 1983.

281. de Jong RH: Toxic effects of local anesthetics, JAMA 239:1166, 1978.

282. Incaudo G et al: Administration of local anesthesia to patients with a history of adverse reaction, J Allergy Clin Immunol 61:339, 1978.

283. Thomas RM: Local anesthetic agents and regional anesthesia of the face, J Assoc Military Dermatol 8:28, 1982.

284. Fregert S, Tegner E, and Thelin I: Contact allergy to lidocaine, Contact Dermatitis 5:185, 1979.

285. Covino BG and Vassallo HG: Local anesthetics: mechanisms of action and clinical use, New York, 1976, Grune & Stratton.

286. Eriksson E: Illustrated handbook of local anesthesia, ed 2, Philadelphia, 1980, WB Saunders.

287. Baker JD and Blackmon BB: Local anesthesia, Clin Plast Surg 12:25, 1985.

288. Kennedy KS and Cave RH: Anaphylactic reaction to lidocaine, Arch Otolaryngol Head Neck Surg 112:671, 1986.

289. Promisloff RA and Dupont D: Death from ARDS and cardiovascular collapse following lidocaine administration, Chest 83:585, 1983.

290. Aldrete JA: Sensitivity to lidocaine, Anesth Intensive Care 7:73, 1979.

291. Gill C and Michaelides PL: Dental drugs and anaphylactic reactions: report of a case, Oral Surg 50:30, 1980.

292. Chin TM and Fellner MJ: Allergic hypersensitivity to lidocaine hydrochloride, Int J Dermatol 19:147, 1980.

293. Ravindranathan N: Allergic reaction to lidocaine: a case report, Br Dent J 111:101, 1975.

294. Lehner T: Lidocaine hypersensitivity, Lancet 1:1245, 1971.

295. Fischer MM and Pennington JC: Allergy to local anaesthesia, Br J Anaesth 54:893, 1982.

296. Garber N: A criticism of present-day methods in the treatment of varicose veins, S Afr Med J 21:338, 1947.

297. Ogilvie WH: Some applications of the surgical lessons of war to civil practice, Br Med J 1:619, 1945.

298. Fegan WG: The complications of compression sclerotherapy, Practitioner 207:797, 1971.

299. Sigg K: The treatment of varicosities and accompanying complications, Angiology 3:355, 1952.

300. Plate G et al: Deep vein thrombosis, pulmonary embolism and acute surgery in thrombophlebitis of the long saphenous vein, Acta Chir Scand 151:241, 1985.

301. Gjores JE: Surgical therapy of ascending thrombophlebitis in the saphenous system, Angiology 13:241, 1962.

302. Bergqvist D and Lindblad B: A 30-year survey of pulmonary embolism verified at autopsy: an analysis of 1274 surgical patients, Br J Surg 72:105, 1985.

303. Bergqvist D and Jaroszewski H: Deep vein thrombosis in patients with superficial thrombophlebitis of the leg, Br Med J 292:658, 1986.

304. Galloway JMD, Karmody AM, and Mavor GE: Thrombophlebitis of the long saphenous vein complicated by pulmonary embolism, Br J Surg 56:360, 1969.

305. From our legal correspondent: Hazards of compression sclerotherapy, Br Med J 3:714, 1975.

306. Goldstein M: Les complications de la sclerotherapie, Phlébologie 32:221, 1979.

307. Oesch A, Stirnemann P, and Mahler F: Das akute ischamiesyndrom des Fusses nach Varizenverodung, Schweiz Med Wschr 114:1155, 1984.

308. MacGowan WAL: Sclerotherapy: prevention of accidents: a review, J R Soc Med 78:136, 1985.

309. Cockett FB: Arterial complications during surgery and sclerotherapy of varicose veins, Phlebology 1:3, 1986.

310. Biegeleisen K, Neilsen RD, and O'Shaughnessy A: Inadvertent intra-arterial injection complicating ordinary and ultrasound-guided sclerotherapy, J Dermatol Surg Oncol 19:953, 1993.

311. Natali J, Maraval M, and Carrance F: Recent statistics on complications of sclerotherapy. Presented at the Annual Meeting of the North American Society of Phlebology, Maui, February 21, 1994.

312. MacGowan WAL et al: The local effects of intra-arterial injections of sodium tetradecyl sulphate (STD) 3%, Br J Surg 59:101, 1972.

313. Staubesand J and Seydewitz V: Ultrastructural changes following perivascular and intra-arterial injection of sclerosing agents: an experimental contribution to the problem of iatrogenic damage, Phlébologie 20:1, 1991.

314. Matsen FA et al: A model compartmental syndrome in man with particular reference to the quantification of nerve function, J Bone Joint Surg 59A:648, 1977.

315. Orbach J: A new look at sclerotherapy, Folia Angiologia 25:181, 1977.

316. Benhamou AC and Natali J: Les accidents des traitements sclerosant et chirurgical des varices des membres inferieurs: a propos de 90 cas, Phlébologie 34:41, 1981.

317. Somer-Leroy R de, Wang A, and Ouvry P: Echographie du creux poplite recherche d'une arteriole petite saphene avant sclerotherapie, Phlébologie 44:69, 1991.

318. Sternbergh WC III, Makhoul RG, and Adelman B: Heparin prevents postischemic endothelial cell dysfunction by a mechanism independent of its anticoagulant activity, J Vasc Surg 17:318, 1993.

319. Lantz M et al: On the binding of tumor necrosis factor (TNF) to heparin and the release in vivo of the TNF-binding protein I by heparin, J Clin Invest 88:2026, 1991.

320. Bounumeaux H et al: Severe ischemia of the hand following intra-arterial promazine injection: effects of vasodilatation, anticoagulation, and local thrombolysis with tissue type plasminogen activator, Vasa 19:68, 1990.

321. Feied CF: Deep vein thrombosis: the risks of sclerotherapy in hypercoagullable states, Semin Dermatol 12:135, 1993.

322. Kistner RL: Incidence of pulmonary embolism in the coarse of thrombophlebitis of the lower extremities, Am J Surg 124:169, 1972.

323. Coon WW: Venous thromboembolism—prevalence: risk factors and prevention, Clin Chest Med 5:391, 1984.

324. Dalen JE and Alpert JS: Natural history of pulmonary embolism, Prog Cardiovasc Dis 17:259, 1975.

325. Kakkar VV et al: Deep vein thrombosis of the leg, Am J Surg 120:527, 1970.

326. Evans DS and Cockett FB: Diagnosis of deep-vein thrombosis with ultrasonic Doppler technique, Br J Med 28:802, 1969.

327. Milne RM et al: Postoperative deep venous thrombosis. A comparison of diagnostic techniques, Lancet 2:445, 1971.

328. Burrow M and Goldson H: Postoperative venous thrombosis. Evaluation of five methods of treatment, Am J Surg 141:245, 1981.

329. Smith L and Johnson MA: Incidence of pulmonary embolism after venous sclerosing therapy, Minn Med 31:270, 1948.

330. Natali J and Marmasse J: Enquete sur le traitement chirugical des varices, Phlébologie 15:232, 1962.

331. Barber THT: Modern treatment of varicose veins, Br Med J 1:219, 1930.

332. Kern MM and Angle LW: The chemical obliteration of varicose veins: a clinical and experimental study, JAMA 93:595, 1929.

333. Linser P and Vohwinkel H: Moderne Therapie der Varizen, Hamorrhoiden und Varicocele, Stuttgart, 1942, Ferdinand Enke.

334. Sigg K: Zur Behandlung der Varicen der Phlebitis und ihrer Komplikationen, Hautarzt 1-2:443, 1950.

335. Marmasse J: Enquete sur les embolies pulmonaires au cours du traitement sclerosant, Phlébologie 16, 1964.

336. Stevenson IM, Seddon JA, and Parry EW: The occurrence of deep venous thrombosis following compression sclerotherapy, Angiology 27:311, 1976.
337. Williams RA and Wilson SE: Sclerosant treatment of varicose veins and deep vein thrombosis, Arch Surg 119:1283, 1984.
338. Van Der Molen HR: Le risque de thrombose profunde lors des injections intra-variqueuses pourquoi est-il quasi inexisstant? Phlébologie 42:137, 1989.
339. Cepelak V: Effect of sclerosing agents on platelet aggregation, Folia Angiologia 30-31:363, 1982.
340. Zelikowski A et al: Compression sclerotherapy of varicose veins. A few observations and some practical suggestions, Folia Angiologia 26:61, 1978.
341. Virchow R: Cellular pathology as based on physiological and pathological histology, London, 1860, Churchill Livingstone.
342. Schneider W and Fischer H: Fixierung und bindegewebige Organisation artefizieller Thromben bei der Varizenverodung, Dtsch Med Wschr 89:2410, 1964.
343. Atlas LN: Hazards connected with the treatment of varicose veins, Surg Gynecol Obstet 77:136, 1943.
344. Bohler-Sommeregger K et al: Do telangiectases communicate with the deep venous system? J Dermatol Surg Oncol 18:403, 1992.
345. McPheeters HO and Rice CO: Varicose veins—the circulation and direction of venous flow, Surg Gynecol Obstet 49:29, 1929.
346. Muller JHA, Petter O, and Kostler H: Kinematographische Untersuchugen bei der Varizenverodungstherapie, Z Arztl Fortbild 78:345, 1984.
347. Moser KM et al: Frequent asymptomatic pulmonary embolism in patients with deep venous thrombosis, JAMA 271:223, 1994.
348. D'addato M: Gangrene of a limb with complete thrombosis of the venous system, J Cardiovasc Surg 7:434, 1966.
349. Goor W, Leu HJ, and Mahler F: Thrombosen in tiefen Venen und in Arterian nach Varizensklerosierung, Vasa 16:124, 1987.
350. Askar O and Abullah S: The veins of the foot, J Cardiovas Surg 16:53, 1975.
351. Tretbar LL and Pattisson PH: Injection-compression treatment of varicose veins, Am J Surg 120:539, 1970.
352. Thomas JH: Pathogenesis, diagnosis and treatment of thrombosis, Am J Surg 160:547, 1990.
353. Kakkar VV, Howe CT, Nicolaides AN, et al : Deep vein thrombosis of the leg: Is there a high-risk group? Am J Surg 120:527, 1970.
354. Samlaska CP and James WD: Superficial thrombophlebitis. II. Secondary hypercoagulable states, J Am Acad Dermatol 23:1, 1990.
355. Schafer AI: The hypercoagulable states, Ann Intern Med 102:814, 1985.
356. Kaplan NM: Cardiovascular complications of oral contraceptives, Ann Rev Med 29:31, 1978.
357. Durand JL and Bressler R: Clinical pharmacology of the steroidal oral contraceptives, Adv Intern Med 24:97, 1979.
358. Stooley PD et al: Thrombosis with low-estrogen oral contraceptives, Am J Epidemiol 102:197, 1975.
359. Vessey M et al: Oral contraceptives and venous thromboembolism: findings in a large prospective study, Br J Med 292:526, 1986.
360. Helmrich SP et al: Venous thromboembolism in relation to oral contraceptive use, Obstet Gynecol 69:91, 1987.
361. Seigel DG: Pregnancy, the puerperium and the steroid contraceptive, Milbank Mem Fund Q 50(suppl 2):15, 1972.
362. Boston collaborative drug surveillance program: oral contraceptives and venous thromboembolic disease, surgically confirmed gallbladder disease, and breast tumours, Lancet 1:1439, 1973.
363. Quinn DA et al: A prospective investigation of pulmonary embolism in women and men, JAMA 29:1689, 1992.
364. Realini JP and Goldzieher JW: Oral contraceptives and cardiovascular disease: a critique of the epidemiologic studies, Am J Obstet Gynecol 152:729, 1985.
365. Stadel BV: Oral contraceptives and cardiovascular disease, N Engl J Med 305:612, 1981.
366. Alkjaersig N, Fletcher A, and Burstein R: Association between oral contraceptive use and thromboembolism: a new approach to its investigation based on plasma fibrinogen chromatography, Am J Obstet Gynecol 122:199, 1975.
367. Siegbahn A and Ruusuvaara L: Age dependence of blood fibrinolytic components and the effects of low-dose oral contraceptives on coagulation and fibrinolysis in teenagers, Thromb Haemost 60:301, 1988.
368. Srinivasan S et al: The alteration of surface charge characteristics of the vascular system by oral contraceptive steroids, Contraception 9:291, 1974.

369. Oski FA, Lubin B, and Buchert ED: Reduced red cell filterability with oral contraceptive agents, Ann Intern Med 77:417, 1972.

370. Aronson HB, Magora F, and Schenker JG: Effect of oral contraceptives on blood viscosity, Am J Obstet Gynecol 110:997, 1971.

371. Dreyer NA and Pizzo SV: Blood coagulation and idiopathic thromboembolism among fertile women, Contraception 22:123, 1980.

372. Sagar S et al: Oral contraceptives, antithrombin-III activity, and postoperative deep-vein thrombosis, Lancet 1:509, 1976.

373. von Kaulla E and von Kaulla KN: Oral contraceptives and low antithrombin-III activity, Lancet 1:36, 1970.

374. Pizzo SV: Venous thrombosis. In Koepke JA, editor: Laboratory hematology, vol 2, New York, 1984, Churchill Livingstone.

375. Miller KE and Pizzo SV: Venous and arterial thromboembolic disease in women using oral contraceptives, Am J Obstet Gynecol 144:824, 1982.

376. Astedt B et al: Thrombosis and oral contraceptives: possible predisposition, Br Med J 4:631, 1973.

377. Judd HL et al: Estrogen replacement therapy: indications and complications, Ann Intern Med 98:195, 1983.

378. Goodrich SM and Wood JE: Peripheral venous distensibility and velocity of venous blood flow during pregnancy or during oral contraceptive therapy, Am J Obstet Gynecol 90:740, 1964.

379. Alkjaersig N et al: Blood coagulation in postmenopausal women given estrogen treatment: comparison of transdermal and oral administration, J Lab Clin Med 111:224, 1988.

380. Lipton A, Harvey HA, and Hamilton RW: Venous thrombosis as a side effect of tamoxifen treatment, Cancer Treat Rev 68:887, 1984.

381. Fisher B et al: A randomized clinical trial evaluating tamoxifen in the treatment of patients with node-negative breast cancer who have estrogen-receptor-positive tumors, N Engl J Med 320:479, 1989.

382. Jordan VC, Fritz NF, and Tormey DC: Long-term adjuvant therapy with tamoxifen: effects on sex hormone binding globulin and antithrombin III, Cancer Res 47:4517, 1987.

383. Love RR, Surawicz TS, and Williams EC: Antithrombin III level, fibrinogen level, and platelet count changes with adjuvant tamoxifen therapy, Arch Intern Med 152:317, 1992.

384. Auger MJ and Mackie MJ: Effects of tamoxifen on blood coagulation, Cancer 61:1316, 1988.

385. Bertelli G et al: Adjuvant tamoxifen in primary breast cancer: influence on plasma lipids and antithrombin III levels, Breast Cancer Res Treat 12:307, 1988.

386. Pare A: Cited by Ritchie A: Edinburgh Med J 1:157, 1933.

387. Hamilton HG, Pittam RF, and Higgins RS: Active therapy of varicose veins in pregnancy, South Med J 42:608, 1949.

388. Finley BE: Acute coagulopathy in pregnancy, Med Clin North Am 73:723, 1989.

389. Aaro LA, Johnson TR, and Juergens JL: Acute deep venous thrombosis associated with pregnancy, Obstet Gynecol 28:553, 1966.

390. Beller FK: Thromboembolic disease in pregnancy. In Anderson A, editor: Thromboembolic disorders, New York, 1968, Harper & Row.

391. Bonnar J: Hemostatic function and coagulopathy during pregnancy, Obstet Gynecol Annu 7:195, 1978.

392. Bonnar J, McNicol GP, and Douglas AS: Fibrinolytic enzyme system and pregnancy, Br Med J 3:387, 1969.

393. Comp PC et al: Functional and immunologic protein levels are decreased during pregnancy, Blood 68:881, 1986.

394. Miletich J, Sherman L, and Broze G Jr: Absence of thrombosis in patients with heterozygous protein C deficiency, N Engl J Med 317:991, 1987.

395. Engesser L et al: Hereditary protein S deficiency: clinical manifestations, Ann Intern Med 106:677, 1987.

396. Rick ME: Protein C and protein S: vitamin K–dependent inhibitors of blood coagulation, JAMA 263:701, 1990.

397. Bauer KA: Pathobiology of the hypercoagulable state: clinical features, laboratory evaluation, and management. In Hoffman R et al, editors: Hematology: basic principles and clinical practice, New York, 1991, Churchill Livingstone.

398. Svensson PJ and Dahlback B: Resistance to activated protein C as a basis for venous thrombosis, N Engl J Med 330:517, 1994.

399. D'Angelo A et al: Brief report: autoimmune protein S deficiency in a boy with severe thromboembolic disease, N Engl J Med 328:1753, 1993.

400. Fair DS, Marlar RA, and Levin EG: Human endothelial cells synthesize protein S, Blood 67:1168, 1986.

401. Collen D et al: Metabolism of antithrombin III (heparin cofactor) in man: effects of venous thrombosis and of heparin administration, Eur J Clin Invest 7:27, 1977.

402. Odegaard OR and Abildgaard U: Antithrombin III: critical review of assay methods. Significance of variations in health and disease, Haemostasis 7:127, 1978.

403. Towne JB: Hypercoagulable states and unexplained vascular graft thrombosis. In Bernhard VM and Towne JB, editors: Complications in vascular surgery, St Louis, 1991, Quality Medical Publishing, Inc.

404. Espinoza LR and Hartmann RC: Significance of the lupus anticoagulant, Am J Haematol 22:331, 1986.

405. Tabechnik-Schor NF and Lipton SA: Association of lupus-like anticoagulant and nonvasculitic cerebral infarction, Arch Neurol 43:851, 1986.

406. Shi W et al: Prevalence of lupus anticoagulant and anticardiolipin antibodies in a healthy population, Aust N Z J Med 20:231, 1990.

407. Mueh JR, Herbst KD, and Rapaport SI: Thrombosis in patients with the lupus anticoagulant, Ann Intern Med 92:156, 1980.

408. Elias M and Eldor A: Thromboembolism in patients with the "lupus" type circulating anticoagulant, Arch Intern Med 144:510, 1984.

409. Kiely PE: A phlebographic study of the soleal sinuses, Angiology 24:230, 1973.

410. Fegan WG: Continuous compression technique of injecting varicose veins, Lancet 2:109, 1963.

411. Crandon AJ et al: Postoperative deep vein thrombosis: identifying high-risk patients, Br Med J 281:343, 1980.

412. Sue-Ling HM et al: Pre-operative identification of patients at high risk of deep vein thrombosis after major abdominal surgery, Lancet 1:1173, 1986.

413. Coon WW: Epidemiology of venous thromboembolism, Ann Surg 186:149, 1977.

414. Schina Jr et al: Influence of age on venous physiologic parameters, J Vasc Surg 18:749, 1993.

415. McMaster P and Everett WG: Fatal pulmonary embolism following compression sclerotherapy for varicose veins, Postgrad Med J 49:517, 1973.

416. Arneson H and Hoseth A: Streptokinase or heparin in the treatment of deep vein thrombosis, follow-up results of a prospective study, Acta Med Scand 211:65, 1982.

417. Schulman S and Lockner D: Local venous infusion of streptokinase in DVT, Thromb Res 34:213, 1984.

418. Orbach EJ: Sclerotherapy of varicose veins: utilization of intravenous air block, Am J Surg 66:362, 1944.

419. Orbach EJ: Clinical evaluation of a new technic in the sclerotherapy of varicose veins, J Int Coll Surg 11:396, 1948.

420. Richardson HF, Coles BC, and Hall GE: Experimental air embolism, Can Med J 36:584, 1937.

421. Yen D, Robison DL, and Tschen J: Multiple tender, erythematous subcutaneous nodules on the lower extremities, Arch Dermatol 129:1331, 1993.

CLINICAL METHODS FOR SCLEROTHERAPY OF VARICOSE VEINS

"WE FEEL FROM OUR THREE AND ONE-HALF YEARS' EXPERIENCE THAT THE SURGEON WHO BELIEVES THAT THERE IS NOTHING MORE REQUIRED THAN A SYRINGE, SOME SOLUTION, AND A PATIENT TO EFFECT PERMANENT OBLITERATION OF VARICOSE VEINS, STILL HAS MUCH TO LEARN."[1]

This timeless quotation from Henry Faxon, Assistant in Surgery at Harvard Medical School in 1933, resulted from a careful analysis of 314 cases from the peripheral circulatory clinic of the Massachusetts General Hospital. Unfortunately, this quotation is timeless in that only through a continual careful evaluation of past results and review of our colleagues' experience can sclerotherapy treatment be provided in an optimal manner.

Varicose veins represent tortuous dilations of existing superficial veins. They arise because of multiple factors but are always associated with a relatively elevated venous pressure.[2] Therefore treatment initially consists of cutting off the point of high-pressure inflow to the veins (either through surgical or sclerotherapeutic methods) before treating the varicose veins themselves.[3,4]

Because varicose veins are not life threatening, their treatment should be efficacious, cosmetic, relatively free of adverse sequelae and complications, and without significant pain. Caius Marius, the Roman tyrant, was in extreme pain both while and after his varicose veins were treated with surgery. When the same surgeon recommended the same treatment for the other leg, which was also involved with venous disease, Caius Marius refused treatment and was quoted as saying, "I see the cure is not worth the pain." This chapter describes sclerotherapy treatment of varicose veins that our patients will submit to and even request for further therapy when recommended.

HISTORICAL REVIEW OF TECHNIQUES
Tournay (French) Technique

The Tournay procedure encompasses the basic principle of "French phlebology" developed by Tournay et al.[5]: treating varicose veins "from high to low" ("*de haut en bas*").[4] The rationale for this technique is in first eliminating high-pressure reflux blood flow at the point of occurrence. Treating from proximal to distal sites also eliminates the weight of the column of blood on the sclerosed point. This has the advantage of minimizing thrombosis and the extravasation of red blood cells (RBCs) from a sclerosed vein segment. The French school advocates placement of very few injections at this "high (proximal)" point before treating more distal veins or sections of the same vein at a later date. This same philosophy toward treatment was also reported from the Mayo Clinic in 1941 by Heyerdale and Stalker.[6] The principle of eliminating reflux from the saphenofemoral junction (SFJ) was espoused even earlier by Moszkowicz[7] in Germany in 1927 and by de Takats and Quint[8] in the United States in 1930. Thus the "French technique" is multicultural in its origin.

In addition to developing a treatment regimen with this tenet in mind, it is critical to obliterate the SFJ accurately because its location and anatomy are so variable (see Chapter 1). To determine the origin of high pressure in the varicose vein, a noninvasive diagnostic evaluation of the patient should be performed first (see Chapter 5). The handheld Doppler device helps detect points of reflux from the deep to the superficial veins, either through incompetent saphenofemoral or saphenopopliteal junctions or perforating veins. In certain circumstances additional testing may be required. If any points of reflux are detected, they should be treated first. After the high-pressure flow has been eliminated, treatment should proceed first with injection of the largest varicose veins, then injection of the reticular feeding veins, and finally treatment of the remaining "spider" veins.

In defense of the logic of the French technique, de Groot[4] pointed out that any vein in the leg belongs to either the greater saphenous "system" or the lesser saphenous "system" (Fig. 9-1). This concept implies that a vein within the defined area of the greater saphenous vein (GSV) eventually drains into the GSV. Therefore reflux in that vein is derived from reflux at the SFJ. This concept directs treatment toward the reflux point. Unfortunately, clinical examination of the location of a vein does not always correctly determine the point of reflux. Therefore the clinical examination must be correlated with a noninvasive examination to establish the optimal order of therapy.

Sigg (Swiss) Technique

In contrast to the French technique, the Swiss technique of Sigg[9] and the modification by Dodd and Cockett[10] advocate total sclerosation of the entire varicose vein, including incompetent perforator veins and the SFJ. This technique has also been adopted by some physicians who modify Fegan's technique of sclerotherapy of the incompetent perforator veins (described in the following section). Included in this school are Reid and Rothnie[11] who treated 1358 legs of 974 patients and found that selective injection of perforator veins was ineffective, requiring multi-

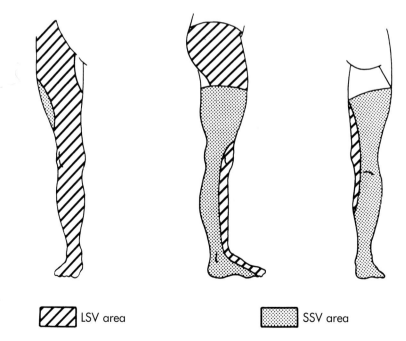

LSV area   SSV area

Fig. 9-1 Diagram of the greater and lesser saphenous vein "systems." (Redrawn from de Groot WP: J Dermatol Surg Oncol 15:191, 1989.)

ple additional treatments of the entire vein. They evolved a technique of placing multiple injections at intervals along the varicose veins to produce diffuse sclerosis and have reported very favorable results. This latter technique is called the *total-vein sclerotherapy technique.*

Fegan Technique

Fegan, Fitzgerald, and Milliken[12] proposed a view opposite the previously mentioned one, namely that saphenofemoral incompetence could occur as a result of perforator incompetence alone. They reached this conclusion by demonstrating that the calf muscle pump is more powerful than the abdominal or femoral muscles in regard to venous flow in the leg. They proposed that sclerotherapy of the incompetent perforator veins should be performed first to restore normal function. Fegan's examination of the SFJ and GSV with phlebography after sclerotherapy of incompetent perforator veins showed narrowing of the vessel lumen in 9 of 11 patients.[13] However, surgical exploration of clinically diagnosed areas of perforator vein incompetence has found at best a 60% incidence of perforator veins being correctly identified clinically.[14] In addition, phlebographic examination performed on 112 patients with clinically suspected incompetent perforators showed that the clinical examination correctly identified only 38% of perforator veins below the knee and only 17% of thigh perforators.[15] An additional study of 180 limbs with primary varicose veins studied with clinical examination, ascending deep-to-superficial venography, Doppler ultrasound, and ambulatory venous pressure measurements showed that only 40% of these patients had evidence of perforator incompetence. Of them, 30% had no hemodynamic significance to the perforator veins.[16] Thus the rationale for Fegan's technique is open to dispute.

Despite the lack of accuracy of clinical diagnosis of incompetent perforating veins, many authors have found Fegan's technique gives excellent results. Tolins[17] reported favorable results using Fegan's technique; he injected varicose veins in areas of fascial defects with 0.5 ml of sodium tetradecyl sulfate (STS) solution at up to 23 sites per leg. Although this many injections may seem similar to the number with total vein sclerotherapy, three quarters of the patients had two to five injections. Doran and White[18] concluded after 2 years of follow-up that there was no difference between the results from Fegan's technique and ligation and stripping procedures for varicose veins. Hobbs[19] concluded from his comparative study of sclerotherapy with Fegan's technique versus traditional surgery that the best treatment of nontruncal varicose veins and incompetent perforator veins of the lower leg is sclerotherapy. Tretbar and Pattisson[20] have found in their follow-up examinations of 264 patients treated with Fegan's technique that treatment failures usually occurred in patients with very large or fat legs with varicosities originating above the knee. They believed this failure was caused by the difficulty of placing injections accurately within the veins of these patients and maintaining adequate compression. Sladen[21] analyzed 263 limbs with up to 7 years of follow-up and found that more than 95% of his patients were satisfied with the treatment and said they would have it repeated. He estimated a retreatment rate of approximately 5% per year. His patients average 3.6 to 5.25 injections per treatment session, and 46% to 74% required one treatment session only. In agreement with Hobbs, Sladen found that all patients with saphenofemoral reflux eventually required surgery. Therefore, although varicose veins treated with Fegan's technique respond well to treatment, the supposition of Fegan's technique, that sclerosis of the incompetent perforator veins is of primary importance and may reverse the remaining pathology in the GSV system, may not be universally correct.

Hobbs[22] has also provided evidence that when saphenofemoral and perforator incompetence occur together, both abnormalities should be corrected. Kerner and Schultz-Ehrenburg[23,24] studied the functional effects of sclerotherapy with photoplethysmography (PPG) and concluded that the greatest functional improvement occurred with obliteration of the SFJ. Obliteration of the incompetent perforator veins of the lower legs was of variable importance. Treatment of perforator veins of the upper leg had no functional significance that could be ascertained with PPG.

Treatment of Reflux from the Saphenofemoral Junction

There are at least three schools of thought regarding which type of therapy is appropriate for initial treatment of the junctional points of reflux: surgical ligation (with or without limited stripping) of the SFJ versus sclerotherapy of the SFJ versus sclerotherapy of incompetent perforator veins alone. Bergan (see Chapter 10), Goldman,[25] Hobbs,[19,26] and others argue that surgical treatment of the junctions is the most appropriate and successful mode of treatment. Neglan,[27] in a comprehensive review, determined that with proper follow-up, including functional testing at 5 years, surgical therapy of the GSV in a patient with incompetence of the SFJ is significantly better than sclerotherapy.[27] Color-flow duplex evaluation from 3 to 55 months after treatment (mean 27.5 months) of 89 limbs in 55 patients with an incompetent SFJ treated with the Sigg technique found that only 6% of veins remained sclerosed despite improvement in symptoms in 50%.[28] Butie[29] has shown that sclerotherapy of the SFJ is difficult and unreliable with the use of STS 3%, which is the strongest sclerosing agent approved for use by the United States Food and Drug Administration (FDA). This has been confirmed even when sclerotherapy was performed at the SFJ under angioscopic guidance (see below).[30] In this case 12 GSVs were occluded at the SFJ through angioscopically guided sclerotherapy with STS 3%. A total of 2 to 5 ml was injected into the GSV just below the junction, which was occluded by manual pressure. Nine veins were evaluated at follow-up and all were reopened and incompetent between 1 and 12 months. Although these carefully performed, unbiased studies have only recently been done, this opinion is not new. As far back as 1934, Cooper,[31] in a series of more than 85,000 injections in more than 3000 patients, documented that the number of sclerosing injections required to produce obliteration of the varicose vein was markedly decreased after ligation of the SFJ.

In addition to its lack of consistent success, sclerotherapy of the SFJ has the inherent risk of damaging the deep venous system and the femoral vein when sclerosing solution is injected in the upper thigh region. This has been demonstrated by radiologic examination showing the rapid flow of contrast media from a varicose GSV into the femoral vein when injections are performed in the upper thigh.[32] With incompetence of the SFJ, it is recommended that sclerotherapy be used for treating residual varicosities after surgery.

Multiple phlebologists, however, have demonstrated that the junctions can be successfully closed with sclerotherapy alone in 50% to 91% of patients.[33-39] A comprehensive illustrated discussion of the technique is presented elsewhere.[40] The difficulty in properly evaluating these conclusions is due to the natural evolution of varicose veins, which obscures the results of both surgical and sclerotherapy treatment. It is sometimes difficult to distinguish between a recanalized vein and a new vein. Results also depend on the type of follow-up examinations (i.e., clinical or objective with duplex or Doppler ultrasound) of patients. One study with *clinical* 6-year follow-up has demonstrated a nearly 90% success rate with sclerotherapy.[33] By whatever method, closure of the SFJ has been shown in

Table 9-1 Summary of "schools" of sclerotherapy

School	Injection site	Compression	Instructions prescribed after procedure
Tournay	Proximal to distal	No	None
Sigg	Entire varicosity	Yes	Walking
Fegan	Perforating vein	Yes (6-week minimum)	Walking

pressure studies to prevent retrograde flow in the saphenous and perforator systems.[41] This suggests that incompetence of the perforator veins occurs as a result of a primary development of saphenofemoral reflux. Therefore when the GSV or its tributaries are involved, the SFJ, when incompetent, should be the first area treated.

Treating incompetence of the SFJ may differ from treating an incompetent saphenopopliteal junction (SPJ). The lesser saphenous vein (LSV) has a variable termination (see Chapter 1) that is often difficult to approach surgically. Ligation alone at the SPJ has a 95% failure rate at 1 year.[42] Sclerotherapy is much more effective, perhaps because of the larger extent of destruction of abnormal feeding veins into this region.[42]

In summary, long-term comparative studies with objective methods for evaluating outcome of the various techniques are lacking. The literature consists mainly of anecdotal reports and clinical studies with short follow-up periods. A comparison of three independent observers regarding treatment outcome of varicose vein surgery shows 60% agreement in assessing visual improvement, with 30% agreement between observers when symptomatic response and visual impression are compared.[43] It is my opinion that no one "school" is absolute but that the correct order of treatment should be individualized for each patient. Some patients have only perforator incompetence and a normal SFJ; thus Fegan's technique would be adequate. Patients with saphenofemoral incompetence require treatment of that junction before treatment is initiated elsewhere. Still other patients have no obvious hemodynamic cause for the origin of their varicose veins, thus directing treatment toward the entire varicosity as described by Sigg.[44] A careful workup of all patients is necessary before beginning therapy. Besides deciding on the sequence of treatment, the physician must consider the various modifications of the injection procedure that some physicians profess have various benefits. Again comparative, objective studies of these treatment modifications have not been reported. This chapter discusses sclerotherapy treatment of varicose veins, perforator veins, and the SFJ and reviews the available literature. Variations in treatment are addressed and illustrative cases are presented. A summary of the three schools of sclerotherapy is found in Table 9-1.

INJECTION TECHNIQUE
Patient Position

Standing. Although the previous description of the treatment of varicose veins seems simplistic, the actual treatment methods for achieving effective sclerotherapy are numerous. Until the 1950s sclerotherapy was performed with the patient standing throughout the procedure. The purpose was both to distend the varicose vein, allowing easier needle insertion, and to produce firm thrombosis of the treated vein.[45] Multiple disadvantages of varicose thrombosis were realized (see Chapter 8), and various methods were devised to limit

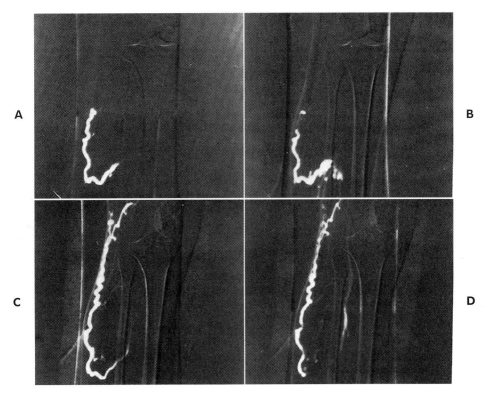

Fig. 9-2   Injected contrast media, 1.5 ml, shown $9\frac{1}{2}$ seconds, **A**, and $18\frac{1}{2}$ seconds, **B**, after injection into a varicose vein while the patient was standing. Injected contrast media, 1.5 ml, shown $9\frac{1}{2}$ seconds, **C**, and 18 seconds, **D**, after injection into a varicose vein while the patient was supine. (Courtesy George Heyn, M.D., Department of Vascular Surgery, DDR-Berlin.)

postsclerotherapy thrombosis. In addition, injecting sclerosing solution while the patient is standing forces the injection to occur against the hydrostatic pressure of a large column of blood. This may cause the solution to seep along the needle into the perivenous tissues, possibly leading to a chemical phlebitis or tissue necrosis.[46]

Another disadvantage of the total standing technique is that the sclerosing solution may escape through a perforator vein and damage the deep veins, especially if more than 1.5 ml of sclerosing solution is injected in a single site.[47] Another radiographic study has shown that an injection of 0.5 ml of contrast media travels rapidly (in 5 seconds) 8 cm distal to the injection site.[48] Also, this amount of contrast did not completely fill the vein. Another radiographic study of the standing position, using Amipaque 150 as the contrast media (diluted to an isomolarity and specific gravity similar to that of polidocanol), showed that the injection of 1.5 ml remained in contact with a convoluted varicosity for approximately 10 seconds before flowing rapidly into the deep venous system through a presumed perforator vein (Fig. 9-2, *A* and *B*).[49] In contrast, when the patient was supine, the contrast media extended proximally along the varicosity and remained relatively undiluted for more than 18 seconds (Fig. 9-2, *C* and *D*).[49] However, injections in some patients, when using the latter technique, also resulted in the contrast media's remaining in contact with the varicosity for a longer period with the patient in the standing position (Fig. 9-3). Therefore multiple variables, including the type of varicosity, its location, the location of associated perforator veins, and the movements of the patient (with associated calf and foot muscle contraction) while standing, may all affect the distribution of the sclerosing solution.

Standing and reclining. A modification of the standing technique, the standing and reclining technique, was described in 1926 by Meisen.[50] In the standing position the needle was inserted while the vein was distended. With the needle still in the vein, the patient reclined on a table, and the leg was elevated. This produced a relative emptying of blood from the vein. The sclerosing solution was then injected into an "empty" vein that was immediately compressed to prevent or minimize thrombosis.

One of the earliest methods used to limit thrombosis was that of isolating the injected vein segment with pressure placed above and below the needle insertion site after first milking the blood out of the vein.[51] One of the first textbooks on sclerotherapy treatment of varicose veins is subtitled *and Their Treatment by "Empty Vein" Injection.*[52] In this text Ronald Thornhill of London detailed his success with injection of a quinine solution into the elevated leg. He massaged the solution throughout the vein, injecting from distal to proximal. He even sclerosed "hair veins" with dilute solution. Unfortunately, he did not use compression except when ulcers were present, and his patients thus had to endure weeks of tender veins until they resolved in approximately 12 months.

The importance of these empty vein injections was emphasized in a histologic evaluation of treated veins by Lufkin and McPheeters[53] in 1932, and the significance of compressing the vein to minimize thrombosis has been stressed by Orbach[54] since 1943. Thus these modifications are not new. They result both in improved efficacy and in decreased incidence of complications when treatment is directed at the SFJ.[18] The improved efficacy may be the result of a longer length of sclerosis of the varicose vein caused by gravitational flow of the sclerosing solution. However, recent evaluations comparing standing and reclining methods of treating varicose veins below the SFJ have not been performed.

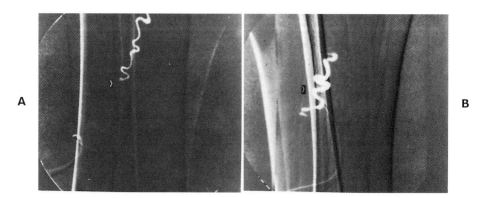

Fig. 9-3 **A,** Contrast media, 1.5 ml, shown 10 seconds after injection into a varicose vein while the patient was supine. Note the distribution of the contrast media proximally within the varicose vein. **B,** Contrast media, 1.5 ml, shown 10 seconds after injection into a varicose vein while the patient was standing. Note the contrast media remains for a relatively long time within the venous convolution. (Courtesy George Heyn, M.D., Department of Vascular Surgery, DDR-Berlin.)

Leg elevated (Fegan). Another obvious disadvantage of the standing technique is the vasovagal reaction (see Chapter 8). To prevent the sequelae of a vasovagal reaction, Fegan[55] recommends that patients sit at the end of the examining table with their legs hanging down while the physician, sitting in front on a low stool, inserts the needle. The leg is then raised while the patient fully reclines for 1 to 2 minutes to empty it of blood. The physician stands to support the raised leg, which is rested on the shoulder or against the chest, and the varicose veins are injected. With this or any technique that moves the patient after the needle is inserted, it is important to ensure that the needle is not displaced from the vein, either by fixing it to the skin with tape (if butterfly catheters or needles attached to syringes are used) or by holding the needle while the leg is raised. Since the varicose veins will collapse when the leg is raised, checking for blood withdrawal must be done as soon as possible after the leg is raised to ensure that the needle has not slipped out of the vein. The lack of spontaneous pulsatile flow from the needle without an attached syringe is proof of nonarterial placement of the needle.

To ensure that the sclerosing solution acts on the intended vein segment during injection, Fegan[55] applies pressure with his fingers a few centimeters proximal and distal to the injection point. Finger pressure is maintained for 30 to 60 seconds, and the leg is then bandaged from the toes to the injection site. With this method injections are made only at the points of fascial defects (which are thought to represent sites of incompetent perforator veins). Injections proceed from distal to proximal sites, with each vein segment or fascial defect treated.

After injecting varicose veins in the elevated leg, compression should be applied immediately to prevent the vein's filling with blood. This can be easily performed using the following method. Before inserting the needle, a compression stocking is placed over the foot and heel and allowed to bunch up at the ankle. After the needle is inserted into the varicosity, the leg is raised. Proper placement is then confirmed through blood withdrawal, and the sclerosing solution is injected. A foam pad is placed over the injection site and secured in place with foam or elastic tape. The compression bandage can then be advanced over the injection site and foam pad in a distal to proximal manner (Fig. 9-4). With this technique, radiographic studies after injection of 0.5 ml of contrast medium show that when the leg is raised above the horizontal plane, the contrast medium travels rapidly for 30 cm before reaching the deep venous system.[48] The sclerosing solution is diluted and probably inactivated by the time it reaches the deep venous system (see Chapter 7). With this technique it may not be necessary to repeat injections every few centimeters in the varicose vein.

With the leg-raising technique, the varicose vein would be presumed empty of blood—this is not the case. Duplex examination demonstrates that the GSV is not totally emptied of blood, even with an 80-degree incline, although tributaries to the GSV are emptied at 45 degrees.[56] In "huge" varicosities, as much as 18 ml of blood can be withdrawn when the leg is raised 45 degrees above the horizontal.[57] Therefore Perchuk[57] developed a method for ensuring an "empty" vein. His method consists of inserting the needle into the varicose vein, elevating the leg 45 degrees, and then withdrawing blood through that needle into a syringe until further blood withdrawal is impossible. Then a syringe with sclerosing solution is attached to the needle, and the injection is made, followed by application of local pressure for 5 minutes. The use of compression bandages or stockings after treatment was not mentioned. A two-way stopcock may also be used for this technique. Perchuk, in an evaluation of 84 patients, found that this technique produced excellent results and limited all complications. Pigmentation, thrombophlebitis, and recurrence were very rare. Fegan,[58] however, disagrees with

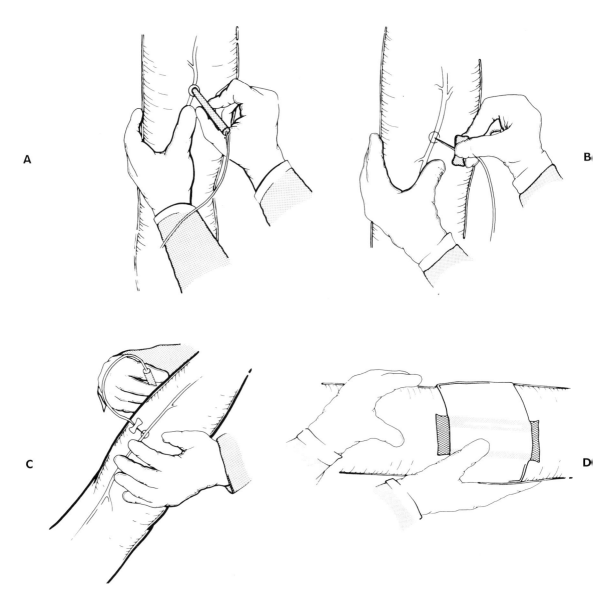

Fig. 9-4 **A,** Localization of an incompetent perforator vein through the use of a hand-held Doppler device. **B,** Cannulation of the incompetent perforator vein with a 26-gauge butterfly needle. **C,** The leg is elevated 45 degrees, and 0.5 to 1.0 ml of sclerosing solution is placed into the now empty perforator vein under minimal pressure. Note placement of a finger distal to the injection site to feel for extravasation of solution (which would indicate improper placement of the needle and necessitate immediate discontinuance of treatment and infiltration of the injection site with lidocaine 1%). **D,** Immediate compression of the treated vessel with an sodium tetradecyl sulfate (STD) foam pad and tape dressing.

Perchuk's conclusions and states that the vein would empty of blood if raised for a longer time and at a more acute angle.

Two-phase (Sigg) technique. A variation on the method described previously is the two-phase technique of Sigg.[9] The variation involves the way in which the needle is inserted into the vein. Sigg recommends that the needle be passed through the vein with the syringe unattached or with a finger placed over the hub and then slowly drawn back until the escape of blood indicates proper placement. The needle is left open and unobstructed while an assistant places a basin beneath it to catch the dripping blood. The leg is then raised above the horizontal plane, and bleeding stops. A syringe is then attached, and blood is withdrawn. After proper placement is confirmed by withdrawal of venous blood and the vein is emptied of blood, the sclerosing solution is injected and the vein compressed, as described above, with a stocking or bandage or both. Since Sigg uses mainly iodinated iodine solutions, he developed this technique to ensure continual intravascular placement of the sclerosing solution (see Chapters 7 and 8).

For both the Fegan and Sigg methods described, either the needles are all positioned and inserted while the varicose veins are distended or each needle is inserted separately, one at a time before each injection. When the latter is performed, distal compression prevents dilation of the preceding vein segment when the leg is lowered for each subsequent needle insertion.

Reclining. Another method for injection advocated since the 1920s is that of having the patient remain horizontal throughout the procedure.[59] If the varicose veins easily collapse in this position, they can be marked with indelible ink before the procedure, while the patient is standing. Radiologic study has shown that a 0.5-ml bolus of contrast medium injected into a varicose tributary of the GSV travels proximally 8 cm and remains within the vessel for approximately 2 minutes before being drawn into the deep venous system.[48] The relaxation of the calf muscles permits the injected fluid to stay within the vein since blood flow in this position is slow. Thus this position produces the longest lasting and most uniform contact between the injected solution and the vein wall.

To produce a relatively bloodless vein during injection in the horizontal position, some authors advocate rubbing along the vein in both a proximal and distal direction away from the injection site.[59] Manual compression is then maintained at the proximal and distal sites along the vein to prevent the vein segment from refilling with blood. After the injection a compression pad and bandage are immediately applied to the treated vein segment.

Variations on Injection Technique

Air bolus. The air-bolus technique was first advocated by Orbach[59] to ensure that sclerotherapy treatment of varicose veins occurred with minimal thrombosis. The rationale for instilling air before injecting the sclerosing solution is that clearing the vessel of blood allows undiluted contact to occur between the solution and the vessel wall. This procedure was thought to minimize the concentration and quantity of solution required to produce endothelial injury. A comparative evaluation of this technique demonstrated enhanced efficacy of treatment regardless of the type of sclerosing agent used.[60] In reality, the potential complications of air embolism as addressed in Chapter 8 are nil. A disadvantage of this technique is that air proximal to the sclerosing solution in the syringe will cause compression of the solution, producing leakage of solution from the needle after depression of the plunger has stopped. This may result in extravasation of solution upon needle withdrawal.

Radiologic studies have shown air-bolus injections into large varicose veins in the area of the GSV are ineffective in clearing the vessel of blood, even when 0.5 ml of air is injected immediately before the injection of contrast medium.[48] In addition, the air inhibits complete and even filling of the varix both proximal and distal to the injection site. In smaller varicosities injected air forms several bubbles and does not act as a bolus. It also moves independently of the position of the patient and is not totally under the influence of gravity. Therefore the air-bolus technique may not be advantageous for use in treating varicose veins.

Foam sclerotherapy. Shaking a solution of STS in the syringe to produce foam increases the thrombogenic activity of the sclerosing solution fourfold.[61] STS foam is made by shaking a vial of STS 3% for 30 seconds. The foam is then aspirated into a syringe. The amount of solution needed to make 1 ml of foam is approximately 0.05 ml.[62] The advantage of the foam is believed to be the result of the STS concentration in the walls of the bubbles, which continually bombard the intima and exert a continuous corroding effect on the vein wall. Unlike injection of a solution that is rapidly carried away and diluted in the bloodstream, the foam acts longer at the point of injection.[62] A comparison of this technique versus the air-block technique has not been performed.

Use of a tourniquet. The use of a tourniquet is not recommended as an aid to injection. Although it may distend the vein for easier cannulation, the increased pressure in the varicose vein may force sclerosing solution into normal veins. In addition, the tourniquet will also impede flow in the normal vein, thus limiting the normal dilution of sclerosing solution. However, the tourniquet may be used to facilitate placement of the needle into the vein. It is then removed, ensuring that the intended vein has been cannulated, and the solution is then injected.

Ultrasound-guided injection. Ultrasound is a useful tool to help visualize injection of a varicose vein in patients who have deeply situated perforator veins, in the obese patient in whom the varicose vein is not easily palpable, in patients with recurrent varicose veins, and in patients with an unusual or complex anatomy that makes finding the point of maximal reflux difficult. Ultrasonic guidance alone does not compensate for lack of dexterity or experience. In fact, injection may be riskier because of the complex reasons that require its use. Initial experience has shown a high level of complications, especially arterial injection with loss of significant amounts of tissue (see Chapter 8).[63]

This technique was first described in 1989 and is a natural extension of the use of ultrasound in patient evaluation.[64-68] The technique for injection is similar to that for standard sclerotherapy except that the needle used is usually longer and of larger diameter. I generally use a $1\frac{1}{2}$-inch 22-gauge needle that is sufficiently large to be echogenic. Smaller needles (25 gauge) cannot usually be seen in the ultrasound image.

The needle is introduced into the vein open (not attached to a syringe) to ensure venous placement because arterial injection is not uncommon (Fig. 9-5, *A*) (see Chapter 8). Injection of the sclerosing solution is seen as echogenic flow (Fig. 9-5, *C*). The injection continues until the vein goes into spasm or thrombosis occurs (Fig. 9-5, *D*).

To provide an even safer method for injection, Grondin and Soriano[69] advocate the use of a 20-gauge, 44-mm Teflon or radiopaque catheter to cannulize the vein under ultrasound guidance to further enhance accurate visualization of proper needle placement. Their reported rate of complications in 500 patients is 19.4% postinjection pain, 6.4% superficial phlebitis, and no cases of intraarterial injection, pulmonary emboli, deep vein thrombosis, or extravasation necrosis.

Finally, a Doppler ultrasound–guided 18- or 20-gauge ($2\frac{3}{4}$ inch or $1\frac{1}{2}$ inch, respectively) introducer needle (SmartNeedle,® Advanced Cardiovascular Systems, Inc., Temecula, Calif.) is now commercially available. This device has the

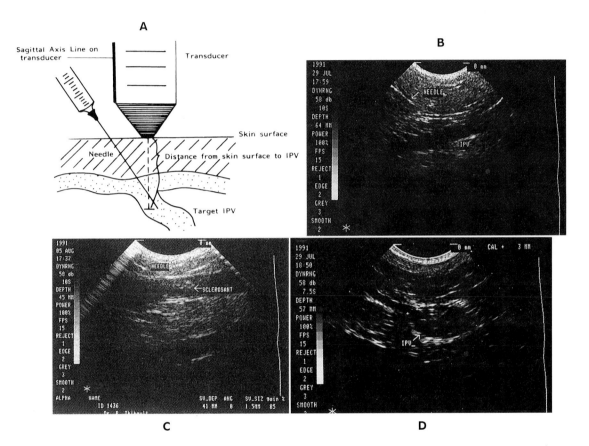

Fig. 9-5 **A,** Needle is inserted close to the transducer tip and along the sagittal plane of the transducer. Depth of target incompetent perforator vein (IPV) is measured on the B-mode image from skin surface to segment of IPV. **B,** B-mode ultrasound image showing needle approaching IPV. **C,** B-mode ultrasound image of needle located in vein with sclerosant flowing in the vein. **D,** Postinjection B-mode image of IPV showing vessel spasm. (From Thibault PK and Lewis WA: J Dermatol Surg Oncol 18:895, 1992.)

proposed benefit of allowing distinction of arterial from venous flow before treatment and has been used to prevent erroneous arterial puncture during placement of a central venous catheter.[70]

Duplex ultrasound is also useful in assessing the response to initial treatment. When patients return for follow-up examination, duplex evaluation can guide subsequent injections to sections of the vein that have not fully sclerosed or to a previously unrecognized area of reflux. When sclerotherapy is successful, the venous wall appears thickened, particularly at the intimal layer, with ultrasound (Fig. 9-6). The vein is noncompressible. When endofibrosis is subtherapeutic, the lumen is open with partial intravascular thrombosis. These findings indicate the need for a further sclerotherapy injection. Incomplete sclerosis appears as a series of multiple echoes represented as intraluminal white dots.[64] Superficial thrombophlebitis appears as an enlarged luminal diameter with minimal parietal changes, partial compressibility, echogenic blood flow, and a lumen partially filled with echogenic material.[71]

Thibault and Lewis[72] have found that incompetent perforating veins comprise the most common site of reflux from deep to superficial veins in patients with recurrent postsurgical varicose veins. In their series of 122 limbs in 76 patients, after ligation and stripping of the SFJ or SPJ, 71.3% of patients had recurrent incompetent superficial thigh veins in the distribution of the GSV. Thirty-two percent of patients had incompetent veins in the distribution of the LSV. These veins can then be injected with sclerosing solution.[68] In this setting ultrasound-guided injection is particularly helpful since an obvious varicosity does not always occur over an incompetent perforator.[73] In addition, surgical exploration for the perforator in this setting is often difficult.[74] Thirty-six patients (38 limbs) with incompetent perforator veins after surgical stripping were injected with 0.5 to 1 ml of STS 3% under ultrasound guidance.[68] Repeat injections were required at 6 to 8 weeks in six patients. Thirty-six of 38 limbs were successfully closed at 6- and 12-month follow-up without notable complications.

Doppler-guided injection. When a duplex ultrasound device is not available, a handheld Doppler probe may just as easily guide accurate placement of the sclerosing solution. The Doppler probe is used to determine the point of maximal reflux and is positioned approximately 1 cm distal or proximal to that point. While an assistant holds the Doppler probe in place, the needle or syringe is advanced toward the vein with slight negative pressure on the plunger. Puncture of the vessel is heard as a tinkling sound, and the syringe fills with venous blood. Injection is heard as a flushing sound.

Cornu-Thenard[75] has found that approximately 20% of varicose veins change their position by 1 cm or more when patients move from a standing to a supine position. Therefore preinjection markings of varicose veins with the patient standing are not reliable. Doppler evaluation is important when the patient is supine to ensure accurate needle placement.

Endoscopic injection. Venous endoscopy is also useful when injecting the SFJ or perforator veins.[30,76] This technique was first presented by Van Cleef[77] in 1989 for treatment of the GSV at the SFJ. This technique uses an angioscope inserted through an 11-French Seldinger introducing set (USCI-Bard, Billerica, Me) while the patient is either standing or in a reverse Trendelenburg position. Endoscopes used have a diameter of 0.85 mm. Irreversible spasm may occur if the introduction occurs with the patient supine.[30]

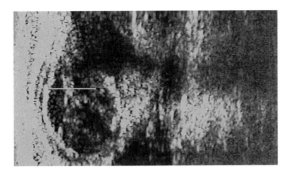

Fig. 9-6 Duplex ultrasound transverse image of the GSV after sclerotherapy. Note presence of adherent heterogeneous material within the lumen and thickening of the endothelium. (From Raymond-Martimbeau P: Semin Dermatol 12:123, 1993.)

The saphenous vein is cannulated with a 16-gauge needle, with the dilator and 11-French sheath inserted over a guide wire after the needle is removed. The angioscope is advanced with visualization helped by 5% dextrose solution infusion at 37° C and manual compression of the refluxing SFJ while the patient is supine. The endoscope is brought to within 2 to 3 cm of the ostial valves, and the sclerosing solution is injected through the infusion channel. Manual compression of both the injection site and the angioscope insertion site is maintained until vessel spasm is complete. After 5 minutes the venous lumen is irrigated and observed for endothelial destruction, which is noted as a change from the normal pearly-white color to a reddish grey. A compression dressing is then applied. At this time visualized endovenous changes have not been correlated with outcome. Therefore at this writing sclerotherapy under endoscopic control is in the experimental stage.

Intravascular ultrasound–controlled injection. Intravascular ultrasound (IVUS) provides a unique perspective to evaluate vessel walls before, during, and after therapeutic interventions. Echographic data processing and computerized image manipulation can produce accuate luminal and transmural images of blood vessels. Electronically switched array devices use frequencies of 12 to 25 MHz in no. 4 to 12 French catheters to produce cross-sectional images of vascular segments. However, with present probes a bright circumferential artifact known as a *ring down* surrounds the catheter and prevents imaging of structures in the area immediately surrounding the catheter.[78]

IVUS is accurate in determining the luminal and vessel wall morphology of normal and minimally diseased vessels, with a dimensional accuracy of 0.05 mm.[79-81] This device can visualize calcified and noncalcified arterial lesions and intimal tears or flaps and can distinguish between the media, intima, and adventitial layers of the vessel wall. Until now this technology has primarily been used in evaluating arterial lesions. Future devices may combine the benefits of angiography, angioscopy, and intravascular ultrasound in a single compact unit.

Raymond-Martimbeau[82] has reported injection through an IVUS probe. This technique allows injection to continue while the vein wall is resonated by the ultrasound probe until sclerosis is visualized by sclerosis of the entire vein wall (Fig. 9-7). The advantage of this technique is the assurance of complete destruction of the vein wall. The concentration or quantity of solution can be varied until effective endosclerosis is seen.

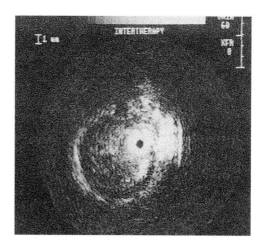

Fig. 9-7 Intravascular ultrasound cross-sectional image from a segment of the GSV after injection of iodine sodium iodide. Note presence of intimal thickening and intimal destruction at 12 o'clock position. (From Raymond-Martimbeau P: Role of sclerotherapy in greater saphenous vein incompetance. In Bergan JJ and Goldman MP, editors: Varicose veins and telangiectasias: diagnosis and treatment, St. Louis, 1993, Quality Medical Publishing, Inc.)

DOES THE MENSTRUAL CYCLE INFLUENCE SCLEROTHERAPY?

The actions of estrogens and progestins on venous distensibility have been discussed previously (see Chapters 3 and 4). Theoretically, sclerotherapy should be performed when the venous system is in its most contracted state so that post-treatment thrombosis is minimized. Since limb volume and venous distensibility are at their least during and just after menses and at their highest during ovulation, the optimal window for sclerotherapy treatment is when estrogen levels are lowest.[83] However, until appropriate studies are performed to test this hypothesis, no absolute recommendation can be made.

RECOMMENDED SCLEROSING SOLUTION AMOUNTS AND CONCENTRATIONS

Although the exact concentration of sclerosing solution depends on the caliber and location of the varicose vein, the following suggestions can serve as an initial guide to therapy. When diluting nonosmotic sclerosing solutions, dilution with sterile water will cause the sclerosing agent to sting with injection. Thus dilutions should be performed with bacteriostatic normal saline solution, which will not impart an additional sting.

The *first principle* of determining solution amounts and concentrations is that the concentrations should be strongest at the highest point of reflux. With saphenofemoral reflux, the concentration should be strongest at the upper thigh and weakest at the ankle. With ankle or calf perforating veins, the concentration should be highest at the perforator. For example, Vin[84] recommends that 1 ml of STS 1.0% be used at the proximal thigh, 0.5 ml of STS 1.0% be used at the medial thigh, and 0.3 ml of STS 0.5% be used at the medial knee to treat a moderately sized varicose vein.

The *second principle,* as described by Tournay in 1949, is, "It is not the concentration of the sclerosing agent in the syringe that matters, but the concentration within the vein."[85] The importance of this statement was discussed in Chapter 7. In short, for sclerotherapy to be effective the entire vein wall must be dam-

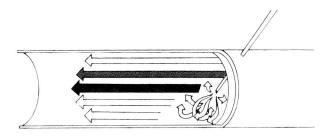

Fig. 9-8 Turbulent flow is produced with injection of solution at the point of discharge of sclerosant from the needle cannula. (From Green D: Semin Dermatol 12:88, 1993.)

aged, and the entire intraluminal volume of the segment of the vein to be obliterated must be destroyed. This is important because the smooth muscle portion of the vein wall can theoretically regenerate endothelium, and endothelial cells can migrate long distances to reestablish a functional conduit. Sackmann[86] expanded on this principle by demonstrating in polyvinyl tubes that the local conditions of "time and space" regarding contact of the sclerosing solution with the vessel wall were also important. He demonstrated that the zone of contact diminishes as the caliber of the vessel increases. In tubes with a diameter less than or equal to 4 mm, the liquid flowed in a laminar fashion. In tubes with a diameter greater than or equal to 8 mm, turbulent flow was produced. In tubes 6 mm in diameter a mixed flow occurred, with a transition between a laminar and turbulent appearance (Fig. 9-8). In contrast, the caliber and position of the needle, the speed of injection, and the viscosity of the solution did not seem to influence the time of contact of the sclerosing solution with the tube.

Green[87] has used Poiseuille's formula to describe resistance to fluid flow in a varicose vein:

$$R = \frac{8\kappa n^1}{\pi\, r^4}$$

where

R = Resistance
κn = Viscosity of the solution
1 = Length of the vein
r = Radius of the vein

From this formula it is apparent that the most important factor in determining resistance of flow is the vessel diameter (radius). At the point of injection into an empty vein, expected flow of sclerosing solution would be nonlaminar (see Fig. 9-8). This may account (along with increased localized concentration; see below) for a greater incidence of vessel damage and blowout at the point of injection (see Chapter 8). Nonlaminar flow also occurs downstream of injection in an empty vein in which resistance is still high since the pressure generated by the physician on the syringe plunger is much greater than intravascular pressure, which would approach zero in an empty vein, especially if the limb were elevated (Fig. 9-9).[88]

Guex[88] has calculated that the concentration of sclerosing solution can be calculated based on the diameter of the vein by the formula:

$$Cm = \frac{v \times C \times N}{pi\; R^2}$$

where

Cm = Mean concentration of solution
v = Volume of injected sclerosing solution
C = Concentration of sclerosing solution
N = Number of injections
R = Radius of the injected vein

Thus if 0.5 ml is injected into a varicose vein 2 mm in diameter, the sclerosing solution will fill a 16-cm length of vein. In reality, the concentration of sclerosing solution at the injection site is maximal and decreases with distance from each point when small volumes of solution are injected (Fig. 9-10). The concentration of sclerosing solution along the entire course of the vein can be equalized either by injecting a larger volume in a single site or by injecting small volumes in multiple sites (Figs. 9-11 and 9-12).

A study by Cornu-Thenard[89] suggests the following sclerosing concentrations for varicosities of various diameters:

4 mm = STS 0.25%
5 mm = STS 0.5%
6 mm = STS 1.0%

He recommends 0.5-ml injections be placed every 6 to 10 cm along the varicose vein. Additional recommended concentrations for injection of other sclerosing solutions into various types and diameters of veins are found in Chapter 7.

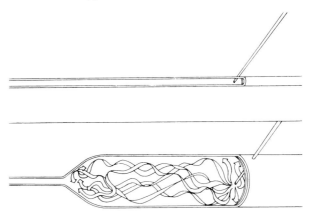

Fig. 9-9 Nonlaminar flow occurs distal to the point of injection in an empty vein. *Top,* Needle inserted into empty vein. *Bottom,* The force of the advancing injected solution dilates the vein and produces turbulent flow. (From Gren D: Semin Dermatol 12:88, 1993.)

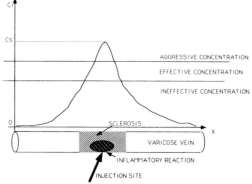

Fig. 9-10 Injection at one site with a high concentration but low volume of sclerosing solution. Note localized excessive concentration. (From Guex J-J: J Dermatol Surg Oncol 19:959, 1993.)

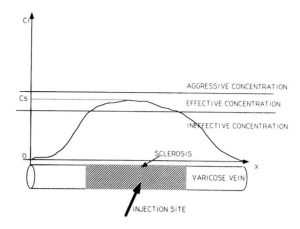

Fig. 9-11   Injection at one site with large volume of a dilute concentration of sclerosing solution. Note that a longer segment of vein is sclerosed without any one point of excessive concentration. (From Guex J-J: J Dermatol Surg Oncol 19:959, 1993.)

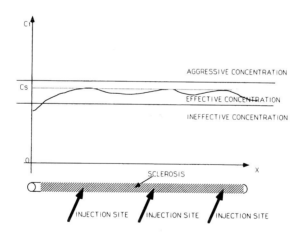

Fig. 9-12   Multiple injections with low volumes of low concentrations of sclerosing solution. This technique theoretically provides the safest method for treating long lengths of veins. (From Guex J-J: J Dermatol Surg Oncol 19:959, 1993.)

The *third principle* is the amount of sclerosing solution injected into a single site should not be more than 1.0 ml (usually 0.5 ml). Venographic studies of direct injections into varicosities of the leg have demonstrated that if more than 1.5 ml of solution is injected at a single site, it is likely to spill over into the deep veins.[48,90] In addition, the patient should not move the leg for a few minutes so that the sclerosing solution can remain in contact with the varicose vein, because any movement of the leg will rapidly move the sclerosing solution into the deep venous system.

Histologic examination of peripheral veins may provide assistance in determining the optimal concentration of sclerosing solution. Corcos et al.[91] have determined through biopsy of the dorsal pedal vein that the degree of intimal thickening, ectasia, muscular hyperplasia, medial fibrosis, fragmentation, and dissociation of the internal elastic membrane and intimal fibrous plaques correlate to the concentration of sclerosing solution necessary to effect endosclerosis of varicose veins.[91] This finding is supported by the theory that varicosis is a systemic disease (see Chapter 3).

POSTSCLEROTHERAPY COMPRESSION

After injections of varicose or telangiectatic veins, the treated veins are immediately compressed to minimize significant thrombosis. The patient is instructed to walk immediately after the injection session to help prevent DVT and reduce venous reflux into the treated veins. Calf muscle movement produces a rapid blood flow in the deep venous system, which dilutes any sclerosing solution that may have migrated into the area.

Postsclerosis compression is perhaps the most important advance in sclerotherapy treatment of varicose veins since the introduction of relatively safe synthetic sclerosing agents in the 1940s. Primarily, compression eliminates a thrombophlebitic reaction and substitutes a "sclerophlebitis" with the production of a firm fibrous cord.[11] The advantages of postsclerotherapy compression are discussed in detail in Chapter 6.

In addition to providing external compression to the treated vessel, one should also try to minimize forces that act to distend the vessel. Since taking hot baths or saunas will dilate the cutaneous venous network, they should be avoided for 2 to 6 weeks after sclerotherapy or until such time as the treated vessel is fully sclerosed. In addition, any activity that increases abdominal pressure may act to force blood in a retrograde manner through the SFJ or incompetent perforator veins, producing venous dilation. Heavy weight lifting therefore must be discouraged, along with any exercises that use the abdominal musculature unless the legs are elevated during abdominal exercise. One such activity that increases abdominal pressure by approximately 22 mm Hg is running, with pressure apparently produced to splint the trunk and pelvis.[92] Therefore aerobic exercises, jogging, and running should be limited for 1 to 2 weeks.

Patients should be examined 2 weeks after injection so that any area of thrombosis can be evacuated early.[93] Each individual area should not be treated again sooner than 6 to 8 weeks after initial injection to allow adequate healing between treatments.

CONTRAINDICATIONS TO TREATMENT
Pregnancy

Besides the risk of absorption of the sclerosing solution by the fetus, pregnancy is associated with dilation of the entire venous system through multiple mechanisms that do not normalize until 3 months postpartum (see Chapter 3).[94,95] Therefore, although sclerotherapy can and has been successfully performed by many physicians on pregnant women,[96-100] the increase in venous distensibility counteracts the desired contraction of the treated varicose vein (see Chapters 3, 4, and 8). Finally, varicose veins may decrease in size and may disappear after delivery (see Chapters 3 and 4).[101] Thus waiting may eliminate the need for the procedure.

One situation that may justify sclerotherapy during pregnancy is the presence of painful vulvar varicosities. Approximately 2% of pregnant women develop significant vulvar varicosities.[102] They usually occur by the second trimester and are more likely in multiparous women. Although they rarely thrombose, they are painful, especially with walking. Bed rest, leg elevation, and localized compression are usually effective in alleviating symptoms, but sclerotherapy may be necessary in severe cases.

Venography has shown vulvar varices arise from any combination of the following: obturator vein, internal pudendal vein, inferior gluteal vein, external iliac, uterine, and ovarian veins, obturator vein, presacral veins, common femoral vein, and the GSV.[103,104] Because of this variable and extensive system of reflux and the thin-walled, fragile nature of these veins, sclerotherapy is preferred over surgical excision or avulsion (see case study 7 on p. 382).

Inability to Ambulate

Walking after treatment is very important because it ensures rapid dilution of the sclerosing solution, which may enter normal deep veins. Walking also lessens the possibility of excessive thrombosis by liberating thrombolytic factors during muscle contraction, thereby avoiding stagnation of blood flow. Walking also decreases physical distention of the vein caused by reflux.

A corollary to this contraindication is performing sclerotherapy during surgical ligation. Although this procedure has been performed by many surgeons and was advocated by de Takats in 1930,[105] it was usually limited to a point distal to the SFJ on the GSV and so was performed on an ambulatory basis. In 1934 Faxon[106] modified this technique to include ligation at the SFJ with retrograde injection of the GSV. He achieved good results (although follow-up was poor) in his series of 117 cases except for one case of fatal pulmonary embolus, which was attributed to faulty technique by a resident surgeon. In more recent times Peter Conrad[107] reports great success with this technique when used in conjunction with ligation at the SFJ. Hubner[108] has reported similar success without mention of complications in 413 patients followed for more than 1 year. Patients treated with polidocanol 4% have a 83% success rate, whereas patients treated with Variglobin 4% have a 94% success rate. However, Hubner separates the two procedures by a few hours to a day because his patients have the ligation performed by a surgeon in a separate office and return to him for sclerotherapy. This later scenario ensures that the patient is ambulatory for both procedures.

In spite of the above-mentioned successful results, there are potential complications that call for separating the two procedures. First, many varicose veins will resolve after surgical treatment of the high-pressure reflux points so that subsequent sclerotherapy is minimized or not necessary.[109] Second, the surgical period is often one of minimal ambulation because of postoperative pain and the use of general or regional anesthesia. The delay in adequate ambulation may allow the sclerosing solution to migrate to the deep venous system where unwanted damage could occur (see Chapter 8).[102] I recommend that postoperative sclerotherapy be delayed for 2 to 3 weeks.

History of Thrombophlebitis and Deep Vein Thrombosis

Patients with a history of certain venous diseases may be predisposed to the development of excessive thrombosis with injection of a sclerosing agent, that is, development of an excessive phlebitic reaction (see Chapter 8). Also, in rare patients the dilated superficial system may serve as a conduit for carrying blood to the heart. Interruption of the superficial system then may increase venous insufficiency. Therefore PPG, both with and without application of a superficial tourniquet or a trial of 30 to 40 mm Hg graduated compression stockings, will help determine which patients will benefit and which may be harmed by sclerotherapy treatment.

Another simple test to determine if the varicosity resulting from DVT is a necessary conduit is a modification of the Perthes' test (see Chapter 5). A tensiometer cuff is inflated to 110 mm Hg, and the patient is asked to walk quickly for 5 minutes. If the patient complains of heavy pain or the leg becomes livid or both, the varicosity is necessary as a collateral channel. This test has allowed surgery on 53 limbs with varicose veins in 52 patients with prior DVT without complication.[110]

Allergic Reaction

Rarely patients are allergic to a sclerosing solution, but a different solution can usually be substituted. If the allergic reaction consists of generalized urticaria, with or without an erythematous papulosquamous appearance, French authors advocate continuing treatment with the offending sclerosing solution with the addition of antihistamines before and after treatment[111] (see Chapter 8).

Infrequently patients develop periorbital edema and a maculopapular cutaneous eruption even with the use of unadulterated hypertonic saline solutions. In this case "allergic reaction" may be the result of histamine release by intravascular basophils or perivascular mast cells that are directly damaged by the sclerosing solution (see Chapter 7).[112] Under this circumstance, administering antihistamines before and after the procedure appears safe while continuing therapy.

Patients Taking Disulfiram

Patients taking disulfiram (Antabuse) should not be treated with polidocanol or Sclerodex since these sclerosing solutions contain ethyl alcohol.

CASE HISTORIES

The following case histories demonstrate my technique of sclerotherapy for different varicose veins (see box below).

SCLEROTHERAPY OF VARICOSE VEINS

SEQUENCE OF EVENTS
1. Physical examination
2. Noninvasive diagnostic examination
3. If findings are abnormal, consider duplex scanning, varicography, or photoplethysmography
4. Eliminate the high-pressure inflow points
   a. Saphenofemoral/saphenopopliteal junction
   b. Incompetent perforators
5. Sclerotherapy of the largest diameter varicose veins
6. Sclerotherapy of perforator or reticular veins that feed "spider" telangiectasia
7. Sclerotherapy of "spider" telangiectasia

CASE STUDY 1: Incompetent perforator veins treated with Fegan's technique

A 35-year-old woman developed varicose veins during the second trimester of her second pregnancy and wore an over-the-counter light compression stocking during the remainder of her pregnancy. At delivery she developed thrombophlebitis that was treated with hot packs only. She came for evaluation and treatment 6 months after delivery. Physical examination showed a 4- to 6-mm varicose tributary of the GSV originating at the medial midthigh and extending to the medial calf with continuation across the anterior tibia (Fig. 9-13, A and B). Venous Doppler examination revealed a continuous venous sound with distal augmentation at the level of the posterior tibial vein at the left ankle. There was no evidence of saphenofemoral reflux or other abnormalities. PPG revealed a normal venous refilling time in the right leg. The venous refilling time was abnormal in the left leg (<20 seconds). The venous refilling time normalized with placement of a tourniquet at the level of the left upper calf and left lower thigh. Therefore the physical and noninvasive examinations were consistent, showing incompetence of the Hunterian vein.

Because of the localized abnormality (incompetent perforator veins) producing the varicose vein, Fegan's technique of perforator interruption was used. Sclerotherapy was performed with the injection of 0.5 to 1.0 ml of STS 1.0% at the midthigh, medial superior calf, and anterior distal tibial point of fascial depression. The needles were inserted with the patient standing, and the patient then assumed the supine position with the leg elevated to 45 degrees. After aspiration to confirm proper needle placement, the sclerosing solution was injected while proximal pressure was maintained. STD E-foam pads were placed over the entire course of the varicose vein and secured with 3M Microfoam tape. A 30 to 40 mm Hg graduated compression stocking was applied and worn continuously for 7 days, after which it was worn for an additional week only while the patient was ambulatory.

The patient was next seen 2 weeks later, at which time physical examination revealed total resolution of the varicosity at the midthigh (Fig. 9-13, C) and persistence of a thrombosed varicosity at the anterior tibial level (Fig. 9-13, D). It was drained, and the pressure

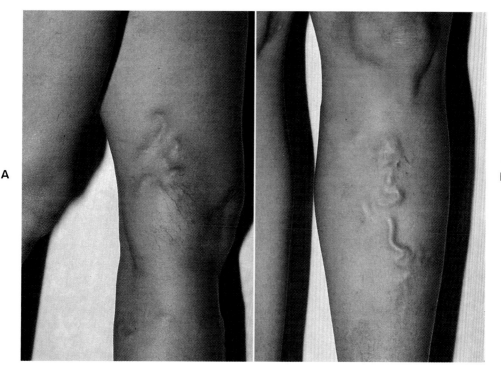

A   B

Fig. 9-13 Varicose tributary of LSV originating at medial midthigh, **A**, and extending to medial calf and continuing across anterior tibia, **B**. *Continued.*

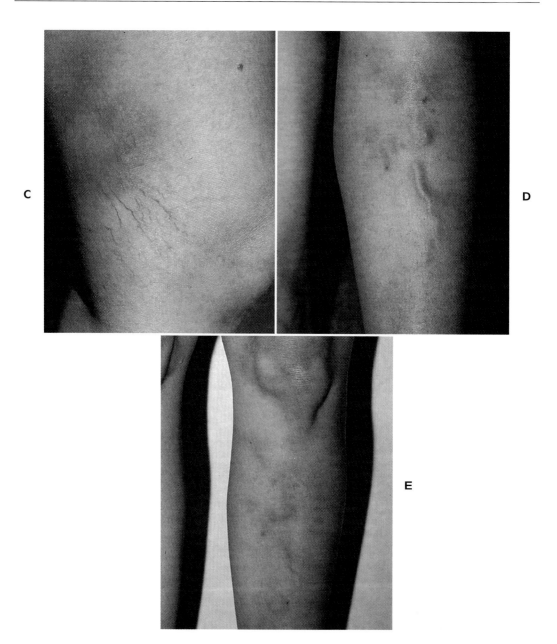

Fig. 9-13, cont'd   C, Two weeks after sclerotherapy total resolution of varicosity is shown at midthigh, but, **D,** persistence of thrombosed varicosity is visible at anterior tibial level. **E,** Complete resolution 6 weeks after sclerotherapy.   *Continued.*

stocking was prescribed for use while the patient was ambulatory for another week. On follow-up examination 6 weeks later the vessel had resolved (Fig. 9-13, E). One-year follow-up demonstrated total obliteration of the varicosity and posttreatment hyperpigmentation (Fig. 9-13, F and G). This case illustrates Fegan's principle that interruption of the incompetent perforator veins alone will result in normalization of the entire varicose vein.

One year later (2 years after her initial sclerotherapy) the patient became pregnant with her third child and noted the development of new varicose and telangiectatic leg veins during her first trimester. Despite wearing 30 to 40 mm Hg graduated support stockings for much of her pregnancy, she developed incompetence of the SFJ bilaterally, with new incompetent GSV bilaterally and new vulvar varicosities. Interestingly, the previously sclerosed veins just above the medial knee and on the anterior tibial surface did not reappear

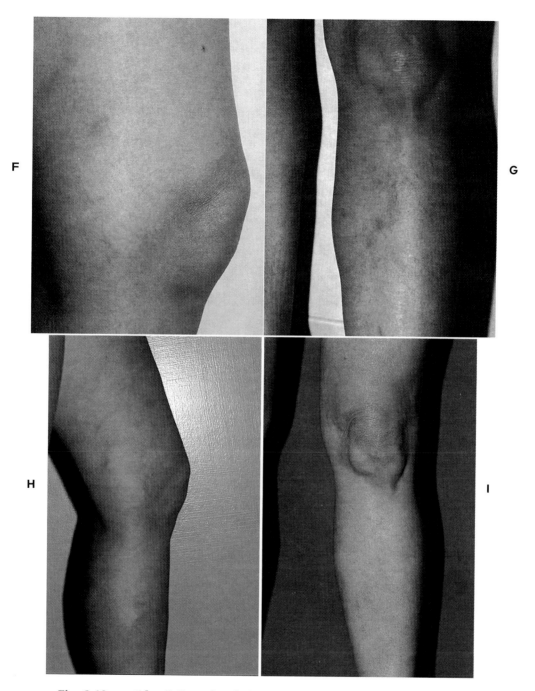

Fig. 9-13, cont'd   F, Lateral and, **G,** anterior views of vein normalization 1 year after treatment. **H and I,** New varicose GSV from an incompetent SFJ. Note that previously treated veins remain sclerosed.

(Fig. 9-13, H and I). Ligation and stripping were performed 18 months postpartum when breast-feeding was discontinued, followed 2 weeks later with sclerotherapy of reticular veins with excellent results (Fig. 9-13, J).

This patient illustrates many important points. Sclerotherapy is very effective in treating large varicose veins when the SFJs are competent. However, varicose veins represent a disease of the venous system that often is progressive. So initial success may be met with new disease over time, especially if additional aggravating events (pregnancy) occur. Fortunately, treatment is both effective and cosmetic.

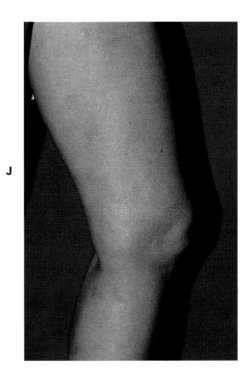

Fig. 9-13, cont'd.   J, Clinical appearance, 6 months after ligation and stripping of GSV followed by sclerotherapy of reticular veins.

CASE STUDY 2: Incompetent perforator vein at the midcalf treated with modified Fegan technique

A 40-year-old woman noticed the gradual development of a varicose vein over 4 years without any predisposing factors. Physical examination showed a varicose tributary of the GSV 3 to 5 mm in diameter extending from the midanterior tibial surface to the medial calf and thigh, ending in the lower anterior thigh (Fig. 9-14, A and B). Venous Doppler examination was remarkable only for an incompetent perforator vein at the right midmedial calf.

Since fascial depressions could not be felt, the classic Fegan technique could not be performed. Therefore 25-gauge butterfly catheters were randomly placed into the varicosity at the level of the anterior midtibia, medial superior tibia, and the lateral knee with the patient standing. After the patient assumed the supine position, STS 0.5% was injected into these sites after proper needle placement was confirmed with blood aspiration. A total of 0.5 ml was injected at the anterior midtibia, 1 ml at the medial superior tibia, and 2 ml at the lateral knee while pressure was maintained on the vein proximally. STD E-foam pads were placed over the entire vessel and were secured with Coban tape applied with moderate pressure. A 30 to 40 mm Hg graduated compression stocking was applied, with two stockings worn on top of each other while the patient was ambulatory and one stocking worn at night for 1 week. During the second week the dressing was removed, and the graduated support stocking was worn for another week only while the patient was ambulatory. The varicosity was completely resolved on follow-up examination at 2 weeks, and a few thrombi were drained. Figure 9-14, C and D, was taken 11 months after treatment.

This latter technique used the principles of Fegan except that the entire area of presumed perforator incompetence was sclerosed. If Sigg's technique had been used, the sclerosing solution would have been more randomly injected throughout the entire course of the varicose veins. The classic Fegan technique could have been performed if the sites of incompetent perforator veins were localized with duplex imaging. Duplex-controlled injections may have limited the quantity of sclerosing solution injection to very specific sites but probably would not have affected the clinical outcome.

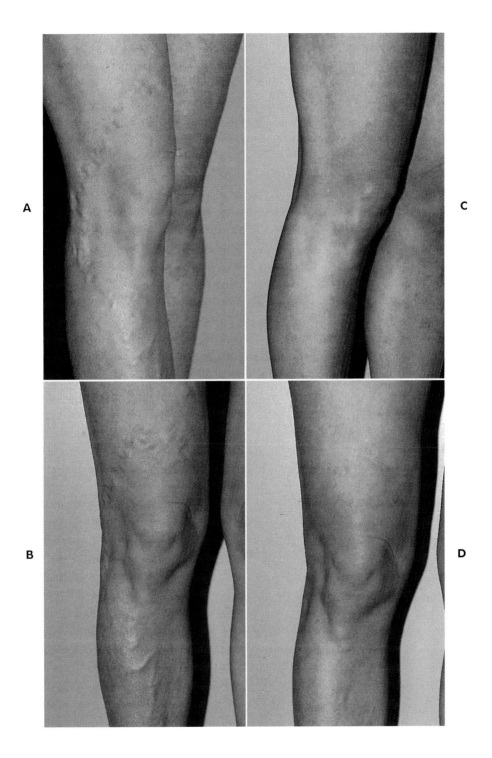

Fig. 9-14   Varicose tributary of GSV extending from midanterior tibial surface, **A,** to medial calf and thigh ending in lower anterior thigh, **B. C,** Midanterior tibial surface and medial calf and thigh and, **D,** lower anterior thigh views of vein normalization 11 months after treatment.

CASE STUDY 3: Reticular varicosities without perforator vein reflux treated with total-vein sclerotherapy (Sigg's technique)

A 34-year-old woman first noticed the appearance of varicose veins with her second pregnancy 3 years before treatment. The veins were symptomatic after prolonged standing and were thought to have enlarged over the past year. Physical examination showed a set of 3- to 4-mm varicose reticular veins coursing from the posterior midthigh to the posterior mid-calf bilaterally (Fig. 9-15, A and B). There was no evidence of incompetence in either the perforator veins or the SFJs on venous Doppler examination.

While the patient was lying horizontal on her abdomen, multiple injections of STS 0.5% were made into the varicose veins. Approximately 0.5 ml was injected into each site every 4 to 6 cm for a total of 8 ml of solution per leg. Continuous compression was maintained for 7 days only with 30 to 40 mm Hg graduated compression stocking overlying STD E-foam pads over the varicose veins. Follow-up examination did not disclose excessive bruising or pigmentation. No thrombosis occurred. Fig. 9-15, C and D, shows the appearance of the treated vessels at 1-year follow-up.

Since points of venous reflux could not be found either at the SFJ or in perforator veins, it was assumed that the varicose vein was essential in nature. Since it was serving no useful function, it was obliterated in its entirety. This forms the rationale for Sigg's technique.

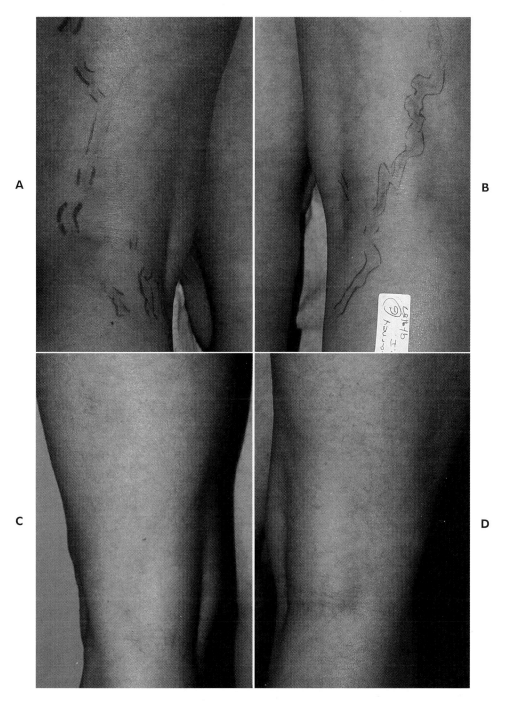

Fig. 9-15   Varicose reticular veins from posterior midthigh, **A**, to posterior midcalf, **B. C**, Posterior midthigh to, **D**, posterior midcalf normalization of veins 1 year after treatment.

CASE STUDY 4: **Posterior thigh varicose GSV tributary associated with an incompetent SFJ treated with sclerotherapy alone using the air-bolus technique**

A 36-year-old woman developed a varicose vein during her second pregnancy, 3 years before my evaluation and treatment. The vein was symptomatic during prolonged standing, and she reported associated ankle edema. Physical examination showed a 5- to 8-mm diameter varicose vein coursing from the midposterior thigh to the midcalf (Fig. 9-16, A). Venous Doppler examination demonstrated gross incompetence of the right SFJ and a positive Trendelenburg test in the lower thigh. The remainder of the examination was normal.

Surgical ligation and limited stripping were recommended but refused by the patient. Therefore sclerotherapy of the involved varicose vein was performed using an air-block technique. The air block was used in an attempt to concentrate the sclerosing solution in the injection site without dilution or inactivation of blood. Butterfly needles, 25-gauge, were placed in the vein at areas of fascial depression—two sites on the thigh and one site on the calf—while the patient was standing. These areas were not found by venous Doppler ultrasound to represent incompetent perforator veins. With the patient lying horizontal with the leg elevated to 45 degrees, 1 ml of STS 1.0% was injected into each site after injection of 0.5 ml of air. STD E-pads were immediately placed and secured with 3M Microfoam tape, and a single 30 to 40 mm Hg graduated compression stocking was worn continuously for 2 weeks. Follow-up examinations at 2 and 6 weeks showed persistent resolution of the vein with a slightly palpable cord. A small amount of coagula was drained at 6 weeks. The vein remained fibrosed 2 years after treatment (Fig. 9-16, B).

Treatment in this patient consisted of a modified Fegan and Sigg technique. The entire varicosity was obliterated using fascial depression areas as injection sites. The French technique with injection of sclerosing solution into the SFJ could have been used. However, this procedure was not performed because of the unavailability of Variglobin. Alternatively, STS 3% could have been injected under duplex control at the SFJ. Refer to the articles by Raymond-Martimbeau[33] and Schultz-Ehrenburg, Weindorf, and Tourbier[39] for a description of these latter techniques.

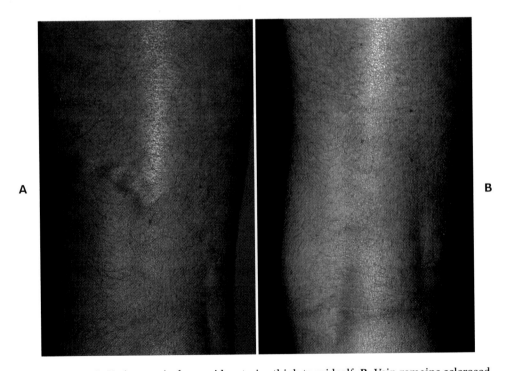

Fig. 9-16   A, Varicose vein from midposterior thigh to midcalf. B, Vein remains sclerosed 2 years after treatment.

CASE STUDY 5: **Incompetent GSV varicose tributaries treated with total-vein sclerotherapy alone**

A 31-year-old woman noted the onset of varicose veins over the right lower leg at 10 years of age. With each of her succeeding three pregnancies, the veins enlarged and became more painful while she was standing. Physical examination showed a clustered varicose vein 5 to 10 mm in diameter over the right anterior and medial calf (Fig. 9-17, A). Venous Doppler examination demonstrated marked reflux of the right GSV throughout the varicosity.

The patient refused surgical ligation and limited stripping. Therefore sclerotherapy with STS 1.0% was performed while the patient was horizontal. One milliliter of solution was slowly injected at each of nine separate locations, followed by application of STD foam pads and a double layer of 30 to 40 mm Hg graduated compression stockings, which were worn continuously while the patient was ambulatory for 2 weeks. One stocking was removed while she was sleeping. A mild phlebitic reaction was clinically apparent 2 weeks after injection (Fig. 9-17, B), and compression was maintained another 2 weeks. Four weeks after the first injection, multiple thrombi were drained from the medial calf, and two more injections of STS 1%, 1 ml each, were made into persistent varicose dilations on the medial and anterior superior calf (Fig. 9-17, C). At 1-year follow-up the leg remained pain free and showed persistent resolution of the treated veins (Fig. 9-17, D). Venous Doppler examination disclosed an incompetent 4-mm diameter varicose vein just below the right anterior tibia and another incompetent varicosis over the inferior midposterior calf. These veins were successfully sclerosed with STS 1%. At 2 years' follow-up the multiple new varicosities became apparent after resolution of sclerotherapy-induced hyperpigmentation. The patient has remained pain free and is very happy with the results of treatment. Her wish is to continue sclerotherapy treatment, even with the understanding that new or recurrent varicose veins may later occur.

This patient represents two common findings in my practice. First, many patients would rather undergo multiple (perpetual?) sclerotherapy treatments rather than limited surgical ligations or strippings. Second, the resolution of symptoms, which is very important to patients, may occur despite a reappearance of the varicose vein. It appears that in many patients incomplete treatment is enough to alleviate symptoms.

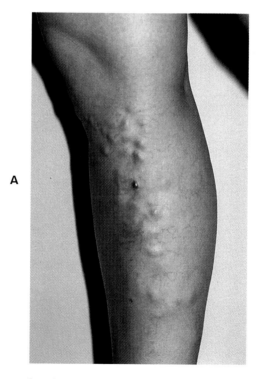

A

Fig. 9-17   A, Clustered varicose vein over right anterior and medial calf.   *Continued.*

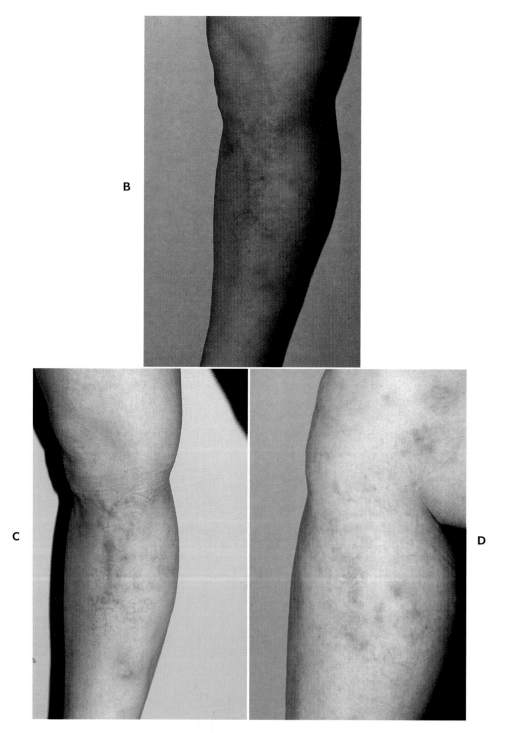

Fig. 9-17, cont'd. **B,** Mild phlebitic reaction 2 weeks after treatment. **C,** Further treatment 4 weeks after first injection. **D,** Resolution of vein continues at 1 year after treatment.

CASE STUDY 6: Incompetent perforator vein underlying ankle ulceration

A 27-year-old woman sought treatment after a 3-year history of cutaneous ulceration over the right medial mallear region (Fig. 9-18, A). The patient had been seen previously by a physician from the infectious disease service and was prescribed multiple courses of systemic antibiotic treatments that did not produce significant change in the appearance of the ulceration. She was also evaluated by a physician in the plastic surgery department and had been treated with the placement of full-thickness pinch grafts, which did not heal. Physical examination was remarkable for pedal edema extending to the midcalf and associated truncal varicosities. Venous Doppler examination demonstrated a normal deep venous system and saphenofemoral and popliteal junctions and an incompetent perforator vein at the base of the ulcer (marked X in Fig. 9-18, A). The perforator vein was injected through the ulcer. A 23-gauge butterfly needle was inserted into the perforator vein while the patient was standing, and the leg was elevated while the patient reclined. STS 1.0%, 1 ml, was slowly injected while the leg was blocked proximally and distally with hand pressure 3 cm in either direction. Immediately afterward compression was applied with an STD foam pad under Microfoam tape and two 30 to 40 mm Hg graduated compression stockings. The stockings were worn for 2 weeks. Double stockings were worn during the day, and the outer stocking was removed when the patient was supine.

Follow-up examination at 3 months showed complete healing of the ulceration and resolution of associated venous stasis changes (Fig. 9-18, B). The patient remained free of ulceration 2 years after treatment.

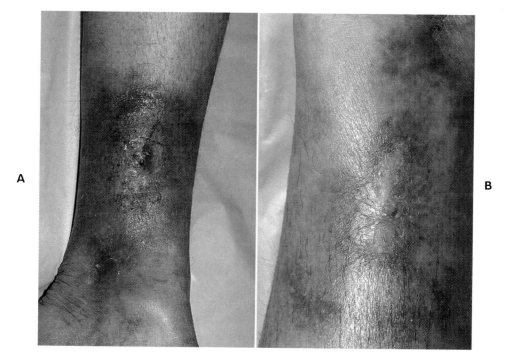

A

B

Fig. 9-18   A, Cutaneous ulceration over right medial mallear region. B, Complete healing of ulceration and resolution of venous stasis changes 3 months after treatment.

CASE STUDY 7: Sclerotherapy of vulvar varicosities

A 40-year-old woman developed vulvar varices with her first pregnancy at age 18. She noted aching and pelvic fullness during her menstrual period and when standing for prolonged periods of time. Physical examination showed a prominent varicose vein 6 to 8 mm in diameter extending from the vulvar region into the GSV. The vein was incompetent throughout its entire length from the midposterior calf to the most superior aspect of the vulva according to venous Doppler examination. Two incompetent perforator veins underlying fascial defects were present at the medial knee and midposterior calf. There was no evidence of incompetence with the Valsalva maneuver. Her SFJ was competent according to venous Doppler examination. Scattered reticular veins 3 mm in diameter were noted on the anterior thigh. Scattered venules 0.4 mm in diameter were present on the anterior and lateral calf. The opposite leg was free of varicose or telangiectatic veins (Fig. 9-19, A).

With the patient lying in a slight reverse Trendelenburg position, a total of 2 ml of STS 1.5% was injected into the two perforator veins at the medial knee and posterior calf. These areas were immediately compressed with an STD E-foam pad and 3M Microfoam tape. A total of 4 ml of STS 1.0% was injected into the network of vulvar and superior thigh varicosities, and a figure #8 wrap over foam pads was used to compress the vulvar varices. This was followed by injection of 4 ml of STS 0.5% into the remaining reticular veins and venulectases. A 30 to 40 mm Hg graduated thigh-high compression stocking was worn continuously for 7 days. When the patient returned 1 month later, all veins were sclerosed and without audible flow during venous Doppler examination. Multiple coagula were drained through 22-gauge needle punctures. Clinical appearance 2 months after treatment was excellent (Fig. 9-19, B). Clinical appearance 3 years after treatment was still excellent, with the patient showing no evidence of recurrence in any of the treated veins (Figs. 9-19, C).

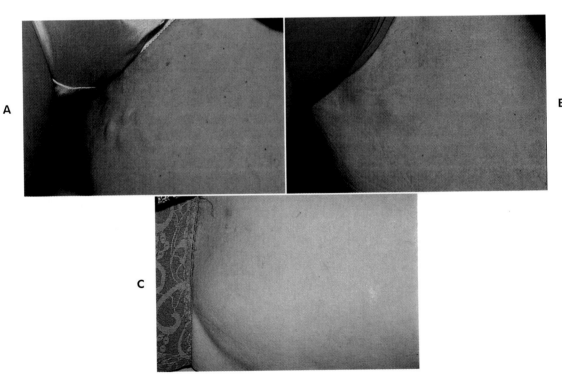

Fig. 9-19   A, Vulvar varices before treatment. B, Vulvar varices 2 months after treatment. C, Vulvar varices resolved 3 years after first treatment.

CASE STUDY 8: Large varicose vein from incompetent perforator veins

After her second pregnancy a 40-year-old woman developed varicose veins in the left lower leg, which increased in severity with her third pregnancy. Six years after her second pregnancy she developed pain in the left calf with associated leg swelling. The pain increased with exercising and resolved with leg elevation. She also complained of resting pain and a generalized tired feeling in the leg. There was a positive history of varicose veins in her mother. PPG was normal, with a venous refilling time of 43 seconds and good calf muscle pump function. Venous Doppler examination demonstrated two incompetent perforator veins at the left lateral knee and left medial posterior thigh without reflux from the SFJ. The vein measured 8 to 10 mm in diameter (Fig. 9-20, A).

She was treated with a Fegan-Sigg technique. A 25-gauge butterfly needle was placed just distal to each of the two perforator veins, and the leg was elevated 45 degrees. A total of 2 ml of STS 1% solution was injected, with the perforator points rapidly compressed with STD foam pads and 3M Microfoam tape. An additional 1.5 ml of STS 1% was injected into distal aspects of the varicose vein in three separate sites. A double layer of 30 to 40 mm Hg compression stockings was worn while she was ambulatory for 1 week, with the outer stocking removed when she was supine. A single 30 to 40 mm Hg stocking was worn for an additional 2 weeks only while she was ambulatory. Thrombus was drained 2 weeks later, and an additional 1 ml of STS 1% was given to a nonsclerosed segment of the vein. Six weeks after the first injection session the vein was entirely sclerosed, and additional coagula were drained (Fig. 9-12, B). She has remained symptom free without evidence of recurrence 2½ years after the first injection session (Fig. 9-20, C).

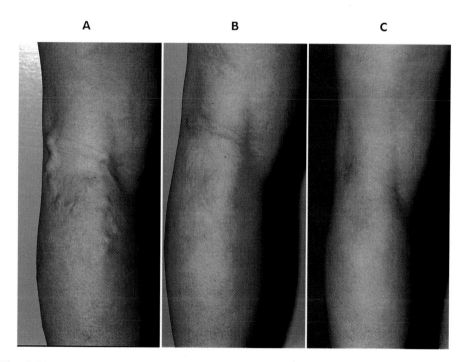

A   B   C

Fig. 9-20   A, Varicose veins before treatment. **B,** Varicose vein 6 weeks after treatment. **C,** Clinical appearance 2½ years after sclerotherapy treatment.

CASE STUDY 9: Extensive varicosities of GSV and GSV tributaries

A 56-year-old woman noted the development of varicose veins during her second pregnancy at age 30. They were entirely asymptomatic, and she was initially seen for cosmetic treatment. There was a family history of varicose veins in her father. Physical examination showed a dilated GSV 6 mm in diameter with vulvar varices 4 mm in diameter and an anterior saphenous varicosity 6 mm in diameter. All varicose veins were incompetent throughout their length as demonstrated by venous Doppler examination but without Valsalva-induced reflux and without reflux across the SFJ (Fig. 9-21, A and B).

With the patient supine, the entire varicose system was treated using a total of 11 ml of STS 1%. A double layer of 30 to 40 mm Hg graduated compression stockings was worn during the day, with the outer stocking removed at night for 1 week. A single 30 to 40 mm Hg stocking was worn during the day for the second week. Six weeks later reticular veins 2 to 3 mm in diameter were treated with a total of 4 ml of POL 0.75%, and telangiectasia was treated with a total of 10 ml POL 0.5%. One year later additional reticular veins were treated with 8 ml of POL 0.75%, and telangiectasia was treated with 4 ml of POL 0.5%. Fig. 9-21, C and D, shows the clinical appearance 2 years after initial treatment with resolution of all varicose, reticular, and telangiectatic leg veins.

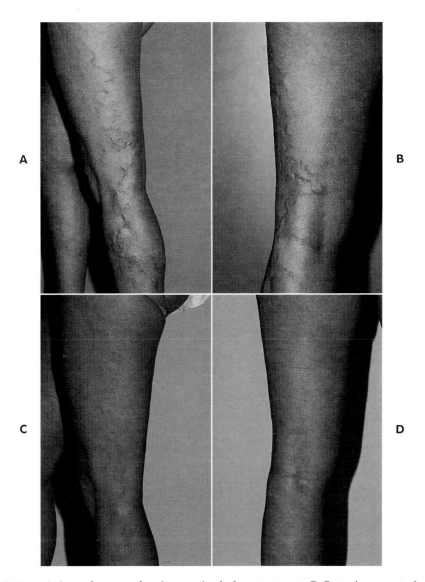

Fig. 9-21   A, Lateral aspect of varicose veins before treatment. **B**, Posterior aspect of varicose veins before treatment. **C**, Lateral aspect of varicose veins 2 years after initial treatment. **D**, Posterior aspect of varicose veins 2 years after initial treatment.

CASE STUDY 10: Development of SFJ incompetence after initial successful treatment of varicose GSV and tributaries

A 34-year-old woman was initially seen at age 27 years with the development of painful varicose veins during her first of four term pregnancies. The varicosities increased in size during each pregnancy, with the largest increase during her second pregnancy. The leg pain was throbbing, especially just before menses, with resolution 3 days into her menstrual period. Throbbing was relieved with leg elevation or by wearing graduated compression stockings. The family history included varicose veins in her mother, aunt, and sister. Physical examination showed a 6-mm diameter incompetent GSV with an incompetent Hunterian perforator vein without Valsalva-induced incompetence. The SFJ was competent (Fig. 9-22, A and B).

With the patient supine, the varicose veins were injected with 2 ml of STS 1% just distal to the Hunterian perforator vein, followed by a total of 16 ml of STS 0.5% to the remaining varicosities, with approximately 0.5 ml injected every 5 cm or so. A double layer of 30 to 40 mm Hg graduated compression stockings was worn for 1 week while the patient was ambulatory, with the outer stocking removed when she was supine, and a single stocking was worn for a second week when she was ambulatory. The patient became completely asymptomatic 1 month after the first sclerotherapy treatment (and remained so 3 years later). Nine months later an additional 16 ml of STS 0.5% was injected into multiple varicose and reticular veins that had not resolved or were newly present, followed by an identical posttreatment compression regimen. One year after the second sclerotherapy treatment there was complete resolution of all visible varicose and reticular leg veins (Fig. 9-22, C and D). Despite no new predisposing factors, new varicose veins were noted 3 years after the first sclerotherapy session. At this time the SFJ was incompetent bilaterally to venous Doppler examination, and the patient was referred for ligation and stripping of the GSV at the SFJ bilaterally (Fig. 9-22, E and F).

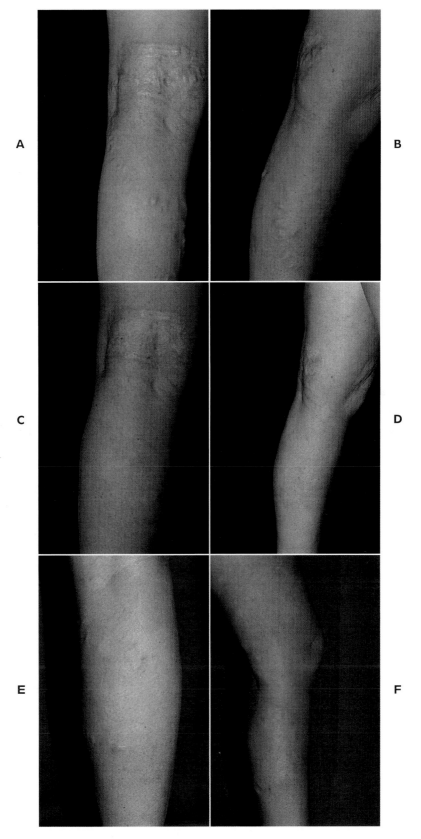

Fig. 9-22 A, Posterior aspect of varicose veins before treatment. B, Medial aspect of varicose veins before treatment. C, Posterior aspect of varicose veins 2 years after initial treatment. D, Medial aspect of varicose veins 2 years after initial treatment. E, F, Development of new varicose veins after initial treatment and resolution. The SFJ is now incompetent bilaterally.

CASE STUDY 11: Symptomatic clinically inapparent varicose vein treated with duplex-controlled sclerotherapy

A 60-year-old woman was initially seen with a complaint of pain in the medial knee and calf area for the last 6 months. She had previously undergone ligation and stripping of the GSV from the SFJ 30 years previously for treatment of varicose veins that occurred during her only pregnancy. Clinical examination did not disclose visible varicose or reticular veins. A color-flow duplex Doppler examination showed normal common femoral and superficial femoral and popliteal veins without evidence of acute or chronic deep vein thrombosis. The deep venous system was without evidence of reflux. An atypical vein was present 5 to 6 cm distal to the area of the SFJ as a remnant or duplicate GSV that coursed down the medial aspect of the thigh, terminating in the area of symptomatology. The vein was markedly incompetent to Valsalva maneuver and thigh and calf compression and communicated with numerous perforator veins along its course (Fig. 9-23, A and B).

Under duplex guidance, 1 ml of STS 3% was injected into the medial thigh varicosity through a 22-gauge needle. Correct position was verified by open-needle insertion. The injection was given slowly until the vein thrombosed (Fig. 9-23, C). An STD E-foam pad was placed with 3M Microfoam compression, and additional injections were given to two additional perforator veins present in the area of greatest symptomatology. The entire procedure was performed with the patient supine. A double layer of graduated 30 to 40 mm Hg compression stocking was worn while the patient was ambulatory for 2 weeks, with the outer stocking removed when the patient was supine. Four weeks later examination showed complete fibrosis and resolution of all symptoms.

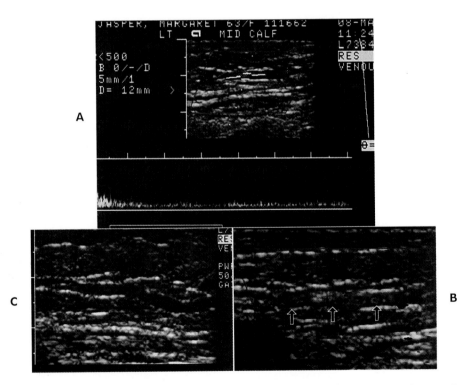

Fig. 9-23   A, Reflux is present in the symptomatic vein before treatment. B, Close-up duplex view of injection site before injection. C, Immediately after sclerotherapy the injected vein is filled with echo-dense material and is noncompressible.

REFERENCES

1. Faxon HH: End results in the injection treatment of varicose veins, N Engl J Med 208:357, 1934.
2. Goldman MP and Fronek A: Anatomy and pathophysiology of varicose veins, J Dermatol Surg Oncol 15:138, 1989.
3. Goldman MP and Bennett RG: Treatment of telangiectasia: a review, J Am Acad Dermatol 17:167, 1987.
4. de Groot WP: Treatment of varicose veins: modern concepts and methods, J Dermatol Surg Oncol 15:191, 1989.
5. Tournay R et al: La sclerose des varices, ed 4, Paris, 1985, Expansion Scientifique Francaise.
6. Heyerdale WW and Stalker LK: Management of varicose veins of the lower extremities, Ann Surg 114:1042, 1941.
7. Moszkowicz L: Behandlung der Krampfadern mit Zuckerinjektionen kombinurt mit Venenligatur, Zentralbl Chir 54:1732, 1927.
8. de Takats G and Quint H: The injection treatment of varicose veins, Surg Gynecol Obstet 50:545, 1930.
9. Sigg K: Neure Gesichtspunkte zur Technik der Varizenbehandlung, Ther Umsch, vol 6, 1949.
10. Dodd H and Cockett FB: The pathology and surgery of the veins of the lower limbs, London, 1956, ES Livingstone, Ltd.
11. Reid RG and Rothnie NG: Treatment of varicose veins by compression sclerotherapy, Br J Surg 55:889, 1968.
12. Fegan WC, Fitzgerald DE, and Milliken JC: The results of simultaneous pressure recordings from the superficial and deep veins of the leg, Ir J Med Sci 6:363, 1964.
13. Quill RD and Fegan WG: Reversibility of femorosaphenous reflux, Br J Surg 55:389, 1971.
14. Schalin L: Arteriovenous communication localized by thermography and identified by operative microscopy, Acta Chir Scand 147:109, 1981.
15. Kakkar VV, Howe CT, and Flanc C: Compression sclerotherapy for varicose veins—a phlebographic study, Br J Surg 56:620, 1969.
16. Zukowski AJ et al: Haemodynamic significance of incompetent calf perforating veins, Br J Surg 78:625, 1991.
17. Tolins SH: Treatment of varicose veins: an update, Am J Surg 145:248, 1983.
18. Doran FSA and White M: A clinical trial designed to discover if the primary treatment of varicose veins should be by Fegan's method or by operation, Br J Surg 62:72, 1975.
19. Hobbs JT: Surgery and sclerotherapy in the treatment of varicose veins: a random trial, Arch Surg 109:793, 1974.
20. Tretbar LL and Pattisson PH: Injection-compression treatment of varicose veins, Am J Surg 120:539, 1970.
21. Sladen JG: Compression sclerotherapy: preparation, technique, complications, and results, Am J Surg 146:228, 1983.
22. Hobbs JT: A random trial of the treatment of varicose veins by surgery and sclerotherapy. In Hobbs JT, editor: The treatment of venous thrombosis, Philadelphia, 1977, JB Lippincott Co.
23. Kerner J and Schultz-Ehrenburg U: Funktionele Auswirkungen unterschiedlicher Angriffspunkte bei der Sklerosierungstherapie, Phlebol Proktol 17:101, 1988.
24. Kerner J and Schultz-Ehrenburg U: Functional meaning of different injection levels in the course of sclerotherapy, Phlebology 4:123, 1989.
25. Goldman MP: Rational treatment of varicose and spider leg veins. In Robins P, editor: Surgical gems in dermatology, vol 2, New York, 1991, Igaku-Shoin Medical Publishers, Inc.
26. Hobbs JT: Surgery or sclerotherapy for varicose veins. In Superificial and deep venous diseases of the lower limbs, 1984, Minerva Medica.
27. Neglan P: Treatment of varicosities of saphenous origin: comparison of ligation, selective excision, and sclerotherapy. In Bergan JJ and Goldman MP, editors: Varicose veins and telangiectasias: diagnosis and treatment, St Louis 1993, Quality Medical Publishing, Inc.
28. Bishop CCR et al: Real-time color duplex scanning after sclerotherapy of the greater saphenous vein, J Vasc Surg 14:505, 1991.
29. Butie A: Experience with injections at the saphenofemoral junction in the United States. In Davy A and Stemmer R, editors: Phlebologie '89, Montrouge, France, 1989, John Libbey Eurotext, Ltd.
30. Biegeleisen K and Nielsen RD: Failure of angioscopically guided sclerotherapy to permanently obliterate greater saphenous varicosity, Phlebology 9:21, 1994.
31. Cooper WM: The treatment of varicose veins, Ann Surg 99:799, 1934.
32. Boyd AM and Robertson DJ: Treatment of varicose veins: possible danger of injection of sclerosing fluids, Br Med J 2:452, 1947.
33. Raymond-Martimbeau P: Two different techniques for sclerosing the incompetent saphenofemoral junction: a comparative study, J Dermatol Surg Oncol 16:626, 1990.

34. Bassi G: Indikationen und Resultate der Sklerotherapie bzw. Chirurgie in der Behandlung der Insuffizienzen, Zbl Phlebol 4:143, 1965.

35. Hordegen K and Sigg K: Krosseverodung der Vena saphena magna. Kasuistischer Beitrag zur Technik der Verodungsinjektion, Phlebol Proktol, 14:231, 1985.

36. Cloutier G and Zummo M: La sclerose des crosses avec compression: resultats a long terme, Phlebologie 39:145, 1986.

37. Leu HJ: Zur Therapie der Saphena-magna-Varikosis. Chirurgie oder Sklerosierung? Praxis 14:491, 1968.

38. Avramovic A and Avramovic M: Statistical evaluation of sclerotherapy of the long saphenous vein and the sapheno-femoral junction. In Raymond-Martimbeau P, Prescott R, and Zummo M, editors: Phlebologie '92, Paris, 1992, John Libbey Eurotext.

39. Schultz-Ehrenburg U, Weindorf N, and Tourbier H: Moderne, hamodynamisch orientierte Richtlinien fur die Sklerosierung der Stamm- und Seitenastvaricosis der V saphena magna und parva, Phlebol Proktol 17:83, 1988.

40. Raymond-Martimbeau P: Role of sclerotherapy in greater saphenous vein incompetence. In Bergan JJ and Goldman MP, editors: Varicose veins and telangiectasias: diagnosis and treatment, St. Louis, 1993, Quality Medical Publishing, Inc.

41. Bjordal RI: Circulation patterns in incompetent perforating veins in the calf and in the saphenous system in primary varicose veins, Acta Chir Scand 138:251, 1972.

42. Trempe J: Long-term results of sclerotherapy and surgical treatment of the varicose short saphenous vein, J Dermatol Surg Oncol 17:597, 1991.

43. McAdam WAF, Horrocks JC, and de Dombal FT: Assessment of the results of surgery for varicose veins, Br J Surg 63:137, 1976.

44. Sigg K: Varizen—ulcus cruris und thrombose, Berlin, 1976, Springer-Verlag.

45. McCaffrey JJ: An approach to the treatment of varicose veins, Med J Aust 1:1379, 1969.

46. Sigg K: The treatment of varicosities and accompanying complications, Angiology 3:355, 1952.

47. Kimmonth JB: Discussion on primary treatment of varicose veins, Proc R Soc London 41:631, 1948.

48. Steinacher J and Kammerhuber F: Weg und Verweildauer eines Kontrastmittels im oberflachlichen Venesystem unter Bedingungender Varicenverodung: Eine Studie zur Technik der Varicenverodung, Zschr Haut-Geschl-Krkh 43:369, 1968.

49. Heyn G, Waigand J, and Tamaschke C: Flow behaviour of sclerosants in the treatment of primary varicose veins. In Davy A and Stemmer R, editors: Phlebologie '89, Montrouge, France, 1989, John Libbey Eurotext, Ltd.

50. Meisen V: A lecture on injection-treatment of varicose veins and their sequelae (eczema and ulcus cruris), clinically and experimentally, Acta Chir Scand 60:435, 1926.

51. Foote RR: Varicose veins, St Louis, 1949, The CV Mosby Co.

52. Thornhill R: Varicose veins and their treatment by "empty vein" injection, London, 1929, Balliere, Tindall, & Cox.

53. Lufkin H and McPheeters HQ: Pathological studies on injected varicose veins, Surg Gynecol Obstet 54:511, 1932.

54. Orbach EJ: A new approach to the sclerotherapy of varicose veins, Angiology 1:302, 1950.

55. Fegan WG: Continuous compression technique of injecting varicose veins, Lancet 2:109, 1963.

56. Foley DP, Forrestal MD: A comparative evaluation of the empty vein utilizing duplex ultrasonography. In Raymond-Martimbeau P, Prescott R, and Zummo M editors: Phlebology '92, Paris, 1992, John Libbey Eurotext, Ltd.

57. Perchuk E: Injection therapy of varicose veins: a method of oblitering huge varicosities with small doses of sclerosing agent, Angiology 25:393, 1974.

58. Fegan WG: Personal communication, 1990.

59. Orbach EJ: Sclerotherapy of varicose veins: utilization of intravenous air block, Am J Surg 66:362, 1944.

60. Orbach EJ: Clinical evaluation of a new technique in the sclerotherapy of varicose veins, J Int Coll Surg 11:396, 1948.

61. Orbach EJ and Petretti AK: Thrombogenic property of foam synthetic anionic detergent (sodium tetradecyl sulfate, NNR), Angiology 1:237, 1950.

62. Orbach EJ: Has injection treatment of varicose veins become obsolete? JAMA 166:1964, 1958.

63. Knight RM: Treatment of superficial venous disease with accurate sclerotherapy. Proceedings of the Canadian Society of Phlebology, 1991, Whistler, British Columbia, Canada.

64. Raymond-Martimbeau P: Advanced sclerotherapy treatment of varicose veins with duplex ultrasonographic guidance, Semin Dermatol 12:123, 1993.

65. Knight RM, Vin F, and Zygmunt JA: Ultrasonic guidance of injections into the superficial system. In Davy A and Stemmer R, editors: Phlebologie '89. Montrouge, France, 1989, John Libbey Eurotext, Ltd.

66. Misery G, Reinharez D, and Ecalard P: Sclerose sous echographie dans certaines zones a risques, Phlebologie 44:84, 1991.

67. Cornu-Thenard A and Boivin P: Treatment of varicose veins by sclerotherapy: an overview. In Bergan JJ and Goldman MP, editors: Varicose veins and telangiectasias: diagnosis and treatment, St Louis, 1993, Quality Medical Publishing, Inc.

68. Thibault PK and Lewis WA: Recurrent varicose veins: Part 2: Injection of incompetent perforating veins using ultrasound guidance, J Dermatol Surg Oncol 18:895, 1992.

69. Grondin L and Soriano J: Echosclerotherapy, a Canadian study. In Raymond-Martimbeau P, Prescott R, and Zummo M, editors: Paris, 1992, John Libbey Eurotext, Ltd.

70. Oishi AJ, Zietlow SP, and Sarr MG: Erroneous arterial placement of a central venous catheter, Mayo Clin Proc 69:287, 1994.

71. Grondin L and Raymond-Martimbeau P: Superficial venous disease disorders. In Leclerc JR, editor: Venous thrombo-embolic disorders, Philadelphia, 1991, Lea & Febiger.

72. Thibault PK and Lewis WA: Recurrent varicose veins. Part 1: Evaluation utilizing duplex venous imaging, J Dermatol Surg Oncol 18:618, 1992.

73. Royle JP: Recurrent varicose veins, World J Surg 10:944, 1986.

74. Doran FSA and Barkat S: The management of recurrent varicose veins, Ann R Coll Surg Engl 63:432, 1981.

75. Cornu-Thenard A: Sclerotherapy: doppler guided injection. Presented at the Annual Meeting of the North American Society of Phlebology, Maui, Hawaii, February 23, 1994.

76. Van Cleef JF et al: Sclerose de la saphene externe sous controle endoscopique, Phlebologie 44:131, 1991.

77. Van Cleef JF: Sclerotherapy of the external saphenous vein under endoscopic control. Presented at the World Congress of Phlebology, Strasbourg, France, 1989.

78. Cavaye DM et al: Intravascular ultrasound imaging: the new standard for guidance and assessment of endovascular interventions? J Clin Laser Med Surg 10:349, 1992.

79. Gussenhoven WJ, Essed CE, and Lancee CT: Arterial wall characteristics determined by intravascular ultrasound imaging: an in vitro study, J Am Coll Cardiol 14:947, 1989.

80. Mallery JAS et al: Assessment of normal and atherosclerotic arterial wall thickness within intravascular ultrasound imaging catheter, Am Heart J 119:1392, 1990.

81. Nissen SE et al: Application of a new phased-array ultrasound imaging catheter in the assessment of vascular dimensions, Circulation 81:660, 1990.

82. Raymond-Martimbeau P: Role of sclerotherapy in greater saphenous vein incompetance. In Bergan JJ and Goldman MP, editors: Varicose veins and telangiectasias: diagnosis and treatment, St Louis, 1993, Quality Medical Publishing, Inc.

83. Keates JS and Fitzgerald DE: Limb volume and blood flow changes during the menstrual cycle, Angiology 20:618, 1969.

84. Vin F: Principles, technique, and results of treatment of the greater saphenous vein by sclerotherapy. Paper presented at the second annual International Congress of the North American Society of Phlebology, New Orleans, February 25, 1989.

85. Merlen JF et al: Histologic study of a sclerosed vein, Phlebologie 31:17, 1978.

86. Sackmann LA: Etude physique de l'injection sclerosante, Soc Fr Phlebol 22:149, 1969.

87. Green D: Mechanism of action of sclerotherapy, Semin Dermatol 12:88, 1993.

88. Guex J-J: Indications for the sclerosing agent polidocanol, J Dermatol Surg Oncol 19:959, 1993.

89. Cornu-Thenard A: Sclerotherapy of varicose veins: value of measurement of vessel diameter before the first injection. Paper presented at the second annual International Congress of the North American Society of Phlebology, New Orleans, February 25, 1989.

90. Kinmonth JB and Robertson DJ: Injection treatment of varicose veins: radiological and histological investigations of methods, Br J Surg 36:294, 1949.

91. Corcos L et al: Peripheral venous biopsy: significance, limitations, indications and clinical applications, Phlebology 4:271, 1989.

92. Stegall HF: Muscle pumping in the dependent leg, Circ Res 19:180, 1966.

93. Orbach EJ: The importance of removal of postinjection coagula during the course of sclerotherapy of varicose veins, Vasa 3:475, 1974.

94. Barwin BN and Roddie IC: Venous distensibility during pregnancy determined by graded venous congestion, Am J Obstet Gynecol 125:921, 1976.

95. Skudder PA Jr et al: Venous dysfunction of late pregnancy persists after delivery, J Cardiovasc Surg 31:748, 1990.

96. McPheeters HO: Prophylactic injection treatment of varicose veins during pregnancy, Lancet 51:589, 1931.

97. Kilbourne NJ: Varicose veins of pregnancy, Am J Obstet Gynecol 25:104, 1933.

98. Mullane DJ: Varicose veins of pregnancy, Am J Obstet Gynecol 63:620, 1952.

99. McCausland AM: Varicose veins in pregnancy, West J Surg 47:81, 1939.
100. Fegan G: Varicose veins: compression therapy, London, 1967, Heinemann Medical.
101. Mantse L: The treatment of varicose veins with compression sclerotherapy: technique, containdications, complications, Am J Cosmetic Surg 3:47, 1986.
102. Dodd H and Payling Wright H: Vulval varicose veins in pregnancy, Br Med J 1:831, 1959.
103. Tibbs DJ: Varicose veins and related disorders, Oxford, 1992, Butterworth-Heinemann, Ltd.
104. Rabe E et al: Die pudendale Varicosis, Phlebologie 20:222, 1991.
105. de Takats G: Ambulatory ligation of the saphenous vein, JAMA 94:1194, 1930.
106. Faxon HH: Treatment of varicosities, Arch Surg 29:794, 1934.
107. Conrad P: Sclerostripping—a "new" procedure for the treatment of varicose veins, Med J Aust 2:42, 1975.
108. Hubner K: The out-patient therapy of trunk varicosis of the greater saphenous vein by means of ligation and sclerotherapy, J Dermatol Surg Oncol 17:818, 1991.
109. de Groot WP: Practical phlebology: sclerotherapy of large veins, J Dermatol Surg Oncol 17:589, 1991.
110. Bihari I: Can varicetomy be performed if deep veins are occluded? J Dermatol Surg Oncol 16:806, 1990.
111. Passas H: One case of tetradecyl-sodium sulfate allergy with general symptoms, Soc Fr Phlebol 25:19, 1972.
112. Stroncek DF et al: Sodium morrhuate stimulates granulocytes and damages erythrocytes and endothelial cells: probable mechanism of an adverse reaction during sclerotherapy, J Lab Clin Med 106:498, 1985.

THE ROLE OF SURGERY IN TREATMENT OF VARICOSE VEINS AND VENOUS TELANGIECTASIAS

John J. Bergan

Jean Van der Stricht called attention to the fact that some observations made in the late nineteenth century are applicable to treatment of varicose veins in the late twentieth century. Specifically, he has cited Quenu who said in 1890, ". . . the continuation of the disorder is inevitable. . . . The only real cure is the treatment which would restore the normal structure to the vascular walls."

Before 1900, at the time of Quenu, the various therapeutic possibilities included elastic compression, sclerotherapy, and surgery. They remain mainstays of treatment today.

Another observation from the 1890s discussed sclerotherapy particularly and said that "any method whose main characteristic is that it provokes phlebitis is bad." Surgical therapy then was treated no more kindly by opinions, that said "most varicose vein patients do not need surgery." Finally, the overall conclusion of workers in the field that treated venous stasis 100 years ago was that "the surgical solution is perhaps only palliative."

With the above observations in mind, it is possible in this chapter to touch on the current contribution of surgery to the care of patients with varicose veins and cutaneous telangiectasias.

HISTORICAL LESSONS

For many years after 1950 the monumental contribution by Harold Dodd and Frank Cockett, *Pathology and Surgery of the Veins of the Lower Limbs,* was the bible and textbook for varicose vein surgery. The foreword was written by R.R. Linton, and thus the three most famous names in vein surgery were linked inseparably.[1] That text was greatly concerned with the techniques of operative surgery. Detailed results of operations developed in the first half of this century are found there and are still relevant to present-day surgery.

Types of Operations Performed

The operations detailed in Dodd and Cockett's text include proximal ligation and division of the saphenous vein at the groin, ligation of the saphenous vein in the groin combined with retrograde injection of sclerosing solution, ligation of the saphenous vein above the knee either with or without distal sclerosing injections, and operative injection of sclerosing solutions into various segments of the greater saphenous vein (GSV) alone. Interestingly, among the sclerosing solutions used was hypertonic saline (30%), recently rediscovered in its 23.4% incarnation. Finally, it can be emphasized that after 1950, stripping of the GSV was by far ". . . the most satisfactory after three to eight years' follow-up." The operation, as depicted in photographs and drawings, was the standard surgical procedure from that time until approximately 1980.

Greater and Lesser Saphenous Vein Stripping

Lessons learned from the standard greater and lesser saphenous stripping operation are as follows. First, the long incisions at groin, ankle, and over large varicosities in the thighs and legs were anticosmetic. Even as late as 1983 at least one author advocated a "6- to 8-cm incision placed 3 to 4 cm below and lateral to the pubic tubercle." This was too much incision placed too low. Its saving grace was that its length allowed wide exploration, but the resulting scar was simply too obvious. Next, passing the stripper internally was frequently quite easy; consequently, the surgeon was able to remove long lengths of vein from the body. Unfortunately, these veins were often found to have competent valves, absence of dilation, and absence of elongation and tortuosity—in short, they were normal saphenous veins.

Recurrent Varicosities

It became apparent to many physicians that a large body of literature on the subject of recurrent varicose veins was accumulating. The only logical conclusion to draw from such an expanse of literature was that the vein stripping operation, which often removed a normal vein, failed to cure the patient of the condition for which it was designed. It is that operation, now greatly modified and to some extent abandoned, that is the subject of criticism by nonsurgeons today.

MODERN SURGERY
Stripping and Stab Avulsion Varicectomy

As a reaction to those lessons, many surgeons modified techniques of varicose vein removal. The newer objectives were to preserve normal axial veins while achieving effective ablation of malfunctioning veins, the varicosities. Some pressures came from cardiac and arterial surgeons who decried stripping because it removed a vein that might be used as an arterial substitute.

After surgical evaluation, which includes the use of the handheld, continuous-wave Doppler instrument, the modern operation begins with additional assessment of the limb as needed using the noninvasive techniques described in Chapter 5. The objective of this assessment is to identify or verify saphenofemoral and saphenopopliteal junctional reflux and to ascertain the status of the deep venous system. When this is done, a conservative operation can be planned, specifically designed to remove the offending varicosities and other sources of venous hypertension while preserving normal functioning veins.

Ultimately the present-day operation has resolved into three stages: (1) preoperative evaluation as mentioned, which includes the history taking and requisite supplemental testing of the functioning of the deep and superficial veins; (2) accurate marking of the varicosities to allow removal of virtually all abnormal veins as results of the operation are correlated directly with the totality of ablation of varicosities[2]; and (3) the operation itself. This is done in as cosmetic a fashion as possible, usually with the patient's legs elevated to reduce blood loss and frequently under tourniquet control.[3] Incisions are limited in length and are made with a fine-bladed, narrow scalpel. Varicosities are avulsed, and skin closure is accomplished. Tape strips reinforce the closure.[4-6]

High-Tie and Distal Sclerotherapy

There has been a tendency in recent years to avoid stripping the greater saphenous vein (GSV). Some surgeons still advocate proximal division without stripping. Some add compression sclerotherapy to this maneuver. This technique of groin tie and compression sclerotherapy leads to very satisfactory results when assessed early, but this salutary outcome deteriorates so that at 5 years only 40% of such operations have a satisfactory result.[7]

A mid-1990's review of this subject is important because it demonstrates economic pressures cause simple proximal ligation and distal sclerotherapy to look attractive to controlled care. In a prospective, partially randomized study with a 5-year follow-up, 78 lower limbs received compression sclerotherapy, 74 received saphenous stripping and stab avulsion of varices, and 63 received proximal saphenous ligation and compression sclerotherapy. Although the patients' perception of the simpler procedures remained good throughout the study period, objective evaluation with laboratory techniques revealed the sclerotherapy group showed deterioration by as early as 6 months so that by 5 years, less than 5% remained cured and more than 50% had failed. In the group with high tie and sclerotherapy, 12% were cured at 5 years, 68% were improved, and 20% had failed. Five-year objective results were best in the radical surgery group, with 60% cured, 35% improved, and only 5% failed. The author's summary statement was, "Radical surgery is superior to compression sclerotherapy alone or in combination with high tie in the treatment of varicose veins with saphenous incompetence."[8]

Of equal importance is the report from the Middlesex Hospital group (England). They performed a prospective, randomized study in which proximal saphenous ligation was compared to saphenous vein stripping to below the knee.[9] Both groups of limbs also had stab avulsion removal of varicose clusters. Persistent saphenous vein reflux at calf level was found in 45% of the ligation group and in only 18% of the saphenous vein stripping group. Neither of the study groups experienced increased rates of hematoma, wound infection, or paresthesias. The authors concluded that stripping of the saphenous vein to the upper calf combined with multiple avulsions of varices resulted in fewer veins with residual reflux and a better functional outcome.

Telangiectasias and Their Treatment

Intradermal, dilated venules and arterioles (termed *telangiectasias*), alone and in combination, are of great concern to many patients. Being common, they are known by many names, including "spider veins," "spider web veins," "rocket bursts," "starbursts," "venous stars," and "arborizing telangiectases." They are described elsewhere in this volume. Many are asymptomatic, but at least an equal number produce local aching, heaviness, and fatigue. These symptoms more likely are caused by deeper veins that, being unsupported, have dilated under the pressures of hormonal cycling, pregnancy, aging, and upright posture. They, in turn, transmit their hypertension to their feeding dermal venules. These venules dilate to the point of disrupting the capillary barrier, thus allowing exertion of arteriolar pressure on primary dermal venules. When symptomatic, this vascular arborization can be treated by sclerotherapy, and such therapy may be effective for the dermal tip of the "iceberg" and the iceberg itself, the subcutaneous, blue, incompetent perforator vein. The "glacier," to continue the metaphor, is incurable. Surgery cannot treat the intradermal dilated vessels but may in some instances remove the subcutaneous 2- to 4-mm veins that are in direct continuity with the dermal reticular blemishes.

PREOPERATIVE PREPARATION

Preoperative evaluations are as important as surgical technique; they consist of photoplethysmography (PPG), varicography, Doppler examination, and skin marking.

Photoplethysmography and Light Reflection Rheography

PPG and light reflection rheography (LRG) use the fact that the subdermal tangle of blood vessels is largely a venous pool. Infrared light beamed through the epidermis into this pool can be reflected back and give a semiquantitative evaluation of the emptying of that pool and its refilling. Refill time, as assessed by PPG and

LRG, has correlated with venous pressure refill time. When performing the examination with the patient in a comfortable sitting position (legs dependent), in a warm room, and with tourniquets placed at below-knee and above-knee positions, differentiation between deep venous reflux and superficial venous reflux can be ascertained. This is the entire purpose of this examination. If only superficial incompetence is present, the patient can be cured. The effect of tourniquets on reflux gives an estimate of beneficial effects of superficial venous stripping.[10] Accuracy of tourniquet testing has been challenged and is generally believed imprecise.

Duplex Testing

Axial venous insufficiency is diagnosed by clinical examination aided by the Doppler study. However, the examination has its shortcomings. The continuous-wave Doppler device cannot clearly isolate reflux in the individual veins, one from another. It detects the velocity of blood flow from any vein lying in the path of the ultrasound beam. Thus at groin level the reflux might be in the saphenous vein, the femoral vein, or a major tributary to the saphenous vein. Because venous anomalies are common, the handheld Doppler device cannot identify these anomalies or detect duplicated greater or lesser saphenous systems. Neither can the termination of the lesser saphenous vein be identified clearly.

It is duplex ultrasound scanning that gives precision to the clinical evaluation and allows more accurate planning of ablative therapy.[11] An attempt to standardize venous reflux testing was made by two groups almost simultaneously in 1989.[12,13] This method of testing has not yet received uniform standardization. However, there is no doubt that duplex venous imaging greatly aids in evaluating patients before treatment. It uncovers unsuspected deep venous insufficiency when only superficial venous incompetence is suspected and has even revealed correction of deep venous reflux after superficial vein stripping.[14] It is clear that duplex scanning has its greatest value in studying patients with recurrent varicose veins.

Duplex imaging has emphasized several facts that previous studies could not show. Chief among them is a demonstration of regional venous reflux. Of greatest clinical importance in this regard is the reflux in the greater saphenous system limited to the upper anteromedial calf in which both the anterior and posterior tributaries may become varicose without proximal greater saphenous incompetence. Also, limited saphenous reflux may be revealed by duplex scanning when the source of this reflux is a midthigh or Hunterian perforator vein. In addition, incompetence of the GSV is now found to be more often segmental than total. This leads to removal of only the proximal refluxing portion of this vein.

Saphenous Vein Angioscopy

As vascular surgical technology progressed, angioscopes became a common feature of the vascular operating room. Use of the angioscope in saphenous vein surgery has been limited but informative.[15] In patients selected for saphenous vein surgery by duplex scanning, incompetence of the terminal or subterminal valve was expected and has been confirmed by the angioscope. Because anatomic studies have shown a number of valves are present in the saphenous vein, it was surprising to find with the angioscope that long segments of valveless greater saphenous veins (GSVs) were regularly encountered. This clinical finding at saphenous surgery confirmed the observation of Cotton[16] who also reported long segments of avalvular GSV in patients with varices. This finding achieves greater importance as experimental surgery attempts to preserve the saphenous vein by creating competence of the proximal saphenous valve.

Varicography

Varicography is planned and used only when the surgical situation is complex. Several indications for this procedure are (1) after previous major vein stripping, (2) in the presence of massive, recurrent varicose veins, (3) in identifying tributaries to the lesser saphenous system, and (4) in identifying popliteal fossa and gastrocnemius veins described below. Furthermore, identification of the termination of the lesser saphenous vein (LSV) at the popliteal vein is well accomplished with on-table varicography if preoperative duplex imaging has failed to reveal this junction.

Doppler Examination

Surgery is also preceded by Doppler examination. The patient is examined standing, supported by an adjacent chair or table. The Doppler probe is placed on the GSV in the thigh, at the femoral vein, the LSV, and the popliteal vein sequentially. The patient is asked to breathe deeply, cough, and perform the Valsalva maneuver as each site is examined. Reflux during inspiration, coughing, or Valsalva maneuver is a reliable index of reflux. If GSV reflux is present, this vein must be removed to achieve long-lasting surgical benefit.

Marking Varicosities

Preoperative marking is done with a felt-tipped, indelible marking pen; the relative size of the varix is indicated by the breadth of the line, and individual palpable fascial defects are marked by circles (Fig. 10-1). Accurate marking is an absolute requisite to successful varicosity removal. Subsequently, during the surgical procedure such markings may dictate the placement of surgical incisions.

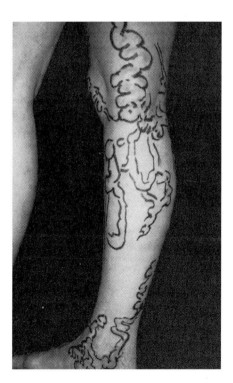

Fig. 10-1 Preoperative marking of the varicosities as completely as possible ensures operative incisions are placed exactly where desired and all offending varicosities are removed. In this instance a limited GSV stripping to the below-knee position was planned with stab avulsion of varicose clusters. The LSV was found to be competent and was left intact.

SURGICAL TECHNIQUE
Greater Saphenous Vein Stripping

At surgery the GSV and LSV are ignored if Doppler studies show their terminations are competent. This point deserves emphasis because surgical literature contains many descriptions of removal of the saphenous veins and very few details of preservation of these structures.

Surgeons have no difficulty identifying the GSV termination when viewed through a short, oblique groin incision made at the groin crease in patients who do need removal of this vein. The incision is begun at the medial edge of the femoral pulse and is carried medially as far as is necessary (2 to 3 cm). Distal stripping extends only to the distal thigh or upper anteromedial calf as indicated previously (Fig. 10-2). Removal of the saphenous vein below the upper calf level is usually unnecessary and is occasionally associated with damage to the saphenous nerve. Removal of the GSV for gross incompetence automatically removes the midthigh perforator veins (Hunterian perforators), which are a source for recurrent venous insufficiency. A short incision in the upper anteromedial calf allows removal of the stripping instrument from the lumen of the vein at this point. The vein is fixed to the stripper at the upper end, and the stripper and the inverted vein are removed distally. Inversion stripping is illustrated in Fig. 10-3.

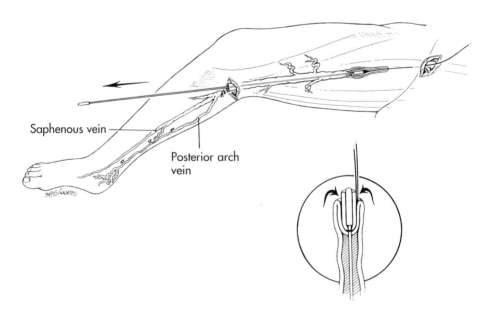

Saphenous vein

Posterior arch
vein

Fig. 10-2   Surgical removal of the GSV through a proximal groin and distal upper calf incision is illustrated in these diagrams. In practice, the proximal incision is 3 cm in length, and the distal incision is 4 mm. The inset drawing details the method of inversion and shows the ligature which may be used to place a hemostatic pack. (Note the anatomical arrangement of distal perforationg veins and the posterior arch vein.)

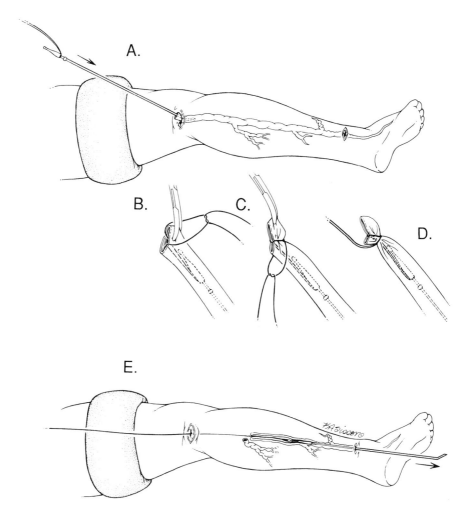

Fig. 10-3 Prior to performance of the SSV stripping shown here, demonstration of saphenopopliteal incompetence is requisite. Precise location of the termination of the SSV by duplex scan or operative varicography is also mandatory.

The Oesch stripper illustrated here has considerably eased SSV stripping. It is introduced through the proximal incision and may exit through a short 2 mm incision anywhere distal to mid-calf. The vein is fixed to the stripper as illustrated in **B** and **C**, and firmly tied in place as emphasized in **D**. Inversion stripping from above downward is shown in **E**, and the use of an inflatable tourniquet is shown in **A** and **E**. Such a tourniquet may be used in the procedure illustrated in Fig. 10-2.

Lesser Saphenous Vein Stripping

Stripping of the LSV is required in a minority of cases and should always be preceded by identification of the termination of the LSV by duplex color-flow imaging or by intraoperative varicography.

Care must be taken in dissection of the LSV in the popliteal fossa, and the vein should never be ligated until the surgeon has seen the popliteal junction clearly. This dissection may be difficult and complicated by large tributaries. Some of them join the LSV from above, and some may come from varicosities within the nerve. It is essential that the popliteal vein and peroneal nerve be carefully preserved during this part of the dissection.

Stab Avulsion (Ambulatory Phlebectomy)

When greater and lesser saphenous stripping was abandoned as the cornerstone of the operation for varicosities, it was replaced by the stab avulsion technique of varicosity removal. Because of the meticulous marking that precedes the surgical procedure today, each of the varicose veins, singly or in clusters, can be removed through minimal incisions. Associated incompetent perforator veins are not necessarily ligated. The incisions are made with a sharp-pointed blade directly over the vein, and the varicosity is lifted through the wound with a fine instrument (Fig. 10-4, *A*). After surrounding fat is cleared away, the loop of vein that appears through the wound is doubly clamped and divided (Fig. 10-4, *B*). Each end is teased out through the incision as the areolar tissue on the surface is dissected off (Fig. 10-4, *C*). The forceps are always placed close to the skin to prevent the vein from breaking. Traction on the skin itself allows breaking of tributaries and removal of greater lengths of the varicosity. Observation has shown that varicosities may be divided clinically into two types—those that are white on their surface

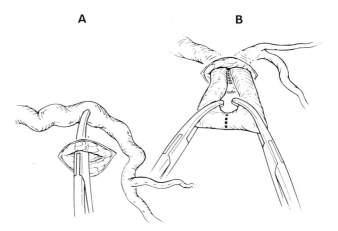

A   **B**

Fig. 10-4 **A,** Grasping of previously marked varicosities. The incision is a 2- to 3-mm stab made with a no. 11 blade. After the varicosity is exteriorized, **B,** it is divided and each end is carefully avulsed to remove as much varix as possible.

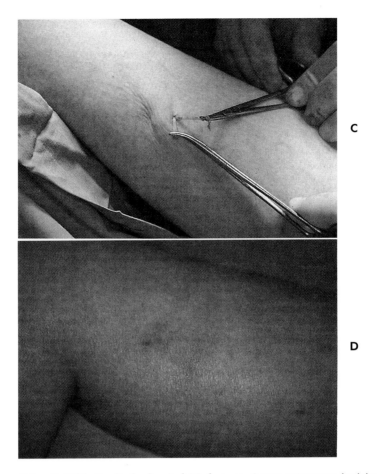

Fig. 10-4, cont'd   C, With the limb elevated 30 degrees, 2-mm cutaneous incisions can be made, the varicosity can be brought to the surface by the hook technique, and after division of the vein each end can be avulsed selectively. Placement of subsequent incisions will depend on the length of varicosity excised. **D,** This photograph, taken 10 days after surgery, shows the location of a distal medial calf incision through which the GSV has been stripped from the groin to this level.

avulse well and those that are blue often tear easily. Distal or proximal incisions are made within the markings to ensure that total removal of offending varicosities is accomplished. Varicosities removed by this technique are inevitably tributaries to axial veins and do not require ligation except if they terminate into the axial vein itself and that vein is to be left in place. Perforator veins identified with clusters of varices may be ligated. Incisions made for local varicosity removal are made small enough that sutures are unnecessary and tape closure can be used. If an individual incision is made longer than the average, it can be closed by an inverted, absorbable suture and covered over with the usual tape closure. Fig. 10-4, *D,* shows the appearance 10 days after surgery.

Recurrent Varicosities

Surgery has a definite place in the treatment regimen for removal of recurrent varicose veins. These veins may be residual varicosities left as a result of incomplete sclerotherapy, new veins not treated at sclerotherapy or a previous operation, or residual veins overlooked at prior surgery. It would be most correct to refer to varicose veins present after therapy as being either residual veins missed at the time of original therapy or recurrent veins that were formerly normal and then became varicose because of an underlying genetic or physiologic abnormality that was not corrected.

Varicography or duplex scanning may be very important for accurate removal of residual or recurrent varicosities. Complications introduced by prior surgery can be diagnosed by using such direct imaging of offending incompetent veins. At the groin level a number of causes of recurrence have been identified. They include failure to complete flush ligation of the saphenous vein, failure to remove terminal tributaries to the saphenous vein, failure to identify duplicated saphenous veins or their tributaries, and failure to remove the termination of the saphenous vein, thus allowing midthigh perforator veins to develop recurrent saphenous incompetence. In Darke's careful study of varicose recurrence after surgery,[17] a retained and incompetent saphenous vein was the single most important culprit.[17] At the popliteal level recurrent varicosities frequently develop in scar tissue through transgastrocnemius perforator veins not ligated at the initial operation and also through secondary muscular perforator veins. Isolated, recurrent, superficial varicosities are also a major reason for failures of primary therapy. They are best managed by careful marking and simple avulsion as indicated above or through sclerotherapy as described elsewhere in this volume.

It should be emphasized that not all recurrent veins are caused by inadequate primary operations or sclerotherapy. Clearly, new abnormal veins can develop after primary therapy; they can even develop in the absence of deep venous abnormalities. The stab avulsion surgical technique lends itself well to treatment of such veins.

Perforator Veins

Surgery on the perforator veins is not simple surgery. Planning surgery on major perforator veins in cases of severe chronic venous insufficiency should not be undertaken lightly. Underlying difficulties in judgment is the startling fact that from 15% to 50% of such operations are failures. Even when failure is judged by the harshest criteria, recurrence of venous ulcer, this fact is true.

Principles that act as a guide in deciding whether to perform perforator interruption include the following: (1) classic anatomic studies by surgeons in the first half of the twentieth century are informative but inaccurate,[18] for the perforator veins tributary to the posterior arch vein, so carefully mapped out in such studies, are extremely variable in importance and location; (2) surgery performed to interrupt such perforator veins and remove associated varicosities is plagued by wound healing failure and secondary infection; (3) classic subfascial perforator interruptions produce a formidable operative procedure frequently followed by immediate wound complications and later ulcer recurrence; and (4) the subcutaneous or Cockett approach causes skin slough if undermining is performed.

Recognizing both the hazards of the Linton procedure and the successes of it in preventing recurrent venous ulceration in 75% to 85% of cases led surgeons to explore other methods of accomplishing the objectives of the procedure. In Germany and Switzerland minimally invasive perforator interruption was developed using endoscopic techniques.[19,20] Various manufacturers responded by creating specialized instruments, which are now generally available.

The new operation consists of making a small incision posterior to the tibia in the proximal third of the leg. A space is created between the deep fascia and the flexor muscles, and the two proximal perforator veins approximately 24 cm from the heel pass through this base. Normal perforator veins can be distinguished from incompetent perforators. The normal perforator is narrow and straight and consists of two parallel, fine veins with an accompanying artery. The incompetent perforator is thick, often passes transversely, can appear white in the bloodless-limb technique, or may look like an ordinary varicose vein. Parallel electrocoagulating forceps are applied and activated. The specialized scissor divides the vein, and the two stumps can be seen in the avascular plane.

The importance of this technique is that the proximal incision is distant from the potentially or actually damaged distal liposclerotic, heavily pigmented skin. The liabilities of the endoscopic perforator interruption technique include potential damage in the retromalleolar area to the tibial nerves. This space is narrow but important. Further, paratibial perforator veins must be searched for carefully, and in some cases the deep posterior fascial compartment must be opened to expose them. Subfascial hematomas may develop and cause pain and an Achilles tendon contracture until the hematoma is resolved. Despite these hazards, subfascial endoscopic perforator interruption is especially valuable in the presence of distal ulceration or severe trophic changes. The offending perforator vein can be diagnosed and treated at the same setting.

ALTERNATIVE OPERATIONS
Babcock Internal Stripping

When Babcock of Philadelphia described his new operation for removal of varicose veins in 1907, he said, "The cause of varicose veins is pressure acting upon imperfect or damaged venous walls." How prescient that statement has been demonstrated over the years. New information has only confirmed Babcock's observations.[21]

Babcock described the previous methods of varicose vein extraction, including that of Schede, in which an incision was made circumcising the leg down to the muscular aponeurosis at the junction of the middle and upper thirds of the thigh. Predictably, the superficial venous circulation was reestablished after that operation by collateral venous anastomoses, and the scar produced disconcerting areas of anesthesia, paresthesia, and sometimes even ischemia of the foot. Subsequently the same operation was accomplished by making interrupted incisions, leaving bridges of undivided skin, and eventually by extracting long axial venous trunks by raising large flaps of skin.

Mayo External Stripping

Later Charles Mayo described the external vein stripper; the instrument, shaped like a dull ring, was pushed down over the vein, tearing it free from adjacent tissues and venous branches.

Although Mayo's external stripper is still in use, Babcock described its shortcomings by saying, "In our own experience, the method is valuable. But fragile, very tortuous or adherent vessels often embarrass the operator."

Keller Inversion Stripping

Babcock went on to describe Keller's method. Stripping the saphenous vein was described before 1910 by Keller[21] and then cited by Rivlin[22] in 1975 and by Van der Stricht[23] in 1982. Nevertheless, the procedure is still unfamiliar to most surgeons in North America. Keller's method consisted of passing a stout thread through the vein by means of a probe or twisted wire, tying it firmly to one of the divided ends, and then pulling the other end of the thread, causing the vein to be turned inside out and then removed through the upper or lower incision. Saphenous stripping by invagination is ingenious and has great theoretic appeal.

However, Babcock said this method was disadvantaged because, "Unfortunately, the vein often tears in two before the inversion has proceeded very far." The article concluded with a long description of the intraluminal vein stripper similar to that in use today.

The article, in the style of the early 1900s, described 11 cases in which this method had been used, gave the author's address, and no supporting references. Despite this, it was a truly landmark article and set the stage for surgical treatment of varicose veins for the next 50 years.

Myers' Internal Stripper

By 1954 varicose vein surgery had been consolidated into intraluminal stripping supplemented by extraluminal stripping and injection of residual venous radicals.[24] At that time T.T. Myers, writing from the "Section of Peripheral Vein Surgery" of the Mayo Clinic, described his experience with an instrument modestly named the Myers' vein stripper. His device took advantage of technology developed during World War II: flexible steel aircraft cables were developed that were extremely strong and of small external diameter. The procedure performed was essentially the one Babcock described 40 years earlier. As was typical of descriptions of procedures in the 1950s, no objective data about results were provided, and application of statistical methods was unheard of.

Proximal Ligation and Distal Injection

Even as late as 1970, the surgical fashion was to describe operations without giving accurate, observational, objective data and without applying critical statistical methods, and it is for these reasons that varicose vein surgery remained crude and anticosmetic. For example, in Nabatoff's presentation,[25] operations on 3000 patients were described in which "all incompetent saphenous veins had been stripped out and all other incompetent perforating veins ligated flush with the deep veins." These are objectives impossible to accomplish when one considers there are more than 120 identified perforator veins. The thesis of his presentation was that this procedure could be done on a semiambulatory basis. Our present-day focus is not on the advantages of no hospitalization because that is taken for granted. Instead, emphasis is placed on minimizing morbidity and providing the patient with a cosmetic surgical result.

Attempts to apply the principles espoused by Babcock, Myers, Nabatoff, and others and to perform the operation in a cosmetic fashion were being undertaken simultaneously in the 1970s. Stanley Rivlin's presentation[22] in 1975 describes in detail just how this could be accomplished. To achieve better cosmetic results, emphasis was placed on the belief that ". . . a prime requisite of successful varicose vein surgery is a detailed clinical examination." From such examinations would come the knowledge that lesser saphenous system varicosities caused by lesser saphenous valvular incompetence were present in as many as 14% of patients operated on.

Furthermore, by the time of Rivlin's 1975 report, it was recognized that the standard operations then in vogue, which consisted of GSV vein stripping from groin to ankle, produced dramatic short-term effects but contributed very little to long-term success. Rivlin pointed out correctly that removal of the GSV was only necessary from groin to within 1 cm of the tibial tuberosity at the knee where the upper calf perforator vein contributed to anteromedial leg varicosities. Rivlin's observations have been corroborated in subsequent experiences.

Discussion of varicose vein operations performed before 1980 would be incomplete without a mention of Geza de Takats.[26] His contributions were intellectual and philosophical and were couched in excellent English even though it was his third or fourth language. It may be said that de Takats introduced intelligence into the surgery of varicose veins.

Disappointment with results of saphenous vein stripping as referred to by Rivlin led to the combination of proximal ligation and retrograde injection of varicosities and ligation and stripping combined with injection of residual varicosities as referred to earlier in this chapter.[27,28]

OBJECTIVE EVALUATION OF RESULTS

During the military lull between World War II and the Korean War, operations for removal of varicose veins included GSV stripping from groin to ankle; LSV stripping from knee to ankle, alone or in combination with ligation and division of perforator veins; and excision of varicosities with or without intraoperative, retrograde sclerosing injections, supplemented by postoperative transcutaneous sclerosing injections with or without permanent wearing of elastic support stockings. A complex series of choices indeed. Clearly there was a need for evaluation of techniques and standardization of operations.

Lofgren, Ribisi, and Myers[29] provided an evaluation in the late 1950s, but their analytic methods were flawed by lack of objective data collection. As scientific evaluation of surgical results became more sophisticated through the 1970s and as techniques of measurement of venous dynamics became available, objective data were obtained.[30] Data collection and evaluation by statistical methods were then applied to the two radically opposing forms of treatment so that conclusions could be drawn. John Hobbs[31] of London early on contributed his trial of surgery versus sclerotherapy in treatment of varicose veins, and his observations were later confirmed by Jakobsen[32] of Copenhagen.

A précis of Jakobsen's observations suffices to summarize the experience of the two studies. In his study 516 patients were divided into three treatment groups. Those in the first underwent a radical operation while under full anesthesia, those in the second were treated with saphenous vein ligation and division followed by injection compression, and those in the third group were treated by injection compression alone. The radical operation required more than 1 hour of anesthesia for bilateral procedures and an average of eight incisions. The minor procedures varied from patient to patient but consisted of proximal ligation, usually with distal perforator interruption but without full-length stripping. Injection compression was applied according to the Swiss method of Sigg.[33]

Objective evaluation of the results was done at 3 months and 3 years. It was found that the best results occurred after combined treatment; the worst results occurred with injection compression therapy alone.

When saphenofemoral valvular incompetence was present, all authors agreed that the GSV should be ligated and divided at the groin. However, disagreement occurred with regard to the necessity for distal stripping. Dormandy, operating at St. George's Hospital, performed a prospective, randomized study to determine whether stripping the GSV was essential. His 200 patients were randomly allocated to have either high saphenous ligation with stripping of the GSV and avulsion of calf varices or high saphenous ligation and thigh perforator ligation only. Residual varicosities were treated by injection sclerotherapy. The conclusion of the study was that "there was no subjective or objective advantage to stripping the LSV [i.e., greater saphenous vein] in management of primary varicose veins."[34]

Dormandy's presentation was vigorously criticized at the time, but the criticism had to do mostly with technique rather than follow-up. In fact, no answers were provided about the fundamental question: Is there need of or any value in performing high ligation combined with limited stripping to the knee region?

This question was addressed in the early 1980s when a double-blind control trial of surgery for varicose veins was completed.[35] By using accurate data collection and objective evaluation and applying statistical methods to a study of randomly allocated patients, acceptable conclusions could be drawn. Unfortunately, full stripping to the ankle was used, not the limited stripping advocated by Hobbs and by Rivlin.

In summary, this study showed that ". . . stripping conferred a significant advantage, but the incidence of paresthesia and pain biased patient opinions against stripping." Pain and paresthesias occurred in the region of the saphenous nerve distal to the tibial tuberosity, thus confirming Rivlin's observation made 10 years earlier. In fact, stripping needs to be carried out only to knee level before the nerve becomes intimately associated with the saphenous vein at the upper calf.[36]

More recent evaluations of high ligation versus limited stripping have also supported the limited stripping operation strongly advocated first by Rivlin. The surgical group at Lund, Sweden, for example, compared compression sclerotherapy with high ligation with division and limited stripping of the incompetent GSV.[37,38] These studies can all be summarized in a quotation from the latter article. "The results emphasize the importance in following patients for at least five years and compression sclerotherapy combined with high tie cannot replace surgery (saphenous vein removal) in patients with mainstem insufficiency."

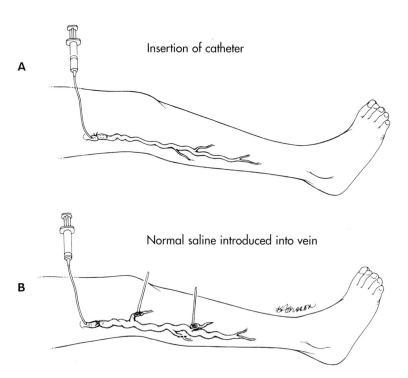

Fig. 10-5 Simkin advocates stab avulsion as illustrated in Fig. 10-4, *A* and *B*. However, he eases the technique by the performance of intraluminal cannulation and distention of the veins using normal saline solution as shown in this figure. **A**, Insertion of the catheter. **B**, Distention of the vein for removal by crochet-hook technique or by stab avulsion with hemostats.

Although there is now agreement that limited saphenous vein stripping is a contribution to treatment in patients with saphenofemoral incompetence and LSV division is a contribution to patients with saphenopopliteal incompetence, there is no agreement on the actual methods of removal of the saphenous vein. In practice, both the intraluminal and extraluminal stripping techniques can be used.

The intraluminal invagination technique has some potential. It has been modified and used extensively by Paul Ouvry of Dieppe. In his modification a gauze strip, 5 to 10 cm wide, is inserted with the invagination so that the risk of breaking and tearing the vein is decreased. Ouvry describes directing the stripper in the GSV from groin to the upper leg. This stripper is then attached to a gauze strip with fishline. A 10-cm wide strip is used for large saphenous veins and a 5-cm strip for moderate or small saphenous veins. As the vein is stripped, the gauze strip remains in the venous pathway until the very end of the operation. In this way it aids in hemostasis, decreasing hematoma formation. Residual varicose veins untreated by the stab avulsion or stripping technique are then treated by sclerotherapy beginning 3 weeks after the operation.

Other techniques of varix removal are less well known. Fig. 10-5 shows the method advocated by Simkin.[39] In his method the varicosities are enlarged by injection before avulsion by the stab-avulsion techniques.

Modern alternatives to vein stripping include plication of the vein wall at the proximal incompetent valve to restore valve competency.[40,41] Although there is no doubt that valve competency can be restored, it is doubtful that this technique will allow long-term successful eradication of distal varicosities either by compression sclerotherapy or satisfactory stab avulsion.

REFERENCES

1. Dodd H and Cockett FB, editors: Pathology and surgery of the veins of the lower limbs, Edinburgh, 1956, E&S Livingstone, Ltd.
2. Large J: Surgical treatment of saphenous varices with preservation of the main saphenous trunk, J Vasc Surg 2:886, 1985.
3. Corbett R and Njayakumar K: Cleanup varicose vein surgery—use a tourniquet, Ann R Coll Surg Engl 71:57, 1989.
4. Samuels PB: Technique of varicose vein surgery, Am J Surg 142:239, 1981.
5. Royle JP: Recurrent varicose veins, World J Surg 10:944, 1986.
6. Haeger K : The anatomy of the veins of the leg. In Hobb JT, editor: The treatment of venous disorders, Lancaster, England, 1977, MTP Press, Ltd.
7. Jakobsen BH: The value of different forms of treatment for varicose veins, Br J Surg 66:182, 1979.
8. Neglen P, Einarsson E, and Eklof B: The functional long-term value of different types of treatment for saphenous vein incompetence, J Cardiovasc Surg 34:295, 1993.
9. Sarin S, Scurr JH, and Coleridge-Smith PD: Assessment of stripping the long saphenous vein in the treatment of primary varicose veins, Br J Surg 79:889, 1992.
10. van Bemmelen PS and Bergan JJ: Quantitative measurement of venous incompetence, Austin, Tex, 1992, RG Landes Co.
11. Bergan JJ, Moulton SL, and Poppitti R: Patient selection for surgery of varicose veins using venous quantification. In Veith FJ, editor: Critical problems in vascular surgery, St Louis, 1992, Quality Medical Publishers.
12. Vasdekis SN, Clarke GH, and Nicolaides AN: Quantification of venous reflux by means of duplex scanning, J Vasc Surg 10:670, 1989.
13. van Bemmelen PS et al: Quantitative segmental evaluation of venous valvular reflux with ultrasound scanning, J Vasc Surg 10:425, 1989.
14. Walsh JC et al: Femoral venous reflux is abolished by greater saphenous vein stripping, Ann Vasc Surg 1994 (in press).
15. Gradman WS, Segalowitz J, and Grundfest W: Venoscopy in varicose veins surgery: initial experience, Phlebology 8:145, 1993.
16. Cotton LT: Varicose veins: gross anatomy and development, Br J Surg 48:589, 1961.
17. Darke SG: The morphology of recurrent varicose veins, Eur J Vasc Surg 6:512, 1992.

18. Sherman RS: Varicose veins: further findings based on anatomic and surgical dissections, Ann Surg 130:219, 1949.

19. Jugenheimer M and Junginger TH: Endoscopic subfascial sectioning of incompetent perforating veins in treatment of primary varicosis, World J Surg 16:971, 1992.

20. Fischer R: Erfahrungen mit der endosckopischen Perforantensanierung, Phlebologie 21:224, 1992.

21. Babcock WW: A new operation for extirpation of varicose veins, NY Med J 86:1553, 1907.

22. Rivlin S: Surgical care of primary varicose veins, Br J Surg 62:913, 1975.

23. Van der Stricht J: Saphenectomie, Presse Med 71:1081, 1963.

24. Myers TT and Cooley JC: Varicose vein surgery in management of the postphlebitic limb, Surg Gynecol Obstet 99:733, 1954.

25. Nabatoff RA: 3000 operations for varicose veins, Surg Gynecol Obstet 130:497, 1970.

26. de Takats G: Ambulatory ligation of the saphenous vein, JAMA 94:1194, 1930.

27. McPheeters HO and Anderson JK: Injection treatment of varicose veins, Surg Gynecol Obstet 81:355, 1945.

28. Waugh JM: Ligation and injection of great saphenous veins, Proc Staff Meet Mayo Clin 16:832, 1941.

29. Lofgren KA, Ribisi AP, and Myers TT: An evaluation of stripping versus ligation for varicose veins, Arch Surg 76:310, 1958.

30. Norgren L: Foot volumetry before and after surgical treatment of patients with varicose veins, Acta Chir Scand 141:129, 1975.

31. Hobbs JT: Surgery and sclerotherapy in treatment of varicose veins, Arch Surg 109:793, 1974.

32. Jakobsen BH: The value of different forms of treatment for varicose veins, Br J Surg 66:182, 1979.

33. Sigg K: Treatment of varicose veins by injection sclerotherapy. In Hobbs JT, editor: Treatment of venous disorders, Lancaster, England, 1977, MTP Press.

34. Woodyer AB et al: Should we strip the long saphenous vein? In Negus D and Jantet G, editors: Phlebology '85, London, 1986, John Libbey & Co, Ltd.

35. Munn SR et al: To strip or not to strip the long saphenous vein? A varicose vein trial, Br J Surg 68:426, 1981.

36. Holme JB, Holme K, and Schmidt-Sorenson L: Anatomic relationship between the long saphenous vein and saphenous nerve, Acta Chir Scan 154:631, 1988.

37. Einarsson E, Eklof B, and Norgren L: Compression sclerotherapy or operation for primary varicose veins? Proceedings of seventh International Congress of Phlebology, vol 1, Copenhagen, 1980.

38. Neglen P, Einarsson E, and Eklof B: High tie with sclerotherapy for saphenous vein insufficiency, Phlebology 1:105, 1986.

39. Simkin R: Enfermeda des enfermedades venosas, Buenos Aires, 1979, Lopez Liberos.

40. Jones JW, Elliot F, and Kerstein MD: Triangular venous valvuloplasty, Arch Surg 117:1250, 1982.

41. Belcaro G: Plication of the saphenofemoral junction: an alternative to ligation and stripping? Vasa 18:296, 1989.

11   CLINICAL METHODS FOR SCLEROTHERAPY OF TELANGIECTASIAS

HISTORICAL REVIEW OF TECHNIQUES

Sclerosing treatment for telangiectasias was ignored until the 1930s when Biegeleisen[1] injected sclerosing agents intradermally or subcutaneously into the general area of capillary enlargement. However, this procedure resulted in severe necrosis and lack of effect on the telangiectasias. Biegeleisen then developed and popularized a method of "micro-injection" of telangiectasias with sclerosing agents through the use of an "extremely fine metal needle" (later described as a handmade 32- or 33-gauge needle).[2] Unfortunately, he used sodium morrhuate (SM) in the treatment of these fragile small vessels, which produced multiple complications, including pigmentation, cutaneous necrosis, and allergic reactions. Thereafter sclerotherapy treatment of leg telangiectasias was thought of disparagingly by most practitioners[3] until the 1970s when Alderman,[4] Foley,[5] Tretbar,[6] and Shields and Jansen[7] published reports of procedures that had achieved excellent results with few adverse sequelae. In these procedures solutions less caustic to the telangiectasia were used (hypertonic saline [HS] with or without heparin and lidocaine [15% to 30%] and sodium tetradecyl sulfate 1% [STS]), as were techniques that ensured accurate placement of the solution into the blood vessels (use of 30-gauge needles).

INDICATION

Microsclerotherapy is theoretically indicated for any small telangiectatic vessel or venule on the cutaneous surface. Best results are obtained on superficial linear or radiating vessels on the lower extremities. Telangiectasias on the face are less reliably responsive to microsclerotherapy because they probably have more of an arteriolar component and result from active vasodilation, but they can be successfully treated (see Chapter 4).[8,9] In addition, bright-red telangiectasias on the leg that have a rapid refilling time after diascopy (applying pressure with a glass slide) (Fig. 11-1) are probably also supplied through arteriolar flow.[10] These vessels are relatively recalcitrant to usual therapy and tend to recur after treatment. More importantly, these arteriolar leg veins are more likely to develop overlying cutaneous necrosis if sclerosing solutions reach the arteriolar feeding loop (see Chapter 8). They may be more effectively treated with the pulsed laser or light sources (see Chapter 12).

The description in Chapter 9 of the injection of varicose veins by first closing off the high-pressure reflux points with sclerosing solution followed by sclerotherapy of remaining abnormal vessels forms the basis for rational compression sclerotherapy of varicose veins. The treatment of "spider" leg veins can be just as rational.

In the vast majority of cases spider veins connect to underlying varicose veins either directly or through tributaries.[11] Doppler examination shows that almost all visible blue reticular veins are connected to telangiectasia.[12,13] Therefore, as with varicose veins, treatment should first be directed at "plugging" the leaking high-pressure outflow at its point of origin. An appropriate analogy is to think

409

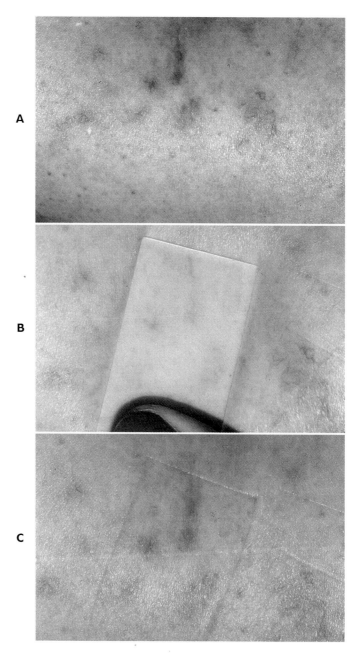

Fig. 11-1 Bright red telangiectasias may have an arteriolar origin. In this series the telangiectasia was located on the medial thigh. **A,** Appearance while the leg is raised 45 degrees. **B,** Blanching with pressure under a glass slide. **C,** Immediate reappearance on removal of the glass slide while the leg is still elevated.

of spider veins as the "fingers" and of the feeding varicose vein as the "arm." Treatment should first be directed to the feeding arm and then, only if necessary, to the spider fingers. There are a number of advantages to this systematic approach to sclerotherapy. When sclerotherapy is performed in this manner, the spider veins often disappear without direct treatment or decrease markedly in size, thus limiting the number of injections into the patient. The larger feeding vein is both easier to cannulate and less likely to rupture when injected with the sclerosing solution, thus minimizing the extent of extravasated red blood cells (RBCs) and solution. Theoretically, this method also should minimize the development after sclerotherapy of hyperpigmentation, cutaneous necrosis, telangiectatic matting, and recurrence (see Chapter 8).

INJECTION TECHNIQUE
Preinjection Procedure

After a physical examination, including the use of noninvasive diagnostic techniques when appropriate (see Chapter 5), the patient is scheduled for a sclerotherapy session and given a questionnaire (Appendix C), consent form (Appendix D), and instructional material (Appendix G) to read and complete at home. Questions about the procedure are answered and all possible complications and adverse sequelae addressed. An estimate of the approximate number of treatment sessions and the cost of treatment is given in writing to prevent any future misunderstandings (Appendix I). Insurance reimbursement policies are discussed and documented (Appendix J). Documentation of the relief of symptoms with compression stockings is helpful in gaining preauthorization of treatment from insurance companies, but in most cases insurance companies decide on the medical necessity for treatment based on size and type of vessel, not symptoms. Since graduated compression stockings should be worn in most cases after treatment, they are fitted at this time and given to the patient to wear before treatment. If the stockings produce a resolution of symptoms, one can be assured that successful sclerotherapy will give the same result. In addition, wearing the stockings before treatment helps answer any requestions about their fit to ensure they will be worn for the prescribed length of time after treatment.

On the day of treatment legs should not be shaved because a burning sensation may result when alcohol is applied to the areas that will be treated. Moisturizers also should not be applied the day of treatment since they cause unnecessary slipperiness of the skin. Patients are instructed to eat a light meal or drink juice an hour or so before the procedure in an effort to prevent a vasovagal reaction. Shorts, a bathing suit, or a leotard should be worn during the procedure since some vessels may be near the groin.

With the patient standing on a low stool, a complete set of photographs of the legs is taken from four different views, and the individual areas that will be treated are photographed close up (Fig. 11-2). Photographic documentation is important because patients often will not remember exactly how their legs appeared before treatment. Any pretreatment pigmentation irregularities and scars may later be blamed on the sclerotherapy treatment since patients usually look more closely at their legs once treatment has begun.

An easy method for measuring the diameter of the telangiectasia was shown to me by Jerry Garden, M.D. (Chicago, IL) He uses various-sized needles to compare diameters.

Gauge	External diameter (mm)
30	0.3
27	0.41
26	0.46
25	0.51
22	0.71
20	0.89
18	1.27

At the end of the treatment session, the treated areas are recorded on a diagrammatic chart to help check progress at follow-up examinations (see Appendix

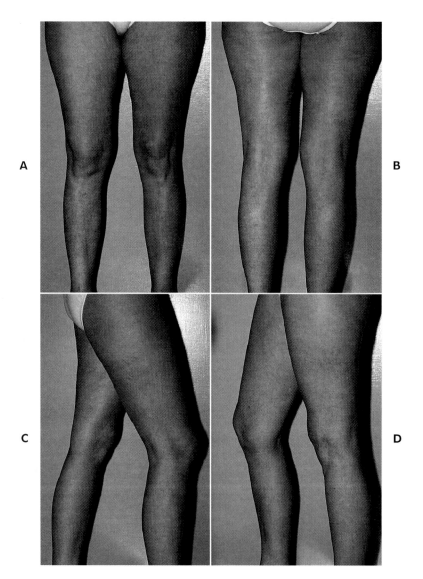

Fig. 11-2 Standard photographs taken before treatment begins to allow accurate determinations of treatment outcome. Four standard views are taken at an F-stop of F8; close-up views are taken at an F-stop of F11, with macro-close-ups taken at an F-stop of F16. All photos are taken with Kodachrome ASA 64 film as described in Chapter 13. **A,** Frontal view. **B,** Rear view. **C,** Right side (the right foot is always in front of the left foot). The right knee is slightly bent so the left inner thigh is better visualized. **D,** Left side (again with the right foot in front of the left).

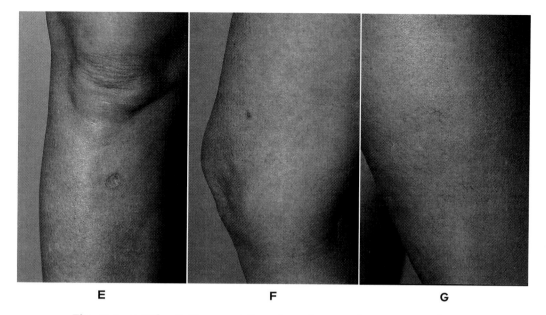

E F G

Fig. 11-2, cont'd   E, Documentation of scar from previous treatment for a verruca on the right anterior tibial area, which could later be thought of as a treatment scar. F, Documentation of dermatofibroma on the right medial knee area, which could later be thought of as punctate pigmentation from treatment. G, Close-up view of telangiectasia and venules (0.2 to 0.6 mm in diameter) on the right lateral thigh, along with pretreatment nonspecific light-brown pigmentation, which could later be thought of as postsclerotherapy hemosiderin pigmentation.

E). Patients are given written postoperative instructions about activity and the disposition of their graduated compression stockings and/or bandages (Appendices K and L).

Preparation and Visualization of the Vessels

Microsclerotherapy of spider veins is performed with the patient in the supine position. Gravitational dilation of telangiectasias is usually unnecessary. The skin is wiped with alcohol, making the telangiectasias more visible because of a change in the index of refraction of the skin. The glistening effect of alcohol renders the skin more transparent and helps clean the injection site. In addition, alcohol may cause some vasodilation of the telangiectasias. Alternatively, Sadick[14] recommends that the skin be wiped with a solution of 70% isopropyl alcohol with 0.5% acetic acid. He finds this solution improves the angle of refraction better than alcohol alone. Scarborough and Bisaccia[15] recommend rubbing a few drops of the sclerosing solution on the skin overlying the venules with a gloved finger. They use polidocanol (POL), which also contains alcohol in water as the dilutent. I agree that visualization is enhanced with this technique once the initial effects of the isopropyl alcohol have worn off through evaporation. To further enhance visualization of the vessels, I recommend the use of magnifiers from $\times 2^{1}/_{4}$ to $\times 5$ (see Chapter 13).

If the vessels are too small to inject, having the patient stand for approximately 5 minutes and then placing him or her in a reverse Trendelenburg position may result in some vessel dilation. Alternatively, inflating a blood pressure cuff to approximately 40 mm Hg proximal to the injection site may also result in some distention of the vessels.

Equipment

Needle and syringe. Although visualization of the vessel is important in ensuring proper needle placement, one actually enters the vessel "by feel." This is particularly true when injecting reticular varices. In this situation it is best to pierce the skin rapidly and advance the needle superficially over the vessel at a slight angle. Penetration of the vessel is "felt," even when one uses a 30-gauge needle. Some authors state that the "feel" is enhanced with the use of a 26- or 27-gauge needle.[16] In this regard the use of a glass syringe would best reflect an impedance to flow if a vessel were not properly cannulated. However, glass syringes are more cumbersome to use. With the availability of high-quality plastic syringes, a good feel can be obtained, and the risk of transmitting blood-borne diseases obviated (see Chapter 13).

Ideally the goal of microsclerotherapy is to cannulate the vessel, injecting sclerosing solution within and not outside of the vessel wall. Usually a 30-gauge needle will suffice for most vessels, although some physicians recommend the use of a 32- to 33-gauge needle to decrease the likelihood of inadvertent perivenular injection in the treatment of the smallest diameter vessels.[17-20] The disadvantages of using a 32-gauge needle are that it is not disposable, dulls rather quickly, and easily bends (see Chapter 13). Boxes of needles sometimes contain dull needles, which gives a "scratchy" sensation to the tip, or needles without honed tips. One should never hesitate to change needles if a vein cannot be cannulated easily. It is usually not the "tough skin" of the patient but a dull needle that makes injection difficult.

One-half inch 30-gauge needles, although 0.3 mm in diameter, are honed to an oblique bevel that permits cannulation of vessels <0.1 mm in diameter. Needles longer than $1/2$ inch are too flexible for reliable and accurate cannulation.

I find the use of a 3-ml syringe filled with 2 ml of sclerosing solution is ideal. This syringe fits well in the palm of the hand and can be easily manipulated. In addition, the quantity of solution is usually satisfactory for injecting either larger venules with 0.5 ml each or multiple smaller vessels. Alternatively, for those with small hands, a 1-ml syringe filled with 0.5 ml may be easier to handle, although a large number of syringes will be needed per treatment session. One theoretical disadvantage to multiple injections with the same needle is that it will become dull.[18] However, this was found not to occur on microscopic examination of the needle tips after eight injections into the skin (see Chapter 13).

Table and lighting. Direct lighting should be avoided during treatment since it may produce a glare from the alcohol-soaked skin. Indirect lighting allows the best visualization.

The ideal treatment table is one that can be easily raised or lowered to provide a comfortable position for the physician to ensure injection accuracy. It is helpful if the physician can easily maneuver around the table on a stool so the best approach to a given vessel is attainable. Tables that can be positioned in Trendelenburg or reverse Trendelenburg positions can help in the treatment of an early vasovagal reaction and in effecting vessel dilation or contraction.

Skin Tension

To facilitate cannulation of the vessel the skin must be taut. This can be accomplished with the help of an assistant who stretches the patient's skin in at least two directions. Alternatively, with proper hand placement, three-point tension can be produced by the physician alone. Fig. 11-3 illustrates my recommended technique for injection. The nondominant hand is used to stretch the skin adja-

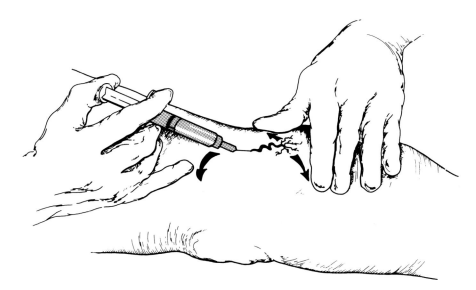

Fig. 11-3 Proper hand placement to exert three-point traction to aid in needle insertion. Injection is made into the feeding "arm" of the "fingers" of the spider vein.

cent to the treated vessel in two directions. Then the fifth finger of the dominant hand exerts countertraction in a third direction. With a little practice, even the most lax skin such as that on the thighs can be brought under tension with this technique. Skin laxity varies with patient age, adiposity, and location on the leg.

Depth of Injection

The location of most leg telangiectasias is in the upper dermis (see Chapter 1). The most common error in technique is to place the needle tip deep to the vessel. To enter the vessel at a less acute angle almost parallel to the skin surface, the needle should be bent to 145 degrees with the bevel up (Fig. 11-4).[21] If the needle is not within the vessel, the solution will either leak out onto the skin or produce an immediate superficial wheal. At times gentle upward traction can be applied as the needle is advanced to ensure superficial placement.

Injecting with the bevel of the needle up has the advantage of minimizing the chance of transsecting the vessel. Inserting the needle bevel down may be easier, probably as the result of the vacuum produced by the bevel on the skin surface.

When using a sclerosing solution that does not cause cutaneous necrosis on extravasation (e.g., STS 0.1% to 0.25%, POL 0.25% to 1.0%, and chromated glycerin [CG]), one can inject as the needle is being inserted into the vessel. As soon as the bevel is within the vessel, the telangiectasia blanches. This technique allows the injection of vessels with diameters smaller than the diameter of the needle because the tip of the bevel is thinner than the needle shaft and with injection the telangiectasia dilates, allowing complete insertion to occur.

Air-Bolus (Block) or Foam Technique

The air-bolus technique, injecting a small amount of air to clear the vessel before instilling the sclerosing solution, is recommended by multiple physicians.[4,5,16] It is thought to minimize the risk of inadvertent intradermal injection. This, however, may not occur since once the vessel is cleared of blood, it is more difficult to see the progress of the sclerosing solution within its lumen. Therefore many other physicians and I have abandoned this technique.[18,20] Another theoretical advantage of the air-bolus technique is the decreased risk of intravascular

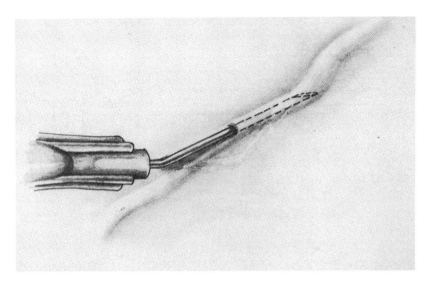

Fig. 11-4   Needle is bent to 145 degrees with the bevel up to facilitate accurate insertion into the superficial telangiectasia. (From Goldman MP and Bennett RG: J Am Acad Dermatol 17:167, 1987.)

thrombosis. It is thought that if the vessel is cleared of blood by first injecting air, the risk of extravasation of RBCs may also be minimized. However, antegrade and retrograde filling of the treated vessel occurs after the injection. Thus the air-bolus technique may not prevent or lessen the incidence of postsclerosis pigmentation.

Another variant of the air-bolus technique that helps visualize clearing of the vessels is that of creating a foamy solution before injection. This can be achieved with the use of any "detergent" class of sclerosing solution such as STS or POL (see Chapter 7). Another method described by Green and Morgan[22] is to add Haemacel to STS to accentuate bubble formation. It is also thought that the foam causes the sclerosing agent to interact more efficiently with endothelium (see Chapter 9).

Quantity of Sclerosing Solution per Injection Site

The maximum quantity of sclerosing solution that can be safely injected into a single site when treating varicose veins is detailed in Chapter 9. In short, one should not inject a volume that would easily travel undiluted into the deep venous system. This is especially important since flow of contrast material from telangiectasias has been noted to flow directly into the deep venous system in 2 of 13 patients (13.3%) with digital subtraction phlebography (Fig. 11-5).[23] The maximum amount of sclerosing solution that can be injected into leg telangiectasias is unclear. Although Duffy[18] places little emphasis on limiting the amount of solution injected at a single site and Lary[24] recommends the injection of up to 3 ml at a single site when injecting a reticular 3-mm diameter vein, multiple complications can and do occur from this technique. Excessive inflammation and inadvertent flow of the solution into a feeding varicose vein or arteriole can produce ulceration with injection and damage to the deep venous system. Thrombosis and emboli can occur when amounts greater than 1 ml are injected in a single site. For example, injection of 0.5 ml of solution into a 2-mm diameter vessel will fill a length of 16 cm (see Chapter 8).

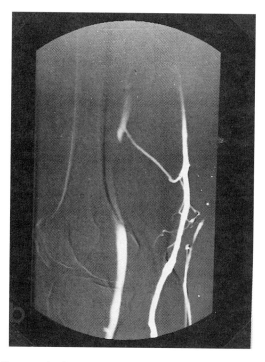

Fig. 11-5   Main collector of telangiectatic vessels *(small arrow)* drains into the femoral vein *(arrow head)* via a perforator vein. (*Large arrow,* Great saphenous vein.) (From Bohler-Sommeregger K et al: J Dermatol Surg Oncol 18:403, 1992.)

Ouvry and Davy[25] recommend that the amount injected should be sufficient to produce blanching of vessels 1 to 2 cm around the point of injection. No more than 0.5 ml should be used to avoid the risk of initiating the formation of new telangiectasias around the edge of the treated area because of excessive inflammation. In this regard the same area should not be retreated more often than every 4 to 6 weeks. In my practice it appears that telangiectatic matting occurs more frequently if reinjections are given to a previously treated area that is still undergoing resolution. This unresolved state can be appreciated clinically by slight inflammation and evidence of microthrombosis of vessels.

In addition to limiting the inflammatory reaction of sclerotherapy treatment, limiting the amount of solution may also prevent pain and cramping when hypertonic solutions are used. Sadick[14] has found that volumes greater than 0.3 ml of HS 23.4% caused the most pain and cramping.

Some areas, especially the ankles, should not be injected with more than 1 ml of any sclerosing solution. In this area the skin is thinnest, the distance between the deep and superficial venous system is the least, and swelling after treatment is common (see Chapter 8).

Concentration and Strength of Sclerosing Solutions

Sclerosing solution concentration and strength are discussed in detail in Chapter 7, but a few points should be mentioned here. The most important concept in sclerotherapy is that of achieving optimal destruction of the blood vessel wall with the minimal concentration of sclerosing solution necessary; too much will lead to excessive complications and adverse sequelae, and too little will lead to ineffective sclerosis or recurrence from recanalization (see Chapter 8). One should always estimate conservatively when choosing the concentration and type of sclerosing solution.

Three randomized double-blind, paired comparative human studies evaluated the results of different sclerosing solutions and concentrations in the treatment of leg telangiectasia. Carlin and Ratz[26] tested POL 0.25%; STS 0.5%; and HS 20% with heparin, 100 U/ml (Heparsal), in the treatment of leg telangiectasia and found that whereas HS and STS gave quicker clearing of telangiectasia with fewer injections, the overall level of improvement was identical for all agents. POL was the best-tolerated sclerosing solution with the fewest number of adverse sequelae. In a follow-up study comparing POL in four concentrations—0.25%, 0.5%, 0.75%, and 1.0%—Norris, Carlin, and Ratz[27] found that all concentrations were equally effective in treating leg telangiectasia. POL 0.5% was ideal, with the least number of adverse effects and the most rapid clearing in their patients with leg telangiectasias 0.2 to 1.0 mm in diameter. Sadick[28] compared HS in three concentrations—23.4%, 11.7% and 5.8%—and found that HS 11.7% was the minimal concentration of saline that produced the most effective vein sclerosis of vessels 1.0 mm in diameter while producing the least discomfort and morbidity.

I recommend that leg telangiectasias less than 1.0 mm diameter be treated with either POL 0.5%, STS 0.25%, CG, or HS 11.7%. Vessels between 1.0 and 3.0 mm should be treated with POL 0.75%, STS 0.5%, or HS 23.4%. The treatment of larger vessels is discussed in Chapter 9.

Pressure of Injection

Another variable of technique is the pressure and rapidity of injection. If leg telangiectasias are injected under excessive force, they may rupture and result in extravasation of solution (see Chapter 8). Therefore injections should be made with minimal pressure. This may be difficult when injecting sclerosing solutions of high viscosity, such as CG, since more pressure is required to push them through a 30-gauge needle. Duffy[18] likens the proper injection pressure to that which is needed to fix a postage stamp to an envelope. In addition, the slower the injection, the longer the solution will be in contact with the vessel wall. Finally, injection pressure (with equal force applied to the piston) is inversely proportional to the square of the piston radius: $P = F/S = F/\pi R^2$; $P1/P2 = (R2/R1)^2$*. If the approximate piston radius of a 2-ml syringe is 8 mm and is 5 mm for a 1-ml syringe, the applied force is 250 g or 180 mm Hg for a 2-ml syringe and more than 300 mm Hg for a 1-ml syringe.[29]

When treating varicose veins, patient position and movement determine the length of time the solution will be in contact with the endothelium (see Chapter 9). But with the injection of telangiectasias, the blood flow is not determined by muscle movement or body position but by many other factors, including environmental temperature, nervous stress, and the telangiectasias' association with arterioles and underlying veins. Therefore injections should be made slowly enough that it takes approximately 5 to 10 seconds to fill the vessel. Many times the vessel will remain filled with sclerosing solution if the plunger of the syringe is held with almost zero force while the needle remains motionless.

POSTTREATMENT TECHNIQUES

Immediately after injection of the sclerosing solution the perivascular tissues may swell, producing a clinically visible occlusion of the vessel, or the vessels may go into spasm. This usually occurs if the injection is given slowly and if the sclerosing solution is of adequate strength. Indeed several of us recommend that a given vessel be treated until such an effect occurs.[16] This may require a second injection

---

*P = pressure, F = force, S = cross-section of the vein, R = radius.

of a more concentrated solution (+25%) into the same vessel during the same sclerotherapy session.

After hypertonic solutions are injected, the injected area should be massaged to minimize the stinging and help alleviate the associated muscle cramping by rapidly diluting the hyperosmotic solution outside of the treated vessel.[18-20,30] The slower the injection, the less cramping occurs. When withdrawing the needle, a small amount of sclerosing solution may be deposited under the skin, causing a burning sensation. This usually occurs only with hypertonic solutions and CG. Massaging for 30 to 60 seconds alleviates the pain and prevents necrosis from the hypertonic saline solution.[19]

All sclerosing solutions, even unadulterated HS (see Chapter 8), will produce some degree of erythema or urtication or both with injection. Pruritus may be associated with this effect, especially when associated with urticarial lesions. This probably occurs as a result of histamine release caused by perivascular release of mast cell mediators because of perivascular irritation or as a result of intravascular degranulation of basophils and other white blood cells destroyed by the direct toxic effects of the sclerosing solution. This reaction and its associated pruritus can be minimized by the application of a potent topical corticosteroid cream, thereby providing relief to the patient, especially if injected areas will be occluded with compression pads and/or stockings.

For telangiectasias that do not respond to standard compression sclerotherapy, added vasoconstriction induced by cold temperature may be helpful. Orbach[31] finds that vessels respond better to the injection of refrigerated sclerosing solution. Marteau and Marteau,[32] using similar logic, advise applying cold compression pads after injection. Although these two techniques seem logical, I have not found them helpful.

POSTTREATMENT COMPRESSION

Compression of the sclerosed vessel with a 30 to 40 mm Hg graduated compression stocking should be maintained for a minimum of 24 to 72 hours after treatment of leg telangiectasias. Postsclerosis compression serves a number of purposes. First, the pressure helps seal the irritated vascular lumen. Second, the pressure helps decrease the likelihood of recanalization of the sclerosed vessel, especially if compression is maintained for 1 to 2 weeks. Third, the possibility of clinical and symptomatic thrombosis is minimized, thus minimizing hyperpigmentation, telangiectatic matting, and recanalization after sclerosis. Although some physicians do not advocate postsclerosis compression,[7,14,19,29,32,33] the procedure is so simple and the benefits theoretically so great that its routine use is recommended. In addition, most patients actually like the feel of the compression stocking while they are ambulatory. (A complete discussion on the use of compression in the treatment of varicose and telangiectatic leg veins is presented in Chapter 6.)

REPEAT TREATMENT SESSIONS

All patients are informed that successful treatment of a given telangiectasia may require more than one treatment. As previously mentioned, the same vessel or the immediate area is not retreated for 4 to 6 weeks to allow resolution of the endosclerosis or controlled phlebitis to occur. Waiting also allows appreciation of the effectiveness of treatment with a given solution and concentration. If little change is apparent 6 weeks after injection, the second treatment can be performed with a stronger sclerosing agent or more concentrated solution. Different areas can be treated as often as every day, but the venous system of the leg is a complex interwoven network so that treatment of only one part may not prevent reflux pressure from another part from promoting continued blood flow through the treated area (see Chapter 1). This will lead to an increased incidence of complications from blood flow through a damaged endothelial system (see Chapter 8). Thus when treating superficial reticular and telangiectatic leg veins, the only real limiting factor is patient and physician motivation for treatment and adherence to using the maximal daily recommended amounts of sclerosing solution that can be injected (see Chapter 7). In addition, if compression is used, it may be best to wait until the pressure stocking has been removed for a few days before continuing treatment on the same leg.

Although we as physicians think of medicine as a science, it is also an art. Therefore the sclerotherapy technique just mentioned should not be perceived as dogma. Rather it should serve as a logical outline for the physician in planning individualized treatment.

CASE HISTORIES

CASE STUDY 1: Traumatic telangiectatic patch

A 46-year-old woman was accidentally hit by a tennis ball while she was "playing the net." A telangiectatic patch on the posterior medial thigh developed after resolution of the bruise 4 to 6 weeks after the initial injury and did not change in size or color over the following 4 years (Fig. 11-6, A). The patch was treated one time only with injections of POL 0.5% in three locations to blanch the lesion completely. A total of 1 ml was used. A localized pressure dressing with an STD foam pad was placed and secured with Medi-Rip tape for 3 days. Fig. 11-6, B, shows the same area 10 months after initial treatment.

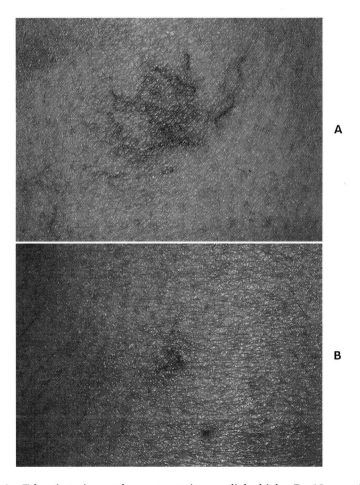

Fig. 11-6 **A,** Telangiectatic patch on posterior medial thigh. **B,** 10 months after treatment.

CASE STUDY 2: Unassociated telangiectasia

Fig. 11-7, A, shows the appearance of linear telangiectasia on the medial thigh of a 46-year-old woman that was noted during her second pregnancy 22 years previously. The area was asymptomatic, and treatment was requested for cosmetic improvement. The appearance 6 months after a single treatment using approximately 3 ml of POL 0.5% is shown in Fig. 11-7, B. A 30 to 40 mm Hg graduated compression stocking was worn for 3 days after the injection. Note there is some mild hyperpigmentation in one of the treated vessels.

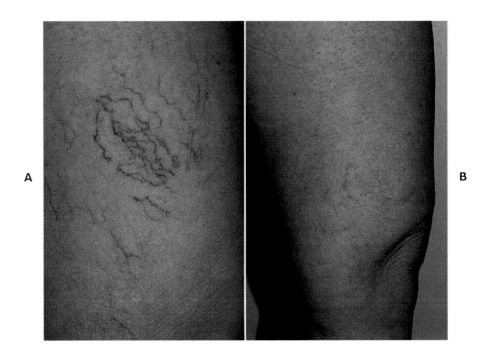

Fig. 11-7   A, Linear telangiectasia on medial thigh. **B,** 6 months after treatment.

CASE STUDY 3: Reticular vein unassociated with the saphenous system

Appearance of a reticular vein 2 to 3 mm in diameter on the popliteal fossa in a 32-year-old woman is shown in Fig. 11-8, A. The same area 18 months after one treatment with 1 ml of POL 0.75% is shown in Fig. 11-8, B. The area was compressed for 72 hours after treatment with an STD foam pad under a 30 to 40 mm Hg graduated compression stocking, after which the compression stocking alone was worn for 1 more week while the patient was ambulatory. In the intervening 18 months the patient wore a 20 mm Hg graduated compression stocking on a fairly consistent basis while she was ambulatory.

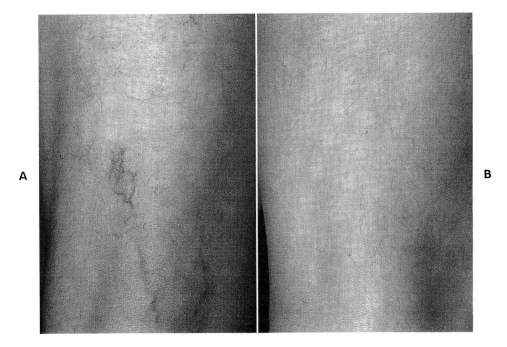

Fig. 11-8   A, Reticular vein on popliteal fossa. B, 18 months after treatment.

CASE STUDY 4: Mixed reticular and telangiectatic veins

Reticular veins approximately 2 mm in diameter, associated with multiple telangiectasias on the lateral distal thigh in a 32-year-old woman, appeared during her second pregnancy 10 years previously (Fig. 11-9, A). The patient requested treatment because of a dull aching that occurred in the area during menses and after prolonged standing. The treated veins are shown immediately after a total injection with 0.5 ml of POL 0.75% in Fig. 11-9, B. Fig. 11-9, C, shows the treated area 1 day after injection after removal of the STD pad and 30 to 40 mm Hg graduated compression stocking. Note the ecchymosis induced by the pressure dressing. Fig. 11-9, D, shows the area 1 week after injection. Intravascular thrombi were noted and drained at that time. Eight weeks after injection the vessels were almost totally resolved. Some mild pigmentation was present in the distal aspect where thrombosis was most extensive (Fig. 11-9, E). Fig. 11-9, F, shows the area 22 months after initial treatment, demonstrating sustained resolution of the telangiectasia, reticular veins, and pigmentation.

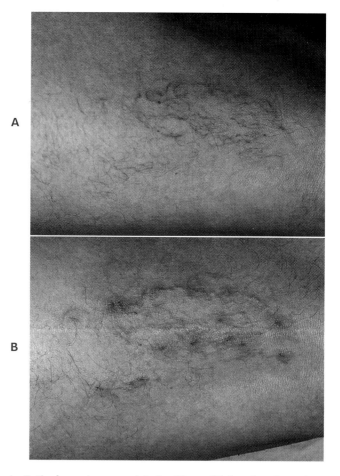

Fig. 11-9   A, Reticular veins associated with multiple telangiectasias on lateral distal thigh. B, Immediately after injection. C, 1 day after injection and removal of pad and graduated pressure stocking. D, 1 week after injection. E, 8 weeks after injection. F, 22 months after treatment with complete resolution.

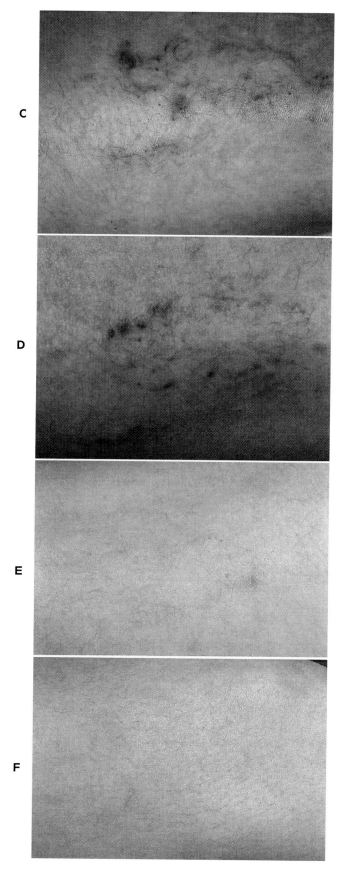

Fig. 11-9, cont'd   For legend see opposite page.

CASE STUDY 5: Extensive reticular and telangiectatic veins

A 53-year-old woman had a 30-year history of asymptomatic reticular and telangiectatic leg veins that had been stable in appearance since her last of two pregnancies 20 years previously. She sought treatment for cosmetic reasons (Fig. 11-10, A). A total of 10 ml of POL 0.75% was injected into all feeding reticular veins on the proximal and distal lateral thigh. POL 0.5%, 2 ml, was injected into the portion of the telangiectatic mats on the lateral calf and knee, which did not blanch with the previous injection. STD foam pads were placed under a 30 to 40 mm Hg graduated support stocking that was worn continually for 7 days after the procedure. When the stocking was removed, multiple small thrombi were drained. Fig. 11-10, B, shows the appearance of the treated area 25 months after the single treatment session.

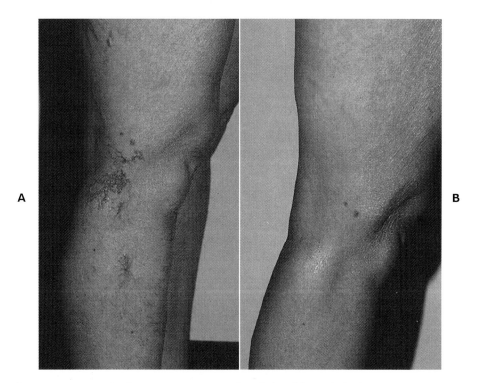

A   **B**

Fig. 11-10 A, Reticular veins on proximal and distal lateral thigh. B, 25 months after treatment.

CASE STUDY 6: Treatment of cherry hemangiomas
A 48-year-old woman had multiple cherry hemangiomas on her abdomen and thighs and a 4-mm diameter hemangioma located on her anterior thigh (Fig. 11-11, A). Fig. 11-11, B, shows the appearance 5 months after injection with 0.1 ml of POL 0.75%. Note the slightly indented and hypopigmented scar, which was acceptable to the patient.

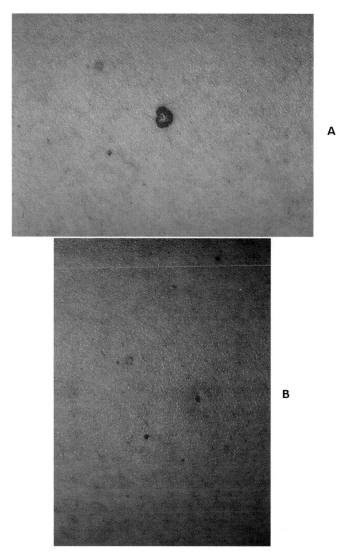

Fig. 11-11   A, Multiple cherry hemangiomas on anterior thigh. B, 5 months after injection.

CASE STUDY 7: Lateral subdermal plexis

A 59-year-old woman was initially seen with a leg ache from the lateral thigh veins that had been increasing in severity over the last 2 years. Reticular and telangiectatic veins had been present since age 16. The lateral subdermal plexis, noted as having 2- to 3-mm diameter reticular veins, was incompetent to venous Doppler examination (Fig. 11-12, A). Sclerotherapy began with injection of a total of 4 ml of POL 0.75% to all reticular veins on the left leg while the patient was supine. All telangiectasias that did not become inflamed after reticular vein injection were then sclerosed with a total of 6 ml of POL 0.5%. The leg was compressed for 72 hours with a 30 to 40 mm Hg graduated compression stocking. A second treatment to the same leg was given 4 months later with 4 ml of POL 0.75% injected into reticular veins and 2 ml of POL 0.5% injected into remaining telangiectasias. The leg was compressed as previously described, and all veins and bruising resolved within 2 months. Fig. 11-12, B, shows total resolution of all veins 1 year after the second treatment.

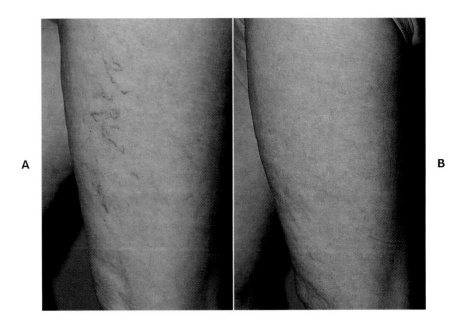

A   B

Fig. 11-12   **A,** Clinical appearance before sclerotherapy. **B,** Clinical appearance 1 year after treatment (see text for details).

CASE STUDY 8: Treatment of telangiectasia and resulting telangiectatic matting

A 66-year-old woman was initially seen with extensive telangiectasias and venules 0.2 to 0.6 mm in diameter over the left lateral knee (Fig. 11-13, A). These veins developed when she was near 40 years of age after she began estrogen replacement therapy. There was no previous family history of varicose veins. In addition to the cosmetic appearance that was disturbing when she wore shorts while playing golf, her legs ached continuously, especially over the telangiectasias. These vessels were treated with POL 0.5%, 2 ml, with the development of telangiectatic matting 4 weeks after treatment (Fig. 11-13, B). Examination 3 months after initial treatment showed a "feeding" reticular vein in the telangiectatic area. The feeding reticular vein, 2 mm in diameter, was treated with POL 0.75%, 1 ml, and the telangiectatic matting vessels were then treated with chromated glycerin mixed 1:1 with 1% lidocaine and with epinephrine, 1 ml, with resolution occurring in approximately 4 weeks. When the woman was examined 1 year later, the telangiectasia and leg pain had both resolved (Fig. 11-13, C).

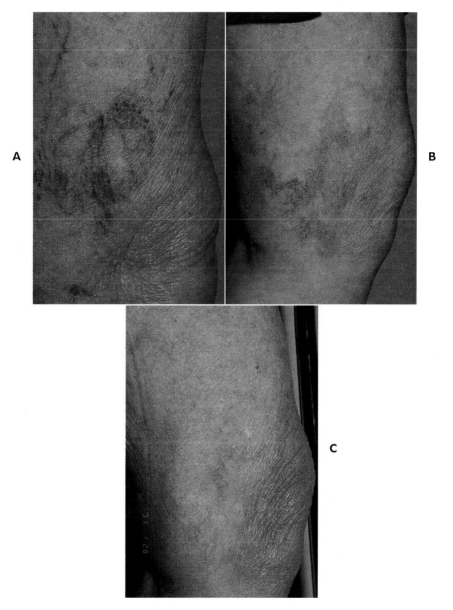

Fig. 11-13   **A,** Clinical appearance before sclerotherapy. **B,** Developmental of telangiectatic matting after sclerotherapy. **C,** Resolution of telangiectasia 1 year after treatment (see text for details).

REFERENCES

1. Biegeleisen HI: Telangiectasia associated with varicose veins: treatment by a micro-injection technique, JAMA 102:2092, 1934.
2. Biegeleisen HI: Varicose veins, related diseases, and sclerotherapy: a guide for practitioners, Canada, 1984, Eden Press.
3. Higgins TT and Kittel PB: Injection treatment with sodium morrhuate, Lancet 1:68, 1930.
4. Alderman DB: Therapy for essential cutaneous telangiectasias, Postgrad Med 61:91, 1977.
5. Foley WT: The eradication of venous blemishes, Cutis 15:665, 1975.
6. Tretbar LL: Spider angiomata: treatment with sclerosant injections, J Kans Med Soc 79:198, 1978.
7. Shields JL and Jansen GT: Therapy for superficial telangiectasias of the lower extremities, J Dermatol Surg Oncol 8:857, 1982.
8. Goldman MP et al: Treatment of fascial telangiectasia with sclerotherapy, laser surgery, and/or electrodesiccation: a review, J Dermatol Surg Oncol 19:899, 1993.
9. Prescott R: Treatment of fascial telangiectasias by sclerotherapy. In Raymond-Martimbeau P, Prescott R, and Zummo M, editors: Phlebologie '92, Paris, 1992, John Libbey Eurotext, Ltd.
10. Merlen JF: Red telangiectasias, blue telangiectasia, Soc Fr Phlebol 22:167, 1970.
11. de Faria JL and Moraes IN: Histopathology of the telangiectasias associated with varicose veins, Dermatologia 127:321, 1963.
12. Tretbar LL: The origin of reflux in incompetent blue reticular/telangiectasia veins. In Davy A and Stemmer R, editors: Phlebologie '89, Montrouge, France, 1989, John Libbey Eurotext, Ltd.
13. Weiss RA and Weiss MA: Doppler ultrasound findings in reticular veins of the thigh subdermic lateral venous system and implications for sclerotherapy, J Dermatol Surg Oncol 19:947, 1993.
14. Sadick N: Treatment of varicose and telangiectatic leg veins with hypertonic saline: a comparative study of heparin and saline, J Dermatol Surg Oncol 16:24, 1990.
15. Scarborough DA and Bisaccia E: Sclerotherapy—translucidation of the skin prior to injection, J Dermatol Surg Oncol 15:498, 1989.
16. Marley W: Low dose sotradecol for small vessel sclerotherapy, Newsletter North Am Soc Phlebol 3:3, 1989.
17. Eichenberger H: Results of phlebosclerosation with hydroxy-polyethoxydodecane, Zentralbl Phlebol 8:181, 1969.
18. Duffy DM: Small vessel sclerotherapy: an overview. In Callen et al, editors: Advances in dermatology, vol 3, Chicago, 1988, Year Book Medical Publishers, Inc.
19. Bodian E: Sclerotherapy, Dialogues in Dermatology 13(3), 1983.
20. Green D: Compression sclerotherapy techniques, Dermatol Clin 7:137, 1989.
21. Goldman MP and Bennett RG: Treatment of telangiectasia: a review, J Am Acad Dermatol 17:167, 1987.
22. Green AR and Morgan BDG: Sclerotherapy for venous flare, Br J Plast Surg 38:241, 1985.
23. Bohler-Sommeregger K et al: Do telangiectases communicate with the deep venous system? J Dermatol Surg Oncol 18:403, 1992.
24. Lary BG: Varicose veins and intracutaneous telangiectasia: combined treatment in 1500 cases, South Med J 80:1105, 1987.
25. Ouvry P and Davy A: Le traitement sclerosant des telangiectasies des membres inferieurs, Phlebologie 35:349, 1982.
26. Carlin MC and Ratz JL: Treatment of telangiectasia: comparison of sclerosing agents, J Dermatol Surg Oncol 13:1181, 1987.
27. Norris MJ, Carlin MC, and Ratz JL: Treatment of essential telangiectasia: effects of increasing concentrations of polidocanol, J Am Acad Dermatol 20:643, 1989.
28. Sadick N: Sclerotherapy of varicose and telangiectatic leg veins: minimal sclerosant concentration of hypertonic saline and HS relationship to vessel diameter, J Dermatol Surg Oncol 17:65, 1991.
29. Guex J-J: Indications for the sclerosing agent polidocanol, J Dermatol Surg Oncol 19:959, 1993.
30. Weiss R and Weiss M: Resolution of pain associated with varicose and telangiectatic leg veins after compression sclerotherapy, J Dermatol Surg Oncol 16:333, 1990.
31. Orbach J: A new look at sclerotherapy, Folia Angiologia 25:181, 1977.
32. Marteau J and Marteau J: Contribution de la cryotherapie en phlebologie, Phlebologie 31:191, 1978.
33. Chrisman BB: Treatment of venous ectasias with hypertonic saline, Hawaii Med J 41:406, 1982.

LASER AND NONCOHERENT PULSED LIGHT TREATMENT OF LEG TELANGIECTASIAS AND VENULES

The laser was first conceived in the imagination of H.G. Wells who described the use of a light gun in 1896 as an outer-space weapon. Albert Einstein then transformed imagination into a theoretical possibility in the early 1900s. He described the process of stimulated emission as an offshoot in his quest to show the inherent singular nature of the four basic forces of the universe. However, it was not until 1960 that the first laser was actually constructed (ruby laser).

The acronym *LASER* stands for *Light Amplification by the Stimulated Emission of Radiation*. In short, a laser emits a beam of monochromic, coherent, collimated photons of a specific wavelength. The emitted wavelength is produced by exciting an atom or molecule to release particles, or photons, at a wavelength specific for that type of molecule. This ability to produce a laser light at a specific wavelength is one key factor in producing selective damage. By tuning the laser to the absorption wavelength of a particular substance such as oxygenated hemoglobin, only that substance will theoretically be affected by the laser energy.

With proper usage, lasers are very safe and have not been associated with long-term side effects. Laser radiation used in medicine is in or near the range of visible light in the electromagnetic spectrum. Therefore its radiant energy level is at a much longer wavelength than the high-energy ionizing type of radiation associated with x-rays or radiation therapy and is not associated with the commonly perceived radiation hazards.[1] In addition, the wavelength determines the depth of penetration of each type of laser (Fig. 12-1). (A complete practical discussion of laser physics can be found in other sources.[1])

Lasers have been used to treat leg telangiectasia for various reasons. First, lasers have a futuristic appeal. By virtue of their high technology, they are perceived as "state-of-the-art" and are sought by the general public because "high tech" is thought of as safer and better. Unfortunately, as described below, this perception by both the general public and the physician has often resulted in unanticipated adverse sequelae (scarring).

In addition, lasers have theoretical advantages compared to sclerotherapy for treating leg telangiectasia. Sclerotherapy-induced pigmentation is secondary to hemosiderin deposition through extravasated erythrocytes (see Chapter 8). Laser coagulation of vessels should not have this effect. In the rabbit ear model approximately 50% of vessels treated with an effective concentration of sclerosing solution demonstrated extravasated erythrocytes, compared to a 30% incidence when treated with the flashlamp pumped pulsed dye laser (FLPDL) (Goldman MP, unpublished observations). Telangiectatic matting (TM) has also not been associated with laser treatment of any vascular condition and occurs in a significant percent of sclerotherapy-treated patients. Finally, specific allergenic effects of the sclerosing solution do not occur with laser treatment.

Four types of lasers have been used to treat leg telangiectasias: carbon dioxide (CO_2); neodymium: yttrium-aluminum-garnet (Nd:YAG); argon; and 577 to 585 nm flashlamp pumped pulsed dye and continuous wave lasers. In addition, a

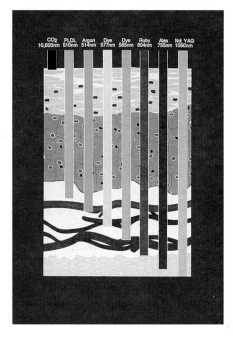

Fig. 12-1 Diagram representing approximate levels of penetration for various lasers. (*FLPDL*, Candela pigment lesion laser; *Nd:YAG*, neodymium:yttrium-aluminum-garnet; *CO₂*, carbon dioxide.) (From Goldman MP and Fitzpatrick RE: Cutaneous laser surgery, St Louis, 1994, Mosby.)

novel, noncoherent pulsed light, Photoderm VL light source (Energy Systems Corporation, Newton, Mass.), effectively thermocoagulates leg telangiectasias, venules, and reticular veins up to 3 mm in diameter. They each act in a different manner to effect vessel destruction. CO_2, Nd:YAG, argon, and continuous wave dye lasers are not entirely specific for vascular tissue because of both wavelength and pulse durations that are outside of the thermal relaxation time of the treated vessel. Their energy therefore affects perivascular and cutaneous tissue, causing nonspecific damage. However, various methods have been devised to allow these nonspecific lasers to be somewhat useful. The FLPDL acts within the thermal relaxation times of blood vessels to produce specific destruction of vessels less than 0.2 mm in diameter. The Photoderm VL was developed to treat vessels up to 3 mm in diameter 2 mm beneath the epidermis. This chapter reviews and evaluates the use of these nonspecific and specific laser and light systems in the treatment of leg venules and telangiectasias.

LASER MODALITIES
Carbon Dioxide

The CO_2 laser, developed in 1964, has been used for the obliteration of venules and telangiectatic vessels.[2-5] The CO_2 laser emits light energy at 10,600 nm in the infrared portion of the electromagnetic spectrum. At this wavelength vaporization occurs through a conversion of intracellular and intravascular water to steam. Thus the CO_2 laser produces total vaporization of all targeted tissue.

The rationale for using the CO_2 laser in the treatment of telangiectasias is that it can produce a precise vaporization of a blood vessel without causing significant damage to tissue structures adjacent to the penetrating laser beam. However,

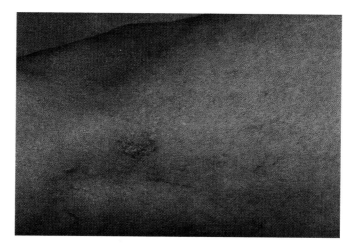

Fig. 12-2   Hypopigmented scars with skin textural changes 5 years after treatment of leg telangiectasia with the CO_2 laser.

DISADVANTAGES OF CARBON DIOXIDE LASER TREATMENT

Nonselective tissue damage	Possibility of brisk bleeding
Hypopigmented punctate scars	Painful procedure

---

since tissue destruction is nonselective when produced by vaporization of water within cells, the skin surface and the dermis overlying the blood vessel are also destroyed. CO_2 laser penetration of vessels has also been reported to cause occasional brisk bleeding from the vessel, which required the use of pressure bandages for 48 hours.[4] Pain during treatment is moderate to severe but of short duration.

All reported studies of the CO_2 laser demonstrate unsatisfactory cosmetic results. Treated areas show multiple hypopigmented punctate scars with either minimal resolution of the treated vessel or neovascularization adjacent to the treatment site (Fig. 12-2). Because of this nonselective action, the CO_2 laser has no advantage over the electrodesiccation needle and has not been used successfully in treating telangiectasias on the leg. When given a choice, patients prefer sclerotherapy to CO_2 laser therapy.[5] The box above summarizes the disadvantages of the CO_2 laser.

Nd:YAG

The Nd:YAG laser has been used to treat leg telangiectasias.[4] This laser light has a wavelength of 1060 nm, which is not absorbed well by melanin, hemoglobin, or any cutaneous chromophore but is absorbed much better by water. Just as with the CO_2 laser, tissue damage is relatively nonspecific. The average depth of penetration of this laser in human skin is 0.75 mm; a reduction of the incident power to 10% occurs at a depth of 3.7 mm.[6] Thus this laser is able to treat blood vessels only to the depth of the middermis.

When used to treat facial vascular lesions, the tissue destruction that occurs requires up to 4 weeks to heal. In addition, scar formation is more likely to occur with this laser than when similar lesions are treated with the argon laser.[7]

DISADVANTAGES OF NEODYMIUM-YAG LASER TREATMENT

Relatively nonselective tissue damage   Hypopigmented linear scars
Significant risk of scar formation   Painful procedure

Apfelberg et al.[4] treated leg telangiectasias with a Nd:YAG laser equipped with a 1.5-mm sapphire contact probe. Problems encountered included linear hypopigmentation and depressions overlying the skin of the treated vessel and the need to retreat the vessels at 6-week intervals. Also the cost of the procedure is high because the disposable sapphire tips are expensive. In summary, as reported with the CO_2 laser, this modality produces unsatisfactory cosmetic results and is not yet useful in treating leg telangiectasias. The disadvantages of the Nd:YAG laser are summarized in the box above.

Argon

The argon laser theoretically is better suited for treating telangiectasias than the modalities previously mentioned. The blue-green light of this laser emits 80% of its energy at 488 and 514 nm. The red-purple oxygenated hemoglobin located in the superficial dermal ectatic blood vessels 0.05 mm in diameter 0.2 mm below the dermal-epidermal junction has absorption peaks at 418, 542, and 577 nm and, for the most part, is selectively absorbed by the argon laser spectrum (Fig. 12-3). However, the argon laser light is not entirely hemoglobin specific. The epidermis absorbs the 488- and 514-nm wavelengths approximately half as strongly as blood does and is therefore nontransparent.[8] Epidermal melanin also absorbs a variable portion of argon laser light. This may result in hypopigmentation of the treated areas. Thus the specificity of argon laser-induced damage apparently is much lower than originally hypothesized (Fig. 12-4). (See box on p. 435.)

In addition to the relative nonspecificity of the argon laser wavelength for oxygenated hemoglobin, presently available argon lasers deliver energy exposures with pulse durations as short as only 20 to 50 ms. This minimal exposure still allows time for extensive radial diffusion and dissipation of heat generated in the treated blood vessels, thereby resulting in a relatively nonselective thermal destruction.[9] In practice, for the argon laser to produce clinically effective results, pulses are delivered until tissue whitening occurs.[10] This whitening represents nonspecific thermal damage to the epidermis and dermis and not simply blanching of the vascular bed. In fact, there is no clinical difference between continuous-wave therapy and 50-ms pulse therapy.[10] Thus there is a risk of hypertrophic or atrophic scarring caused by nonspecific epidermal and upper dermal necrosis and subsequent fibrosis. This is noted clinically by epidermal sloughing postoperatively followed by crusting and gradual reepithelialization over 1 to 2 weeks.[11] This effect may be minimized through the use of lower laser energies.

Although satisfactory treatment results have been reported with the use of the argon laser for facial telangiectasias, a number of adverse effects also occur. Typically, pitted, hypertrophic, and depressed scars have been observed.[12-20] "Unexpected pigmentary changes" have been noted by 43% of physicians using the argon laser.[21] Hypopigmentation has been reported to occur in up to 32% of women having port-wine stain treatment.[12] Hyperpigmentation, occurring in up to 20% of patients, has been demonstrated as a result of an increased production of melanin by a normal population of melanocytes.[22] The authors speculate that this pigmentation is induced by thermal stimulation of melanocytes as the argon

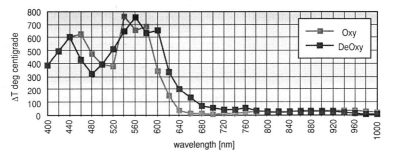

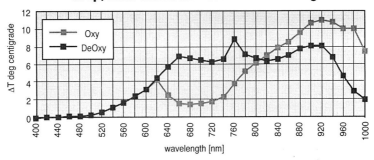

ESC Inc. Newton, Ma, USA

Fig. 12-3　Average temperature increase across a cutaneous vessel as a function of wavelength for two cases: a shallow capillary vessel (similar to those found in a port-wine vascular malformation) and a deeper (2 mm), larger (1 mm) vessel typical of a leg venule. The calculated curves are generated assuming that the main light-absorbing chromophore in the blood is either oxygenated or deoxygenated hemoglobin. The calculation is carried out for a 10 J/cm^2 fluence and does not take into account cooling by heat conductivity. Note the dramatic shift in the optimal wavelength as a function of vessel depth and diameter. Also note the difference between oxygenated and deoxygenated hemoglobin. (Courtesy Shimon Eckhouse, Ph.D., Energy Systems Corporation, Inc., Newton, Mass.; from Goldman MP and Fitzpatrick RE: Cutaneous laser surgery, St Louis, 1994, Mosby.)

DISADVANTAGES OF ARGON LASER TREATMENT

Partially selective vascular damage
Hypopigmentation and hyperpigmentation after treatment

Atrophic and hypertrophic scarring
Painful procedure

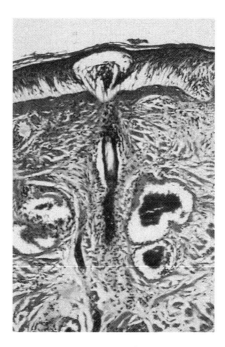

Fig. 12-4 Biopsy of a port-wine vascular malformation on the cheek of a 40-year-old man immediately after argon laser treatment at 15 J/cm², 1-mm spot diameter, which produced clinical epidermal whitening. Note coagulation of ectatic vessels in the middle and deep dermis with smudging of perivascular collagen. The overlying epidermis shows marked thermal effects with streaming of the epidermal cells and coagulation necrosis of the superficial papillary dermis. (Hematoxylin-eosin ×200). (From Goldman MP and Fitzpatrick RE: Cutaneous laser surgery, St Louis, 1994, Mosby.)

laser produces a superficial burn. Again these adverse sequelae are decreased somewhat with the use of lower laser energies.

A number of techniques have been developed in an attempt to limit thermal-induced complications. A grid or checkerboard pattern of treatment has been shown by some to offer no advantage[23] but may be of some benefit when produced through a robotized scanning laser handpiece.[24] Apfelberg et al.[12] have reported on the use of a stripping technique that produces unacceptable sequelae. Apfelberg et al.[25] also have described a dot or pointillistic method that may offer some improvement over standard treatment techniques, but it still produced scarring in 3 of 8 patients treated on the upper or lower extremity and in 2 of 25 evaluable patients with treatments on the upper lip or nasolabial folds. Thus variations in treatment technique have failed to minimize the complications of argon laser treatment significantly.

Telangiectasias or superficial varicosities of the lower extremities are much less responsive than are facial lesions to argon laser treatment. Apfelberg and McBurney[26] and Craig et al.[27] caution that the treated areas in this location usually appear purple or depressed, often leaving a worse cosmetic appearance than the untreated condition. In a report of 38 patients treated by Apfelberg et al.,[28] 49% had either poor or no results from treatment; only 16% had excellent or good results. In addition, almost half of the patients had hemosiderin bruising.[28] In another series Dixon, Rotering, and Huether[29] noted significant improvement in only 49% of patients. They speculated that after initial improvement, incomplete thrombosis, recanalization, or new vein formation produced reappearance of the vessels after 6 to 12 months.[30] Thus use of the argon laser has been demon-

Fig. 12-5 Hypopigmented scars with skin textural changes 4 years after treatment of leg telangiectasia with the argon laser (specific laser parameters unknown).

Table 12-1 Results of treatment of leg telangiectasias with argon laser

Study	No. of sites treated	< 90% faded (%)	100% faded	Adverse sequelae
Arndt (1982)[17]	8	37	27%	37%
Dixon (1984)[18]	24*	48	None	4+ %
Apfelberg (1984)[3]	38	89	11%	6+ %
Craig (1985)[27]	4	100†	None	None

*51% of patients would not undergo additional treatment.
†"Poor response."

strated to result in a relatively high percentage of unsatisfactory treatment outcomes when used to treat leg telangiectasias (Table 12-1; Fig. 12-5).

Tissue Cooling

Argon laser light passes through the skin surface into the upper reticular dermis for a distance of approximately 1 mm in white skin.[31] The depth of laser absorption can be increased by, cooling the tissue. When experimentally excised tissue is cooled, the depth of effective vascular coagulation increases from 1.7 to 3.5 mm.[32] Chilling of port-wine stain vascular malformations before argon laser treatment has been found to improve treatment results.[33,34] But this beneficial effect has not been reported universally. Multiple investigators have found that before and after treatment cooling of the skin offers no improvement in the rate of frank hypertrophic scarring.[33,35-36] Tissue cooling may also affect thermal energy absorption so that high laser energies are necessary to effect tissue destruction. Thus the increased laser energy required to offset the decrease in efficiency of thermal damage to the targeted tissues may result in nonselective tissue damage.

In an effort to refine tissue cooling effects further, a novel device for simultaneously cooling the skin while lasing leg telangiectasia was recently evaluated in 30 leg telangiectasias in 13 patients.[37] Patients with telangiectasias approximately 1 mm in diameter were treated with either an argon 577-nm or an argon 585-nm continuous wave dye laser through a "cool laser optics" (CLO) device that consists of a plastic box $1\frac{1}{4}$ inches deep filled with ice cold water (Fig. 12-6). The

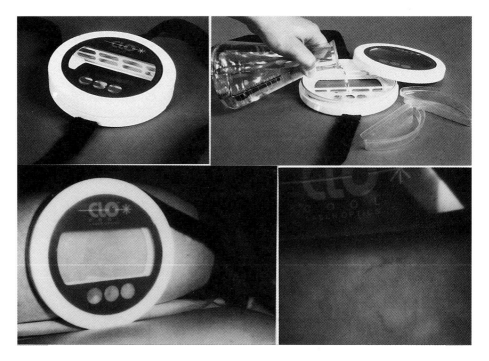

Fig. 12-6 Cool laser optics (CLO) device. *Upper left,* Appearance of device. *Upper right,* Open unit being filled with ice water. Half-moon–shaped plastic forms to make ice blocks for lateral compartments of the unit. *Lower left,* CLO unit attached with Velcro straps to the patient's left thigh over telangiectasia. *Lower right,* Close up of telangiectasia viewed through the CLO unit before treatment. (Courtesy Cyruc Chess, M.D.)

author/inventor calculates an energy transmittance of approximately 80% through this device. The treated site is chilled by placing the device on it for 2 minutes; then the laser handpiece is held perpendicular to the outer wall and is aimed at the vessel target. Laser energy is delivered until the vessels become indiscernible. Irradiance for argon-treated vessels ranged from 1301 to 1954 W/cm² and 124 to 2516 for dye treatments, with energy fluence ranging from 173 to 867 J/cm² and from 62 to 242 J/cm² for argon and dye lasers, respectively. Treatment time varied from 5 to 30 minutes, depending on the diameter and extent of telangiectasia.

This treatment modality resulted in 30% of vessels completely clearing (five with one treatment and five requiring two treatments). Partial clearing (20% to 70% fading) occurred in 10 sites, and 10 sites showed no changes. Two sites (7%) developed temporary hyperpigmentation, and one patient developed permanent hypopigmentation. The authors state no recurrence of faded vessels at 3-year follow-up. The success in eliminating these vessels is only minimally better than that achieved with the similar use of lasers without tissue cooling. But the extent of adverse sequelae is much improved with tissue cooling; therefore minimizing nonspecific thermal damage with tissue cooling is beneficial.

Fiber-guided Laser Coagulation

Trelles and coworkers (Institute Medico Vilafortuny, Cambrils, Spain) reported another method for treating leg veins with fiberoptic transmission of argon or tunable dye laser into the vessel (International Society of Cosmetic Laser Surgeons, Palm Desert, Calif., February 1993). With this technique, a vessel is cannulated with an 0.8 × 40 mm hypodermic needle, and a 200-μm optical fiber is passed through the needle into the vein. Two to four pulses of laser light (514, 570, 585, 620 nm) are delivered with a pulse duration of 100 to 300 ms at 1.5 to 5 W. The pulse duration and energy are adjusted to coagulate the vessel. Because of non-specific thermal heating related to long pulse durations, they cool the skin with ethyl chloride. One-hundred eleven of 175 patients were satisfied with treatment, with nine developing a depressed or pigmented scar. This technique is tedious and time-consuming to perform.

Contact Probe Delivery

Another method for more selective delivery of nonspecific laser energy is pro-duced by directing the laser energy to the target vessel. Keller has reported on the use of a microcontact argon laser probe to treat "spray telangiectasias" of the leg.[38] Fifteen patients were treated with this device using an argon laser energy of 1 to 2 W with a pulse duration of 0.1 seconds. This treatment was performed as "spot welding" along the course of the blood vessel; 100% effectiveness and no notable complications were reported. We have not achieved the same success rate as Keller,[39] and further reports of this novel form of therapy have not occurred. Thus at the present time argon laser therapy apparently is a satisfactory method for treating selected facial telangiectasias but is much less effective in treating leg telangiectasias. A summary of the disadvantages of the argon laser treatment ap-pears in the box on p. 435.

532-nm Krypton Laser

Smith et al.[40] reported on the use of a 532-nm green laser beam treatment on "nonpalpable," smooth, fine-linear, purple-to-red leg telangiectasias. The 100-mm spot-size beam was directed along the vessel in a continuous mode until tissue whitening appeared. Moderate-to-severe pain during the procedure and a 1- to 2-week wound healing time were observed, and only 50% of patients received a sat-isfactory result. The incidence of postlaser scarring and pigmentation was not de-scribed; the diameter of the treated vessels was also omitted. Compression was not used after treatment.

577- to 585-nm Dye Laser and Flashlamp-pumped Pulsed Dye Laser

In an effort to produce highly selective laser destruction with less interference from overlying melanin, lasers using various dyes at wavelengths at the longer oxygenated hemoglobin absorption peaks were developed. The main chro-mophore in the blood vessel is oxyhemoglobin.[41] The oxyhemoglobin absorption spectrum has three major bands calculated for 50-μm vessels 0.2 mm deep, the largest at 418 nm and the two smaller peaks at 542 and 577 nm. Although there are stronger oxyhemoglobin bands at shorter wavelengths, competing absorption by epidermal melanin overlying the dermal vessels tends to dominate.[42] However, when tuned to 577 nm, corresponding to the alpha band of oxyhemoglobin, the laser energy penetrates to the depth of dermal blood vessels,[41,43] with little inter-fering absorption by melanin in light skin types.[44,45]

A restriction of the application of the 577-nm wavelength in the treatment of vascular lesions has been its penetration to only approximately 0.5 mm in depth from the dermal-epidermal junction.[46] However, the depth of vascular dam-age increases from 0.5 to 1.2 mm by changing the wavelength from 577 to 585 nm while maintaining the same degree of vascular selectivity as that previ-ously described for 577-nm irradiation.[47,48] This change in wavelength from 577 to 585 nm results in a more complete clearance of vascular cutaneous lesions in patients.[49] Increasing the wavelength of the FLPDL to 600 nm has also been shown histologically to give deeper thermocoagulation than with a 585-nm

FLPDL.[50] Thus longer wavelengths may be desirable when treating deeper blood vessels.

Besides matching the wavelength of the laser to the target tissue, it is ideal to limit the laser energy absorption and contain it within the targeted structure. This is accomplished by pulsing the laser. Limiting the duration of laser exposure ensures that highly specific laser energy is delivered in a period of time less than that required for the cooling of the target vessel, that is, less than the thermal relaxation time.

For superficial cutaneous blood vessels, thermal relaxation times range from 0.1 to 10 ms, depending on the size and type of the vessel,[41,51] an average of 1.2 ms[41] (Table 12-2). A pulsed dye laser has been developed in an attempt to perfect selective vascular injury. Experimentally, a 1.5-ms pulse is absorbed almost entirely by the erythrocyte, resulting in microvaporization with endothelial and pericyte damage, vessel rupture, and hemorrhage.[46,52] In contrast to the destruction in these specific cellular structures, mast cells, fibroblasts, and even collagen fibers in the perivascular tissues remain unaltered.[46] Multiple studies have found that the ideal pulse duration to produce endothelial damage without microvessel rupture is 20 to 450 ms.[52-54] Because of technical production limitations, a 450-ms machine was developed (FLPDL).

In addition to thermal damage produced by the absorption of the 577-nm wavelength, photoacoustic "shock-wave" damage resulting from rapid absorption of energy by the oxyhemoglobin molecules has also been demonstrated.[45,46,55] In vitro studies[53,56] have demonstrated that the 577-nm pulsed dye laser produces a direct destructive effect on endothelial cell cultures. Therefore, in addition to thermal absorption of laser energy by erythrocytes, that results in shock-wave and thermal-induced destruction of the blood vessel, direct laser effects on endothelial cells may also contribute to the highly specific vessel damage. This shock wave promotes the undesirable purpuric response commonly seen with the FLPDL, which may take 1 to 3 weeks to resolve completely. Thus its nonspecific endothelial effect may not be more beneficial than its side effect.

The advantage of using longer pulse durations that are still within the thermal relaxation times for the targeted blood vessels is that larger diameter blood vessels may be treated. The average diameter of blood vessels in the upper dermis is 40 to 60 μm; in deeper dermis, 100 to 400 μm; and in subcutaneous tissue, 1 to 3 mm (see Chapter 1). In addition, longer pulses may prevent the shock-wave effect, thus preventing purpura. Studies are presently underway to test even longer pulse durations with the hope of extending treatment to larger diameter vessels (see the following paragraphs).

Table 12-2 Thermal relaxation time of laser targets

	Approximate diameter (μm)	Thermal relaxation time (r)
Epidermis	60	2 ms
Basal layer	20	400 μs
Melanosome	1	0.2 μs
Microvessels	20	140 μs
	50	1.2 ms
	100	3.6 ms
	300	
Erythrocyte	5	5 μs

Studies using a 577-nm dye laser with a 300-μs pulse demonstrate minimal perivascular or epidermal damage.[54,57,58] In fact, multiple studies note no evidence of scarring after the treatment of patients with port-wine stains, including using a number of retreatments.[53,59] However, although facial port-wine hemangiomas, telangiectasias, spider ectasia, and capillary hemangiomas have been treated effectively,[58-61] telangiectasias over the lower extremities have not responded as well; they show less lightening and more hyperpigmentation after therapy.[62] Polla et al.[63] treated 35 superficial leg telangiectasias with the FLPDL. The exact laser parameters were not given except for information that vessels were treated an average of 2.1 times with a maximum of four separate treatments. These vessels were described as either red-purple and raised or blue and flat. No mention was made about the association of reticular or varicose veins or about the vessel diameter. Of vessels treated, 15% had greater than 75% clearing, and 73% of treated areas showed little response to treatment. The only lesions that responded at all were the red or pink "tiny" telangiectasias. Almost 50% of the treated patients developed a persistent hypopigmentation or hyperpigmentation of treated sites (Fig. 12-7). Table 12-3 lists the advantages and disadvantages of the FLPDL.

Table 12-3 Pulsed dye laser treatment of leg telangiectasias

Advantages	Disadvantages
Extremely selective vascular destruction	Variable success rate (high energies necessary)
Rare temporary pigmentary changes	Only effective on small-diameter blood vessels
No telangiectatic matting	Expensive
No scarring	Mildly painful

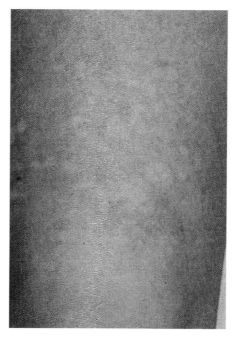

Fig. 12-7 Temporary hypopigmentation that lasted for 6 months developed in this 32-year-old woman with type 3 tan skin treated on the anterior thigh with the FLPDL at 7.5 J/cm^2.

Unfortunately, it is difficult to compare the clinical and experimental studies of laser treatment of leg telangiectasias with that of port-wine stains. Laser studies on the treatment of leg telangiectasias typically do not report the diameter, location, or type of vessel treated. In addition, no mention is made of "feeding" perforator or reticular veins or of postlaser compression. Therefore we systematically examined the clinical effects of various powers of the FLPDL in specific leg telangiectasias. We chose type 1 red telangiectasia less than 0.2 mm in diameter and vessels arising as a function of telangiectatic matting for examination since these vessels are the most difficult to treat with standard sclerotherapy techniques.

In addition, we hypothesized that the use of subtherapeutic concentrations of sclerosing solutions in combination with highly specific laser-induced endothelial damage would result in an enhanced efficacy with laser treatment of larger blood vessels. The combination of FLPDL and sclerotherapy technique (FLPDL/SCL) was hypothesized to result in a decreased incidence of extravasation of erythrocytes and a decrease in perivascular inflammation. Thus FLPDL/SCL would result in a decreased incidence of adverse sequelae (postsclerotherapy hyperpigmentation and TM).

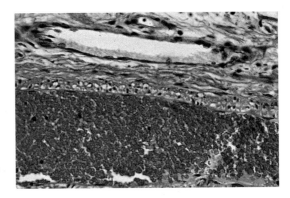

Fig. 12-8   Vessel 1 hour after treatment with FLPDL alone at 8 J/cm². Endothelium is vacuolated. (Hematoxylin-eosin, original magnification ×200.) (Goldman MP et al: J Am Acad Dermatol 23:23, 1990.)

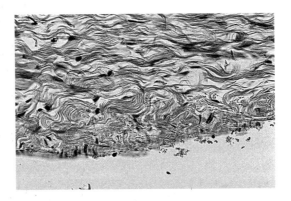

Fig. 12-9   Vessel 1 hour after treatment with FLPDL alone at 9.5 J/cm². There is focal endothelial necrosis with adherence of platelets to damaged endothelium. (Hematoxylin-eosin, original magnification ×400.) (Goldman MP et al: J Am Acad Dermatol 23:23, 1990.)

To demonstrate this novel form of treatment was efficacious, an experimental analysis of the clinical and histologic effects of both FLPDL alone and FLPDL/SCL in the rabbit ear vein was performed. Using this animal model had previously been demonstrated as an accurate method of comparing different sclerosing solutions and concentrations, and it was used also as a guide in choosing the most clinically appropriate laser parameters.[64] The results of these experimental and clinical studies have been reported.[65,66]

All vessels in the rabbit ear vein model treated with the FLPDL alone demonstrated an immediate clinical thrombosis. After 10 days vessels treated with 8 to 9.5 J/cm^2 returned to a clinically normal appearance. Only the vessels treated with 10 J/cm^2 remained clinically sclerosed at 45 days.

Histologically, no evidence of laser-induced vascular damage was apparent at 1 hour or at 2 days in vessels treated with FLPDL at 8 and 8.5 J/cm^2 except for some mild endothelial vacuolization (Fig. 12-8). At 9.0 and 9.5 J/cm^2, focal endothelial necrosis was apparent with intravascular fibrin deposition, thrombosis, and adherence of platelets to the damaged endothelium (Fig. 12-9). At 10 J/cm^2, perivascular heat denaturization of collagen was demonstrated (Fig. 12-10; Table 12-4).

At the study's conclusion on day 45, vessels treated with 8 and 9 J/cm^2 were histologically normal. The vessel treated with 8.5 J/cm^2 showed endosclerosis with microangiopathic recanalization. Endosclerosis and full recanalization were present in the vessel treated with 9.5 J/cm^2 (Fig. 12-11), and complete endosclerosis was present in the vessel treated with 10 J/cm^2 (Fig. 12-12; Table 12-5).

The FLPDL produces vascular injury in a histologic pattern that is different from that produced by sclerotherapy (see box on page 444). An examination of

Table 12-4 FLPDL treatment of 0.4-mm diameter rabbit ear vein: immediate effects

Laser energy (J/cm^2)	Immediate histologic effects
8-8.5	Endothelial vacuolization
9-9.5	Focal endothelial destruction
10	Perivascular thermal effects

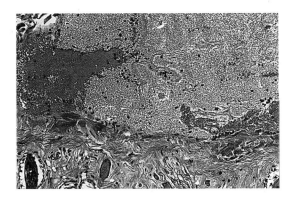

Fig. 12-10   Vessel 1 hour after treatment with FLPDL alone at 10 J/cm^2. Perivascular heat denaturization of collagen is apparent. Also there is extensive homogenization of red blood cells with intravascular fibrin deposition. (Hematoxylin-eosin, original magnification ×200.) (Goldman MP et al: J Am Acad Dermatol 23:23, 1990.)

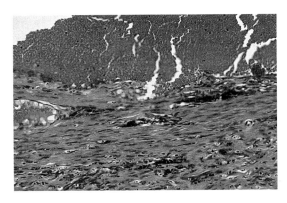

Fig. 12-11   Vessel 2 days after treatment with FLPDL alone at 9.5 J/cm². Focal endothelial necrosis and thrombus formation are present along with margination of white blood cells. (Hematoxylin-eosin, original magnification × 200.) (Goldman MP et al: J Am Acad Dermatol 23:23, 1990.)

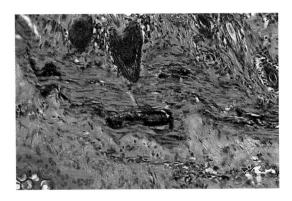

Fig. 12-12   Vessel shown 10 days after treatment with FLPDL alone at 10 J/cm². Advanced endosclerosis is present within organizing thrombosis. (Hematoxylin-eosin, original magnification ×200.) (Goldman MP et al: J Am Acad Dermatol 23:23, 1990.)

Table 12-5   FLPDL treatment of 0.4-mm diameter rabbit ear vein: effects after 48 hours

Laser energy (J/cm²)	Histologic effects after 48 hours
8-10	Intravascular fibrin strands
8-10	Minimal perivascular inflammation
9-10	Thrombosis
10	Endosclerosis

SPECIFIC HISTOLOGIC EFFECTS OF PULSED DYE LASER TREATMENT IN THE RABBIT EAR VEIN

Platelet adherence to endothelium
Perivascular heat denaturization of collagen
Intravascular fibrin strands

Relative decrease in perivascular inflammation
Relative decrease in extravasated red blood cells

the FLPDL-specific histologic effects may explain its theoretically enhanced clinical efficacy. We hypothesized two advantages to gain from this form of treatment: a decreased incidence and/or extent of postsclerosis pigmentation and a decreased incidence and/or extent of telangiectatic matting.

FLPDL TREATMENT OF LEG TELANGIECTASIA: CLINICAL STUDIES

Patients with red leg telangiectasias less than 0.2 mm in diameter were treated with a Candela FLPDL tuned to 585 nm with a pulse duration of 450 μs at energies ranging from 6.0 to 8.5 J/cm^2 delivered through a 5-mm spot size to the entire length of the telangiectasia. Laser impacts were overlapped slightly, with every effort made to treat the entire vessel.

Patients were initially evaluated approximately 2 to 4 weeks after treatment and had a follow-up visit at 4 to 16 months. Garden, Polla, and Tan[59] have discussed the difficulty of objective evaluation of lesional lightening either by the investigator or patient and with or without the use of photographic documentation. Since we have found it is difficult to reproduce identical quality photographs of lesions accurately for comparison by independent investigators, we have elected to use rigid criteria in judging successful outcome of treatment (Fig. 12-13). Therefore patients and investigators graded the response to therapy as 90% to 100% faded, <90% faded, or no change. Pigmentation was also noted. This basic yes-or-no question is a more accurate way for both investigator and patient to evaluate treatment outcome. In truth, patients usually are not satisfied with only partial resolution of their leg veins. Therefore these all-or-none criteria appear practical for the practicing clinician.

Complications

The most significant outcome of FLPDL treatment of leg telangiectasias was the relative lack of adverse sequelae and complications. With FLPDL treatment alone, there were no episodes of TM in the 101 treated sites. (As of this writing we have treated more than 1000 sites of leg telangiectasia, still with no evidence of TM or complications other than those as described.) All patients with hyperpigmentation induced by FLPDL experienced complete resolution within 4 months. There were no episodes of cutaneous ulceration, thrombophlebitis, or other complications (Fig. 12-14).

Effective Energy Levels

Unlike the effective FLPDL energy requirement for the successful treatment of rabbit ear veins, FLPDL treatment of human telangiectasias demonstrates that the most effective laser energy is that between 7.0 and 8.0 J/cm^2 (Table 12-6). At these laser parameters, 48% to 67% of telangiectatic patches totally fade within 4 months.

The percentage of telangiectasias that totally fade increases when only vessels without reticular feeding veins are considered (Table 12-7; Figs. 12-15 and 12-16). There apparently is no difference in the response to FLPDL in TM vessels (Fig. 12-17).

Vessel Location

Many physicians have found that vessel location can affect treatment outcome, with vessels on the medial thigh the most difficult to resolve completely.[67-69] However, with the FLPDL, vessel location apparently is unrelated to treatment outcome if telangiectatic patches with untreated feeding reticular veins are excluded (Table 12-8; Fig. 12-18).   *Text continues on p. 452*

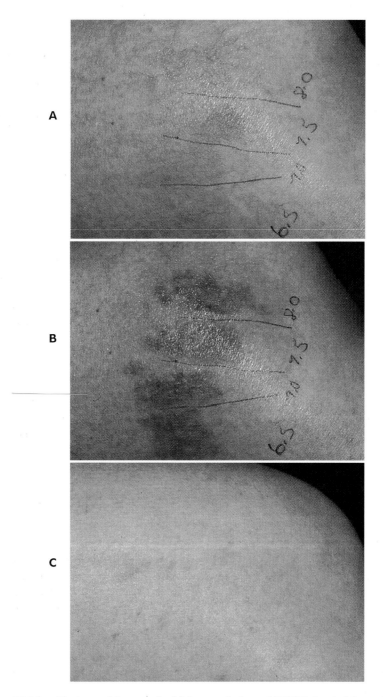

Fig. 12-13 Photographic record of false resolution of FLPDL-treated leg veins. **A,** Treatment site at medial distal thigh with parameters of experimental treatment marked. **B,** Immediately after FLPDL treatment; note extent of purpura. **C,** Same treatment site immediately before marking the skin with laser parameters (taken at different F-stop exposure). Note "false" clearing of vessels.

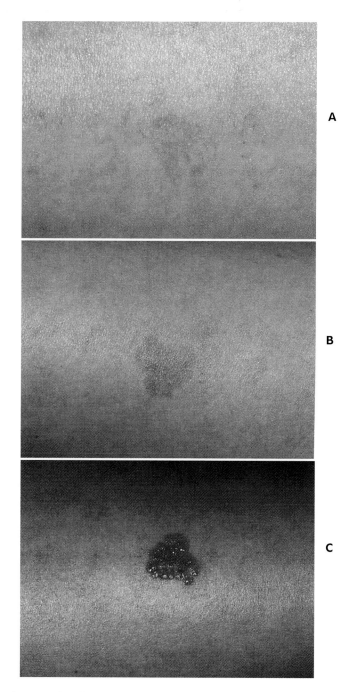

Fig. 12-14 Photographic follow-up of telangiectatic patch on the medial thigh treated with the FLPDL at 7.5 J/cm^2, 15 pulses. **A,** Immediately before treatment. **B,** Immediately after treatment. **C,** 2 days after treatment. Note some nonspecific vesiculation of the skin.

Continued.

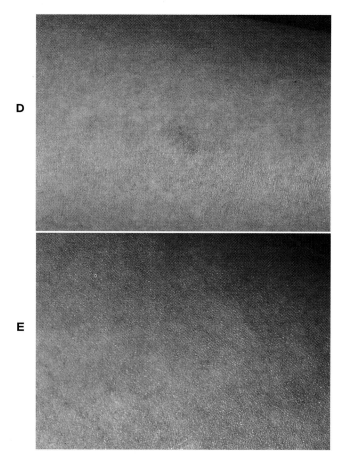

Fig. 12-14, cont'd   D, Vessel shown 11 days after treatment. Note some hypopigmentation and fading of the telangiectasia; purpura no longer present. E, 11 months after treatment showing complete vessel elimination without pigmentary or textural skin changes.

Table 12-6   Results of pulsed dye laser treatment of leg telangiectasia

Laser energy (J/cm²)	No. of sites treated	No change (%)	< 90% faded (%)	Total fade (%)
6.0	1	100		
6.5	4	25	50	25
6.75	7	42	16	42
7.0	25	24	28	48
7.25	30	10	23	67
7.5	23	13	39	48
7.75	6	17	33	50
8.0	3	23		67
8.5	2	100		

Modified from Goldman MP and Fitzpatrick RE: J Dermatol Surg Oncol 16:338, 1990.

Table 12-7 FLPDL treatment of leg telangiectasia: results of vessels without reticular veins

Laser energy (J/cm²)	No. of sites treated	No change (%)	<90% faded (%)	Total fade (%)
7.0	22	23	23	54
7.25	27	11	15	74
7.5	20	10	35	55
7.75	3	0	0	100
8.0	2			100
	—	—	—	—
TOTAL	74	13	19	68

Modified from Goldman MP and Fitzpatrick RE: J Dermatol Surg Oncol 16:338, 1990.

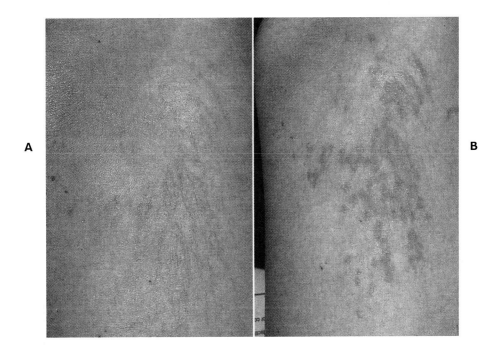

Fig. 12-15 Photographic follow-up of telangiectatic flair on the lateral thigh treated with FLPDL at 7 J/cm², 125 pulses. **A,** Immediately before treatment. **B,** Immediately after treatment. *Continued.*

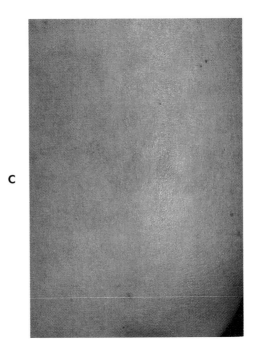

Fig. 12-15, cont'd   C, 6 weeks after treatment; note slight hyperpigmentation and total resolution of telangiectasia. Pigmentation completely faded after 2 to 4 more weeks.

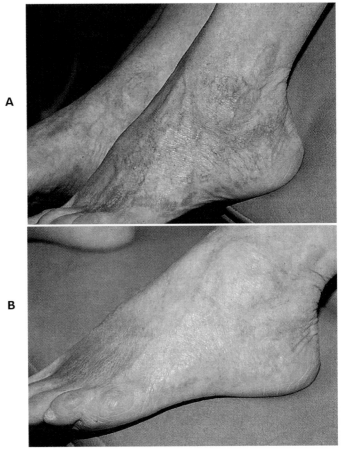

Fig. 12-16   Photographic follow-up of extensive pedal telangiectasia treated on two occasions with the FLPDL at 7.25 J/cm², 84 pulses and 115 pulses. A, Before treatment. B, 6 months after initial treatment; 3 months after second treatment. (Courtesy Richard Fitzpatrick, M.D.)

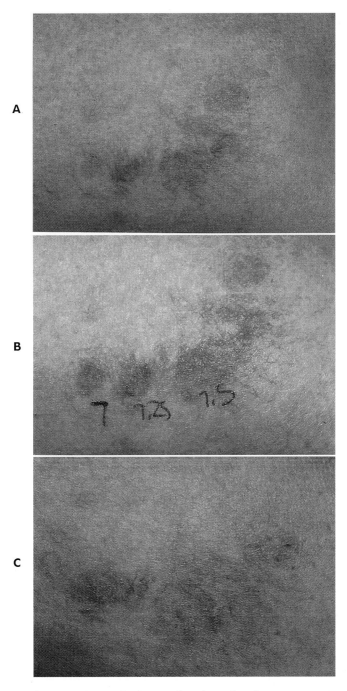

Fig. 12-17   Telangiectatic matting 9 months after sclerotherapy treatment of leg telangiectasia on the medial thigh. **A,** Immediately before treatment. **B,** Immediately after patch tests were performed with the FLPDL, 9 pulses to each site. **C,** 2 months after patch test treatment; note complete vessel resolution in areas treated at laser parameters of 7.25 and 7.5 J/cm^2. Only partial resolution occurred at 7.0 J/cm^2. Some hyperpigmentation is noted.

Continued.

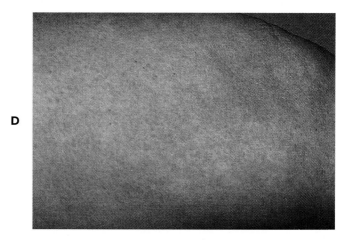

Fig. 12-17, cont'd **D,** 1 year after treatment of the entire area with FLPDL at 7.25 J/cm², 46 pulses; note complete resolution of the telangiectatic mat without pigmentary or textural skin changes.

Table 12-8 Results of pulsed dye laser treatment by vessel location of leg telangiectasia (laser energy: 7-7.75 J/cm²)

Vessel location	No. of sites treated	No change (%)	<90% faded (%)	Total fade (%)
Thigh	35	26	40	34
Thigh*	22	15	20	65
Knee	9	11	11	78
Calf	28	14	18	68
Ankle	6	0	50	50
Foot	13	23	8	69
TOTAL	91	19	25	56

Modified from Goldman MP and Fitzpatrick RE: J Dermatol Surg Oncol 16:338, 1990.
*Minus patients with untreated feeding reticular veins.

Compression

Goldman[70] hypothesized and Goldman et al.[71] found that compression of telangiectatic leg veins improves sclerotherapy treatment outcome and promotes a decreased incidence of adverse sequelae. With FLPDL treatment, no obvious difference appeared in treatment efficacy between telangiectatic patches that were treated with compression and those that were not (Table 12-9).

Conclusions

In conclusion, the FLPDL at 585 nm is an effective modality for treatment of red leg telangiectasia less than or equal to 0.2 mm in diameter. FLPDL treatment is efficacious for both essential telangiectasia and vessels that arise through the phenomenon of TM. This form of treatment used alone has a remarkably low incidence of adverse sequelae.

The optimal clinically useful laser energy in the treatment of red, 0.2-mm diameter telangiectatic mats is between 7.0 and 8.0 J/cm². Treatment is most efficacious if all vessels larger than 0.2 mm in diameter, especially varicose and reticular feeding veins, are treated first. Treatment results are not affected by vessel location. Compression of the vessels after treatment appears unnecessary.

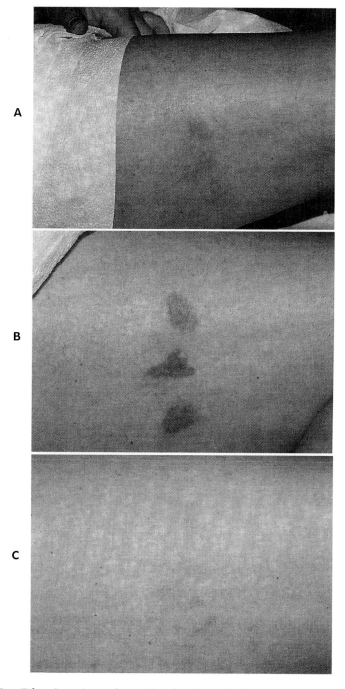

Fig. 12-18   Telangiectatic patches with a feeding reticular vein 2 mm in diameter on the lateral thigh. **A,** Immediately before treatment. **B,** Immediately after treatment with the FLPDL, 20 pulses to each patch: 7.25 J/cm^2, superior patch; 7.5 J/cm^2, medial patch; 7.75 J/cm^2, inferior patch. **C,** 9 months after treatment. Note only partial resolution of the treated areas with persistence of the untreated reticular vein. (Courtesy Richard Fitzpatrick, M.D.)

Table 12-9 Effect of compression combined with pulsed dye laser treatment (laser energy: 7.0-8.0 J/cm²)

	No. of sites treated	No change (%)	<90% faded (%)	Total fade (%)
Compression	39	26	20	54
No compression	44	4	23	73

Modified from Goldman MP and Fitzpatrick RE: J Dermatol Surg Oncol 16:338, 1990.

COMBINED LASER AND SCLEROTHERAPY TREATMENT
Experimental Evaluation of the Clinical and Histologic Effects of Combined FLPDL and Sclerotherapy in the Rabbit Ear Vein Model

Combined FLPDL/SCL therapy has two theoretical advantages: an increase in efficacy of treatment, allowing for successful sclerosis of blood vessels with a diameter >0.2 mm, and a decrease in the most common adverse sequelae of sclerotherapy alone (pigmentation and TM). In addition, the combination of FLPDL and SCL treatments, by its synergistic endosclerotic action, may effectively treat previously untreatable cutaneous telangiectasias (those associated with arteriolar feeding vessel communication).

To summarize, FLPDL/SCL produces cumulative damage that leads to an enhanced efficacy of the sclerosing agent. However, a comparison of the degree and type of endothelial damage histologically does not demonstrate a significant difference between treatment with FLPDL and with FLPDL/SCL (Table 12-10).[65] Pilot studies using a combination of sclerotherapy with POL 0.25% and FLPDL with laser energies of 6 and 7 J/cm² demonstrated no endothelial damage in vessels treated with FLPDL alone at 8 days. The combination of FLPDL at 6 and 7 J/cm² with SCL did demonstrate endothelial vacuolization. Thus it is possible that FLPDL energies less than 8 J/cm² may be successfully combined with sclerotherapy in human leg veins to provide effective therapy.

FLPDL Treatment Combined With Sclerotherapy of Leg Telangiectasia

A study was conducted of 27 patients who had either bilaterally symmetrical telangiectatic patches or a large "starburst" telangiectatic flair that could be divided into two separate treatment sites (Fig. 12-19).[66] These patients were treated at one site with only a FLPDL tuned to 585 nm with a pulse duration of 450 μs at energies ranging from 6.0 to 8.5 J/cm² delivered through a 5-mm spot size to the entire length of the telangiectasia. The other site was treated with laser energies of 5.5 to 8.0 J/cm² immediately before injection of the telangiectasia with POL 0.25%, 0.5%, or 0.75%, a volume of 0.1 to 0.25 ml per injection site.

Of areas treated, 44% completely resolved (Table 12-11; Fig. 12-20). There was little difference in efficacy and adverse sequelae produced with concentrations of POL 0.25% and POL 0.5% (Table 12-12). When two areas were treated with POL 0.75%, ulceration occurred at 7.0 J/cm², and <90% fade was noted at 7.5 J/cm². There apparently was an increased efficacy of treatment with laser energies of 7.5 to 7.75 J/cm². As with FLPDL alone, treatment site location did not appear to affect treatment outcome significantly except for an increased incidence of complications in the ankle and knee areas (Table 12-13; Fig. 12-21).

Text continues on p. 458

Table 12-10 Comparison of endothelial damage resulting from FLPDL and FLPDL/SCL (J/cm²)

| | Laser energy used | |
Type of damage	PDL alone (J/cm²)	PDL + SCL with POL 0.25%
Vacuolization	8-8.5	8
Necrosis	9-9.5	8.5-9.5
Perivascular collagen denaturization	10	10

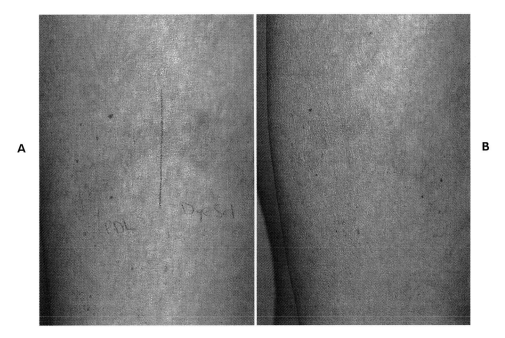

Fig. 12-19 Telangiectatic flair on lateral thigh divided into two treatment sites. Anterior aspect treated with FLPDL at 6 J/cm², 50 pulses, immediately before sclerotherapy with POL 0.25%, 2 ml. Posterior aspect treated with FLPDL at 7 J/cm², 34 pulses. **A**, Immediately before treatment. **B**, 3 months after treatment.

Table 12-11 Results of FLPDL/SCL treatment of leg telangiectasia (all POL concentrations)

Laser energy J/cm²	No. of sites treated	No change (%)	<90% faded (%)	Total fade (%)	Ulceration/ matting (%)
5.5	3		100		
6.0	10	20	30	40	10
7.0	4		25	25	50
7.25	2		50	50	
7.5	7	14	14	72	
7.75	1			100	
	—	—	—	—	—
TOTAL	27	11	33	44	11

Modified from Goldman MP and Fitzpatrick RE: J Dermatol Surg Oncol 16:338, 1990.

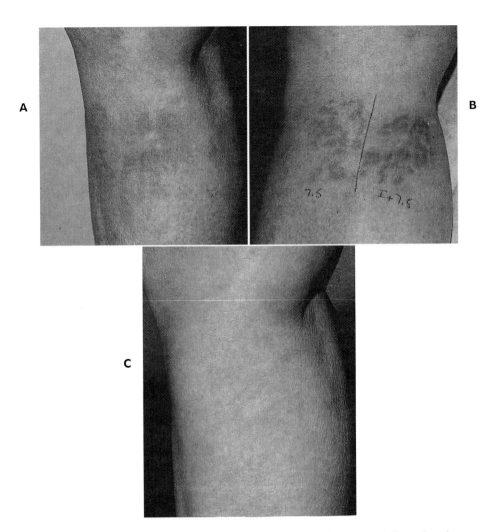

Fig. 12-20 Telangiectatic matting on medial knee and calf 6 months after sclerotherapy. **A,** Immediately before treatment. **B,** Immediately after treatment with FLPDL to anterior aspect at 7.5 J/cm², 51 pulses; posterior aspect treated with FLPDL at 7.5 J/cm², 41 pulses, followed by sclerotherapy with POL0.5%, 1 ml. **C,** 11 months after treatment.

Table 12-12 Results of FLPDL/SCL treatment with FLDPL 0.25% and POL 0.5%

Laser energy J/cm²	No. of sites treated	No change (%)	<90% faded (%)	Total fade (%)	Ulceration/ matting (%)
POL 0.25%					
5.5	1		100		
6.0	6	17	33	33	17
7.0	1			100	
POL 0.5%					
5.5	2		100		
6.0	2	50		50	
7.0	2		50		50
7.25	2		50	50	
7.5	6	17		83	
7.75	1			100	

Modified from Goldman MP and Fitzpatrick RE: J Dermatol Surg Oncol 16:338, 1990.

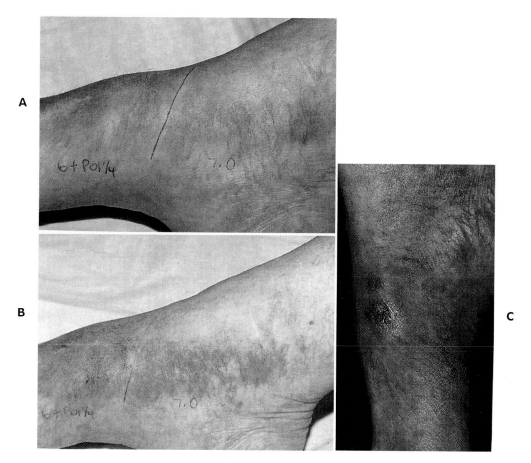

Fig. 12-21 Essential telangiectasia on the feet. Distal aspect treated with FLPDL at 6 J/cm², 114 pulses, immediately followed by sclerotherapy with POL 0.25%, 1 ml. Proximal aspect treated with FLPDL at 7 J/cm², 100 pulses. **A,** Immediately before treatment. **B,** Immediately after treatment. **C,** 4 months after treatment. Note superficial ulceration at the FLPDL/SCL–treated site.

Table 12-13 Results of FLPDL/SCL treatment (all POL concentrations) by vessel location

Vessel location	No. of sites treated	No change (%)	<90% faded (%)	Total fade (%)	Ulceration/ matting (%)
Thigh	8	12	25	63	
Knee	7	28	28	14	28
Calf	7		28	72	
Ankle	3		33	33	33
Foot	1	100			

Modified from Goldman MP and Fitzpatrick RE: J Dermatol Surg Oncol 16:338, 1990.

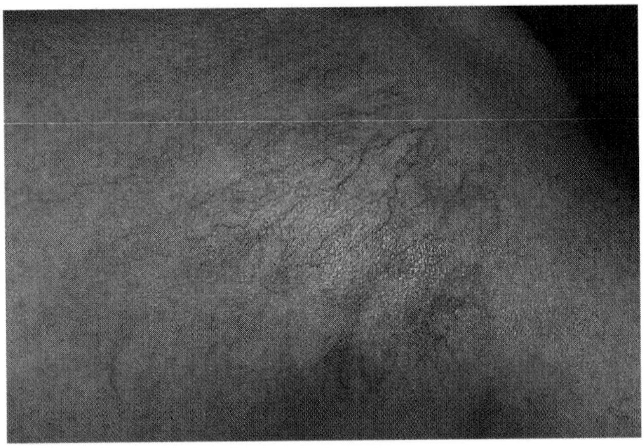

Fig. 12-22 Treatment of telangiectatic matting 7 months after sclerotherapy treatment of telangiectasia on the medial knee. **A,** Immediately before initial sclerotherapy treatment.

Complications

The most significant difference between using FLPDL alone and using FLPDL/SCL was the incidence of complications. With FLPDL/SCL treatment, posttreatment ulceration and TM occurred in 11% of patient treatment areas. Six of 23 nonulcerated treatment sites developed persistent pigmentation that remained unresolved beyond 1 year. Two of 27 sites developed TM that lasted more than 1 year. Four of 27 treatment sites developed superficial ulceration. In these patients with ulceration laser energies were equal to or greater than 6.5 J/cm^2, and POL concentration was equal to or greater than 0.5% (Fig. 12-22).

Conclusions

FLPDL/SCL treatment appears to offer no advantage over FLPDL treatment alone and appears to have a significant degree of complications when treatment is limited to red telangiectasias less than 0.2 mm in diameter. The important points cited for each treatment modality are listed in the boxes on p. 460.

Theoretical evidence suggests that FLPDL/SCL treatment may be more efficacious than either FLPDL or SCL alone in the rabbit ear vein model. However, this result was not demonstrated in human leg telangiectasia less than 0.2 mm in diameter. Future studies on the use of FLPDL/SCL treatment for larger-diameter blood vessels appear necessary. A comparison of the results of both treatment modalities appears in Table 12-14.

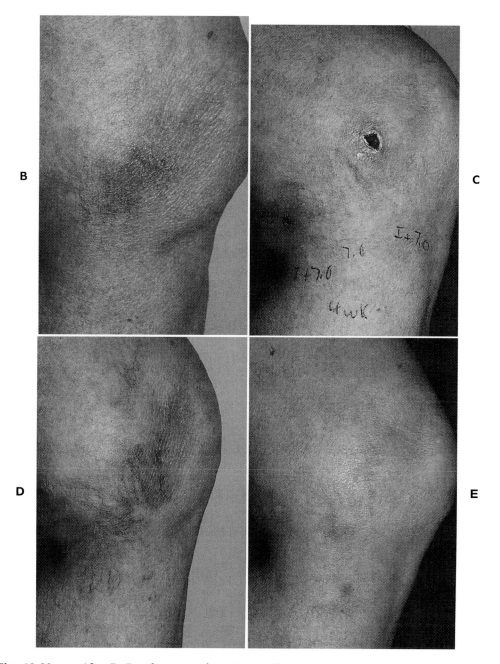

Fig. 12-22, cont'd **B,** Development of persistent telangiectatic matting 7 months after initial treatment. **C,** 3 months after FLPDL and FLPDL/SCL treatment showing the development of a persistent superficial ulceration in the two FLPDL/SCL treatment sites. Anterior site treated with FLPDL at 7 J/cm², 31 pulses, before sclerotherapy with POL 0.5%, 1 ml; medial site treated with FLPDL alone at 7 J/cm², 27 pulses; posterior site treated with FLPDL at 7 J/cm², 31 pulses, before sclerotherapy with POL 0.75, 1 ml. **D,** 7 months after initial FLPDL and FLPDL/SCL treatment showing persistent telangiectatic matting and healing of the ulceration. **E,** 6 months after treatment with chromated glycerin solution (diluted 1:1 with lidocaine 1%), 2 ml. Resolution of the telangiectatic matting has occurred.

FLPDL TREATMENT OF LEG TELANGIECTASIA

Posttreatment pigmentation cleared within 2 to 6 months

No episodes of telangiectatic matting were noted (101 treatment sites)

Optimal laser energy: 7.0 to 8.0 J/cm²

Must treat feeding reticular veins first

Results not affected by treatment location

Compression not necessary

FLPDL/SCLEROTHERAPY TREATMENT OF LEG TELANGIECTASIA

Persistent pigmentation developed in 6 of 34 nonulcerated treatment sites

Persistent telangiectatic matting developed in 2 of 38 sites

Superficial ulceration developed in 4 of 38 sites (Laser energies >6.5 J/cm², polidocanol >0.5%)

Optimal laser energy: 5.5 to 6.0 J/cm²

Optimal polidocanol concentration: 0.25% to 0.5%

Must treat feeding reticular veins first

Results not affected by treatment location

Table 12-14 Results of FLPDL/SCL versus FLPDL alone

Treatment modality	No. of sites treated	No change (%)	<90% faded (%)	Total fade (%)	Ulceration/ matting (%)
FLPDL	91	19	25	56	
FLPDL*	78	15	20	65	
FLPDL/SCL†	27	11	33	44	11

Modified from Goldman MP and Fitzpatrick RE: J Dermatol Surg Oncol 16:338, 1990.
*Minus patients with untreated feeding reticular veins.
†All POL concentrations.

PHOTODERM VL LIGHT SOURCES*

An ideal laser or pulsed light source to treat leg veins should have a wavelength that can penetrate to the full depth of the target blood vessel and deliver sufficient energy to the target vessel to thermocoagulate the entire vessel wall without damage to perivascular tissues or overlying skin. In addition, the energy should be delivered without causing a shock wave to prevent posttreatment purpura. In an effort to maximize efficacy in treating leg veins, a novel pulsed light source has been developed. This new technology is more appropriate for treatment of leg telangiectasia and venules since these vessels are substantially larger and more deeply situated in the skin and have thicker walls than fascial telangiectasia.

*Photoderm VL is a trademark of ESC, Inc., Newton, MA.

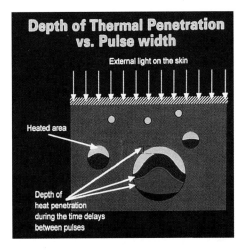

Fig. 12-23   Diagram of the effect of repetitive pulses of the Photoderm light source on a 2-mm vessel 1 mm below the epidermis. (Courtesy Shimon Eckhouse, Ph.D., Energy Systems Corporation, Inc., Newton, Mass.)

To treat larger vessels, energy must be delivered in the range of 3- to 30-ms pulses so absorbed heat from erythrocytes has time to diffuse throughout the vessel circumference. This may require double or triple simultaneous pulses to maximize absorption of light fluence to the vessel while allowing thermal cooling of epidermal and perivascular tissues (Fig. 12-23). To treat deep vascular structures, the wavelength must be long enough to reach not only the top of the vessel beneath the skin, but also the entire diameter of the vessel (Fig. 12-24). A longer wavelength will also minimize coupling to the epidermis, with resulting heat absorption. Finally, because leg telangiectasia and venules have thicker walls than the ectatic vessels of port-wine vascular malformations, higher-energy fluences must be given.

Fortunately, calculated energy absorption for oxygenated and deoxygenated hemoglobin is very different for vessels 1 mm in diameter and 2 mm beneath the dermal-epidermal junction (see Fig. 12-3). In these deeper and larger vessels oxygenated hemoglobin peaks at 920 nm, and deoxygenated hemoglobin has a fairly plateau peak between 660 and 920 nm. Thus using a light source of 600 to 900 nm has the advantage of both penetrating to the proper depth of leg telangiectasia and venules and being selectively absorbed by oxygenated-deoxygenated hemoglobin. This is the basis for the ESC Photoderm VL light source.

The Photoderm VL can deliver energy fluences of 20 to 80 J/cm^2 over 5 to 20 ms and may be repetitively pulsed with delays between pulses of 20 to 1000 ms. This has been demonstrated to thermocoagulate vessels up to 3 mm in diameter 2 mm below the dermal-epidermal junction and telangiectasia 0.2 to 0.6 mm in diameter (Figs. 12-25 and 12-26).

Histologic evaluation demonstrates that the Photoderm VL does not cause vessel rupture, also evidenced by the lack of clinical purpura. Instead, the vessel wall is more slowly heated, producing destruction (Fig. 12-27).

The Photoderm VL delivers its energy through a "footprint" whose size and dimensions can vary based on the requirements of the target vessel. The present machine has a standard footprint, or spot size, of 8 mm $\times$ 35 mm. This permits efficient treatment of large sections of vessels.

To prevent nonspecific damage to overlying skin, clear coupling gel is placed on the skin as a thin layer between the light guide and epidermis. The gel acts as

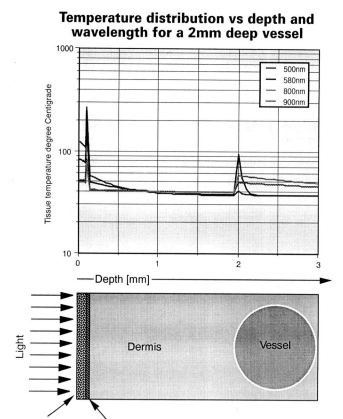

Fig. 12-24 Temperature distribution across skin and blood vessel. A 2-mm deep, 1-mm diameter vessel is assumed. A 10 J/cm² fluence is assumed at 4 different wavelengths. The calculation takes into account scattering effects in the epidermis and dermis and fluence enhancement due to scattering. Note the very high temperature on the skin surface and at the epidermal-dermal junction and the shallow penetration for the shorter wavelengths. (Courtesy of Shimon Eckhouse, Ph.D., ESC, Inc., Newton, Mass.; from Goldman MP and Fitzpatrick RE: Cutaneous laser surgery, St Louis, 1994, Mosby–Year Book.)

a heat sink, absorbing reflected photons from the epidermis to prevent epidermal heating. We have found that the gel must be changed every 5 to 10 pulses, depending on the delivered energy fluence. Spreading a thin layer of gel over the entire treatment area necessitates changing the gel usually once or twice during a treatment session.

At this writing the Photoderm VL is in its final stages of development. Vessels up to 3 mm in diameter have been successfully obliterated without significant adverse sequelae. Patients report less pain as compared with the FLPDL, and treatment sessions are well tolerated. The only noted adverse effect is slight epidermal burning without resultant scarring in patients with Fitzpatrick 3 or greater pigmented skin. Intradermal nevi, lentigines, and other pigmented lesions within the treated area often disappear after treatment.

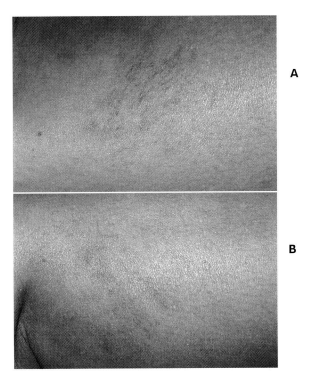

Fig. 12-25 Clinical appearance of telangiectasia on the thigh of a 32-year-old woman. A, Before treatment. B, Clinical appearance 10 weeks after treatment.

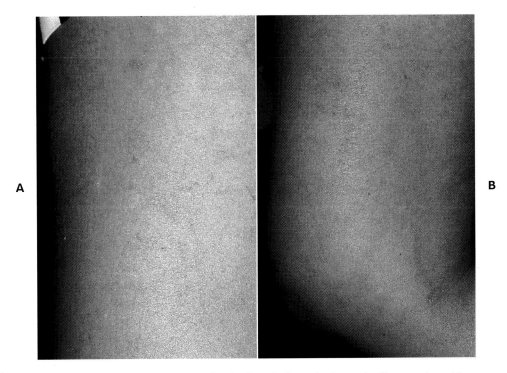

Fig. 12-26 Clinical appearance of a thigh reticular vein 3 mm in diameter in a 40-year-old woman. A, Before treatment. B, 6 weeks after treatment with a 590 nm cutoff filter at a fluence of 44 J/cm^L given in 2 pulses of 6.5 to 15 msec separated by a 100 msec delay.

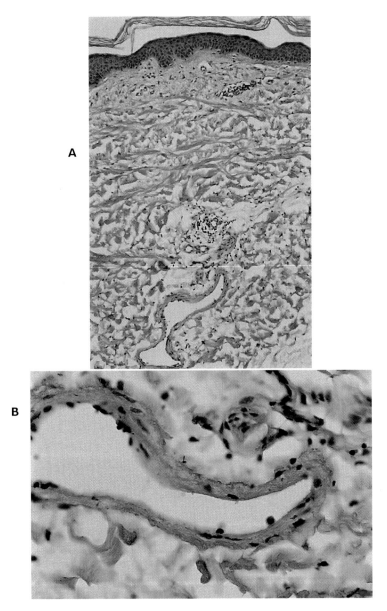

Fig. 12-27   Appearance of venule 1 mm in diameter stained with hematoxylin-eosin 48 hours after treatment with the Photoderm VL at 26 J/cm², delivered in a double pulse 6-ms and 15-ms long separated by 50 ms. **A,** Note size and depth of vessel, which appears collapsed from biopsy and processing artifacts but devoid of blood; original magnification ×50. **B,** Same vessel as in **A.** Note intravascular margination of mast cell and lymphocytes with partial destruction of endothelium and vessel wall; original magnification ×200.

CONCLUSIONS

Laser or light treatment of leg veins has the advantage of being relatively noninvasive (no needles) and nontoxic (no injection of sclerosing solution). Theoretically, decreased inflammation should also prevent the development of TM, and thermocoagulation should prevent extravasation of red blood cells to limit posttreatment hyperpigmentation. However, high-pressure reflux from incompetent perforator, reticular, or varicose veins must first be treated either surgically or with sclerotherapy before laser or photothermocoagulation can be expected to be effective.

REFERENCES

1. Anderson RR: Laser-tissue interactions. In Goldman MP and Fitzpatrick RE, editors: Cutaneous laser surgery, St Louis, 1994, Mosby.
2. Kaplan I and Peled I: The carbon dioxide laser in the treatment of superficial telangiectasias, Br J Plast Surg 28:214, 1975.
3. Apfelberg DB et al: Use of the argon and carbon dioxide lasers for treatment of superficial venous varicosities of the lower extremity, Lasers Surg Med 4:221, 1984.
4. Apfelberg DB et al: Study of three laser systems for treatment of superficial varicosities of the lower extremity, Lasers Surg Med 7:219, 1987.
5. Pfeifer JR and Hawtof GD: Injection sclerotherapy and CO_2 laser sclerotherapy in the ablation of cutaneous spider veins of the lower extremity, Phlebologie 4:231, 1989.
6. Landthaler M et al: Laser therapy of venous lakes (Bean-Walsh) and telangiectasias, Plast Reconstr Surg 73:78, 1984.
7. Dolsky RL: Argon laser skin surgery, Surg Clin North Am 64:861, 1984.
8. van Gemert MJC and Henning JPH: A model approach to laser coagulation of dermal vascular lesions, Arch Dermatol Res 270:429, 1981.
9. Finley JL et al: Argon laser port-wine stain interaction: immediate effects, Arch Dermatol 120:613, 1984.
10. Arndt KA: Treatment techniques in argon laser therapy: comparison of pulsed and continuous exposures, J Am Acad Dermatol 11:90, 1984.
11. Apfelberg DB, Maser MR, and Lash H: Argon laser management of cutaneous vascular deformities: a preliminary report, West J Med 124:99, 1976.
12. Apfelberg DB et al: Analysis of complications of argon laser treatment for port-wine hemangiomas with reference to striped technique, Lasers Surg Med 2:357, 1983.
13. Apfelberg DB, Maser MR, and Lash H: Treatment of nevi aranei by means of an argon laser, J Dermatol Surg Oncol 4:172, 1978.
14. Lyons GD, Owens RE, and Mouney DF: Argon laser destruction of cutaneous telangiectatic lesions, Laryngoscope 91:1322, 1981.
15. Remington BK: Argon laser therapy—rosacea, telangiectasia (letter to the editor), J Dermatol Surg Oncol 9:424, 1983.
16. Goldman L: Application of laser therapy. Paper presented at the Noah Worcester Dermatologic Society, Hilton Head, SC, April 1984.
17. Arndt IA: Argon laser therapy of small cutaneous vascular lesions, Arch Dermatol 118:219, 1982.
18. Dixon JA, Huether S, and Rotering RH: Hypertrophic scarring in argon laser treatment of port-wine stains, Plast Reconstr Surg 73:771, 1984.
19. Ratz JL, Goldman L, and Bauman WE: Post treatment complications of the argon laser, Arch Dermatol 121:714, 1985.
20. Landthaler M et al: Argon laser treatment of naevi flammei, Hautarzt 38:652, 1987.
21. Olbricht SM et al: Complications of cutaneous laser surgery: a survey, Arch Dermatol 123:345, 1987.
22. Bonafe JL et al: Hyperpigmentation induced by argon laser therapy of hemangiomas: optimal and electron microscope studies, Dermatologica 170:225, 1985.
23. Ginsbach G: New aspects in the management of benign cutaneous tumors. Laser 79 H Opto-Electronics, Conference Proc, Munich, West Germany, 1979, International Optical Society.
24. Rotteleur G et al: Robotized scanning laser handpiece for the treatment of port-wine stains and other angiodysplasias, Lasers Surg Med 8:283, 1988.
25. Apfelberg DB et al: Dot or pointillistic method for improvement in results of hypertrophic scarring in the argon laser treatment of port-wine hemangiomas, Lasers Surg Med 6:552, 1987.
26. Apfelberg DB and McBurney E: Use of the argon laser in dermatologic surgery. In Ratz JL, editor: Lasers in cutaneous medicine and surgery, Chicago, 1986, Year Book Medical Publishers, Inc.
27. Craig RDP et al: Argon laser therapy for cutaneous lesions, Br J Plast Surg 38:148, 1985.
28. Apfelberg DB et al: Use of the argon and carbon dioxide lasers for treatment of superficial venous varicosities of the lower extremity, Lasers Surg Med 4:221, 1984.
29. Dixon JA, Rotering RH, and Huether SE: Patient's evaluation of argon laser therapy of port-wine stain, decorative tattoo, and essential telangiectasia, Lasers Surg Med 4:181, 1984.

30. Dixon JA and Gilbertson JJ: Cutaneous laser therapy. In Hightech Medicine (Special Issue), West J Med 143:758, 1985.

31. Greenwald J et al: Comparative histological studies of the tunable dye (577 nm) laser and argon laser: the specific vascular effects of the dye laser, J Invest Dermatol 77:305, 1981.

32. Haina D et al: Comparison of maximum coagulation depth in human skin for different types of medical lasers, Lasers Surg Med 7:355, 1987.

33. Gilchrist BA, Rosen S, and Noe JM: Chilling port-wine stains improves the response to argon laser therapy, Plast Reconstr Surg 69:278, 1982.

34. Dreno B et al: The benefit of chilling in argon laser treatment of port wine stains, Plast Reconstr Surg 75:42, 1985.

35. Welch AJ, Motamedi M, and Gonzales A: Evaluation of cooling techniques for the protection of the epidermis during Nd:YAG laser radiation of the skin. In Joeffe SN, editor: Neodymium-YAG laser in medicine and surgery, New York, 1983, Elsevier.

36. Yanai A et al: Argon laser therapy of port-wine stains: effects and limitations, Plast Reconstr Surg 75:520, 1985.

37. Chess C and Chess Q: Cool laser optics treatment of large telangiectasia of the lower extremities, J Dermatol Surg Oncol 19:74, 1993.

38. Bruck LB: Micro-contact argon laser probe may enhance therapy, Dermatol Times, p 15, October 1988.

39. Fitzpatrick RE: Unpublished observations, 1988.

40. Smith T et al: 532-nanometer green laser beam treatment of superficial varicosities of the lower extremities, Lasers Surg Med 8:130, 1980.

41. Anderson RR and Parrish JA: Microvasculature can be selectively damaged using dye lasers: a basic theory and experimental evidence in human skin, Lasers Surg Med 1:263, 1981.

42. van Gemert MJC, Welch AJ, and Amin AP: Is there an optimal laser treatment for port-wine stains? Lasers Surg Med 6:76, 1986.

43. Hulsbergen Henning JP, van Gemert MJC, and Lahaye CTW: Clinical and histological evaluation of port-wine stain treatment with a microsecond-pulsed dye-laser at 577 nm, Lasers Surg Med 4:375, 1984.

44. Tan OT, Kerschmann R, and Parrish JA: The effect of epidermal pigmentation on selective vascular effects of pulsed laser, Lasers Surg Med 4:365, 1985.

45. Tong AKF et al: Ultrastructure: effects of melanin pigment on target specificity using a pulsed-dye laser (577 nm), J Invest Dermatol 88:747, 1987.

46. Nakagawa H, Tan OT, and Parrish JA: Ultrastructural changes in human skin after exposure to a pulsed laser, J Invest Dermatol 84:396, 1985.

47. Tan OT, Murray S, and Kurban AK: Action spectrum of vascular specific injury using pulsed irradiation, J Invest Dermatol 92:868, 1989.

48. Anderson R and Parrish JA: The optics of human skin, J Invest Dermatol 77:13, 1981.

49. Kurban AK, Sherwood KA, and Tan OT: What are the optimal wavelengths for selective vascular injury? Lasers Surg Med 8:190, 1988.

50. Goldman L et al: 600 nm flash pumped dye laser for fragile telangiectasia of the elderly, Lasers Surg Med 13:227, 1993.

51. Anderson RR and Parrish JA: Selective photothermolysis: precise microsurgery by selective absorption of pulsed radiation, Science 220:524, 1983.

52. Garden JM et al: Effect of dye laser pulse duration on selective cutaneous vascular injury, J Invest Dermatol 87:653, 1986.

53. Glassberg E et al: The flashlamp-pumped 577-nm pulsed tunable dye laser: clonical efficacy and in vitro studies, J Dermatol Surg Oncol 14:1200, 1988.

54. Tan TT et al: Histologic responses of port-wine stains treated by argon, carbon dioxide, and tunable dye lasers: a preliminary report, Arch Dermatol 122:1016, 1986.

55. Gange RW et al: Effect of preirradiation tissue target temperature upon selective vascular damage induced by 577-nm tunable dye laser pulses, Microvasc Res 28:125, 1980.

56. Glassberg E et al: Cellular effects of the pulsed tunable dye laser at 577 nanometers on human endothelial cells, fibroblasts, and erythrocytes: an in vitro study, Lasers Surg Med 3:567, 1988.

57. Anderson RR, Jaenicke KF, and Parrish JA: Mechanisms of selective vascular changes caused by dye lasers, Lasers Surg Med 3:211, 1983.

58. Morelli JG et al: Tunable dye laser (577 nm) treatment of port-wine stains, Lasers Surg Med 6:94, 1986.

59. Garden JM, Polla LL, and Tan OT: The treatment of port-wine stains by the pulsed-dye laser: analysis of pulse duration and long-term therapy, Arch Dermatol 124:889, 1988.

60. Garden JM et al: The pulsed-dye laser for the treatment of port-wine stains, J Dermatol Surg Oncol 12:757, 1986.

61. Garden JM et al: The pulsed-dye laser as a modality for treating cutaneous small blood vesesl disease processes, Lasers Surg Med 6:259, 1986.
62. Garden JM, Tan OT, and Parrish JA: The pulsed-dye laser: its use at 577-nm wavelength, J Dermatol Surg Oncol 13:134, 1987.
63. Polla LL et al: Tunable pulsed dye laser for the treatment of benign cutaneous vascular ectasia, Dermatologica 174:11, 1987.
64. Goldman MP et al: Sclerosing agents in the treatment of telangiectasia: comparison of the clinical and histologic effects of intravascular polidocanol, sodium tetradecyl sulfate, hypertonic saline in the dorsal rabbit ear vein model, Arch Dermatol 123:1196, 1987.
65. Goldman MP et al: Pulsed-dye laser treatment of telangiectases with and without sub-therapeutic sclerotherapy: clinical and histologic examination of the rabbit ear vein model, J Am Acad Dermatol 23:23, 1990.
66. Goldman MP and Fitzpatrick RE: Pulsed-dye laser treatment of leg telangiectasia: with and without simultaneous sclerotherapy, J Dermatol Surg Oncol 16:338, 1990.
67. Duffy DM: Small vessel sclerotherapy: an overview. In Callen JP et al, editors: Advances in dermatology, vol 3, Chicago, 1988, Year Book Medical Publishers, Inc.
68. Green D: Compression sclerotherapy techniques, Dermatol Clin 7:137, 1989.
69. Ouvry PA: Telangiectasia and sclerotherapy, J Dermatol Surg Oncol 15:177, 1989.
70. Goldman MP: Compression in the treatment of leg telangiectasia: theoretical considerations, J Dermatol Surg Oncol 15:184, 1989.
71. Goldman MP et al: Compression in the treatment of leg telangiectasia: a preliminary report, J Dermatol Surg Oncol 16:322, 1990.

13 SETTING UP A SCLEROTHERAPY PRACTICE

DECIDING WHO WILL DELIVER PATIENT CARE

Before proceeding with the practical aspects of establishing a practice, one must decide who will deliver patient care. Most physicians agree that the sclerotherapy procedure should be performed by a physician; however, some clinics use nurses to treat "spider" telangiectasias. A survey of the membership of the North American Society of Phlebology (NASP) found that approximately 25% of the members would allow a registered nurse and 20% would allow a nurse practitioner to perform sclerotherapy on spider veins.[1] Of NASP members surveyed, 10% would allow a registered nurse to perform sclerotherapy on varicose veins versus 7% who would allow nurse practitioners to perform this procedure. Using registered nurses to perform intravenous therapeutic injections is legal in the state of California. Checking with your state licensing board for nursing for the specific requirements in your state is recommended.

The arguments for allowing nurses to render such care are both economic and procedural. An economic benefit is realized for both the patient and the physician if a lower-salaried person performs the sclerotherapy procedure, and in these days of cost containment, this issue does assume importance. Since the injection of spider veins is primarily cosmetic and is rarely fully reimbursable under most insurance plans, cost containment is translated into economic marketing.

Because the cannulation of a blood vessel is relatively easy to perform and there are relatively few serious or life-threatening complications that can arise from sclerotherapy treatment of spider telangiectasias, an argument can be made for using nonphysicians as sclerotherapists. On the other hand, although they are rare, serious complications can occur as a result of injection of spider telangiectasias. Anaphylactic allergic reactions do occur with the use of many sclerosing agents; a fatality was recently reported that occurred as a result of a "trial" injection of sodium tetradecyl sulfate.[2] Pulmonary emboli also have occurred from the injection of a leg telangiectasia (see Chapter 8). Injection into an arteriovenous anastomosis usually produces a cutaneous ulceration, and cutaneous ulceration from sclerotherapy injection (extravasation and/or arteriolar injection) is the most common reason (in sclerotherapy) for medical malpractice litigation. Injection into a superficial artery, especially around the malleoli, theoretically can lead to arterial embolism and pedal gangrene. Thus as with most of medicine, sclerotherapy is not entirely risk free.

In addition to being skilled at sclerotherapy technique, the sclerotherapist must have a thorough knowledge of the anatomy and pathophysiology of venous disease and of the mechanism of action of the procedure, including its potential complications. The ability to appreciate these mechanisms and immediately recognize potential complications and render preventive treatment is critical to maintaining optimal patient care.

The role of the nurse in a sclerotherapy-phlebology practice was recently reviewed.[3] Hallgren et al. defined basic nursing assessment skills and the requirements for transfer of function. In short, for a nurse to function as a sclerotherapist the following must be known:

1. Nature and purpose of the procedure
2. Specific conditions under which the procedure may be performed
3. Complications of the procedure and methods for notifying the physician and stabilizing the patient with immediate countermeasures
4. Knowledge of the mechanism of action and potential side effects of sclerosing solutions
5. Contraindications to sclerotherapy

This knowledge base should also include instruction so that the nurse can do the following:

1. Record appropriate physical findings such as size, location, and type of vein and associated cutaneous manifestations of venous hypertension
2. Recognize and describe the presence and extent of superficial and deep thrombophlebitis and venous ulceration
3. Perform a noninvasive physical examination to include identifying the presence or absence of reflux from the saphenofemoral or saphenopopliteal junctions and/or perforator veins through venous Doppler examination; perform photoplethysmography
4. Photograph the patient's leg in four general views and specific close-up views to document preexisting cutaneous irregularities and the specific area of telangiectasia
5. Complete detailed mapping of the varicose and telangiectatic leg veins
6. Locate pedal pulses; determine the brachial and ankle blood pressures to determine the degree of arterial insufficiency
7. Accurately measure and fit the patient with a graduated compression stocking
8. Apply a graduated compression bandage

In conclusion, nurses who practice phlebology must be actively involved in the practice of nursing when delivering care. They should be able not only to prepare the operating room for the procedure, but also to prepare the patient for the procedure by answering questions, allaying fears, and documenting pretreatment disease. In addition, follow-up treatments allow the nurse the opportunity to reinforce patient teaching so that preventive measures can be emphasized.

EQUIPMENT

Relatively little specialized equipment is required to perform successful sclerotherapy. In the future certain types of lasers may be available for treating specific types of leg veins (see Chapter 12). For now all that is required is a needle, syringe, sclerosing solution, binocular loupe, foam pads, tape, graduated support stockings, and camera. (See Appendix F for information on manufacturers.)

Needles

The injection of telangiectasias requires a fine-gauge needle. It is useful to have a needle with a clear plastic hub instead of a metal hub to allow visualization with aspiration. Although some physicians prefer to use a 32- to 33-gauge or 26- to 27-gauge needle, I prefer the 30-gauge needle. There are two types of 30-gauge needles. One is the Becton-Dickinson (B-D) Precision Glide needle, which has an elongated bevel on a $\frac{1}{2}$-inch needle with a 45-degree angle at the tip. The needle can be easily bent at varying angles to penetrate telangiectasias. In addition, it is relatively sharp and holds up well when used for multiple punctures of the skin. The second type is a tri-bevel tipped needle. The Acuderm and Delasco 30-gauge needles have a $\frac{1}{2}$-inch metal hub and a silicone-coated tri-bevel point. This type is preferred because its silicone coating and more acute angle at the tip allow it to pierce the skin with less pain. In addition, the length of the bevel is shorter than that of the B-D needle. Accordingly, extravasation of solution perivascularly while the needle is in the vessel lumen is less likely. Tri-beveling of the tip also makes it harder so that it retains its sharpness with multiple injections. A comparison of the bevels of all of the recommended needles is shown in Fig. 13-1. However, even with this magnified comparison, the differences between the needle tips cannot be fully appreciated. Clinical trials using each needle type are necessary to discern the subtle differences.

One objection to the use of a 30-gauge needle has been the perception that it dulls after multiple insertions into the skin. Microscopic examination of tri-beveled needles used to pierce the skin up to 15 times in my patients did not show the needle tip had dulled.

Some sclerotherapists advise the use of a 33-gauge needle to cannulate the smallest diameter telangiectasia. Multiple 31- to 33-gauge $\frac{1}{2}$-inch needles have recently become available (Fig. 13-2). These needles have several drawbacks. They are more expensive than 30-gauge needles and must be cleaned and sterilized between patients if they are not disposed of (this is of concern to patients who fear inadequate sterilization with the subsequent risk of blood-borne

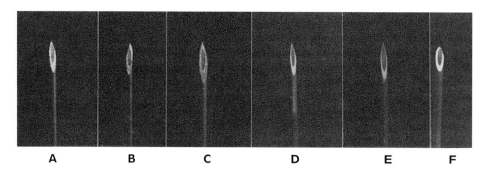

| A | B | C | D | E | F |

Fig. 13-1 Comparison of bevels of recommended needles. **A,** Acuderm needle, 30 gauge. **B,** Becton-Dickinson (B-D) needle, 30 gauge. **C,** Yale needle (B-D), 27 gauge. **D,** Yale needle (B-D), 26 gauge. **E,** Butterfly needle (Abbott), 25 gauge. **F,** Butterfly needle (Abbott), 23 gauge.

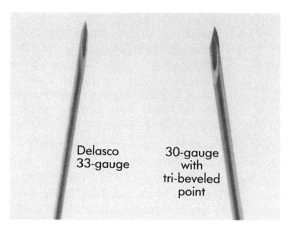

Delasco
33-gauge

30-gauge
with
tri-beveled
point

Fig. 13-2 Comparison of 33-gauge Delasco needle tip with a 30-gauge tri-bevel point. (Courtesy Dermatologic Lab and Supply, Inc.)

pathogens). Repetitive sterilization also dulls the needle point. In addition, the tips of these needles bend and dull more quickly than those of the 30-gauge needles, and the needle shafts are thinner and thus less stable during injections through tough skin. John Phiffer, M.D., (personal communication, 1992) reported recently on the construction of a rigid shaft used to support the 32-gauge needle tip to help stabilize it. However, as mentioned previously (Chapter 11), I find these needles of little use.

Finally, some physicians prefer 26- or 27-gauge needles for injecting telangiectasias. Again the preference arises from a perceived sharpness of the bevel, allowing easier, more painless insertion. The 27-gauge needle comes separately in a $\frac{1}{2}$-inch length as either a Yale hypodermic needle or as an allergy needle-syringe combination fixed to a 1-mm syringe. The benefit of using the 1-mm syringe is the ease of handling perceived by some sclerotherapists. The Yale 26-gauge needle also comes in a $\frac{1}{2}$-inch length and has the advantage of a sturdy, nonbendable shaft. In short, all types have their advantages and disadvantages. The best needle is the one with which the physician is most comfortable.

Larger needles are used most often to inject varicose veins. When injecting varicose veins, it is critical to determine the proper placement of the needle. Therefore the smallest recommended needle size is 25 gauge (23 gauge if there is any doubt whether the vessel to be cannulated is an artery or vein or if a highly caustic sclerosing solution is being used). Larger-bore needles offer no additional advantage. A 25-gauge needle easily allows retrograde blood flow through the inserted needle, which aids in determining if placement is intravenous or intra-arterial.

The surest method of determining proper needle placement is to insert an open needle into the vein. With this technique blood flow from the needle serves as the indicator of arterial versus venous injection. In an effort to avoid blood exposure, some sclerotherapists attach a syringe to the needle and withdraw to determine flow. Still others combine the needle with a glass syringe to "feel" for proper intravascular placement.

To take advantage of the safety of a large-gauge needle without incurring the risk of blood contamination, a 21-, 23-, or 25-gauge butterfly needle may be used. The needle length is $\frac{3}{4}$ inch, and the tubing is 30 cm. The plastic tubing on the proximal end of the needle allows visualization of arterial versus venous flow without risking blood exposure. The tubing takes up 0.41 ml of fluid. Some physicians fill the needle tubing with sclerosing solution to prevent the blood's clotting within the needle tubing. However, if the injection is performed within a few minutes of blood aspiration, this is not necessary.

Syringes

Although glass syringes have been used in the past to allow easy detection of an arterial puncture, modern plastic syringes have a feel comparable to that of glass syringes. The disadvantages of the glass syringe are that it requires practice both to fill and to use smoothly and it must be cleaned and sterilized between patients.

The 3-ml plastic syringe, Luer Lok or nonLuer Lok, is used exclusively in my practice. This syringe allows the use of an ideal quantity of solution, and when filled to a 2-ml capacity, it fits easily in the palm of the hand. A nonLuer-Lok syringe has the advantage of causing the needle hub to separate from the syringe if resistance, which indicates noncannulation of a vessel, is encountered.

If one does not bend the needle to facilitate penetration of the vein, the Plastipak eccentric syringe (Fig. 13-3) is useful. With this syringe, the hub is eccentrically placed at the syringe tip so that it abuts the skin surface. It is available in 1-ml, 2-ml, 5-ml, and 10-ml sizes.

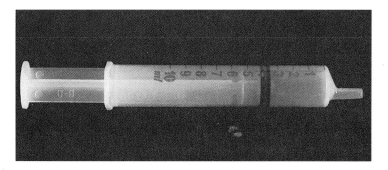

Fig. 13-3 Plastipak eccentric syringe by Becton-Dickinson. Note eccentrically placed hub.

Sclerosing Solutions

The various sclerosing solutions available are discussed in detail in Chapter 7. The addresses of the manufacturers and distributors of these solutions are listed in Appendix B.

Binocular Loupes

Protective eyeglasses are necessary equipment for the physician who performs any surgical procedure. These glasses should be constructed to prevent the splatter or spray of body fluids (blood) from coming in contact with the orbital tissues, thus helping to prevent the physician's contamination with infectious, bloodborne viral or bacterial disease. It is recommended that protective glasses be worn when performing sclerotherapy.

The injection treatment of varicose veins does not require magnification of the surgical field. However, when one is cannulating venulectases or telangiectasias, magnification of the treatment site is important. The enhanced detail that magnification affords allows more accurate placement of the needle within the vessel lumen, which prevents extravasation of the sclerosing solution into extravascular spaces.

To magnify the field of vision, one moves closer to the viewed object to enlarge its field on the retina. Moving closer to an object requires the eyes to refocus and converge more. The consequences of maintaining this close focusing distance are eye strain and back muscle stress. Eye tension and muscle fatigue may then occur, which tends to reduce efficiency. Optical magnification offers an alternative to such strain and allows maintenance of a more comfortable working distance.

The magnifying loupe allows the focusing and converging systems of the eye to relax. The loupe also allows one to switch back and forth between normal vision and magnified vision as necessary. This versatility is relaxing to the eyes. Viewing through magnification for long periods is not harmful and cannot damage vision. The only question is, "How much magnification is necessary?"

The ideal magnifier provides a wide field of view with distortion-free magnification within a reasonably long working distance. Unfortunately, with presently available optics, the higher the magnification, the smaller are the field of view and depth of field. Complex, multilens binocular magnifiers overcome some of the limitations of short working distances. Some of these magnifiers are detailed in Appendix F. An independent evaluation of magnifiers for use in dermatology appears in another source.[4]

Two types of optics are commonly available. Gallilean optics are shorter and lightweight but have a mild distortion (10%) at the periphery. Prismatic optics

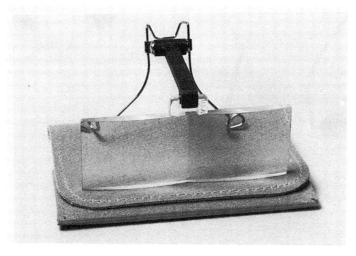

Fig. 13-4   Almore Clip-On Loupe. (Courtesy Almore International.)

Table 13-1   Comparison of loupe magnification

| | Refractive power | | |
Measurement	3 diopters	5 diopters	8 diopters
Magnification	×1.75	×2.25	×3
Lens-to-object distance	8-34 cm	13-20 cm	10 cm
Eye-to-object distance	17-45 cm	22-36 cm	20-25 cm
Field of view	8 cm	4 cm	2 cm
Depth of field	25 cm	8 cm	1 cm

have a narrower field of vision but have no lateral distortion. The prismatic optics require more light than the Gallilean optics because of their increased length.

When choosing the proper magnification, five factors must be addressed: magnification, lens-to-object distance, eye-to-object distance, field of view, and depth of field. Table 13-1 shows a comparison of these factors in regard to a person with normal focusing-converging ability. Note that magnifications greater than 5 diopters decrease the field of view and depth of focusing sufficiently to make their use impractical for sclerotherapy. In my experience lenses with 2× to 3× power provide the ideal combination of focal distance and magnification.

Magnifying glasses

Half-frame clip-on lens are available in multiple powers. The most useful is a 5-diopter, 2.25×-power lens with a 19-cm focal distance. These lenses produce marked peripheral distortion but have a usable field of view of 7 cm for the 3-diopter and 5 cm for the 5-diopter lens. The working distance from lens to object is 17 cm for the 3-diopter and 12 cm for the 5-diopter lens (Fig. 13-4). This type of magnification aid is available from most opticians and department stores.

Headband-mounted simple binocular magnifiers

Headband-mounted magnifiers are available equipped with interchangeable lens plates that provide a range of magnification from 1.5× to 3.5× (Fig. 13-5). These magnifiers can be worn comfortably over prescription eyeglasses. The most

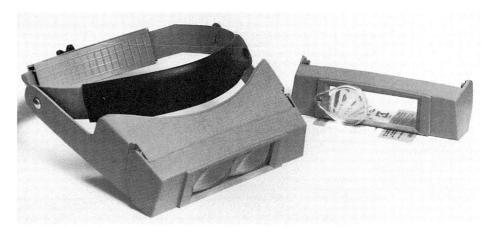

Fig. 13-5   Mark II Magni-Focuser. (Courtesy Edroy Products Co., Inc.)

widely used magnifications with the least peripheral distortion and best working distance are 2× and 2.5×. An optional Optiloupe attachment lens adds 2.5× magnification to any base lens but has a very small field of view without distortion. These magnifiers are available from many manufacturers and vary in price, type of headgear padding, and adjustability; Optivisor and Mark II Magni-focuser are two examples.

Simple binocular loupes

The Precision binocular loupe comes with varying diopter loupes fitted on a double-hinged telescoping rod so that the eye-to-object distance can be adjusted. It also comes with an adjustable bridge-of-nose-to-lens distance of 9 to 21 cm, thus increasing the eye-to-object distance from 19 to 44 cm depending on the diopter used. The 3-diopter lens has a 13-cm usable field of view and a working distance of 16 cm from lens to object. The 5-diopter lens has a 10-cm field of usable view and a working distance of 13 cm from lens to object. It is available with 3-, 5-, or 8-diopter lenses[5] (Fig. 13-6) and is also available as a multidistance headband-mounted loupe. Available powers include 1.5×, 1.75×, 2.25×, and 2.75×, with working distances from 50 to 15 cm, respectively.

Multilens binocular magnifiers

Multilens binocular magnifiers are referred to as *binocular loupes, telescopic magnifiers,* and *surgical telescopes.* They are available in magnifications ranging from 2× to 8× and are designed to provide a working distance of 25 to 40 cm. Their drawback is their significantly higher expense and limited field of view. However, the entire field is usually not distorted; thus the nondistorted portion of the field of view approaches that of lesser-quality magnifiers. Some high-quality binocular loupes have a field of view larger than that of other brand models; therefore one should compare many loupes. These loupes are used exclusively in my practice and are recommended for both sclerotherapy and multiple surgical procedures.

Epstein[4] has found the Designs for Vision loupe best suited for dermatologic examination. The working distance of this loupe is 35 cm for the 3.5× and 40 cm for the 2.5× magnifier.

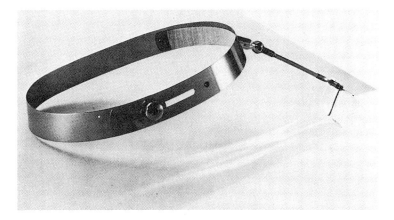

Fig. 13-6   Almore +3-diopter loupe. (Courtesy Almore International.)

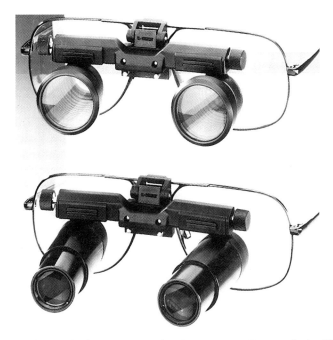

Fig. 13-7   Heine binocular loupe. *Top,* Series G, 2× power. *Bottom,* Series K, 3.5× power. (Courtesy Delasco, Dermatologic Lab and Supply, Inc.)

Heine binocular loupes come in 2×, 2.5×, 3.5×, 4×, and 6× power (Fig. 13-7). The most useful power for sclerotherapy is the 2.5× model, which has a working distance of 340 mm with a field of view of 75 mm. The Gallilean optics are shorter than most other loupes and are lightweight (80 g). They are available on a large or small spectacle frame. Like many other loupes, the Heine loupe has both a asymmetric pupil distance adjustment and two alternate height settings for the optics.

The Keeler panoramic surgical Loupe has the following advantages: optics that can flip up out of view when not needed, lightweight frames, and optics with

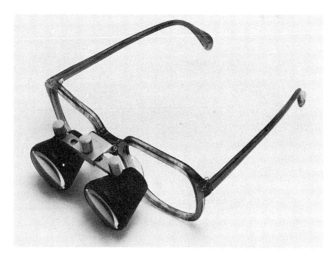

Fig. 13-8   Keeler 2.5× panoramic loupes. (Courtesy Keeler Instruments, Inc.)

an antireflection coating. The 2.5× magnification loupe (Fig. 13-8) has a field size of 9.4 cm and a working distance of 42 cm. A 3× magnifier is available with a working distance of 34 cm and a field size of 6.2 cm or with a working distance of 50 cm and a field size of 7.6 cm.

Orascoptic Research, Inc., has a wide-field loupe of outstanding quality available in 2×, 2.35×, 2.6×, and 3.25× power (Fig. 13-9). There is no distortion across the entire field of view. The depth and field of view are approximately 125 mm for the 2×; 88 mm for the 2.35×; 100 mm for the 2.6×; and 50 mm for the 3.25 loupes. These loupes are ergonomically designed with a downward sightline that can be adjusted to the exact angle that is most useful and comfortable for the physician, allowing a more upright posture, which reduces back and neck strain. A flipup design with autoclavable hand piece makes changing from normal to magnified viewing easy. The lightweight frames come in two sizes with detachable side shields. I personally use the 2.6× loupes and find them ideal for sclerotherapy and dermatologic surgery.

Surgitel loupe from General Scientific Corporation is very similar to the Orascopic loupe. It is available in 2.15×, 2.75×, 3.5×, and 5× power. It also has five adjustments to optimize the viewing angle. The lightweight frames come in two sizes with available side shields. The 2.75× loupe (most useful for sclerotherapy) has a field of view of 58 to 106 mm with a working distance of 250 to 404 mm or a 66- to 136-mm field of view with a 312- to 553-mm working distance, depending on the model type.

Other less expensive models include the N1064 Oculus loupe (Fig. 13-10). Another, the Westco 2× to 2.5× adjustable loupe, is also less expensive and of excellent quality. The lens-to-object working distance is 13 cm with a 3-cm field of view at 2.5×.

The lowest-priced loupe of high quality is the See Better loupe. The magnification is 2.5× with a field of view of 9 cm and an eye-to-working distance of 35 cm.

Foam Pads

Foam compression pads (Fig. 13-11) are manufactured from white latex rubber. They are beveled to produce maximum compression along the line of the injected

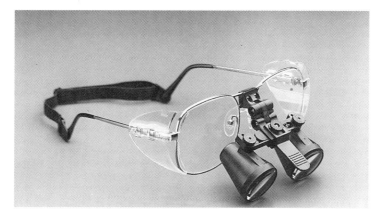

Fig. 13-9   Orascoptic telescope Model OR-2.6 shown with optional side shields and flip-grip autoclavable handle. (Courtesy Orascoptic Research, Inc.)

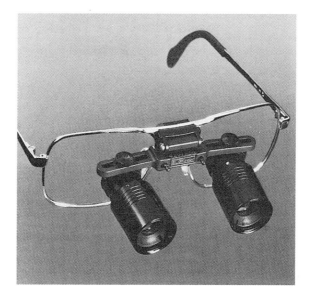

Fig. 13-10   N1064 Oculus loupe. (Courtesy Storz Instrument Company.)

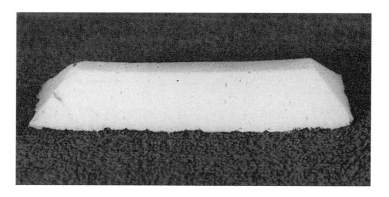

Fig. 13-11   Foam compression pad

vein segment. STD Pharmaceutical distributes two sizes of pads useful for providing additional compression over varicose veins (see Chapter 6). They are:

D pad (5 cm × 13 cm × 2.5 cm high)

E pad (4 cm × 13 cm × 1.75 cm high)

Tape Dressings

To support the placement of foam pads with minimal pressure, three sizes of microfoam surgical tape are recommended:

Size D: 7.5-cm diameter (for legs)

Size E: 8.75-cm diameter (for legs or small thighs)

Size F: 10-cm diameter (for thighs)

To support the placement of pads and/or to apply additional localized pressure, Coban tape or Medi-Rip Bandages are recommended. The Medi-Rip Bandage is a cohesive, tearable, elastic bandage rolled in 1-inch tubes. It is available in 1-, 2-, 3-, 4-, and 6-inch widths and is composed of 99.2% cotton and 0.8% polyurethane with a latex cohesive finish. The cotton-covered rubber threads minimize constriction and control elasticity. The microfine cohesive cover allows it to stick to itself instead of to hair or skin and eliminates slippage.

Graduated Compression Stockings

Information about graduated compression stockings can be found in Chapter 6 and Appendix A.

One useful aid to help support the thigh stocking in the proper position on the leg is a body adhesive called "It Stays!" This body adhesive comes in a roll-on bottle, it does not dry on the skin, and it remains tacky until it comes in contact with water. The product is nontoxic and nonflammable and only rarely causes skin irritation.

Antiseptic

Alcohol-soaked cotton balls are liberally applied to the telangiectatic area before injection to cleanse the area of bacteria and applied oils and grime. Doing so also improves the refraction of light to enhance the appearance of the vessels. The addition of 5% acetic acid (white vinegar) to the alcohol solution may aid visualization but has not been found useful in my practice.

PHOTOGRAPHY

Photographic documentation is recommended when treating any patient with varicose or telangiectatic leg veins. Not only do many insurance companies require photographic documentation before approving reimbursement, but patients often cannot remember later exactly how their leg veins appeared initially. In addition, because varicose telangiectatic leg veins may continue to appear throughout a patient's lifetime, documentation of treated areas will help distinguish between new veins and recurrent veins. Finally, some patients with long-standing varicose veins have hyperpigmentation around the varicosity. Preoperative photographic documentation is thus important (see Chapter 11).

Ideally all photographs should be taken with the same camera, same type of film and processing, same lighting, same F-stop and shutter speed, and same distance and angle of exposure from the camera to the patient. I recommend using a Nikon 2020 fully automatic camera fitted with a Nikon 105-mm macro lens and Sunpak auto 444D Thyrister flash. It is beneficial to replace the factory "split-image" internal lens with a clear lens to aid in close-up focusing. All photographs are taken at standard F-stops; F16 for close up, F11 for half-leg view photos, and

F8 for full-leg vein photos. Photographs are taken at an automatic "through-the-lens" (TTL) setting. Kodachrome ASA 25 or 64 film gives the highest quality reproductions.

PATIENT INFORMATIONAL BROCHURES

To educate patients about sclerotherapy, it is best for the physician to produce a brochure or information sheet that incorporates his or her unique and personalized approach to such treatment. There is no totally right way to perform sclerotherapy, and there are relatively few absolutes regarding preoperative preparation, treatment, and postoperative instructions. However, to produce personalized brochures is expensive. As an alternative, a number of ready-made commercial brochures are available (see Appendix G).

INSURANCE REIMBURSEMENT

Many physicians have expressed frustration in regard to the difficulty in obtaining insurance reimbursement for the treatment of varicose veins with compression sclerotherapy, even though the veins are symptomatic. It appears from a limited review of insurance reimbursement in my practice that there is a marked variability in the amount of reimbursement, not only among different insurance companies but also within the same insurance company from patient to patient and in the same patient from one treatment to the next.

Table 13-2 is a random selection of cases from my practice during 1986 showing insurance reimbursements for sclerotherapy treatment of symptomatic varicose (not spider) veins billed using RVS code 36471 (injection sclerotherapy of varicose vein) plus RVS code 99070 for a surgical tray. The reimbursement prob-

Table 13-2 Insurance reimbursements for sclerotherapy treatment

Insurance company	Amount billed*	Amount paid†
Cigna	$210	$114
Medicare	$200	$34.20
	$150	$54.70
Aetna	$125	$108
Blue Cross of California	$100	$56
	$150	$82
	$100	$80
Greater San Diego Health Plan	$125	$28.34
Admar	$125	$50
New York Life	$150	$37
Champus	$150	$108
Principal Mutual Life	$145	$145
	$130	$51
	$175	$60.50
	$195	$95
Insurnational Insurance	$160	$149
	$250	$250
	$210	$210

*Represents a charge of $125 for 15 minutes or $225 for 30 minutes plus surgical tray charge of either $15, $25, or $30, depending on the quantity of solution, number of compression pads, and number of syringes and butterfly needles used.
†Represents the amount allowed by the insurance company without reflecting the patient's deductible or co-payent fees.

lem has become so illogical and costly that I have not billed insurance companies for treatment in the last 3 years. Patients are told in advance of our office policy and are advised to get preapproval before they proceed with treatment. However, preapproval usually is in the form of a statement that the procedure will be reimbursed at fees "reasonable and customary" as determined by the individual insurance company. I have not yet been able to determine the logic used in defining "reasonable and customary." The wide-ranging variations reflect the enigma of insurance reimbursement for sclerotherapy of varicose veins. Reimbursement of primarily cosmetic or symptomatic spider telangiectasias or venulectases is even more of an enigma. Unfortunately, spider vein reimbursement is made worse by the actions of many physicians.

Most physicians will not submit bills for insurance reimbursement charges for treating purely cosmetic veins. However, some of my colleagues correctly point out that what is perceived as cosmetic by the patient is in reality a normalization of cutaneous blood flow and thus not, strictly speaking, cosmetic. In addition, many colleagues use RVS codes in the 17000 series that indicate destruction of benign lesions for this treatment. Although one may be able to defend this practice, I believe that to use the 17000 codes only serves to confuse the representatives of the insurance companies further and may result in furthering a distrust between the insurance carrier and the sclerotherapist. It is my belief that those who perform sclerotherapy should use the sclerotherapy code; when reimbursement is less than adequate, the insurance claim should be petitioned and the company should be properly educated about the cost effectiveness of sclerotherapy. With this direction, NASP produced a "White Paper" on sclerotherapy that was sent to more than 600 insurance carriers in 1992.[6] This paper was produced as an aid to the physician when submitting bills for reimbursement to educate the insurance company. It defines phlebology, sclerotherapy, and surgical treatments; discusses symptomatology and the medical necessity for treatment of defined disease; and concludes with guidelines for determination of medical necessity. Not one insurance company representative responded to this document even after numerous follow-up letters.

Many methods have been used by colleagues to educate insurance companies on the technique of compression sclerotherapy. Some of us send the insurance companies detailed operative reports with or without summaries of the history of compression sclerotherapy and the cost-effective nature of this treatment versus surgical ligation and strippings (see Appendix H). However, this education process, despite being time-consuming for the physician, is often met with unresponsiveness on the part of insurance companies. Thus each physician must make an individual decision regarding insurance reimbursement.

REFERENCES

1. Butie A and Goldman MP: Preliminary results from the North American Society of Phlebology membership questionnaire, Newsletter North Am Soc Phlebol 2:3, 1988.
2. Food and Drug Administration: Communication under the Freedom of Information Act, 1990.
3. Hallgren R, Fry PD, and Goldman MP: The current and future role of the nurse in phlebology: the Canadian experience, Dermatol Nurs 5:60, 1993.
4. Epstein E: Magnifiers in dermatology: a personal survey, J Am Acad Dermatol 13:687, 1985.
5. Siegel DM: The precision binocular loupe, J Dermatol Surg Oncol 15:388, 1989.
6. Weiss RA, Haegle CR, and Raymond-Martimbeau P: Insurance Advisory Committee report, J Dermatol Surg Oncol 18:609, 1992.

Appendices

A Compression Hosiery

In addition to the large manufacturers and distributors listed, a number of other manufacturers of graduated compression hosiery are in the United States. Many of these companies have a limited sales and distribution region. I have included two such companies in those noted below; they were brought to my attention by physicians who have used their products and were impressed by their quality and price. I have not personally evaluated these stockings, nor have I been able to obtain detailed information about their construction or specifications other than what is provided. With the background provided in Chapter 6 and its appendix, the reader should be able to evaluate each stocking company to decide which brand and type of stocking will be best for his or her practice.

Refer to Tables 6-1 (p. 215) and 6-2 (p. 226) for specific information and specifications about each type of graduated compression stocking.

Camp

All of the Camp models are produced by a circular knitting process and are seamless. Two knitted yarns provide the required longitudinal elasticity, or vertical stretch. A laid-in yarn builds up the necessary lateral compression. This combination of lateral and vertical elasticity provides a two-way stretch fabric. Yarns used in Camp stockings are double wrapped for improved comfort and greater durability. The double wrapping protects the yarn so there is less fraying.

The advantage of the Camp stocking, stated by the manufacturer, is its increased number of stitches per inch to provide greater elasticity, easier application, and increased durability. The company also claims to use a low-modulus, high-elongated yarn that allows greater elasticity without change in compression. The knitting process begins in the toe, so it will not unravel or run.

All panty and maternity stockings have a ventilated cotton crotch piece. All maternity panty stockings have a single seam in back and two in front for greater comfort as the abdomen expands.

Available from:
Camp International, Inc.
P.O. Box 89
Jackson, MI 49204-0089

Elastic Therapy, Inc.

Elastic Therapy, Inc., was referred to me by a physician with an active phlebology practice. He has been using its line for more than 1 year and can attest to its high quality and reasonable price. In addition to lightweight men's socks and ladies' panty hose (22 and 15 mm Hg compression at the ankle, respectively), they manufacture a line of both class II and class III stockings in below-knee and above-knee hose and panty hose with closed and open toes.

Available from:
Elastic Therapy, Inc.
1517 North Fayetteville St.
P.O. Box 4068
Asheboro, NC 27204-4068

Hanes Alive

Haines Alive is a readily available support panty hose that provides a nongraduated compression of 8 mm Hg.

Jobst

Arising from a desire to treat his own venous insufficiency, which resulted in stasis ulceration, Conrad Jobst, inventor and engineer, designed and patented the graduated compression stocking in the 1940s and 1950s in the United States. The original stocking was custom-made from a template-cut bobbinet fabric. The template consisted of a vertical strip of paper to which horizontal strips of paper were attached and then cut to the size of the leg. Graduation was achieved by reducing the length of the horizontal template strips by the appropriate percentage.

Jobst manufactures several types of graduated medical compression stockings. The Jobst Custom Support stocking conforms to the original design concept of Conrad Jobst. Jobst Custom Supports are made with a unique bobbinet fabric. This fabric is composed of either natural rubber or Lycra, cotton, and Dacron. Each stocking is engineered individually to design a garment with precise measurements taken every $1^1/_2$ inches along the leg. Counterpressures are prescribed according to the severity of the condition as described by the physician. Five classes of compression are most often used—25, 30, 35, 40, or 50 mm Hg—commencing at the ankle and decreasing proximally. However, higher or lower compression can be engineered into the supports.

Vairox graduated compression stockings are moderate-weight ready-to-wear seamless support stockings available in four styles: knee length, with or without a zipper; thigh length; thigh length with waist attachment; and waist-high length. They are available in 12 sizes and in two compression ranges: 30 to 40 mm Hg and 40 to 50 mm Hg. Depending on the style, a maximum of five measurements is needed to fit a patient. (Knee-length style requires only three measurements.)

Fast-Fit graduated compression stockings are ready-made and lightweight. They can be obtained without a prescription. The stockings are constructed of a seamless blend of nylon and Lycra. Fast-Fit stockings are available in four styles: knee, thigh, waist, and maternity. Also, they are available as closed- or open-toe stockings in small, medium, and large sizes in a mild (18 to 25 mm Hg) or moderate (25 to 35 mm Hg) compression range at the ankle. Only one leg and foot length is available, limiting its use for some patients.

Ultimate Sheer is the newest ready-made graduated compression stocking from Jobst. It is composed of uncovered Lycra and nylon. This style is available as either a closed-toe knee-high or panty hose with compression of 30 to 40 mm Hg.

> Available from:
> Jobst: A Beiersdorf Company
> P.O. Box 471048
> Charlotte, NC 28247-1048

JuZo

JuZo medical two-way stretch compression stockings have been manufactured for more than 75 years in Germany by Julius Zorn, Inc., and are manufactured and distributed by the same company in the United States. These support stockings are available in seven styles: below-knee stocking, half-thigh stocking, thigh stocking, thigh stocking with hip attachment, thigh stocking with panty part, compression leotard, and compression leotard for maternity. These styles are available in both closed-toe and open-toe designs and are all seamless. They are also available in four compression classes: 25, 35, 45, and 60 mm Hg. As with most large stocking manufacturers, the stocking can also be custom fitted to each patient.

One unique advantage of the JuZo line is the availability of different textile coatings over the compression threads. Standard compression threads are covered with cotton on the inner layer, which comes in contact with the skin (JuZo-Varin cotton style). For an easier and smoother fit, the compression threads of the inner stocking layer are covered with silk in the JuZo-Varin soft-in style. A style with a woolen lining in the knee area is also available to help prevent chaffing.

Another unique aspect of this stocking line is the relative increase in the elastic knit in the upper thigh area of the Varilastic model. This allows maintenance of proper compression in patients with large-diameter thighs and also helps prevent slippage as the patient moves.

Available from:
Julius Zorn, Inc. (JuZo)
80 Chart Road, Northhampton
P.O. Box 1088
Cuyahoga Falls, OH 44223

International Medi-Surgical

International Medi-Surgical distributorship supplies two types of graduated compression stockings: Ibici from Italy and Sirlex Radiante from France.

The Ibici line is available in assorted colors in compression classes 0, I, and II.

The Sirlex Radiante line is also available in assorted colors in compression classes I, II, and III.

Available from:
International Medi-Surgical
P.O. Box 3000187
Houston, TX 77230

Medi

In 1962 Medi developed and patented a new knitting technology for the production of a seamless, ultra-sheer product. The Medi stocking is differentiated from other compression stockings by its use of uncoated spandex threads. Medi uses five leg circumference sizes. The company claims that using a larger number of ankle sizes allows a more accurate fit. In addition, Medi's processing technique uses a spandex thread inlaid into every woven row in its Medi Plus and Medi 75 lines. This technique is said to impart a finer quality to a sheerer stocking. Most other compression stockings use spandex threads in every other row. Finally, Medi offers a size VII stocking to fit legs with a thigh circumference greater than 33 inches. This allows very large people to use ready-made stockings in lieu of made-to-measure stockings.

Medi stockings are all produced with white threads. The final product is then dyed to impart the desired color. Therefore it is available in many colors; nude, off-white, black, and gray are presently available in the United States.

One study found that after 6 weeks 36% of 226 patients with venous outflow disorders treated by 82 practitioners in various specialties discontinued treatment with the Medi stocking as compared to 53% of patients who discontinued treatment in a previous study with another brand of graduated compression stocking.[1]

Medi compression stockings are available in seven styles: below-knee stocking, half-thigh stocking, thigh stocking, thigh stocking with waist attachment, compression leotard, and compression leotard for maternity wear. Medi is the only company that offers a ready-made full-length leotard, with a fly, for men. These styles are available with either a closed toe or an open toe, come in two foot and leg lengths, and are all seamless. They are also available in three compression classes for all styles: 20 to 30 mm Hg, 30 to 40 mm Hg, and 40 to 50 mm Hg. The stockings can also be custom made for each patient.

Available from:
Medi USA (American Weco)
76 W. Seegers Rd.
Arlington Hts., IL 60005

Sigvaris

Sigvaris support stockings are available in six styles: below-knee stocking, half-thigh stocking, thigh stocking, thigh stocking with waist attachment, panty stocking, and maternity panty stocking. These styles are available in both closed-toe and open-toe styles and all are seamless. The four available compression classes are 20 to 30 mm Hg, 30 to 40 mm Hg, 40 to 50 mm Hg, and 50 to 60 mm Hg.

The 500 series is composed of natural rubber threads and nylon and is available in various graduated compression ranges:

503: 30 to 40 mm Hg, available in all styles
504: 40 to 50 mm Hg, available in all but panty styles
505: 50 to 60 mm Hg, available in calf and thigh only

A 601 line is available as a 20 to 30 mm Hg graduated compression calf stocking with synthetic rubber threads covered with nylon.

An 801 line is available as a 20 to 30 mm Hg graduated compression panty hose and maternity panty stocking composed of synthetic rubber with nylon.

An 802 line is available as a calf-length, closed-toe graduated compression stocking in beige or black. The compression is 30 to 40 mm Hg at the ankle. The stocking is composed of synthetic rubber and nylon.

A 902 line is available in calf, thigh, and panty styles in a 30 to 40 mm Hg compression class composed of synthetic rubber threads covered with nylon.

A 202 line with 30 to 40 mm Hg compression is available as a graduated calf-length stocking made of a cotton blend. The synthetic Lycra threads are covered with cotton. This line is softer and easier to put on than the other Sigvaris lines because of its cotton-coated thread lining.

Available from:
Sigvaris
P.O. Box 570
Branford, CT 06405

Venosan

Venosan Medical Therapeutic Compression Stockings and Panty Hose are distributed in the United States by Freeman Manufacturing Co. These support stockings are available in 10 basic ready-to-wear models, including below-knee stocking, over-knee (half-thigh) stocking, thigh stocking, thigh stocking with hip attachment, compression panty hose, and maternity compression panty hose. These stockings are available in closed-toe and open-toe styles and with short or long foot lengths, and all are seamless. There are 60 different styles, 12 sizing options, and 4 compression classes. Each small, medium, and large size has an additional "normal" or "extra" sizing measurement at the midcalf and midthigh levels to optimize fit. The four compression classes include 20 to 30 mm Hg, 30 to 40 mm Hg, 40 to 50 mm Hg, and 50 to 60 mm Hg.

The stockings are manufactured on circular knitting machines. Venosan 2000 stockings have a material content of 60% nylon, 25% Lycra, and 15% cotton. Venosan 1000 stockings are lighter in weight with a material content of 72% nylon and 28% Lycra. The inner lining of cotton, unique to the Venosan 2000 series, adds to the porous nature of the stocking.

COMPRESSION BANDAGES

A complete discussion of the various manufacturers and types of compression bandages is beyond the scope of this text. Dozens of companies, large and small, distribute in the United States. In addition, many veterinary products used for horses are quite useful and cost effective in phlebology. The reader is referred to Chapter 6 for a discussion on the relative uses of short-stretch, long-stretch, and inelastic bandages. Although I use many types of compression bandages for treating venous insufficiency, I only use one short-stretch bandage to supplement compression with graduated support stockings when treating a patient with varicose veins.

Medi-Rip

The Medi-Rip compression bandage is particularly useful in applying localized pressure to a segment of the leg. Since the bandage sticks only to itself, it must be applied circumferentially around the limb. Thus it can be applied only in an approximate graduated manner by the nurse or physician. Graduation in support is achieved by wrapping the bandage either more or less tightly around the leg. In addition, support padding underneath the bandage can provide a localized increase in compression pressure.

It is recommended that this bandage be used when compressing lateral thigh varicosities. A graduated compression stocking applies a limited compression in this proximal location and applies even less compression to the lateral aspect of the limb by virtue of its oval configuration. Therefore applying pads or cotton balls on the lateral thigh and compressing them locally with a bandage will increase the compression strength without unduly compromising the advantage of using graduation in compression.

The composition of the bandage fabric is 99% cotton and 1% polyurethane (spandex). The warp is constructed with longitudinal threads of alternating cotton, twisted spandex thread, and twisted cotton threads in a 3:1 ratio. Threads are twisted 1950 times per meter in an alternating clockwise and counterclockwise manner. An equal number of clockwise and counterclockwise twisted threads maintain proper stability. Fill threads of the weft are woven with 100% cotton for strength and porosity.

A fine latex spray is then applied to the fabric. The unique application of the spray adheres only to the surface of the yarn and does not occlude the openings between, thus maintaining the porosity, breathability, and absorption qualities of the cotton fabric.

Available from:
  Conco Medical Company
  Bridgeport, CT 06610

Tubigrip

Tubigrip is an elasticized surgical tubular bandage knitted from either 100% cotton (flesh shade) or 67% cotton and 33% rayon (natural shade). Covered elastic threads are laid into the material to form continuous spirals. When applied to the affected area, the elastic moves within the bandage, evening pressure over the contours of the body.

Tubigrip is best used as a cover or support bandage for compression pads in patients allergic to adhesive tape or Medi-Rip tape. In these circumstances the compression pad can be held in place before application of the graduated support stocking by a layer of Tubigrip. Using Tubigrip as a support bandage is cumbersome and of doubtful validity as a graduated support stocking because of the ease with which the bandage can migrate with movement of the leg.

The amount of pressure to apply can be selected by choosing the appropriate size of Tubigrip with the aid of the Tubigrip Tension Guide. Because the tension guide measures only the widest diameter of the limb, true graduated compression cannot be obtained. It is recommended that Tubigrip be applied as a double layer with the cut edges uppermost. The second layer should overlap the first by 2 to 3 cm to prevent occlusion.

Tubigrip Shaped Support Bandage is an anatomically shaped compression bandage available in a range of full-leg and below-the-knee sizes that provide a degree of graduated compression to the limbs. The material stretches only in a radial direction, thus providing firm support without slipping. Size choice is determined by measuring the widest diameter of the limb; therefore a "true" graduation in pressure with the greatest pressure at the ankle cannot be obtained.

Available from:
  Se Pro Healthcare, Inc.
  Montgomery, PA 18936

PRESSURE PADS

At times, additional pressure is required in a localized area. The use of foam rubber padding, tightly twisted firm rolls of cotton wool, or cotton balls, as previously mentioned in Chapters 6, 9, 11, and 13, can provide this additional compression. Foam rubber padding may also be required to distribute compression more evenly around the leg. The ankle area (where the greatest degree of compression is applied by a stocking) is the most irregularly contoured part of the leg. Here the medial and lateral malleoli jut out of the smooth plane of the leg, resulting in a concavity posteriorly (see Fig. 6-3). When patients complain about compression stockings, they usually complain about pain in this area. Various pads have been constructed to fill this concavity and more evenly distribute the compression.

Such padding fills the pocket formed by the bridging of elastic material from the malleolus to the Achilles tendon. The padding also creates additional pressure in this area to prevent pooling of fluids (Fig. A-1).

Jobst Stasis Pads

Three types and sizes of Jobst Stasis Pads are available to fit the concavity properly: small crescent, large crescent, and oval. Pads are made of a layer of foam rubber and a layer of polyurethane foam. They are washable and reusable.

Available from:
The Jobst Institute, Inc.
P.O. Box 652
Toledo, OH 43694

JuZo-Helastic

The JuZo-Helastic model 3022 compression stocking is made with a specially designed pressure pad at the lateral malleolar area. The pressure pads are sewn into elastic knitted pockets and connected to the two-way stretch stocking to preserve the two-way stretch properties of the fabric. The pads are composed of silicon.

Available from:
Julius Zorn, Inc. (JuZo)
80 Chart Road, Northhampton
P.O. Box 1088
Cuyahoga Falls, OH 44223

REFERENCE

1. von Beratung U: Die therapie venoser Beinleiden Kompressionstherapie, medikamentos kombiniert? Der Bayerische Internist 1:46, 1987.

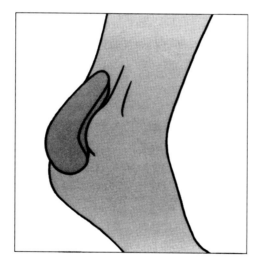

Fig. A-1   Foam pad placed to fill in the concavity behind the lateral malleolus. (Courtesy Julius Zorn, Inc.)

B Manufacturers and Distributors of Sclerosing Solutions

ETHANOLAMINE OLEATE

Available from:
Block Drug Company
1 New England Avenue
Piscataway, NJ 08855

HYPERTONIC SALINE 23.4%

Available from:
Invenex
Gibcol Invenex Division
The Dexter Corporation
Chagrin Falls, OH 44022

American Regent
Laboratories, Inc.
Shirley, NY 11967

Omega Laboratories, Ltd.
11,177 Hamon St.
Montreal, Canada H3M 3E4

POLIDOCANOL

Available from:
Globopharm AQ
P.O. Box 1187
8700 Kusnacht, Switzerland

Chemische Fabrik
Kreussler and Co. GmbH
D-6200 Wiesbaden-Biebrich
Germany

Laboratories Pharmaceutiques
DEXO, S.A.
31 Rue D'Arras
92000 Nanterre, France

POLYIODINATED IODINE

Variglobin from:
Globopharm AQ
P.O. Box 1187
8700 Kusnacht, Switzerland
Sclerodine from:
Omega
Montreal, Canada H3M3A2

CHROMATED GLYCERIN (CHROMEX)

Available from:
Omega Laboratories, Ltd.
11,177 Hamon St.
Montreal, Canada H3M 3E4

Farmacia, Giouami PELLI
via al Furte 3
6900 Lusano, Switzerland

Available from:
Amodont SAS
cia di Camporella 15/A
50019 Sesto Fiorentino
Firenze, Italy

GLYCERIN 70%

Available from:
Amodont SAS
cia di Camporella 15/A
50019 Sesto Fiorentino
Firenze, Italy

SCLERODEX

Available from:
Omega Laboratories, Ltd.
11,177 Hamon St.
Montreal, Canada H3M 3E4

SODIUM MORRHUATE

Available from:
American Regent Laboratories,
Inc.
1 Lutipold Dr.
Shirley, NY 11967
Palisades Pharmaceuticals, Inc.
219 Country Road
Tenafly, NJ 07670

SODIUM TETRADECYL SULFATE

Available from:
Wyeth-Ayerst Laboratories
P.O. Box 8299
Philadelphia, PA 19101

Sample Patient Questionnaire

Date _____

Name _____

Age _____ Sex _____ Blood Type _____

Height _____ Weight _____ Shoe size _____

Referred by _____

PERSONAL MEDICAL HISTORY (CURRENT COMPLAINT)

	No	Yes
1. Are you consulting for		
a. Cosmetic purposes	_____	_____
b. Medical reasons	_____	_____
c. Both	_____	_____

2. How many years have you noticed this problem?   _____

3. Have you ever been treated for this problem?   _____   _____
   By whom and when? _____

   With what method?

      Injection   _____

      Electrocautery _____

      Laser   _____

      Surgery   _____

4. Have you ever been treated for one of the following?

	No	Yes
a. Phlebitis (inflammation of a vein)	_____	_____

   Right leg _____ Left leg _____

   Hospitalization _____

	No	Yes

b. Leg ulcer _____ _____

    Right leg _____ Left leg _____

    Hospitalization _____

c. Pulmonary embolism/blood clots _____ _____

    Hospitalization _____

d. Leg fracture _____ _____

5. When did your veins occur?

    Age _____

    Before pregnancy _____

    During pregnancy _____

    After trauma _____

    After birth control or
       estrogen therapy _____

    Other _____

6. Are you developing new veins? _____ _____

7. Are your present veins getting bigger? _____ _____

8. Indicate which of the following problems you have experienced:

	Right leg	Left leg	How many years?
a. Pain in your			
Lower limbs	_____	_____	_____
Thigh	_____	_____	_____
Calf	_____	_____	_____
Leg	_____	_____	_____
Foot	_____	_____	_____
b. Swelling of the legs	_____	_____	_____
c. Skin or ulcer problems	_____	_____	_____
d. Others	_____	_____	_____

    Specify _____

Continued.

9. If you experience pain in your lower limbs:

a. Is the pain exacerbated by   No   Yes

    Extended periods in standing position   _____   _____

    Heat   _____   _____

    Menstrual periods   _____   _____

    Exercising and/or walking   _____   _____

    Medication   _____   _____

    Others   _____   _____

    Specify _____

b. Is the pain alleviated by

    Elevation of the limbs   _____   _____

    Elastic stockings   _____   _____

    Walking and/or exercising   _____   _____

c. Indicate the type of pain

    Resting pain   _____   _____

    Resting cramps   _____   _____

    Night cramps   _____   _____

    Tiredness   _____   _____

    Heaviness in the legs   _____   _____

    Pain in specific areas _____

    Numbness   _____   _____

    Burning sensation   _____   _____

    Additional comments _____

    _____

10. Do you have a family history of   No   Yes

a. Varicose vein problems   _____   _____

              Family member   _____

b. Phlebitis (inflammation of a vein)   _____   _____

              Family member   _____

c. Blood clots   _____   _____

              Family member   _____

	No	Yes
d. Leg ulcers	_____	_____
Family member		_____
e. Cancer	_____	_____
Family member		_____

11. a. Do you have a history of	No	Yes
Diabetes	_____	_____
High blood pressure	_____	_____
Seizures or convulsions	_____	_____
Fainting or dizzy spells	_____	_____
Stroke	_____	_____
Blood transfusions	_____	_____
Asthma	_____	_____
Hives	_____	_____
Arthritis	_____	_____
Thrombophlebitis	_____	_____
Pulmonary embolus	_____	_____
Deep vein thrombosis	_____	_____
Septicemia	_____	_____
Autoimmune disease (i.e., Lupus)	_____	_____
Hepatitis	_____	_____
Bleeding disorders	_____	_____
Easy bruisability	_____	_____
Heart disease	_____	_____
Migraine headaches	_____	_____
Dark spots after pregnancy, skin injury, or surgery	_____	_____
HIV positive (AIDS test)	_____	_____

b. Do you have a personal history of allergies to medications? (Please list)

_____

_____

_____

_____

Continued.

	No	Yes
c. Allergies to any foods	_____	_____
d. Allergies to nail polish	_____	_____
e. Allergies to cosmetics	_____	_____
f. Allergies or sensitivity to adhesive tape	_____	_____

12. Does your work require a

    a. Prolonged standing position   _____   _____

    b. Prolonged sitting position   _____   _____

13. In the course of a normal day, how much time is spent in a standing position?

    a. 10% of the day   _____

    b. 20% of the day   _____

    c. 30% to 50% of the day _____

    d. More than 50%   _____

14. Does walking or exercise relieve or aggravate the pain?   _____

	No	Yes
15. Do you jog, run, jump rope, or do aerobics?	_____	_____

    How often per week?   _____

16. Are you pregnant or planning a pregnancy soon?   _____   _____

17. Number of past pregnancies and year of births _____

18. Do you spend long hours sitting?   _____   _____

19. Do you smoke cigarettes?   _____   _____

    If yes, how many packs per day?   _____

20. Do you wear elastic support stockings?   _____   _____

    What kind? _____

    How often? _____

21. Have you ever had a blood transfusion?   _____   _____

	No	Yes

22. Are you taking any medication?
    Indicate which of the following you are taking:

    a. Aspirin   _____   _____

    b. Anticoagulants   _____   _____

    c. Hormones or contraceptives (birth control pills)   _____   _____

    d. Chemotherapy for any type of tumor   _____   _____

    e. Thyroid medication   _____   _____

    f. Cortisone   _____   _____

    g. Insulin   _____   _____

    h. Sedatives (sleeping pills)   _____   _____

    i. Tranquilizers   _____   _____

    j. Appetite depressants   _____   _____

    k. Others   _____   _____

       Specify _____

23. Indicate the date of your last

    a. Physical examination _____

    b. Laboratory tests _____

24. Is there any additional information that you would
    consider pertinent?   _____   _____

    If yes, specify _____

    _____

25. Do you wish to be included in our periodic follow-up
    assessment recall list?   _____   _____

    Do you wish to receive our newsletters and educational
    updates on venous disease?   _____   _____

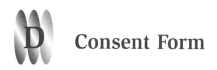

Consent Form

DERMATOLOGY ASSOCIATES OF SAN DIEGO COUNTY, INC.*
Sclerotherapy: Informed Consent Form

This form is designed to provide you with the information you need to make an informed decision on whether or not to have sclerotherapy performed. If you have any questions or do not understand any potential risks, please do not hesitate to ask us.

WHAT IS SCLEROTHERAPY?
Sclerotherapy is a popular method for eliminating varicose veins and superficial telangiectasias ("spider veins") in which a solution, called a "sclerosing agent," is injected into the veins.

DOES SCLEROTHERAPY WORK FOR EVERYONE?
The majority of persons who have sclerotherapy performed will be cleared or at least see good improvement. Unfortunately, however, there is no guarantee that sclerotherapy will be effective in every case. Approximately 10% of patients who undergo sclerotherapy have poor to fair results ("poor results" means that the veins have not totally disappeared after six treatments). In very rare instances the patient's condition may become worse after sclerotherapy treatment.

HOW MANY TREATMENTS WILL I NEED?
The number of treatments needed to clear or improve the condition differs from patient to patient, depending on the extent of varicose and spider veins present. One to six or more treatments may be needed; the average is three to four. Individual veins usually require one to three treatments.

WHAT ARE THE MOST COMMON SIDE EFFECTS?
The most common side effects experienced with sclerotherapy treatment include the following:

1. *Itching.* Depending on the type of solution used, you may experience mild itching along the vein route. This itching normally lasts 1 to 2 hours but may persist for a day or so.

2. *Transient hyperpigmentation.* Approximately 10% of patients who undergo sclerotherapy notice discoloration (light brown streaks) after treatment. In almost every patient the veins become darker immediately after the procedure. In rare instances this darkening of the vein persists for 4 to 12 months.

3. *Sloughing.* Sloughing occurs in less than 1% of the patients who receive sclerotherapy. Sloughing consists of a small ulceration at the injection site that heals slowly over 1 to 2 months. A blister may form, open, and become ulcerated. The scar that follows should return to a normal color. This occurrence usually represents injection into or near a small artery and is not preventable.

4. *Allergic reactions.* Very rarely a patient may have an allergic reaction to the sclerosing agent used. The risk of an allergic reaction is greater in patients who have a history of allergies.

NOTE: Patients must read and sign a new consent form every 6 months.

_____
Patient initial

*Copyright Dermatology Associates, San Diego County, Inc 1994

Continued.

CONSENT FORM
DERMATOLOGY ASSOCIATES OF SAN DIEGO COUNTY, INC.

5. *Pain.* A few patients experience moderate to severe pain and some bruising, usually at the site of the injection. The veins may be tender to the touch after treatment, and an uncomfortable sensation may run along the vein route. This pain is usually temporary, in most cases lasting 1 to at most 7 days.

6. *Telangiectatic mattting.* This refers to the development of new tiny blood vessels in the treated vessel. This temporary phenonmenon occurs 2 to 4 weeks after treatment and usually resolves within 4 to 6 months. It occurs in up to 18% of women receiving estrogen therapy and in 2% to 4% of all patients.

7. *Ankle swelling.* Ankle swelling may occur after treatment of blood vessels in the foot or ankle. It usually resolves in a few days and is lessened by wearing the prescribed support stockings.

8. *Phlebitis.* Phlebitis is a very rare complication, seen in approximately 1 out of every 1000 patients treated for varicose veins greater than 3 to 4 mm in diameter. The possible dangers of phlebitis include the possibility of a pulmonary embolus (a blood clot to the lungs) and postphlebitis syndrome, in which the blood clot is not carried out of the legs, resulting in permanent swelling of the legs.

WHAT ARE THE POSSIBLE COMPLICATIONS IF I DO NOT HAVE SCLEROTHERAPY PERFORMED?
In cases of large varicose veins (greater than 3 to 4 mm in diameter), spontaneous phlebitis and/or thrombosis may occur with the associated risk of possible pulmonary emboli. Additionally, large skin ulcerations may develop in the ankle region of patients with long-standing varicose veins with underlying venous insufficiency. Rarely these ulcers may hemorrhage or become cancerous.

ARE THERE OTHER TYPES OF PROCEDURES TO TREAT VARICOSE VEINS AND TELANGIECTASIAS? WHAT ARE THEIR SIDE EFFECTS?
Because varicose and telangiectatic leg veins are not life-threatening conditions, treatment is not mandatory in every patient. Some patients may get adequate relief of symptoms from wearing graduated support stockings. Ambulatory phlebectomy is a procedure in which certain types of veins can be removed through small surgical incisions. The complications of this procedure are similar to those of sclerotherapy with the addition of small surgical scars that naturally occur with this procedure.

Vein stripping and/or ligation may also be used to treat large varicose veins. This procedure may require a hospital stay and usually is performed while the patient is under general anesthesia. Risks of vein stripping and/or ligation include permanent nerve paralysis in a small percentage of patients, possible pulmonary emboli, infection, and permanent scarring. General anesthesia has some associated serious risks, including the possibility of paralysis, brain damage, and death.

WHAT IF I EXPERIENCE A PROBLEM AFTER RECEIVING SCLEROTHERAPY?
If you notice any type of adverse reaction, please call the doctor immediately.

Patient initial

COMMENTS _____

_____

_____

_____

_____

_____

BY MY INITIALS, I ACKNOWLEDGE THAT I HAVE RECEIVED A COPY OF THIS
SCLEROTHERAPY INFORMED CONSENT FORM. _____

BY SIGNING BELOW, I ACKNOWLEDGE THAT I HAVE READ THE FOREGOING INFORMED
CONSENT FORM AND THAT THE DOCTOR HAS ADEQUATELY INFORMED ME OF THE
RISKS OF SCLEROTHERAPY TREATMENT, ALTERNATIVE METHODS OF TREATMENT, AND
THE RISKS OF NOT TREATING MY CONDITION, AND I HEREBY CONSENT TO SCLERO-
THERAPY TREATMENT PERFORMED BY DR. _____ .

Date _____ , 19_____   Time _____ AM/PM

_____   _____
Patient's Signature   Patient's Representative
                                          (If patient is a minor or is mentally incom-
                                          petent, signature of Parent or Legal Guardian
                                          is required)

_____   _____
Witness   Relationship to Patient

Patient's name _____ Age _____ Initial date _____

Resolution scale

−1 Blue

0 No change   +2 Moderate fade

+1 Mild fade   +3 Total fade

Side effects

E = Edema   M = Matting

P = Pigment   U = Ulcer

Anterior   **Right lateral**   **Left lateral**   **Posterior**

R   L   R   L   R   L   L   R

Date	Location	Type	Diameter	Length	Solution/Amount

1-3 weeks	1-2 months	2-6 months	Over 1 year

F Equipment Sources

Many different manufacturers and distributors for equipment are used in phlebology and sclerotherapy. The following list is not meant to be comprehensive but to provide sources to the reader of a number of products mentioned in the text and with which I am familiar.

NEEDLES
30-Gauge

Acuderm Acu-Needle
Acuderm, Inc.
5370 NW 35 Terrace
Ft. Lauderdale, FL 33309
Henke-Sasse, Wolf (HSW), Germany
Air-Tite of Virginia, Inc.
P.O. Box 9354
Virginia Beach, VA 23450
Precision Glide
Becton-Dickinson and Company
Rutherford, NJ 07070
MPL Solopak
Delasco
Dermatologic Lab and Supply, Inc.
698 13th Ave.
Council Bluffs, IA 51501

31- and 32-Gauge

Misawsa Medical of Japan
Air-Tite of Virginia, Inc.
P.O. Box 9354
Virginia Beach, VA 23450

33-Gauge

Hamilton
Hamilton Company
Reno, Nevada
800/648-5950
Delasco
Dermatologic Lab and Supply, Inc.
698 13th Ave
Council Bluffs, IA 51501

26- or 27-Gauge

Yale
Becton-Dickinson and Company
Ft. Lauderdale, FL 33314

21-, 23-, or 25-Gauge Butterfly

Abbott Hospitals, Inc.
North Chicago, IL 60064
Surflo Winged Infusion Set
Terumo Corporation
Tokyo, Japan

SYRINGES
2.5-ml syringe

Air-Tite of Virginia, Inc.
P.O. Box 9354
Virginia Beach, VA 23450

3-ml syringe

Luer Lok or non–Luer Lok
Becton-Dickinson and Company
Rutherford, NJ 07070
Plastipak eccentric syringe
Becton-Dickinson and Company
Rutherford, NJ 07070

MAGNIFYING GLASSES

Clip-on Loupes
Almore International
Portland, OR 97225
Opticaid
Edroy Products Co., Inc.
Nyack, NY 10960

HEADBAND-MOUNTED SIMPLE BINOCULAR MAGNIFIERS

Optivisor
Donegan Optical Company
15549 West 108th St.
Lenexa, KS 66219
Mark II Magni-Focuser
Edroy Products Co., Inc.
Nyack, NY 10960

SIMPLE BINOCULAR LOUPES

Precision Binocular Loupe
Almore International
Portland, OR 97225
Multidistance Headband Loupe
Edroy Products Co., Inc.
Nyack, NY 10960

499

BINOCULAR LOUPES

Designs for Vision
New York, NY 10010
Surgitel
General Scientific Corporation
77 Enterprise Dr.
Ann Arbor, MI 48103
Heine Binocular Loupes
Heine USA, Ltd.
3500 Regency Park Way
Cary, NC 27511-8569
N1064 Oculus
Storz Instrument Company
St. Louis, MO 63122

Orascoptic Research, Inc.
7 North Pinckney St., Ste 305
Madison, WI 53703

Westco Medical Corporation
7079 Mission Gorge Rd.
Building J
San Diego, CA 92138
See Better Loupe
Edroy Products Co., Inc.
Nyack, NY 10960

FOAM PADS

STD Pharmaceutical
Fields Yard, Plough Lane
Hereford, Esngland HR4 OEL

TAPE DRESSINGS
With Minimal Pressure

3M Microfoam Surgical Tape
Medical Surgical Division/3M
St. Paul, MN 55144
Tubigrip Tubular Support Bandage
Seaton Products, Inc.
Montgomeryville, PA

Additional Localized Pressure

Coban tape
Medical Surgical Division/3M
St. Paul, MN 55144
Medi-Rip Bandage
Conco Medical Company
Bridgeport, CT 06610

BODY ADHESIVE

It Stays!
New Horizons Diversified Interests
Grants Pass, OR 97526

G Patient Brochures

(1) *Spider Vein, Varicose Vein Therapy*

This excellent eight-panel brochure accurately describes the pathogenesis and treatment of both varicose and telangiectatic leg veins (with a heavy concentration on "spider veins"). Operative and before-and-after color photographs are reproduced with excellent quality. The common patient questions are addressed and the common side effects are given.

Source:

American Academy of Dermatology
930 N. Meacham Rd.
P.O. Box 4014
Schaumberg, IL 60168-4014

(2) *Sclerotherapy: Treatment of Leg Veins*

This simple six-panel brochure describes the treatment of spider veins only. There are no color photographs of actual patients, but two-color diagrams of veins and sclerotherapy treatment are included. This brochure can be personalized with your name, address, and some individualized information on the rear panel.

Source:

Contemporary Communications
P.O. Box 71985
Marietta, GA 30007

(3) *Facts for Consumers: Varicose Vein Treatments (#F030421)*

This seven-panel free brochure was prepared with the assistance of the Board of Directors of the American Venous Forum.

Source:

Federal Trade Commission
Bureau of Consumer Protection
Office of Consumer and Business Education
Washington, D.C. 20580

(4) *Treatment of Leg Veins*

This four-panel brochure provides information about sclerotherapy and surgical treatments for varicose veins and is available for purchase. It was developed under the direction of the Board of Directors of the North American Society of Phlebology.

Source:

North American Society of Phlebology
930 N. Meacham Rd.
Schaumberg, IL 60168-4014

(5) *Questions and Answers About Sclerotherapy for Varicose Veins*

This simple brochure provided as a patient education service by the manufacturers of Sotradecol provides answers to 10 commonly asked questions about sclerotherapy. It was prepared with assistance from the Board of Directors of the North American Society of Phlebology.

Source:

Wyeth-Ayerst Laboratories
P.O. Box 8299
Philadelphia, PA 19101

(6) *Treatment of Unwanted Leg Veins (Spider Veins)**

This brochure was developed by my practice, Dermatology Associates of San Diego County, Inc. It is copyright protected, and the following text from the brochure is reproduced only as an aid to those who wish to produce their own individualized products.

Unwanted leg veins (spider veins), known medically as telangiectasias or superficial varicosities, are dilated skin capillaries. These may become unsightly with time and may also lead to a dull aching of the legs after prolonged standing.

Sclerotherapy is the technique of instilling a specific solution into these vessels (tiny capillaries or larger varicose veins), using a small needle. The solution irritates and destroys the inner lining of the blood vessel so it ceases to carry blood. The body then replaces this damaged vessel with an imperceptible scar tissue. *This does not harm the circulation—it improves it by eliminating the abnormal, unnecessary vessel.* Several injections may be needed for a specific *area* of telangiectasia. The procedure is virtually painless. Fading of the vessels is a slow process which takes 1 to 6 months. The goal is to produce a 75% to 90% improvement.

Charges relate to the amount of time spent by the doctor. Actual injection is done only by the doctor, rather than by a nurse or assistant. There is also a one-time purchase charge for compression stockings. The stockings cost from $25 to $75 depending on the type required.

Insurance may cover the procedure in full or in part depending on the type of vessel treated and the type of insurance coverage you have.

Appointments are required in advance. Payment is required at the time of the procedure.

Results of treatment cannot be guaranteed, but most patients are very pleased with the cosmetic and functional improvement.

1. *What causes spider veins?*

   No one is totally sure. Certain families are predisposed to this condition, particularly female relatives. Certain things make spider veins worse: estrogens, pregnancy and birth control pills, tight girdles and garter belts, prolonged standing or sitting, and trauma.

2. *How does sclerotherapy work?*

   The solution destroys the tiny cells which line the blood vessels, without damage to the surrounding tissues.

3. *How soon will the vessels disappear?*

   Each vessel usually requires one to three treatments. The vessels disappear over a period of 2 weeks to 3 months. Recurrences may rarely occur over a period of 1 to 5 years. This treatment does not prevent new telangiectasias from developing.

4. *Are there certain vessels which tend to recur more commonly?*

   Yes. They are the type of vessels which occur in a mat of very fine radiating vessels.

5. *How often can I be treated?*

   The same area should not be injected for 3 to 4 weeks to allow for complete healing. Additional different areas may be treated every week.

6. *How many times does it have to be done?*

   This varies with the number of areas that have to be injected, as well as the response to each injection. It usually takes one to three injections to obliterate any vessel, and 10 to 40 vessels may be treated in any one session.

7. *Are there certain kinds of spider veins that can't be treated?*

   Certain types of large varicose veins may not respond readily to sclerotherapy alone. These vessels may require a minor surgical procedure followed later with sclerotherapy. You may be referred to a vascular surgeon for complete or partial treatment of these specific types of large varicose veins. Some of the extremely small vessels (less than 1/1000 of a millimeter) may require treatment with a Pulsed Dye Laser.

8. *Are there other methods of treating these vessels?*
    Four other methods are used:
  a. Laser surgery
       To date, this method has only been effective for tiny facial blood vessels. The present laser systems tend to produce a greater risk of scarring. The laser is an expensive device, and treatment is thus more costly. We have recently evaluated the use of a new type of laser (Candela Flashlamp Pumped Pulsed Dye Laser) for vessels which do not respond to injection treatment or are too small to be injected. Although more expensive than conventional sclerotherapy, this new laser system is quite effective for treating the tiniest of red blood vessels that may remain after successful treatment of other varicose and telangiectatic leg veins. Finally, I am helping to develop a novel pulsed light source for treating larger telangiectasia and leg veins, Photoderm VL (Energy Systems, Inc.). This new technology should be available for use in the near future. While this or any LASER system will not totally replace sclerotherapy of some surgical techniques for treating varicose and telangiectatic leg veins, they may be helpful in certain patients.
  b. Electrodesiccation
       This method produces a non-specific destruction of both the vessel and overlying skin, thus resulting in a greater incidence of scarring.
  c. Ambulatory phlebectomy
       This operative procedure is often recommended for veins larger than 6 mm in diameter. It results in minimal or even unnoticeable scars along the course of the extracted vein. It is usually performed under local anesthesia and has few complications. It may be recommended that this procedure be performed before sclerotherapy. In this case it will minimize the side effects of sclerotherapy and enhance results.
  d. Surgical ligation and stripping
       This operative procedure always results in a scar although modern techniques limit the extent and number of scars. It is best reserved for large varicose veins. This procedure may be required before other more cosmetically noticeable veins are treated by sclerotherapy to limit the side effects and enhance the results of sclerotherapy.

9. *Is there any way to prevent them?*
    The use of support hose may be helpful. Reducing your weight and regular exercise may also be of help.

10. *What are the side effects of sclerotherapy?*
  a. Slight blistering may occur around the injected vessels and resolves in a day or so.
  b. Ten percent to 30% of patients develop a small freckle-like tan-to-brown spot around the injected vessel. This usually resolves in 80% of these patients within 3 to 6 months. A few patients will have a persistent freckle for up to a year.
  c. Slight stinging or burning may occur with injection of certain types and concentrations of solutions in certain areas.
  d. Sometimes a clot develops at the injection site (especially if the recommended pressure stockings are not worn for the proper amount of time). This clot will never cause internal problems, but its removal within 2 weeks of the injection will speed the healing process and decrease the incidence of "freckling."
  e. Swelling over the injection site may rarely occur. It is particularly common when patients have jobs in which they stand for long periods of time or when vessels in the ankles are injected. The swelling is never dangerous but occasionally must be treated with elevation and compression dressings.
  f. A small superficial ulceration of the skin overlying the injected vessel may occur. This does not usually leave a scar but needs to be seen as soon as possible by your doctor.
  g. Superficial thrombophlebitis, an irritation of the injected vessel, occurs in less than 1 per 1000 patients. It may have to be treated with antiinflammatory agents and compression stockings.

Sample Letter to Insurance Company to Accompany Operative Report

Date line

Insurance Company
Street Address
City, State ZIP CODE

Department of Claim Reimbursement:

The method of sclerotherapy we practice is a combination of the Swiss (Dr. Sigg) and Irish (Dr. Fegan) schools for the treatment of varicose veins. We have been using this method for over 8 years with very good results. In contrast to the older type of treatment, which is still practiced in some places, our approach is based on a concentrated effort to obliterate the diseased vessels in a very limited number of sessions. Depending on the number and extent of varicose veins, the treatment is usually completed in two to four sessions. The treatment of extensive telangiectatic vessels may take a little longer.

Compression sclerotherapy makes it possible to treat even large varicosities successfully, which would otherwise require surgical removal (ligation, vein stripping), except in those patients for whom we recommend surgical treatment. As you are aware, the cost incurred with surgical treatment is extensive: charges for hospitalization, surgeon's fee, anesthesiologist's fee, and operating room, not to mention the loss of work time for the patient as a result of the treatment. In contrast, sclerotherapy, as performed in our clinic, requires only the time needed to perform the examination and treatment. The patient can immediately resume his or her normal everyday activities and is able to return to work the same day. Also, the absence of anesthesia and postincision scars associated with this procedure is not to be underestimated.

As already pointed out, we inject as many varicose veins in one session as is medically indicated (limited only by the amount of injected sclerosing agent), thus further economizing the treatment (limited number of visits). Obviously, if only one or two injections are performed in one session, the time spent with the patient is significantly shorter. We spend an average of 15 to 45 minutes with each patient (including Doppler examination).

Before the therapeutic procedure is initiated, a complete medical history and a physical examination are required to rule out possible contraindications. They are followed by a series of special tests (including Doppler ultrasound) to determine the status of the deep venous system, the presence and location of perforator veins, and the sufficiency of the superficial and deep venous systems.

After mapping out the most suitable injection sites, a small amount of the sclerosing substance is injected to test the patient's sensitivity. Equipment and drugs to use in case of allergic responses must be on hand. Each injection is followed by a special bandaging procedure. After completion of the injection session, in which up to approximately 20 injections can be performed in each leg, the patient is instructed to walk and then report back in 30 minutes, at which time the condition is reassessed.

Sincerely,
Doctor's signature

OPERATIVE REPORT
Compression Sclerotherapy of Superficial Varicosities

Patient

Date

Physician

Treated vessels
(Location-Size-Color-Arborization)

Sclerosing Agent
(Type-Concentration-Quantity)

Procedure:
After signing detailed informed consent and posing for complete photographic documentation of the condition, the patient was examined using venous Doppler and placed in a reverse Trendelenburg position. The area to be injected was prepared with alcohol. Butterfly needles, 23- or 25-gauge, were then inserted into the most appropriate points along the varicose veins beginning with areas of reflux. The leg was then elevated above 180 degrees, and the vein was emptied of blood. An appropriate quantity of sclerosing solution was injected (usually 0.5 ml), and the vessel was immediately compressed using foam rubber pads under a 3- to 4-inch microfoam-tape dressing. The procedure was then repeated using a 26- to 30-gauge needle with the patient supine in a proximal to distal direction, proceeding from larger to smaller vessels. Repeat injections into the same vessel were made at approximately 3- to 5-cm intervals along its path.

Telangiectatic veins were treated after all reticular and varicose veins were sclerosed. Under appropriate magnification using operative loupes, the abnormal vessels were cannulated with a 30-gauge needle fitted to a 3-ml syringe containing 2 ml of the appropriate sclerosing solution.

After the vessels were injected along their entire length, the entire limb was wrapped in a 30- to 40-mm graduated compression stocking.

The compression stocking is to be left in place for _____ days.

The patient was instructed to return to this office in 2 weeks for examination and treatment of any thrombi that may have occurred in the injected vessels.

Complications:

Fee for Leg Vein Sclerotherapy

Name _____ Date _____

- Spider/telangiectatic veins: $ _____ per injection session, requiring a minimum of _____ sessions spaced _____ weeks apart or as needed. This fee is payable at the time of each injection session.

- Varicose/reticular veins:
  $ _____ per injection session, **left leg,** requiring a minimum of _____ sessions.

  $ _____ per injection session, **right leg,** requiring a minimum of _____ sessions.

- Ambulatory phlebectomy: $ _____ per surgical excision.

Varicose vein injection sessions are spaced 1 to 6 weeks apart with follow-up visits 2 weeks and 2 months after the last injection session. You should schedule all "injection sessions" and the "follow-up visits" after the first injection session. You will have to pay in full at the time of each injection session.*

In addition to the doctor's fee, there are additional charges for the following:

_____ Photoplethysmography (PPG)

_____ Doppler ultrasound examination of veins

_____ Spider vein tray @ $ _____ per injection session

_____ Varicose vein tray @ $ _____ per injection session

_____ Pressure garment: below-knee, mid-thigh stockings or panty hose

_____ Shower Safe

*There is a $50.00 charge for "MISSED" or "NO SHOW" varicose vein injection session appointments. NO EXCEPTIONS unless there is a 24-hour cancellation.

I understand and agree to these terms.

Date _____ , 19____   Time _____ AM/PM

_____   _____
PATIENT'S SIGNATURE   PATIENT'S REPRESENTATIVE (IF PATIENT IS A
                                    MINOR OR IS MENTALLY INCOMPETENT, SIG-
                                    NATURE OF PARENT OR LEGAL GUARDIAN IS
                                    REQUIRED)

_____   _____
WITNESS   RELATIONSHIP TO PATIENT

Patient's name

Address

Dear Patient,

Your consultation for varicose veins has revealed a problem that has both a cosmetic component and a "medically necessary component." It is understood that your contracted insurance will *not* cover the cost of the entire procedure; therefore payment is expected at the time of service. The cosmetic portion of the treatment is considered to be performed *outside* of the normal contractual relationship because coverage for cosmetic procedures cannot be expected. You will be given a fee quote that will outline the expected charges incurred.

Upon receipt of payment, each patient will receive an itemized bill. This charge slip will include all information required if you decide to submit to your insurance company on your own.

Many insurance companies require additional information to complete the processing of a claim. Dermatology Associates will provide this information upon receipt of the following charges:

Operation reports, chart notes, copies of the chart, physician's letter (charged for cosmetic procedures only). $25.00

Pictures (cost is incurred for all types of procedures) . . . . $5.00 each

The above fees are to cover our expenses. The policy allows us to provide nonmedically necessary procedures at a cost level for all patients to participate.

Your signature below acknowledges that you have had an opportunity to read the above and your questions concerning this information have been answered.

Signature   Date

Witness   Date

Patient Information

SCLEROTHERAPY

BEFORE YOUR APPOINTMENT

- If you take birth control pills or estrogen, inform the physician about it.
- Do not take aspirin, ibuprofen, or other nonsteroidal antiinflammatory drugs (e.g., arthritis medicine) for 2 days before your treatment because these medications can increase bruising.
- We recommend not to drink alcoholic beverages and not to smoke for 2 days before and 2 days after your treatment because drinking alcohol may impair healing.
- Do not shave your legs the day of your appointment to avoid discomfort.
- Before your appointment, shower and wash your legs thoroughly with an antibacterial soap. Do not apply any cream or lotion to your legs.
- Bring loose-fitting shorts or a leotard to wear during the treatment.
- Eat a light meal or snack $1\frac{1}{2}$ hours before your appointment.

AFTER YOUR TREATMENT

- Immediately after the procedure, you will be required to put on support stockings and walk for 10 to 30 minutes. Be sure to have loose-fitting slacks and comfortable walking shoes with you.
- If traveling more than 30 minutes to the office, have someone else drive you so you can move your feet and legs as the passenger. This is beneficial after the treatment.
- Maintain normal activities. Walk at least 1 hour a day—the more, the better!
- Avoid standing for long periods.
- Avoid hot baths for 2 weeks. Cool your legs with cold water after each shower.
- Wear the support stockings as instructed. After healing, use them for long trips or when your legs ache.
- Avoid strenuous physical activities such as high-impact aerobics or weight lifting for the first 48 to 72 hours.

Postoperative Sclerotherapy Instructions

Patient's name _____ Date _____

_____   Remove brown tape _____

_____   Remove white tape _____

_____   Wear stockings during the day for _____ days.
           (Remove before going to bed.)

_____   Wrap _____ with brown tape while showering.
           (Remove wet tape, and put stocking on after shower.)

_____   Wear stocking 24 hours/day for _____ days.
           (Use shower bag during showers.)

If any sores develop over treated area, please call this office immediately.

INDEX